Vertigo and Dizziness

Springer Nature More Media App

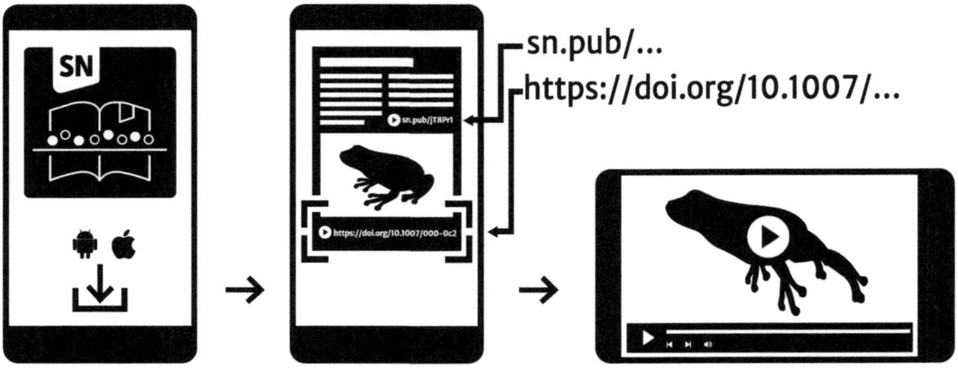

1.
Download

2.
Scan Link

3.
Enjoy Video

Support: customerservice@springernature.com

Michael Strupp • Thomas Brandt • Marianne Dieterich

Vertigo and Dizziness

Common Complaints

Third Edition

Springer

Michael Strupp
Department of Neurology and German
Center for Vertigo and Balance Disorders
Ludwig Maximilians University Munich
Munich, Germany

Thomas Brandt
German Center for Vertigo and Balance
Disorders
Ludwig Maximilians University Munich
Munich, Germany

Marianne Dieterich
Department of Neurology and German
Center for Vertigo and Balance Disorders
Ludwig Maximilians University Munich
Munich, Germany

This work contains media enhancements, which are displayed with a "play" icon. Material in the print book can be viewed on a mobile device by downloading the Springer Nature "More Media" app available in the major app stores. The media enhancements in the online version of the work can be accessed directly by authorized users.

ISBN 978-3-030-78259-7 ISBN 978-3-030-78260-3 (eBook)
https://doi.org/10.1007/978-3-030-78260-3

This Springer imprint is published by the registered company Springer Nature Switzerland AG
The registered company address is: Gewerbestrasse 11, 6330 Cham, Switzerland

Preface to the Third Edition

Since the last edition in 2013, our understanding of the pathophysiology, etiology, diagnosis, terminology, and therapy of peripheral, central, and functional vestibular syndromes has continued to improve. This has a major impact on our daily clinical practice.

Laboratory testing of the function of the semicircular canals can now be easily done using the video head impulse test, which provides valid and quantitative data. The simple measurement of subjective visual vertical has become an important diagnostic procedure, which is now also a part of clinical routine. Genetic testing has improved our understanding of the etiology of acute unilateral vestibulopathy/vestibular neuritis, Menière's disease, and downbeat nystagmus. Vertigo and dizziness in the emergency department has been identified as a very relevant issue, and there are now several studies that show how to discriminate acute peripheral from acute central vestibular syndrome, which has a major impact on clinical practice. Studies have also shown that central spinning vertigo is found mainly in acute unilateral caudal brainstem or cerebellar lesions affecting relevant central vestibular cerebellar areas. Imaging, in particular structural and functional magnetic resonance tomography, has helped to further elucidate the bilateral organization of the central vestibular networks within the brainstem, cerebellum, thalamus, and cortex, which can now be correlated with typical vestibular syndromes and disorders affecting spatial orientation. Higher central vestibular disorders, which, for instance, impair spatial orientation or multisensory attention (neglect), indicate a right-hemispheric lesion, which is compatible with the right-sided thalamocortical dominance of the vestibular system.

Since 2009, the Committee for the International Classification of Vestibular Disorders of the Bárány Society has developed internationally accepted and clinically oriented diagnostic criteria for the most frequent vestibular disorders, which are updated continuously. They are most helpful for clinicians and also for clinical research, in particular for the design of clinical trials. So far, the following vestibular disorders have been reclassified: benign paroxysmal positional vertigo, Menière's disease, bilateral vestibulopathy, presbyvestibulopathy (a new and clinically relevant entity), vestibular paroxysmia, vestibular migraine, persistent perceived postural dizziness (one of the several forms of functional dizziness), orthostatic dizziness, mal de débarquement syndrome, different types of nystagmus vertigo and dizziness in childhood, vascular vertigo as well as acute unilateral vestibulopathy/vestibular neuritis.

Finally, there are several new trials on the treatment of various vestibular disorders: benign paroxysmal positional vertigo, Menière's disease, bilateral vestibulopathy, vestibular paroxysmia, vestibular migraine, and cerebellar dizziness. We would, however, like to point out that there are still considerable deficits, in particular, in terms of treatment of vestibular disorders due to a lack of up-to-date randomized, placebo-controlled treatment trials, for example, for Menière's disease or functional dizziness.

We would like to thank all the doctors and technicians in the Department of Neurology and the German Center for Vertigo and Balance Disorders at Ludwig Maximilian University Munich. We would also particularly like to thank our neuroorthopticians Claudia Frenzel, Miriam Glaser, Cornelia Karch, Nicole Lehrer, Barbara Muschaweckh, Mona Klemm, and Annika Aurbacher for their careful neuroophthalmological examinations, documentation, and video recordings of patients. We are grateful to Dietmar Lauffer and Anna Huppert for the photographs taken to show typical examination techniques and treatment options for vestibular disorders. Our thanks also go to Sabine Esser and Amelie-Christine Strupp for creating figures used in this book; to Prof. Thomas Liebig and Dr. Robert Forbig at the Institute for Neuroradiology at LMU Munich, and Dr. Valerie Kirsch for their contributions to the imaging of the central and peripheral vestibular system; as well as to Prof. Andreas Zwergal for his contribution to the chapter on acute central vertigo and Prof. Julia Dlugaiczyk for her contribution on vestibular evoked myogenic potentials.

Finally, we would also like to thank Springer Nature London for the careful editing of this book.

Michael Strupp
Munich, Germany
January 2023

Thomas Brandt
Munich, Germany

Marianne Dieterich
Munich, Germany

Preface to the Second Edition

The last 10 years following the first edition of our book have witnessed many new findings on epidemiology, diagnostics, pathophysiology, and – especially important – the course and therapy of various illnesses that have the main symptom of dizziness. It was therefore necessary to totally update the original edition, which had been conceived as a practical compendium of treatment strategies for patients with dizziness and balance disorders. Here we briefly highlight a few of the most important new developments.

Today valid epidemiological studies on the prevalence of various illnesses with the symptom of dizziness are available. The long-time course of benign paroxysmal positioning vertigo, vestibular neuritis, bilateral vestibulopathy, vestibular paroxysmia, Menière's disease, and phobic postural vertigo has now been investigated for over 10 years. Moreover, even physicians not specialized in this field are increasingly recognizing the clinical importance of vestibular migraine, bilateral vestibulopathy, vestibular paroxysmia, and the superior canal dehiscence syndrome. The diagnostic criteria have become more precise thanks to fruitful clinical studies. There is a wealth of new findings on the pathophysiology and central compensation of disorders of peripheral and central vestibular function, e.g., in the form of fMRI and PET evidence of plastic changes in cerebral activity. There are new data on higher spatial orientation disorders and on hippocampal atrophy in bilateral vestibulopathy as well as newly discovered vestibular structures and functions. We have covered these in the comprehensiveness needed for the private practice.

The following four findings are of special practical importance for therapy:

1. An important new therapeutic principle is the use of aminopyridine to successfully treat downbeat nystagmus, episodic ataxia type 2, and cerebellar gait disorders.
2. Corticosteroids significantly improve the recovery of peripheral labyrinthine function in patients with acute vestibular neuritis.
3. The most effective drug therapy for Menière's disease is evidently a high-dosage long-term therapy with betahistine.
4. Carbamazepine significantly reduces attacks in the long-term course of vestibular paroxysmia.

The personal experience of the authors has been gathered in the course of their engagement over many years in the multiregional Munich Dizziness Outpatient Unit. In 2010, the BMBF began funding this unit under a new name, the German Center for Vertigo and Balance Disorders (IFB). Its goal is to develop an international referral centre with an interdisciplinary outpatient unit, its own study centre, and a structured course of studies for foreign clinical scientists in the fields of otoneurology and neuro-ophthalmology.

In this second edition we would like to especially thank both medical and nonmedical employees of the Dizziness Outpatient Unit, especially Ms. Sabine Esser and Ms. Ute Appendino for efficiently organizing the annual Munich seminar, "Vertigo," as well as the neuro-orthoptists Nicole Rettinger, Miriam Glaser, and Claudia Frenzel for carefully examining the patients, documenting each case, and compiling the videos. We would also like to express our appreciation to Sabine Esser for the graphic designs, Jenny Linn for her competent contributions to the imaging, and Erich Schneider for his development work on "bed-side" video-oculography. Our thanks also to Joanna Bolesworth of Springer Medicine UK for her pleasant, reliable, and extremely patient cooperation. Finally, we thank Judy Benson for her careful copy-editing of the English edition of this book. The German second edition of the book *Vertigo – Leitsymptom Schwindel* by T. Brandt, M. Dieterich, and M. Strupp was published by Springer–Verlag in 2012.

Thomas Brandt
Munich, Germany

Marianne Dieterich
Munich, Germany

Michael Strupp
Munich, Germany

Preface to the First Edition

There are three convincing arguments why it is important to learn about the management of vertigo:
- After headache, it is the second most common complaint of patients, not only in neurology and ENT departments.
- Most syndromes of vertigo can be correctly diagnosed only by means of a careful medical history and physical examination of the patient.
- The majority of these cases have a benign cause, take a favourable natural course, and respond positively to therapy.

Vertigo and dizziness are not disease entities, but rather unspecific syndromes consisting of various disorders with different causes. For this reason, our clinically oriented book is for physicians of different specialisations who treat patients with vertigo and for medical students. To make the book easy to use, we have provided an overview of the most important syndromes of vertigo and dizziness, each with elucidating clinical descriptions and illustrations.

A general chapter deals with how the vestibular system functions, its disorders, the pathophysiological mechanisms involved, diagnostic signs, history taking, examination procedures, laboratory diagnostics and principles of therapy. The most important clinical syndromes of vertigo are treated in individual chapters organised as follows: patient medical history, clinical aspects and natural course, pathophysiology and principles of therapy, pragmatic therapy, ineffective treatments, as well as differential diagnosis and clinical problems. We have put special emphasis on the various drug, physical, operative or psychotherapeutic treatments available. The book is based on the common experience that we have accumulated over many years working in a multi-regional referral centre for dizziness outpatients. Many parts of the text, tables and figures are updated versions of those in a considerably more detailed monograph on the clinical and scientific aspects of vertigo (Brandt T. *Vertigo: Its Multisensory Syndromes*, 2nd ed. Springer, London, 1999). The accompanying DVD presents typical case histories, results of examinations for the individual syndromes, physical examination techniques and laboratory diagnostics. The book is oriented to daily medical practice, and we hope that it will prove helpful by providing readily accessible information. The whole field of vertigo and dizziness, imbalance and eye movement disorders has been considered extremely difficult because of the variety of its manifestations and its resistance to compartmentalisation. We hope that we have succeeded in making these syndromes more understandable by using clear, anatomical categories and clinical classifications.

We would especially like to express our thanks to the neuroorthoptists Miriam Glaser, Cornelia Karch and Nicole Rettinger for compiling the videos. Our appreciation also to Ms Judy Benson for copyediting the text and to Dr. Steven Russell for carefully reading the manuscript. We also thank Ms Sabine Eßer for designing the graphics and Ms Melissa Morton and Eva Senior of Springer-Verlag London for cooperating on the production of this book in such a pleasant and efficient manner. The German edition of the book, *Vertigo-Leitsymptom Schwindel* by T. Brandt, M. Dieterich and M. Strupp, was published by Steinkopff-Verlag in 2004.

Thomas Brandt
Munich, Germany

Marianne Dieterich
Munich, Germany

Michael Strupp
Munich, Germany

Contents

Vertigo and Dizziness: Frequent Multisensory Symptoms

Contents

M. Strupp et al., *Vertigo and Dizziness*, https://doi.org/10.1007/978-3-030-78260-3_1

1.1 Introduction

Vertigo and dizziness are the leading symptoms of various sensorimotor syndromes of different pathophysiologies, etiologies, and underlying diseases. There are three different forms:

1. Those arising from the peripheral (labyrinth and/or vestibular nerve) or the central vestibular system (mainly brainstem or cerebellum).
2. Functional dizziness, previously also called somatoform or psychogenic dizziness.
3. Other causes and entities, such as orthostatic dizziness, polyneuropathies, reduced visual acuity, side effects of drugs, metabolic disorders, neurodegenerative disorders such as Parkinson's syndrome, multiple system atrophy, or subcortical vascular encephalopathy. Such diseases typically lead to postural imbalance and gait disorders and are associated with a higher risk of falls. They normally do not cause spinning vertigo.

The reported one-year prevalence of vertigo and dizziness is between 6.5% and 11% (Hulse et al. 2019; Corrales and Bhattacharyya 2016). In comparison with non-affected subjects, affected subjects have—after adjustment for age, sex, and other diseases—a 1.7 times higher mortality (Corrales and Bhattacharyya 2016). The lifetime prevalence for moderate-to-severe vertigo and dizziness is around 30% (Neuhauser 2016). About 65% of the patients are female (Hulse et al. 2019).

Physiological vertigo and dizziness (e.g., spinning vertigo on a merry-go-round) and pathological vertigo and dizziness (e.g., acute unilateral vestibulopathy/vestibular neuritis) are characterized by similar signs and symptoms despite the different underlying mechanisms: vertigo/dizziness, nystagmus, postural imbalance, and a tendency to fall and/or nausea/vomiting (◘ Fig. 1.1). These signs and symptoms in the areas of perception (vertigo/dizziness), gaze stabilization (nystagmus), posture and gait (imbalance), and the vegetative nervous system (nausea/vomiting) correspond to the major functions of the vestibular system and can be assigned to different anatomical areas in the nervous system (◘ Fig. 1.2, Brandt and Daroff 1980).

1.2 The Vestibular System

The most important functional structure of the vestibular system is the vestibulo-ocular reflex (VOR). The VOR has three major planes of action:

- Horizontal head rotation about the vertical z-axis (yaw)
- Head extension and flexion about the horizontal, binaural y-axis (pitch)
- Lateral head tilt about the horizontal line of sight, the x-axis (roll)

These three planes represent the three-dimensional (3-D) space in which the vestibular and ocular motor systems responsible for spatial orientation, perception of self-movement, stabilization of gaze, and postural control operate. The neuronal circuitry of the horizontal and vertical semicircular canals and of the otolith organs is based on a sensory convergence that takes place within the VOR (◘ Fig. 1.2). The VOR connects a set of extraocular eye muscles that are aligned by their primary direction of pull with the same particular spatial plane of the horizontal, the anterior, or the posterior canal. The canals of both labyrinths form functional pairs in the horizontal and vertical working planes. In other words, the canals are stimulated and inhibited pairwise:

- The horizontal right and left pair
- The vertical anterior of one side along with the posterior canal of the opposite side and vice versa

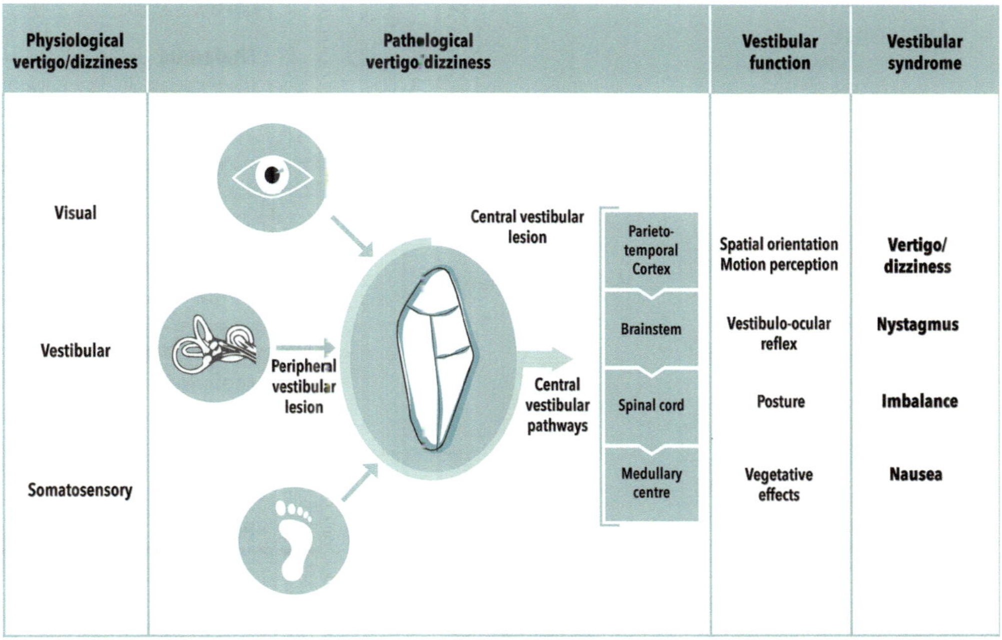

Fig. 1.1 Physiological and pathological vertigo and dizziness. Both are characterized by similar signs and symptoms that derive from the functions of the multisensory vestibular system

The vertical planes of pitch and roll are a result of the wiring, connecting the two vertical canals that are diagonal to the sagittal plane in the head:

- The pairs of canals function as a gauge of angular acceleration and react to the rotational movements of the head in the corresponding plane.
- The otoliths function as a gauge of gravity and linear acceleration.

The leading symptoms of a dysfunction of the semicircular canals are spinning vertigo, a tendency to fall to one side, and/or nausea/vomiting. Clinical examination reveals the following signs depending on the underlying pathophysiology: peripheral vestibular spontaneous nystagmus in the plane of the affected semicircular canal(s) (Ewald's first law) and, if there is a functional deficit, a pathological head impulse test in the plane of the affected semicircular canal(s).

The otolith organs, i.e., the saccule and the utricle, act as sensors for linear acceleration and gravity. Leading symptoms are postural imbalance, dizziness, and/or impairment of gait.

1.3 Peripheral and Central Vestibular Syndromes

The six most frequent forms of peripheral vestibular vertigo are as follows:

- Benign paroxysmal positional vertigo
- Menière's disease
- Acute unilateral vestibulopathy/vestibular neuritis
- Bilateral vestibulopathy
- Vestibular paroxysmia
- Syndrome of the third mobile windows (most often semicircular canal dehiscence, in particular of the anterior canal)

Acute peripheral vestibular syndromes—as a rule—are characterized by an acute, most often spinning vertigo, a peripheral vestibular spontaneous nystagmus with the fast

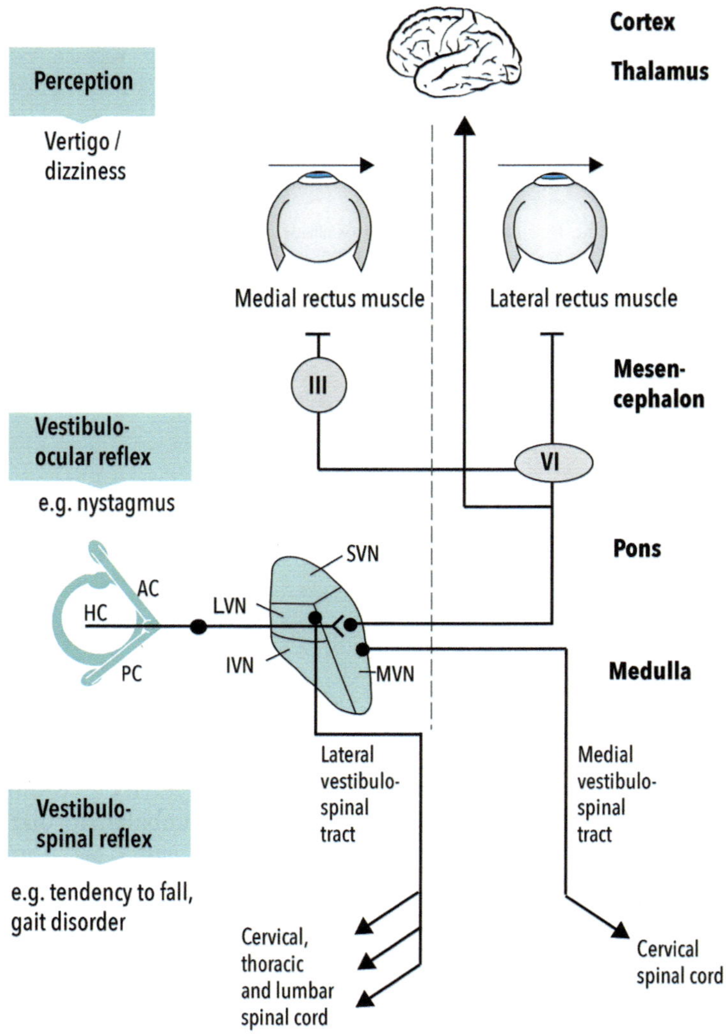

Fig. 1.2 Schematic drawing of the horizontal vestibulo-ocular reflex (VOR). The VOR is part of a complex sensorimotor system, which enables the perception of head position and motion (connections via the thalamus to the vestibular cortex), gaze stability (three-neuron arc to the nuclei of the ocular muscles), as well as head and postural control (vestibulospinal reflexes). AC, HC, and PC anterior, horizontal, and posterior semicircular canals, SVN, LVN, IVN, and MVN superior, lateral, inferior, and medial vestibular nuclei, III and VI oculomotor and abducens nuclei

phase beating toward the relatively more active side, a tendency to fall toward the relatively less active side, and nausea/vomiting.

Central vestibular syndromes arise from a dysfunction/lesion between the entry of the eighth cranial nerve in the brainstem, vestibular nuclei, the cerebellum, other vestibular and ocular motor nuclei, and pathways in the brainstem up to the thalamus and the vestibular cortex (Brandt and Dieterich 2017).

Central vertigo and dizziness can manifest as:

- Part of well-defined infratentorial clinical syndromes with other symptoms or supranuclear/nuclear/fascicular ocular motor disorders and/or other neurological brainstem deficits (e.g., in Wallenberg's syndrome or midbrain lesions)

- Other clinical syndromes of various etiologies such as downbeat or upbeat nystagmus syndromes

The occurrence of these typical ccular motor findings in cerebellar or brainstem lesions also allows their definitive localization.

Clinically, central vestibular syndromes can present as recurrent episodes lasting for seconds or minutes (e.g., paroxysmal brainstem attacks, vestibular migraine), for hours or up to days (e.g., vestibular migraine or episodic ataxia type 2), or with permanent symptoms and signs (e.g., downbeat nystagmus syndrome or other forms of cerebellar dizziness (Feil et al. 2019; Brandt and Dieterich 2017).

1.4 The Frequency of the Various Vestibular Diseases and Syndromes

The following relative frequencies of individual diagnoses are reported in a multiregional interdisciplinary outpatient clinic for dizziness as follows (Table 1.1, Fig. 1.3). Functional dizziness, including secondary functional dizziness, is the most frequent cause, occurring in 17.2% of the patients. The second most frequent diagnosis is BPPV (13.8%), followed by central vestibular syndromes in primarily vascular (stroke) and inflammatory diseases (multiple sclerosis) and neurodegenerative diseases of the cerebellum (cerebellar dizziness) or extrapyramidal system. Vestibular migraine is the most frequent cause of spontaneously recurring episodes of vertigo (12.5%) (Formeister et al. 2018). It has one frequency peak in the second decade and another in the sixth decade; thus, it is by no means only a disease of younger women. As regards total frequency, it now takes the fourth place followed by Menière's disease and acute unilateral vestibulopathy/vestibular neuritis. Bilateral vestibulopathy is characterized by movement-dependent postural imbalance, is still often not diagnosed, and is the most frequent cause of postural imbalance in the elderly. More rare are vestibular paroxysmia and the syndrome of the third mobile windows, of which the most frequent form is superior (anterior) canal dehiscence syndrome.

It is difficult to compare the frequency data of various hospitals and medical specializations, because the definitions of the term and concept "vertigo/dizziness" differ greatly. Some are broader, whereas others are more narrow. Vertigo/dizziness is seen

Table 1.1 Absolute numbers and relative frequency of the various vestibular syndromes and diseases in the multiregional specialized outpatient unit of the German Center for Vertigo and Balance Disorders and the Neurological Clinic of LMU Munich (2019–2021)

Diagnosis	Frequency	
	n	%
1. Functional dizziness	6854	17.2
2. BPPV	5518	13.8
3. Central vestibular vertigo	5067	12.7
4. Vestibular migraine	5012	12.5
5. Menière's disease	4047	10.1
6. Unilateral vestibulopathy	3659	9.2
7. Bilateral vestibulopathy	2584	6.5
8. Vestibular paroxysmia	1234	3.1
9. Third mobile window syndrome	185	0.5
Unknown vertigo syndromes	1823	4.6
Other disorders	3926	9.8
	39,918	

BPPV benign paroxysmal positional vertigo
[a]Other causes of dizziness, such as polyneuropathy and metabolic disorders, non-vestibular dizziness, e.g., in patients with peripheral eye muscle or eye muscle nerve palsies

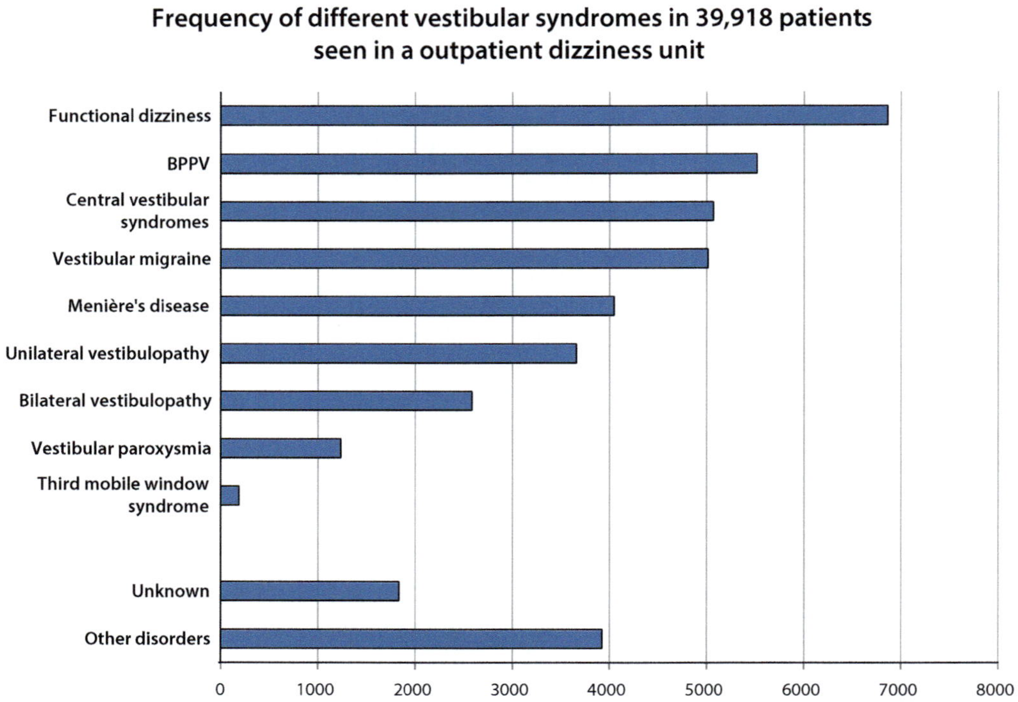

Fig. 1.3 Absolute numbers of the various vestibular syndromes and diseases in the multiregional specialized outpatient unit of the German Center for Vertigo and Balance Disorders and the Neurological Clinic of LMU Munich (1998–2021). BPPV benign paroxysmal positional vertigo

either as a subjective symptom or as a vestibular disorder that can be objectified. Both tendencies are unsatisfactory, as the symptom of vertigo/dizziness is, on the one hand, observed in non-vestibular disturbances (e.g., orthostatic dizziness or movement disorders) and, on the other, central vestibular disturbances (e.g., lateropulsion in Wallenberg's syndrome, thalamic astasia, or cerebellar dizziness) may also occur without any subjective vertigo and dizziness but with imbalance and instability of stance and gait.

Vertigo/dizziness is also frequently seen in emergency situations. A retrospective study of more than 4000 consecutive emergency neurological consultations in 1 year reported that headache (21%) was the most frequent cardinal symptom, followed by motor deficit (13%), dizziness (12%), and epileptic seizure (11%) (Royl et al. 2010). In an emergency situation, one must first and foremost quickly differentiate between central and peripheral causes (Cnyrim et al. 2008; Kattah et al. 2009), since this has immediate diagnostic and therapeutic consequences.

In about 50% of all cases in the emergency room, a discrimination between an acute peripheral and an acute central vestibular syndrome is not achieved (Royl et al. 2010; Tarnutzer et al. 2011). The best approach for the differential diagnosis is taking a systematic patient history and a systematic combined examination of the neurological, in particular the vestibular and ocular motor system to specifically look for central signs, such as prominent skew deviation or gaze-evoked nystagmus (for references, see Zwergal and Dieterich 2020). It is important to note that about 20% of all patients in the emergency room with the leading symptom of vertigo and dizziness have life-threatening diseases; in 4–15%, these are strokes. Imaging in the emergency room is indicated; however, in the acute phase MRI is not very sensitive with false-negative results in up to 50% of patients with vertigo due to small brainstem lesions within the first 48 h (Saber Tehrani et al. 2014).

1.5 Anxiety, Fears, and Vertigo/Dizziness

For syndromal characterization of the various vestibular syndromes, associated fears and anxiety should be considered and patients should be explicitly asked about them, in addition to typical vestibular and ocular motor symptoms. There is increasing evidence, based on animal models and studies in humans, that the vestibular system is connected via reciprocal pathways with the functional areas relevant for fears and anxiety as well as cognitive and emotional effects (Hilber et al. 2019). These pathways between regions relevant for vestibular function and those relevant for fears and anxiety are particularly related to thalamocortical and cerebellar networks (Balaban and Thayer 2001). The functional regulation is based on intrinsic neurotransmitters of the inner ear, thalamocortical and limbic connections as well as serotonergic and non-serotonergic projections from the locus coeruleus and the raphe nuclei (Balaban 2016). The understanding of these vestibular functions, including endocrinological and autonomous stress reactions, requires the knowledge of different neurotransmitter systems For instance, corticotropin-releasing factor—a neuropeptide which is synthesized in the hypothalamic paraventricular nucleus—contributes to stress, fear, and anxiety via the lateral vestibular nucleus (Wang et al. 2019). This example clearly shows the close functional connections between stress, fear, anxiety, and balance, even at the level of the pontomedullary vestibular nuclei of the caudal brainstem.

Clinically, the extent of the fear and anxiety associated with vertigo and dizziness correlates with the type and extent of the impairment of vestibular function: The correlation is strongest in vestibular migraine due to hyperexcitability and minimal in chronic unilateral or bilateral vestibulopathy (Brandt and Dieterich 2020). This was also found in a retrospective analysis using the Vertigo Handicap Questionnaire in 7083 patients from the German Center for Vertigo and Balance Disorders (Decker et al. 2019). The fear and anxiety associated with vertigo and dizziness could also be discriminated from other comorbid anxiety disorders. The reduced or missing associated anxiety in patients with a chronic unilateral or bilateral vestibulopathy raises the question whether an intact vestibular function is essential for the development of fear and anxiety reactions (Brandt and Dieterich 2020).

1.6 Psychiatric Comorbidities in Patients with Vertigo and Dizziness

Several clinical studies consistently found psychiatric comorbidities, such as anxiety disorders or depression, in patients with vertigo, dizziness, or other balance disorders (Eckhardt-Henn et al. 2008; Lahmann et al. 2015; Bigelow et al. 2016). This was also found in patients with fear of heights (Kapfhammer et al. 2015). However, the prevalence of psychiatric comorbidities depends on the underlying disease: The highest rates were found in patients with vestibular migraine and vestibular paroxysmia, whereas the lowest were found in those with bilateral vestibulopathy (Best et al. 2009; Lahmann et al. 2015; Dieterich et al. 2016; Dieterich and Staab

1

2017). Psychiatric comorbidities and psychiatric diseases can often make the diagnosis of vestibular dysfunction more difficult. Again, the patient history is essential for the differentiation of the different vestibular syndromes and the comorbidities, including psychiatric comorbidities.

References

Balaban CD (2016) Neurotransmitters in the vestibular system. Handb Clin Neurol 137:41–55

Balaban CD, Thayer JF (2001) Neurological bases for balance-anxiety links. J Anxiety Disord 15(1-2):53–79

Best C, Eckhardt-Henn A, Tschan R, Dieterich M (2009) Psychiatric morbidity and comorbidity in different vestibular vertigo syndromes. Results of a prospective longitudinal study over one year. J Neurol 256(1):58–65

Bigelow RT, Semenov YR, du Lac S, Hoffman HJ, Agrawal Y (2016) Vestibular vertigo and comorbid cognitive and psychiatric impairment: the 2008 National Health Interview Survey. J Neurol Neurosurg Psychiatry 87(4):367–372

Brandt T, Daroff RB (1980) The multisensory physiological and pathological vertigo syndromes. Ann Neurol 7:195–203

Brandt T, Dieterich M (2017) The dizzy patient: don't forget disorders of the central vestibular system. Nat Rev Neurol 13(6):352–362

Brandt T, Dieterich M (2020) 'Excess anxiety' and 'less anxiety': both depend on vestibular function. Curr Opin Neurol 33(1):136–141

Cnyrim CD, Newman-Toker D, Karch C, Brandt T, Strupp M (2008) Bedside differentiation of vestibular neuritis from central "vestibular pseudoneuritis". J Neurol Neurosurg Psychiatry 79(4):458–460

Corrales CE, Bhattacharyya N (2016) Dizziness and death: an imbalance in mortality. Laryngoscope 126(9):2134–2136

Decker J, Limburg K, Henningsen P, Lahmann C, Brandt T, Dieterich M (2019) Intact vestibular function is relevant for anxiety related to vertigo. J Neurol 266(Suppl 1):89–92

Dieterich M, Staab JP (2017) Functional dizziness: from phobic postural vertigo and chronic subjective dizziness to persistent postural-perceptual dizziness. Curr Opin Neurol 30(1):107–113

Dieterich M, Staab JP, Brandt T (2016) Functional (psychogenic) dizziness. Handb Clin Neurol 139:447–468

Eckhardt-Henn A, Best C, Bense S, Breuer P, Diener G, Tschan R, Dieterich M (2008) Psychiatric comorbidity in different organic vertigo syndromes. J Neurol 255(3):420–428

Feil K, Strobl R, Schindler A, Krafczyk S, Goldschagg N, Frenzel C, Glaser M, Schoberl F, Zwergal A, Strupp M (2019) What is behind cerebellar vertigo and dizziness? Cerebellum 18(3):320–332

Formeister EJ, Rizk HG, Kohn MA, Sharon JD (2018) The epidemiology of vestibular migraine: a population-based survey study. Otol Neurotol 39(8):1037–1044

Hilber P, Cendelin J, Le GA, Machado ML, Tuma J, Besnard S (2019) Cooperation of the vestibular and cerebellar networks in anxiety disorders and depression. Prog Neuro-Psychopharmacol Biol Psychiatry 89:310–321

Hulse R, Biesdorf A, Hormann K, Stuck B, Erhart M, Hulse M, Wenzel A (2019) Peripheral vestibular disorders: an epidemiologic survey in 70 million individuals. Otol Neurotol 40(1):88–95

Kapfhammer HP, Huppert D, Grill E, Fitz W, Brandt T (2015) Visual height intolerance and acrophobia: clinical characteristics and comorbidity patterns. Eur Arch Psychiatry Clin Neurosci 265(5):375–385

Kattah JC, Talkad AV, Wang DZ, Hsieh YH, Newman-Toker DE (2009) HINTS to diagnose stroke in the acute vestibular syndrome: three-step bedside oculomotor examination more sensitive than early MRI diffusion-weighted imaging. Stroke 40(11):3504–3510

Lahmann C, Henningsen P, Brandt T, Strupp M, Jahn K, Dieterich M, Eckhardt-Henn A, Feuerecker R, Dinkel A, Schmid G (2015) Psychiatric comorbidity and psychosocial impairment among patients with vertigo and dizziness. J Neurol Neurosurg Psychiatry 86(3):302–308

Neuhauser HK (2016) The epidemiology of dizziness and vertigo. Handb Clin Neurol 137:67–82

Royl G, Ploner CJ, Mockel M, Leithner C (2010) Neurological chief complaints in an emergency room. Nervenarzt 81(10):1226–1230

Saber Tehrani AS, Kattah JC, Mantokoudis G, Pula JH, Nair D, Blitz A, Ying S, Hanley DF, Zee DS, Newman-Toker DE (2014) Small strokes causing severe vertigo: frequency of false-negative MRIs and nonlacunar mechanisms. Neurology 83(2):169–173

Tarnutzer AA, Berkowitz AL, Robinson KA, Hsieh YH, Newman-Toker DE (2011) Does my dizzy patient have a stroke? A systematic review of bedside diagnosis in acute vestibular syndrome. CMAJ 183(9):E571–E592

Wang Y, Chen ZP, Yang ZQ, Zhang XY, Li JM, Wang JJ, Zhu JN (2019) Corticotropin-releasing factor depolarizes rat lateral vestibular nuclear neurons through activation of CRF receptors 1 and 2. Neuropeptides 76:101934

Zwergal A, Dieterich M (2020) Vertigo and dizziness in the emergency room. Curr Opin Neurol 33(1):117–125

Patient History

Contents

M. Strupp et al., *Vertigo and Dizziness*, https://doi.org/10.1007/978-3-030-78260-3_2

The patient history is, in addition to the combined examination of the vestibular and ocular motor system (▶ Chap. 3), essential for a correct diagnosis when a patient complaints of vertigo, dizziness, or imbalance (Brandt et al. 2014; Welgampola et al. 2019). Vertigo—in the pathological sense—is considered either an unpleasant disturbance of spatial orientation or the illusory perception of a movement of the body (spinning and wobbling) and/or of the surroundings (Bisdorff et al. 2009). Since the patient's complaint of being "vertiginous" or "dizzy" is ambiguous, particular care is necessary when taking the neuro-otological history of the patient. The usual pre-prepared vertigo questionnaire cannot replace it. How important taking the patient history (and the bedside examination) is for differentiating the various dizziness/vertigo syndromes is also reflected by the diagnostic criteria of the ongoing International Classification of Vestibular Disorders (ICVD) (▶ https://www.jvr-web.org/ICVD.html). Videos with typical patient histories are presented in the individual chapters of the specific diseases and syndromes but not in this chapter.

The four most important criteria for differentiating the vestibular syndromes are the "triple **T A**'s":

1. **T**ime course of symptoms
2. **T**ype of symptoms
3. **T**riggers or modulating factors
4. **A**ccompanying symptoms

2.1 Time Course of Symptoms

2.1.1 Attacks or Episodes

Lasting

- Seconds to minutes: e.g., BPPV, vestibular paroxysmia, syndrome of the third mobile windows, paroxysmal brainstem attacks, orthostatic dizziness, transient ischemic attacks (◘ Table 2.1) or

◘ **Table 2.1** Episodic vertigo and dizziness: diseases and disorders with recurrent attacks/episodes (in alphabetical order)

Peripheral vestibular system	Central vestibular system	Peripheral and/or central vestibular systems
Autoimmunological inner ear diseases, e.g., Cogan syndrome BPPV (attacks induced by changes of head or body position relative to gravity) Menière's disease Tumors of the cerebellopontine angle (rare) Syndrome of the third mobile windows (symptoms induced by changes in pressure, e.g., sneezing, coughing, pressing, lifting heavy weights or by sounds, the so-called Tullio phenomenon) Vestibular paroxysmia	Episodic ataxias, most frequently episodic ataxia type 2 Paroxysmal ocular tilt reaction Paroxysmal ataxia/dysarthrophonia (e.g., in multiple sclerosis or after brainstem or cerebellar infarctions) Room tilt illusion Transient vertebrobasilar ischemia Vertebral artery compression/occlusion syndrome Vestibular epilepsy (very rare)	Transient ischemia in the vertebrobasilar artery system, in particular AICA Vestibular migraine

- Many minutes to hours: e.g., Menière's disease, vestibular migraine, and the rare episodic ataxias

Attacks/episodes of vertigo are most often caused by a pathological unilateral excitation, rarely by inhibition of the bilaterally organized peripheral and central vestibular system.

2.1.2 Acute Onset of Symptoms Lasting Many Hours to Weeks: Acute Vestibular Syndrome (AVS)

The symptoms or signs are caused by a unilateral peripheral or central vestibular lesion (Table 2.2), e.g., due to acute unilateral

Table 2.2 Acute vestibular syndrome (AVS) due to peripheral or central vestibular disorders

Peripheral vestibular disorders and diseases	
Infections	Acute unilateral vestibulopathy/vestibular neuritis, most often caused by the reactivation of herpes simplex virus 1 infection Labyrinthitis: due to bacterial or viral (rarely, fungal) infection Otitis media (indirectly due to toxins) Zoster oticus
Autoimmunological inner ear diseases	Cogan syndrome and others
Vascular	Labyrinthine infarction (anterior inferior cerebellar artery (AICA)/labyrinthine artery)
Traumatic	Labyrinthine contusion Fracture of the temporal bone (transverse > longitudinal fractures) Post-traumatic otolith dizziness Syndrome of the third mobile windows
Iatrogenic	Aminoglycosides (systemic or local) Other ototoxic substances (e.g., amiodarone, aspirin, chemotherapeutic agents) Surgery of the inner ear
Central vestibular disorders	
Vascular	AICA infarction Posterior inferior cerebellar artery (PICA) infarction Superior cerebellar artery (SCA) infarction (rare) Hemorrhage in the area of the brainstem or cerebellum
Autoimmunological	MS Autoimmunological encephalitis/cerebellitis Vasculitis
Infections	Cerebellitis Brainstem encephalitis
Traumatic	Brainstem concussion Dissection of the vertebral artery (indirectly via ischemia)

vestibulopathy/vestibular neuritis, labyrinthine contusion, and, in central lesions, due to a brainstem or cerebellar infarction. Pathophysiologically, these symptoms and signs are caused by an acute vestibular tone imbalance, which is compensated over days to weeks.

2.1.3 Symptoms Persisting for More Than 3 Months: Chronic Vertigo or Dizziness

The leading symptoms are most often persisting dizziness, postural imbalance, and impairment of gait. Examples are bilateral vestibulopathy, functional dizziness, neurodegenerative disorders such as cerebellar dizziness, e.g., downbeat nystagmus syndrome or multiple system atrophies, dizziness and postural imbalance, e.g., in movement disorders such as Parkinson's disease, progressive supranuclear palsy or Lewy body dementia, or in other disorders such as normal pressure hydrocephalus. In peripheral vestibular disorders, the symptoms are caused by the sensory deficit. In functional dizziness, the symptoms are caused by permanent self-checking of balance. In central disorders, symptoms are caused by an impairment of coordination, stance, and gait.

2.2 The Type of Symptoms

1. **Spinning vertigo** like riding a merry-go-round (e.g., BPPV or acute unilateral vestibulopathy/vestibular neuritis): Isolated spinning vertigo typically occurs due to a dysfunction of the semicircular canals because, under physiological conditions, they sense angular acceleration. The same sensation can be elicited by a unilateral lesion of the vestibular nerve, as in acute unilateral vestibulopathy, or by a lesion of the vestibular nuclei in the brainstem or vestibular structures in the cerebellum.
2. **Dizziness and postural imbalance** like during boat trips (e.g., bilateral vestibulopathy, post-traumatic otolith dizziness, or functional dizziness): A sensory deficit manifests as movement-dependent postural imbalance (e.g., bilateral vestibulopathy or persisting unilateral vestibular deficit). Dizziness, postural imbalance, and gait disorder are also found in so-called post-traumatic otolith dizziness after successful liberatory maneuvers in BPPV due to the partial repositioning of otoconia to the utricle (Bremova et al. 2013). It is also described by patients with functional dizziness due to selfchecking of balance.
3. **Lightheadedness** (e.g., functional dizziness or side effects of drugs) (◘ Table 2.3).

◘ **Table 2.3** Lightheadedness (causes given in alphabetical order)

Presyncopal lightheadedness	Functional disorders	Metabolic disorders and exogenic noxious agents
Cardiac arrhythmias or other heart diseases	Acrophobia	Alcohol
Hypersensitive carotid sinus	Agoraphobia	Electrolyte disorders (e.g., hypercalcemia, hyponatremia)
Neurocardiogenic (pre-) syncope	Functional dizziness	Hypoglycemia
Orthostatic dizziness	Hyperventilation syndrome	Intoxications
Vasovagal attacks	Panic attacks	Medications (see ◘ Table 17.1)
	Visually induced dizziness	

2.3 Triggers, Exacerbation, Improvement, and Modulating Factors of Symptoms

The patient must be explicitly asked about these features:

1. Do symptoms occur already at rest or spontaneously? E.g., acute unilateral vestibulopathy/vestibular neuritis, brainstem or cerebellar infarction, Menière's disease, vestibular paroxysmia, vestibular migraine, or downbeat nystagmus syndrome. These symptoms are caused by a peripheral or central vestibular tone imbalance and can worsen during movement.
2. Do they occur while standing, walking, or running, and without symptoms while laying or sitting down under static conditions? E.g., bilateral vestibulopathy or persisting unilateral vestibular deficit. These symptoms are caused by a sensory deficit and typically become worse in darkness and during walking on uneven ground. These are very important questions for the differential diagnosis, in particular of a sensory deficit.
3. Other triggers or modulating factors:
   - Head movements (▶ Box 2.1):
     – When changing head position relative to gravity (e.g., BPPV or central positional vertigo)
     – While turning the head to the side (e.g., bilateral vestibulopathy, vestibular paroxysmia, or vertebral artery compression/occlusion syndrome)
   - Context-dependent intensity worsening in certain social or environmental situations with improvement during sport activities or after light alcoholic drinks, e.g., functional dizziness, in particular phobic postural dizziness (Brandt et al. 2015)
   - When coughing, pressing, lifting heavy weights, pressing on one ear, or at loud sounds of a certain frequency—as the Tullio phenomenon (typical for the syndrome of the third mobile windows, often in combination with autophony)
   - Hyperventilation (found in vestibular paroxysmia and vestibular schwannoma)
   - Daytime: In BPPV, typically patients often have their first or their most prominent symptoms in the early morning when they get up. Patients with downbeat nystagmus also have more symptoms in the morning or after bed rest (Spiegel et al. 2010). Patients with functional dizziness typically have fewer symptoms during the first minutes or hours of the day. In bilateral vestibulopathy, there is an increase of symptoms during daytime (Feuerecker et al. 2015).

Box 2.1 Symptoms That Are Induced by or Are More Prominent During Head Movements (in Alphabetical Order)

- Bilateral vestibulopathy
- BPPV (head movements relative to gravity)
- Central positional vertigo and nystagmus (relative to gravity)
- Cerebellar ataxias
- Hypersensitive carotid sinus syndrome
- Intoxication (alcoholic positional nystagmus, head movements relative to gravity)
- Peripheral or central ocular motor disorders
- Persistent unilateral vestibulopathy
- Post-traumatic otolith dizziness
- Syndrome of the third mobile windows
- Vertebral artery compression or occlusion syndrome
- Vestibular paroxysmia (only in a small percentage of patients)

2.4 Accompanying Symptoms

Any further questions should aim to identify possible accompanying symptoms. Here too it is necessary to investigate each possible symptom individually:

1. **Audiological symptoms** (▶ Box 2.2): e.g., hypacusis or tinnitus, which are typical of Menière's disease, but which could also occur in brainstem ischemia and, in particular, an AICA infarction/TIA. Autophony, i.e., patients hear the sounds of their own body unusually loudly, is typically found in the syndrome of the third mobile windows (most frequent form: superior canal dehiscence syndrome).
2. **Potential brainstem and cerebellar symptoms:** e.g., double vision, impaired sensation in the face, problems with swallowing and speaking, facial palsy, unilaterally impaired sensation unilateral weakness, or impaired coordination (for the underlying etiologies, see ▶ Box 2.3). Spinning vertigo occurs mainly in unilateral lesions of the medulla oblongata, pons, and cerebellum. Unilateral lesions of the upper brainstem, i.e., the mesencephalon and the thalamus, lead to postural imbalance, dizziness, and

Box 2.2 Combination of Vestibular and Audiological Symptoms Possible

- Cerebellopontine angle tumour
- Cholesteatoma
- Cogan syndrome or other autoimmune diseases
- Ear/head trauma (labyrinthine contusion)
- Inner ear malformation
- Labyrinthine infarct (AICA, labyrinthine artery)
- Menière's disease
- Neurolabyrinthitis
- Otosclerosis
- Pontomedullary brainstem infarction or MS plaque
- Syndrome of the third mobile windows
- Vestibular paroxysmia
- Zoster oticus

Box 2.3 Vertigo and Dizziness with Additional Brainstem or Cerebellar Symptoms: Examples of Possible Etiologies

- Autoimmune diseases, e.g., MS or brainstem or cerebellar encephalitis
- Craniocervical anomalies (e.g., Arnold-Chiari malformation)
- Episodic ataxias, in particular type 2
- Infarctions of the vertebro-basilar system
- Head trauma
- Hemorrhage
- Intoxication
- Tumors of the cerebellopontine angle with compression of the brainstem or tumors of the brainstem or cerebellum
- Vestibular migraine

impairment of spatial orientation, rarely to spinning vertigo.

3. **Headache, hypersensitivity to light or sound, visual aura, and/or known migraine:** These symptoms are typically found in vestibular migraine. However, headache can also occur in brainstem or cerebellar infarction or hemorrhages (for a summary of possible etiologies, see ▶ Box 2.4).

Box 2.4 Vertigo/Dizziness with Headache

- Brainstem/cerebellar ischemia
- Head trauma (especially transverse temporal bone fracture)
- Infratentorial hemorrhage
- Infratentorial tumour
- Inner/middle ear infections
- Vertebrobasilar dissection
- Vestibular migraine
- Zoster oticus

4. **Illusionary movements of the surroundings (oscillopsia):** With head and body stationary: This is typically found in patients with nystagmus (exception: compensated infantile nystagmus); oscillopsia in patients with nystagmus can increase when the patient is looking in the direction of the fast phase. With head or body movements or during walking: This is typically found in patients with bilateral and persisting unilateral vestibulopathy during fast head turns and during walking because of the VOR deficit; however, less than 50% of these patients have movement-induced oscillopsia for reasons we do not yet know (for possible etiologies of spontaneous oscillopsia, see ▶ Box 2.5).

Box 2.5 Illusionary Movements of the Surroundings (Oscillopsia)

- **With head and body stationary**
  - Acquired fixation pendular nystagmus
  - Congenital/infantile nystagmus (depending on direction of gaze)
  - Convergence-retraction nystagmus
  - Downbeat nystagmus
  - Myokymia of the superior oblique muscle (monocular oscillopsia)
  - Ocular flutter
  - Opsoclonus
  - Paroxysmal ocular tilt reaction
  - Peripheral vestibular spontaneous nystagmus
  - Periodic alternating nystagmus
  - Spasmus nutans (children)
  - Upbeat nystagmus
  - Vestibular paroxysmia
  - Voluntary nystagmus
- **During head or body movements or walking**
  - Bilateral vestibulopathy
  - Unilateral vestibulopathy

5. **Nausea and vomiting**: These are unspecific associated symptoms, which are typically found in acute peripheral and central vestibular syndromes, but can even rarely be reported by patients with functional dizziness.

2.5 Focused or Specific Patient History to Differentiate Between an Acute Peripheral and an Acute Central Vestibular Syndrome

The following symptoms make a central lesion more likely:

1. Acute onset, no triggers, non-episodic symptoms
2. Accompanying symptoms, such as double vision, impaired sensation in the face, facial palsy, dysarthrophonia, or problems with swallowing, unilateral weakness, or impairment of sensation or coordination
3. Known cardiovascular risk factors, such as arterial hypertension, diabetes, smoking, a history of stroke or heart attack, and older age (Navi et al. 2012)
4. Combined vertigo/dizziness and headache or combined vertigo/dizziness and hearing problems (AICA infarction)

Type of symptoms (vertigo, dizziness, imbalance), intensity, and duration are evidently not helpful for the differentiation (Tarnutzer et al. 2017).

Some of these specific aspects of the patient history have been validated by means of the $ABCD^2$ Score or the TriAGe+ Score (for references, see Navi et al. 2012; Kuroda et al. 2017; Zwergal and Dieterich 2020).

2.6 Additional Sources of Information from the Patient

1. Videoing of eye movements during an episode of vertigo or during the diagnostic positioning maneuvers using a mobile/smartphone (Shah et al. 2019; Green et al. 2021; Shaik et al. 2021) or a vestibular event monitor (Young et al. 2019). This has been shown to be helpful for the diagnosis of BPPV to identify the affected side and semicircular canal and for the diagnosis of Menière's disease with change of the direction of the nystagmus during an episode of vertigo as well as vestibular paroxysmia (in particular, to differentiate from a panic attack).
2. Examination of hearing by the patient before, during, and after an attack of vertigo, which can be done using apps (Tse et al. 2019). This is particularly important for the diagnosis of Menière's disease and to differentiate from vestibular migraine because, according to the diagnostic criteria for Menière's disease, an impairment of hearing of at least 30 dB below 2000 Hz related to an attack (ideally ±24 h) is required (Lopez-Escamez et al. 2015).

References

Bisdorff A, von Brevern M, Lempert T, Newman-Toker DE (2009) Classification of vestibular symptoms: towards an international classification of vestibular disorders. J Vestib Res 19(1-2):1–13

Brandt T, Huppert D, Strupp M, Dieterich M (2015) Functional dizziness: diagnostic keys and differential diagnosis. J Neurol 262:1977–1980

Brandt T, Strupp M, Dieterich M (2014) Five keys for diagnosing most vertigo, dizziness, and imbalance syndromes: an expert opinion. J Neurol 261(1):229–231

Bremova T, Bayer O, Agrawal Y, Kremmyda O, Brandt T, Teufel J, Strupp M (2013) Ocular VEMPs indicate repositioning of otoconia to the utricle after successful liberatory maneuvers in benign paroxysmal positioning vertigo. Acta Otolaryngol 133(12):1297–1303

Feuerecker R, Habs M, Dieterich M, Strupp M (2015) Chronic subjective dizziness: fewer symptoms in the early morning–a comparison with bilateral vestibulopathy and downbeat nystagmus syndrome. J Vestib Res 25(2):67–72

Green KE, Pogson JM, Otero-Millan J, Gold DR, Tevzadze N, Saber Tehrani AS, Zee DS, Newman-Toker DE, Kheradmand A (2021) Opinion and Special Articles: Remote Evaluation of Acute Vertigo: Strategies and Technological Considerations. Neurology 96:34–38

Kuroda R, Nakada T, Ojima T, Serizawa M, Imai N, Yagi N, Tasaki A, Aoki M, Oiwa T, Ogane T, Mochizuki K, Kobari M, Miyajima H (2017) The TriAGe+ score for vertigo or dizziness: a diagnostic model for stroke in the emergency department. J Stroke Cerebrovasc Dis 26(5):1144–1153

Lopez-Escamez JA, Carey J, Chung WH, Goebel JA, Magnusson M, Mandala M, Newman-Toker DE, Strupp M, Suzuki M, Trabalzini F, Bisdorff A (2015) Diagnostic criteria for Meniere's disease. J Vestib Res 25(1):1–7

Navi BB, Kamel H, Shah MP, Grossman AW, Wong C, Poisson SN, Whetstone WD, Josephson SA, Johnston SC, Kim AS (2012) Rate and predictors of serious neurologic causes of dizziness in the emergency department. Mayo Clin Proc 87(11):1080–1088

Shah MU, Lotterman S, Roberts D, Eisen M (2019) Smartphone telemedical emergency department consults for screening of nonacute dizziness. Laryngoscope 129(2):466–469

Shaikh AG, Bronstein A, Carmona S, Cha YH, Cho C, Ghasia FF, Gold D, Green KE, Helmchen C, Ibitoye RT, Kattah J, Kim JS, Kothari S, Manto M, Seemungal BM, Straumann D, Strupp M, Szmulewicz D, Tarnutzer A, Tehrani A, Tilikete C, Welgampola M, Zalazar G, Kheradmand A (2021) Consensus on Virtual Management of Vestibular Disorders: Urgent Versus Expedited Care. Cerebellum 20:4–8

Spiegel R, Kalla R, Rettinger N, Schneider E, Straumann D, Marti S, Glasauer S, Brandt T, Strupp M (2010) Head position during resting modifies spontaneous daytime decrease of downbeat nystagmus. Neurology 75(21):1928–1932

Tarnutzer AA, Lee SH, Robinson KA, Wang Z, Edlow JA, Newman-Toker DE (2017) ED misdiagnosis of cerebrovascular events in the era of modern neuroimaging: a meta-analysis. Neurology 88(15): 1468–1477

Tse D, Ramsay T, Lelli DA (2019) Novel use of portable audiometry to track hearing fluctuations in Meniere's disease: a pilot study. Otol Neurotol 40(2):e130–e134

Welgampola MS, Young AS, Pogson JM, Bradshaw AP, Halmagyi GM (2019) Dizziness demystified. Pract Neurol 19(6):492–501

Young AS, Lechner C, Bradshaw AP, MacDougall HG, Black DA, Halmagyi GM, Welgampola MS (2019) Capturing acute vertigo: a vestibular event monitor. Neurology 92(24):e2743–e2753

Zwergal A, Dieterich M (2020) Vertigo and dizziness in the emergency room. Curr Opin Neurol 33(1): 117–125

Combined Neuro-Otological and Neuro-Ophthalmological Bedside Examination

Contents

Supplementary Information The online version contains supplementary material available at [https://doi.org/10.1007/978-3-030-78260-3_3]. The videos can be accessed by scanning the related images with the SN More Media App.

M. Strupp et al., *Vertigo and Dizziness*, https://doi.org/10.1007/978-3-030-78260-3_3

A systematic, combined neuro-otological and neuro-ophthalmological examination is—in addition to the detailed patient history—essential for a correct diagnosis. In the clinical bedside examination, the physician must primarily answer the two following questions:

1. Is there a dysfunction/deficit of the vestibular system?

   This can be achieved by the following five tests: (1) examination for components of the ocular tilt reaction (OTR); (2) looking for a spontaneous nystagmus with and without Frenzel's goggles or M-glasses; (3) performing the head impulse test (HIT, ideally the video-HIT) to look for a VOR deficit; (4) diagnostic positional maneuvers to look for positional nystagmus; and (5) examination of stance by the Romberg test and of gait.
2. Is it a peripheral vestibular or a central vestibular lesion?

   The latter requires a careful neurological, in particular neuro-ophthalmological examination of the various types of eye movements to look for central ocular motor disorders and central types of nystagmus and neurootogical examination, namely the HIT, ideally the video-HIT. Evidence of a central lesion has immediate diagnostic and therapeutic consequences, especially in cases of an acute central vestibular syndrome.

In ◘ Table 3.1 and in ◘ Figs. 3.1, 3.2, 3.3, 3.4, 3.5, 3.6, 3.7, 3.8, 3.9, 3.10, 3.11, 3.12, 3.13, 3.14, 3.15, 3.16, and 3.17, various aspects of the bedside examination with typical findings and their interpretation are summarized. It is important to note that, compared with careful taking of the patient history and careful examination of the vestibular and the ocular motor system, laboratory examinations, with the exception of the video-HIT and caloric testing, are of inferior clinical relevance (see ► Chap. 4).

3.1 Specific Examination of the Vestibular System

3.1.1 Examination for Components of the Ocular Tilt Reaction (OTR)

3.1.1.1 Head Tilt

An ocular tilt reaction (OTR) basically is the triad of head tilt, skew deviation of the eyes (one eye up, the other down), and ocular torsion of both eyes (Westheimer and Blair 1975). In ◘ Fig. 3.1, the examination procedure of head tilt is shown. In OTR, the head is typically tilted toward the side of the lower eye, due to a vestibular tone imbalance in the

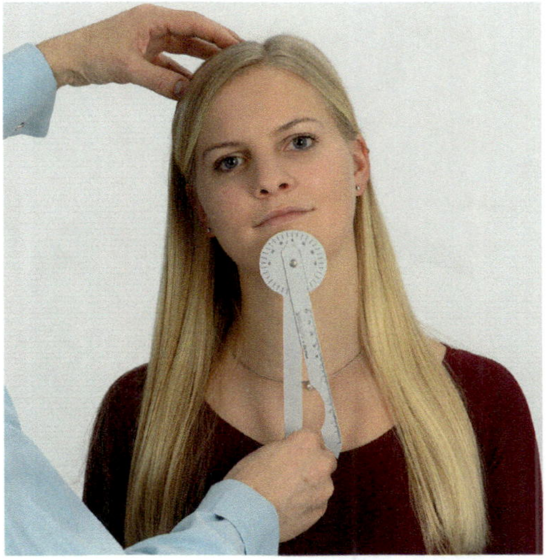

◘ **Fig. 3.1** Measurement of head tilt using the "strabofix"

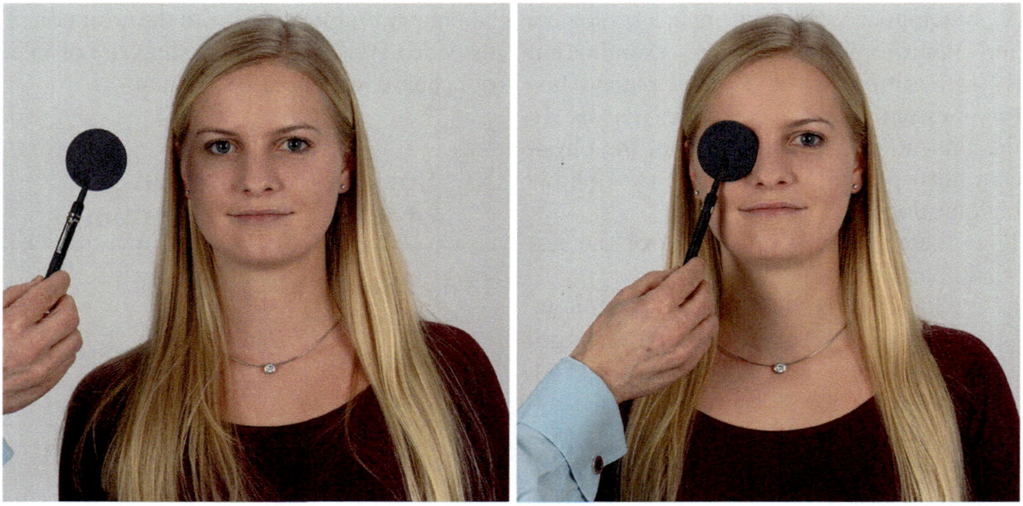

Fig. 3.2 Cover test and uncover test. Examination to detect misalignments of the visual axes, i.e., latent or manifest strabismus and vertical deviation/skew deviation. The prerequisite for all cover tests is the presence of foveal fixation

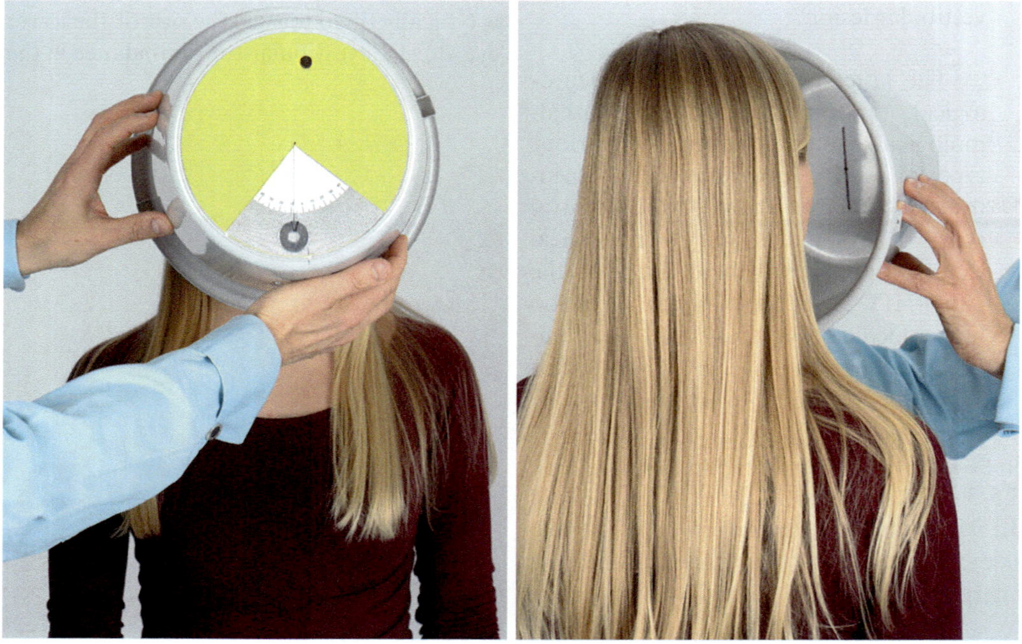

Fig. 3.3 Measurement of the subjective visual vertical (SVV) with the "bucket test." This is a simple bedside test to determine the SVV (Zwergal et al. 2009). Left from the examiner's perspective, right from the patient's point of view. The examiner turns the bucket in a pseudorandomized way seven times to the right and left. The patient looks into the bucket at a line that has been drawn on the bottom and which he/she must get into a vertical position. The examiner then reads the deviation from the actual vertical (perpendicular) and calculates the mean value. The normal range is 0 ± 2.5°

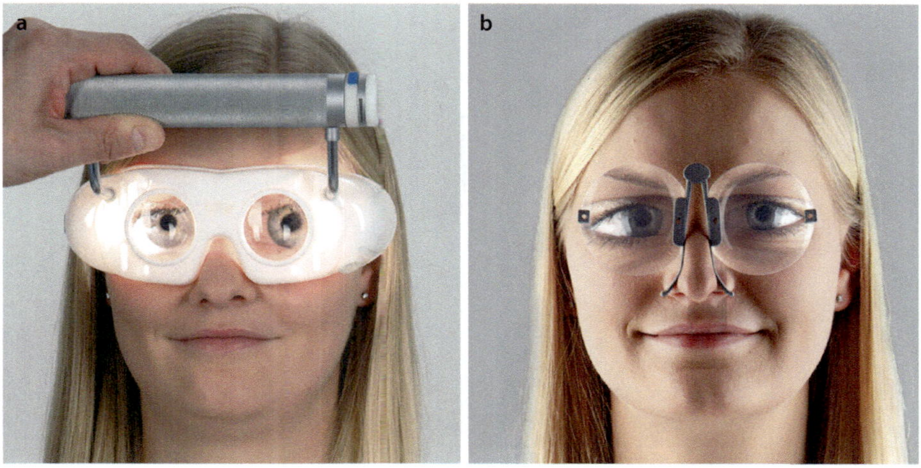

■ **Fig. 3.4** **a**, **b** Clinical examination to look for nystagmus in primary position, i.e., when the patient looks straight ahead. This should be done with fixation and with reduced fixation using **a** Frenzel's goggles or **b** M-glasses. A nystagmus which is *not* reduced by visual fixation is *not* a peripheral vestibular spontaneous nystagmus

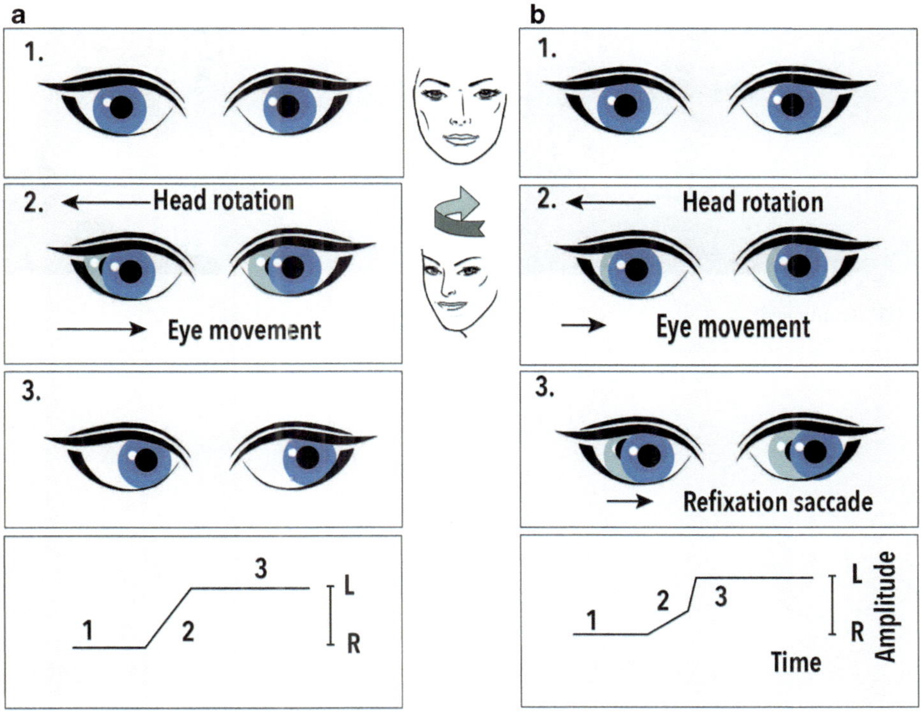

■ **Fig. 3.5** **a–c** Head impulse test: clinical examination of the horizontal vestibulo-ocular reflex (VOR) (Halmagyi and Curthoys 1988). **a** Normal result: The eyes move during rapid rotation of the head with the same angular velocity but in the opposite direction; thus, the eyes remain on the target. **b** Example: Deficit of the right horizontal semicircular canal. In cases of unilateral vestibulopathy on the right side, the eyes move during head rotations to the right with the head, and the patient has to perform a so-called refixation saccade to the left in order to correct and again fixate the target. This is the clinical sign of a deficit of the VOR in the high-frequency range. **c** The examination situation

c

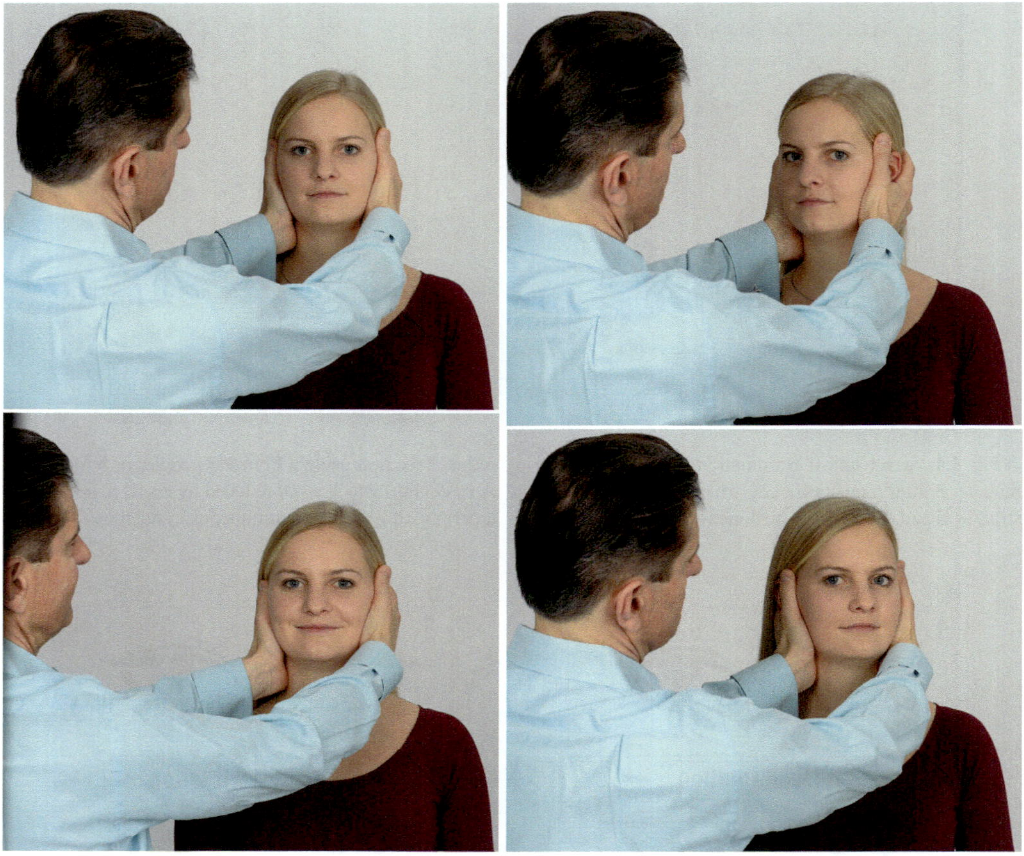

Fig. 3.5 (continued)

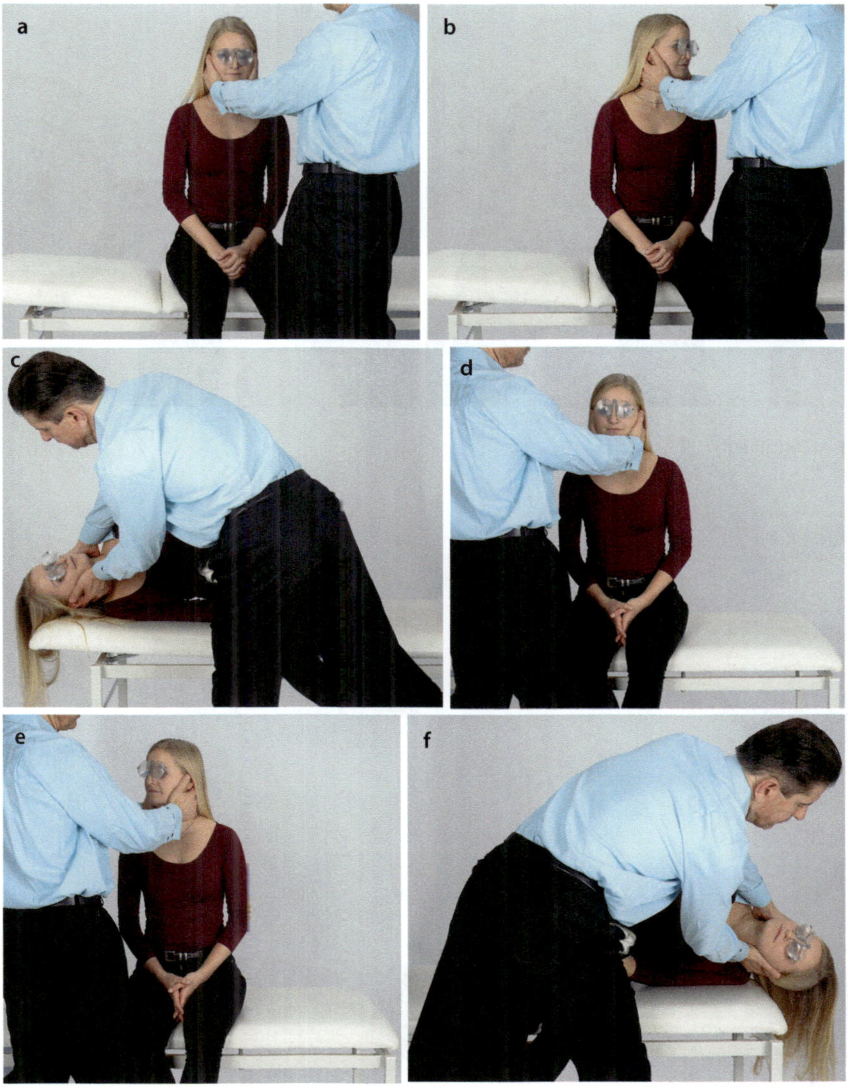

Fig. 3.6 **a**–**h**. Diagnostic Semont maneuver for the right posterior canal (**a**–**c**) and the left posterior canal (**d**–**f**). In the upright position the head is turned by 45° towards one side and the patient moved by 90° towards the other side. Diagnostic SemontPLUS maneuver (**g**: right side, **h**: left side). The difference is that during the last movement the head and body are overextended by at least 60° below earth horizontal with the lower arm abduced and extended

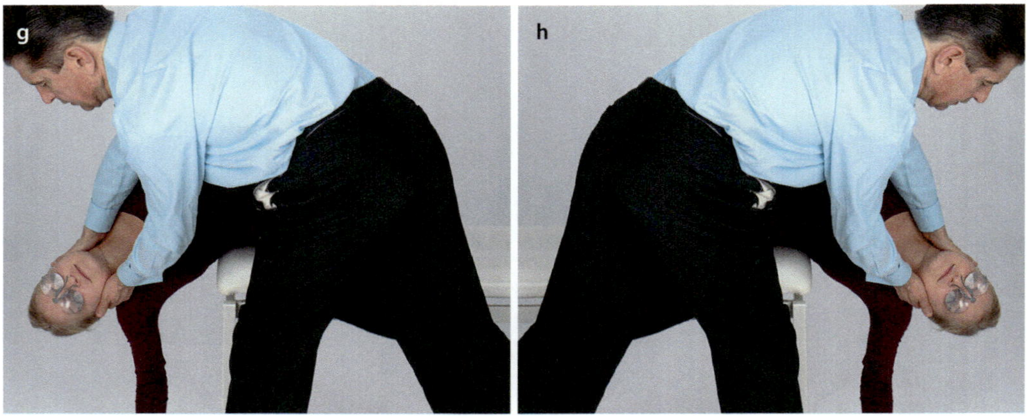

Fig. 3.6 (continued)

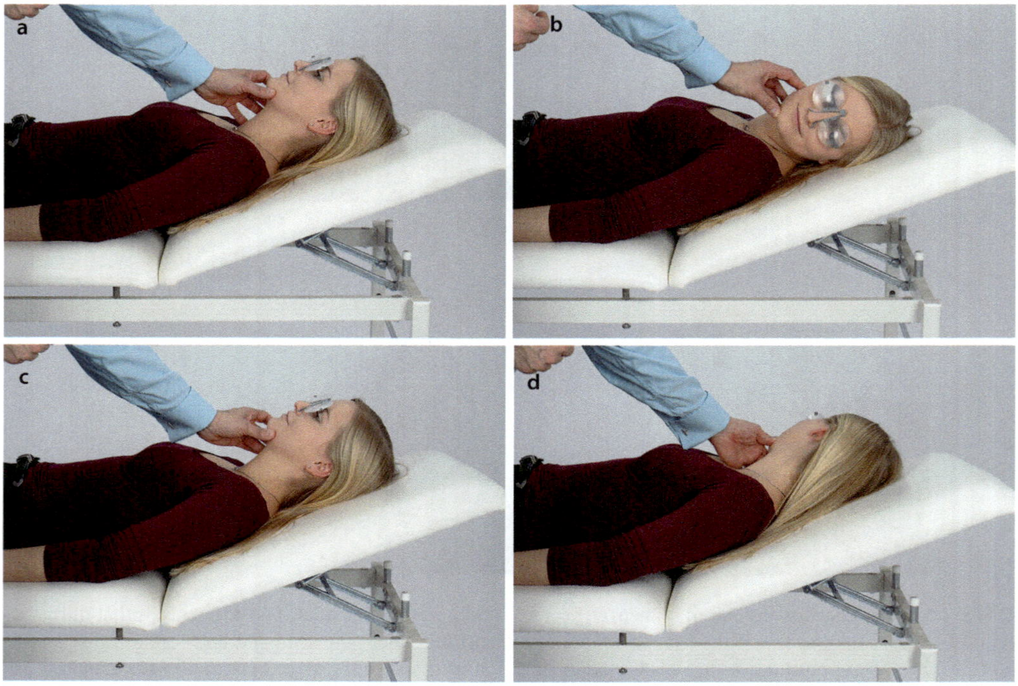

Fig. 3.7 **a–d** Diagnostic positional maneuvers for BPPV of a horizontal canal: the supine roll test. **a** The patient lies supine and the patient's head should be lifted 25° to bring the horizontal canal into a vertical position. **b** Then, the patient's head is tilted 90° toward the right, **c** then back to the midline, and **d** then 90° to the left, while the patient's eye movements are examined using Frenzel's goggles or M-glasses

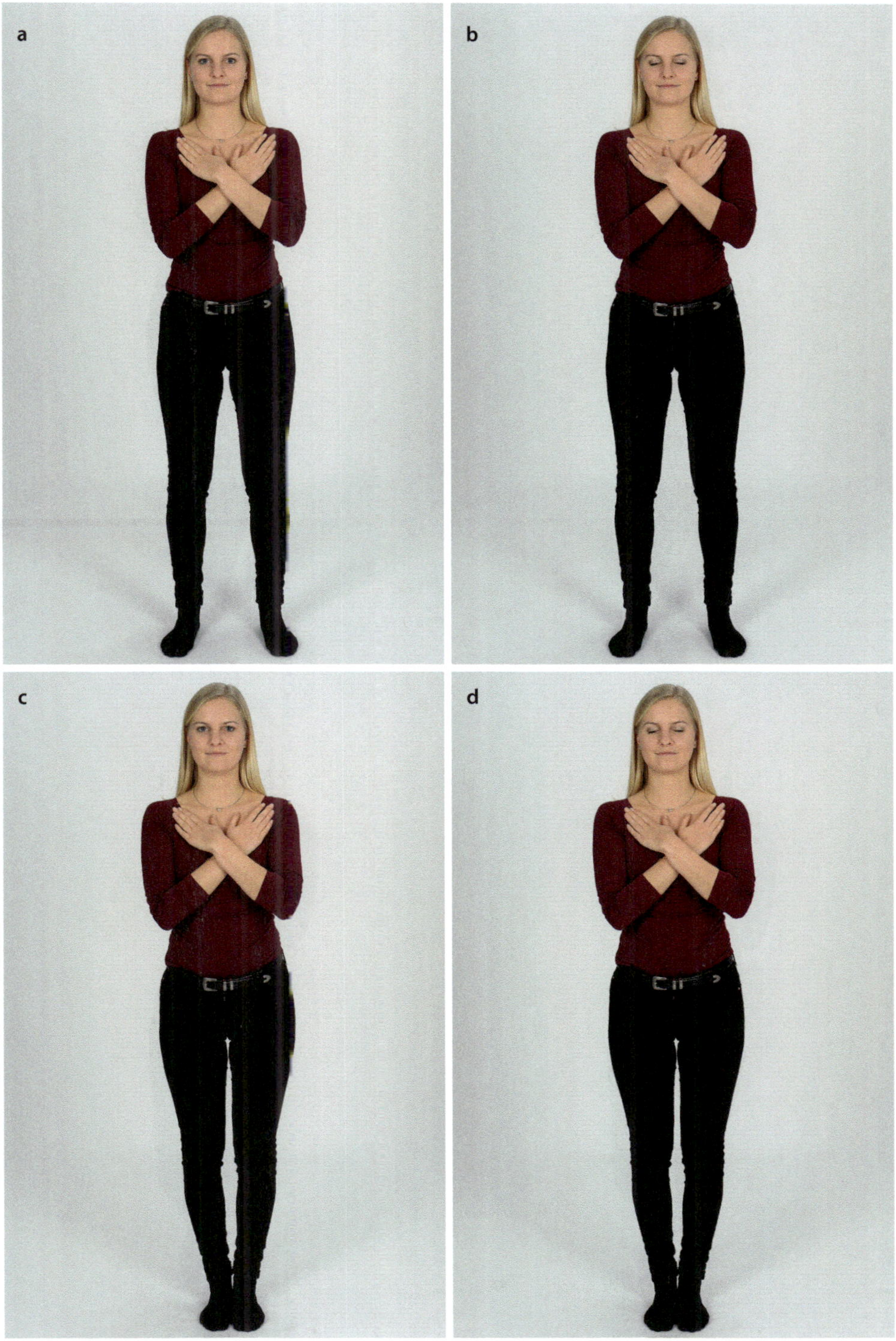

Fig. 3.8 **a–j** Romberg test. Clinical examination of balance under static conditions with eyes open (on the left side: **a**, **c**, **e**, **f**, **i**) and subsequently closed (on the right side: **b**, **d**, **e**, **g**, **j**). Standing (**a**, **b**) with legs wide apart; (**c**, **d**) with legs close together; (**e**, **f**) one foot in front of the other ("tandem Romberg"); (**g**, **h**) on one leg; and (**i**, **j**) distracted state by writing on arm or back or by counting (dual task)

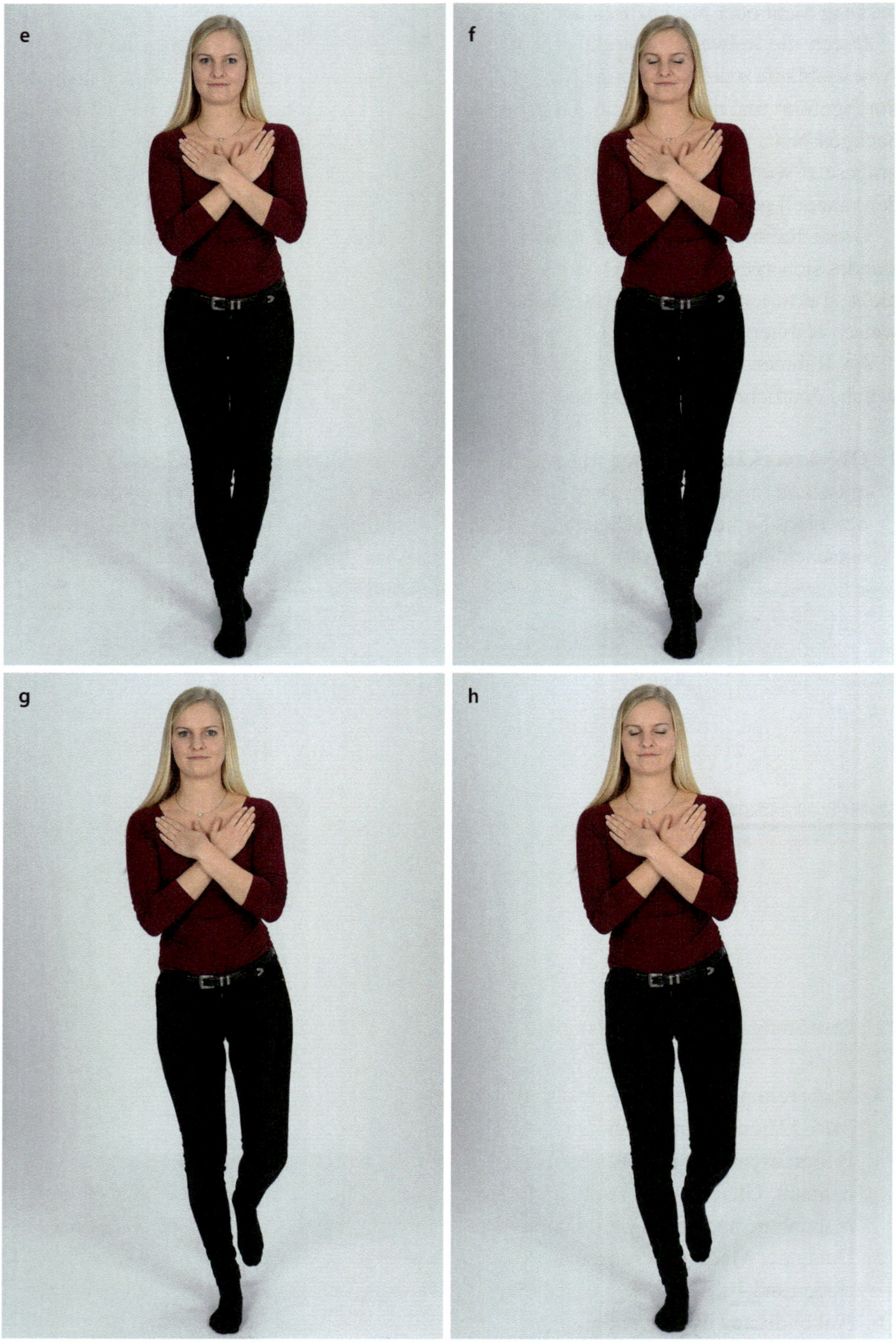

■ **Fig. 3.8** (continued)

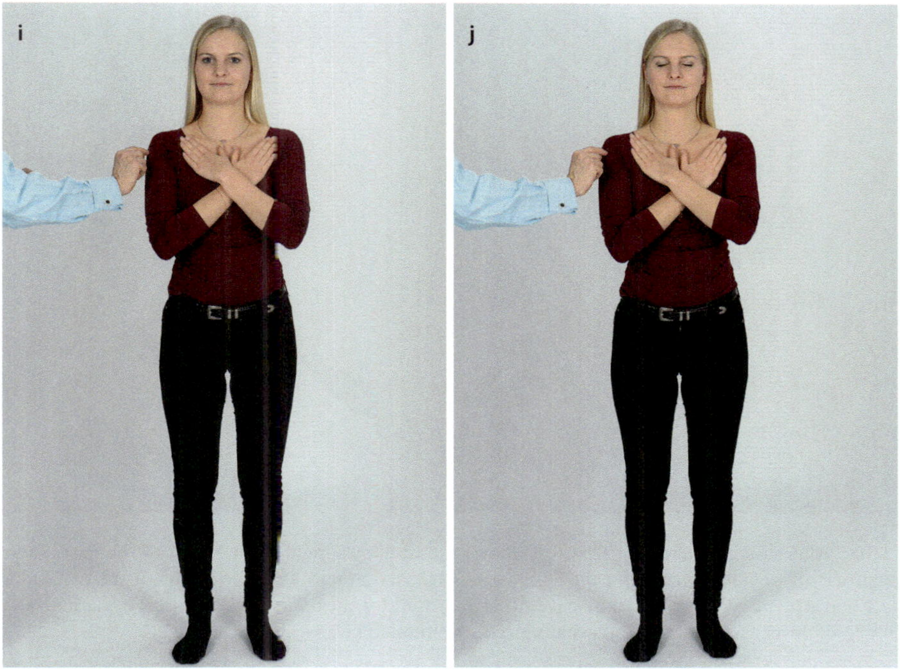

Fig. 3.8 (continued)

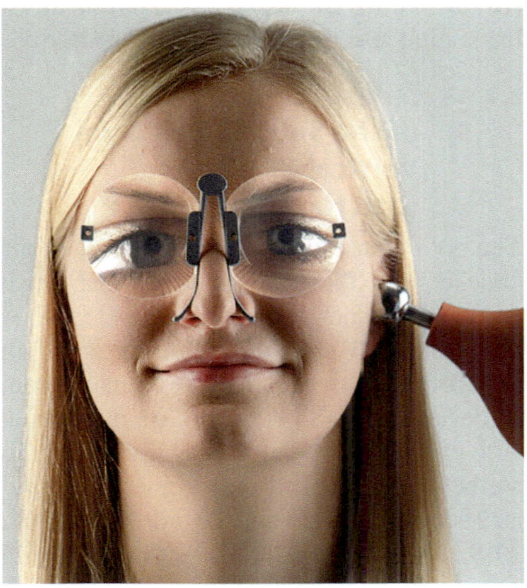

Fig. 3.9 Examination using a Politzer balloon and M-glasses. Positive and negative pressure in the area of the middle ear can be induced using a Politzer balloon. This examination technique is—in addition to the Valsalva maneuvers with pressing against the closed nostrils or the closed vocal cords—an important bedside test to look for signs of the syndrome of the third mobile windows (see ▶ Chap. 12)

role plane. A head tilt toward the side of the deficit either indicates an ipsilateral acute unilateral vestibulopathy or a unilateral lesion in the lower brainstem, as typically found in Wallenberg's syndrome (Dieterich and Brandt 1992). A head tilt can also be observed toward the contralateral side in patients with a pontomesencephalic lesion. Finally, a head tilt is also typically found in trochlear palsy with a head tilt toward the healthy side, which is done by the patient to reduced double vision. (Fig. 3.18).

3.1.1.2 Examination for a Vertical Deviation (VD) of the Eyes (Skew Deviation) Using the Cover and Uncover Test and the Alternating Cover Test

The cover and uncover tests (Fig. 3.2) allow the diagnosis of an ocular misalignment, namely latent or manifest strabismus and, in this context in particular, a vertical deviation/skew deviation. The prereq-

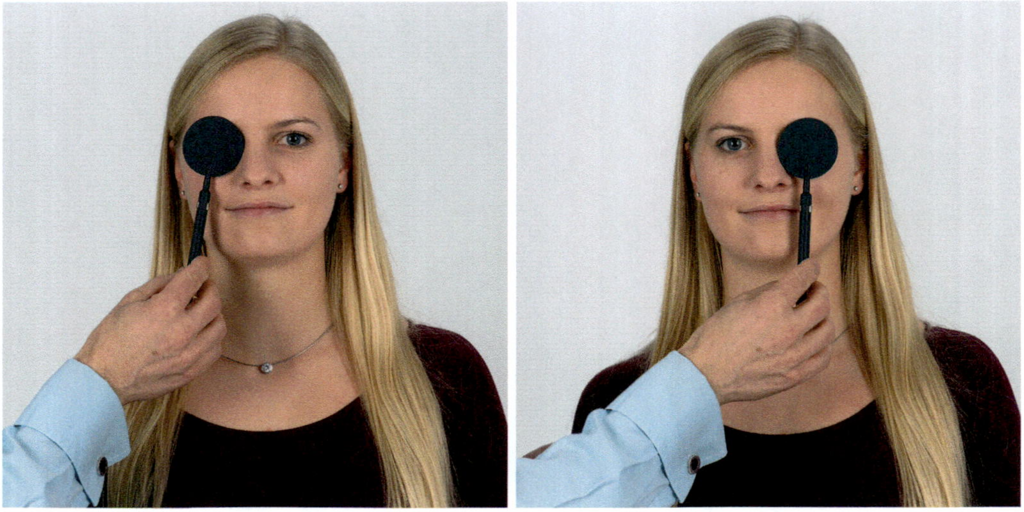

◘ Fig. 3.10 Alternating cover test. This test allows the diagnosis of ocular misalignment (see also ◘ Fig. 3.2 above). The prerequisite for all cover tests is the presence of foveal fixation. The alternating cover test allows the determination of the maximal angle of deviation and has been shown to be particularly relevant for the diagnosis of vertical deviation/skew deviation

uisite for all cover tests is the presence of foveal fixation. The alternating cover test (◘ Fig. 3.10) is useful for determining the maximal misalignment of the eye axes in both a tropia and a phoria. It is particularly helpful when establishing a vestibular vertical deviation/skew deviation (in the context of an OTR) (◘ Fig. 3.19), i.e., a vertical misalignment of the eyes that cannot be explained by an ocular muscle palsy or damage to a peripheral nerve. It is necessary to look for vertical corrective movements, when the cover is switched from one eye to the other (for more details, see ► Sect. 3.2). In contrast to trochlear nerve palsy or superior oblique muscle palsy, in skew deviation as a component of the OTR the vertical misalignment changes little or not at all during different directions of gaze. A prominent vertical deviation (> 3 deg) (Korda et al. 2022) is found virtually only in central vestibular lesions, but not all central vestibular lesions are associated with a vertical deviation: The prevalence in acute brainstem infarction is only 30% (Brandt and Dieterich 1993). That means it has a high specificity, but a low sensitivity.

3.1.1.3 Measurement of the Subjective Visual Vertical (SVV) with the "Bucket Test"

The SVV can be easily measured with the "bucket test" (◘ Figs. 3.3 and 3.20) (Zwergal et al. 2009) which is a simple bedside test. A deviation of SVV is a very sensitive sign of an acute or subacute unilateral vestibular lesion. A deviation of SVV occurs in more than 90% of such cases but it does not differentiate between a central or peripheral vestibular lesion (Dieterich and Brandt 1992, 1993, 2019; Zwergal et al. 2009). In peripheral vestibular and pontomedullary brainstem lesions, there is an ipsiversive deviation, in pontomesencephalic lesions a contraversive deviation (for more details, see ► Sect. 4.4).

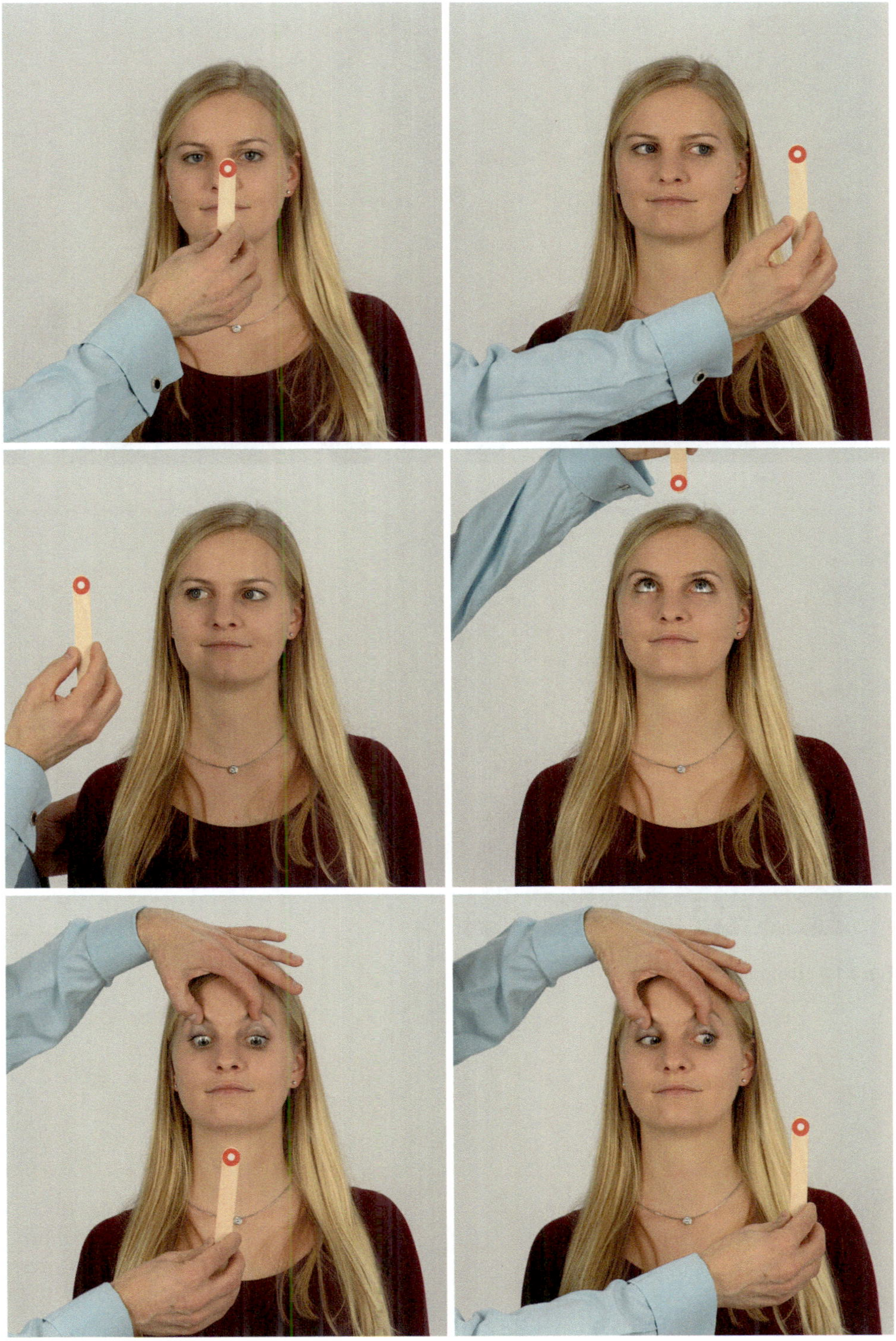

Fig. 3.11 Examination of the eye position and eye motility in the nine different gaze positions: with an object for fixation or a small rod-shaped flashlight

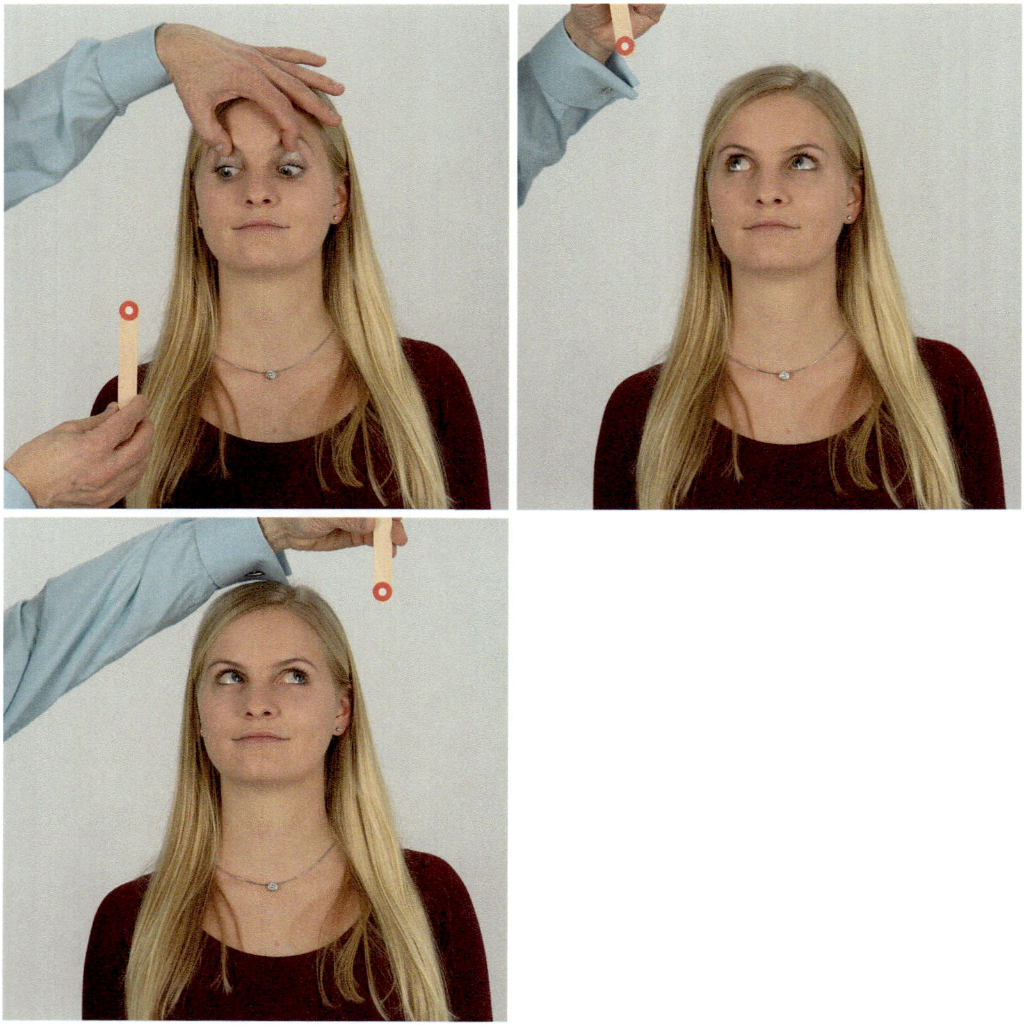

Fig. 3.11 (continued)

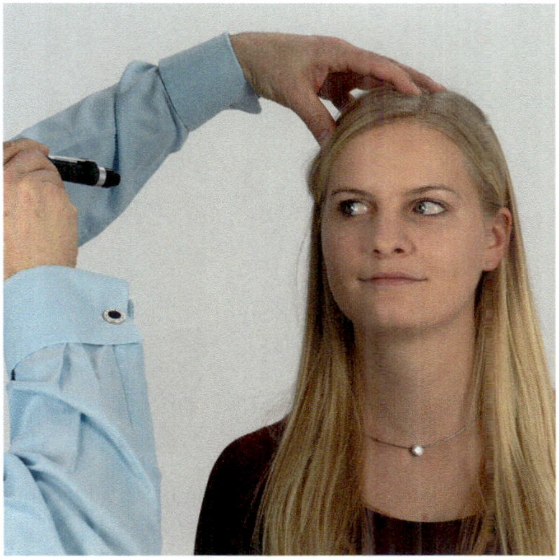

■ **Fig. 3.12** Clinical examination of eye positions and eye movements with an examination flashlight. The examiner checks whether the reflex images on the cornea are on corresponding parts of both eyes, which helps to diagnose ocular misalignment and whether the patient has gaze-evoked nystagmus. Note: it is important to observe the corneal reflex images from the direction of the illumination and to ensure that the patient attentively fixates the object

3.1.2 Examination for Spontaneous Nystagmus

Spontaneous nystagmus (■ Fig. 3.21) is a nystagmus that occurs when the patient looks straight ahead (primary position) without any head movements or other provocative factors (overview and classification in Eggers et al. 2019). The examination is performed in primary position with and without Frenzel goggles or M-glasses (Strupp et al. 2014) (■ Fig. 3.4) (overview in (Halmagyi et al. 2020). The magnification of the lenses (+16 to +20 dpt.) reduces visual fixation suppression. It is important to note that a nystagmus which is *not* reduced by visual fixation is *not* a peripheral nystagmus. This implies that in some patients a central nystagmus can also be at least partially reduced by visual fixation (Mantokoudis et al. 2021). Further, it is important to note that in the very acute phase of an acute unilateral vestibulopathy patients can only partially suppress the spontaneous peripheral nystagmus.

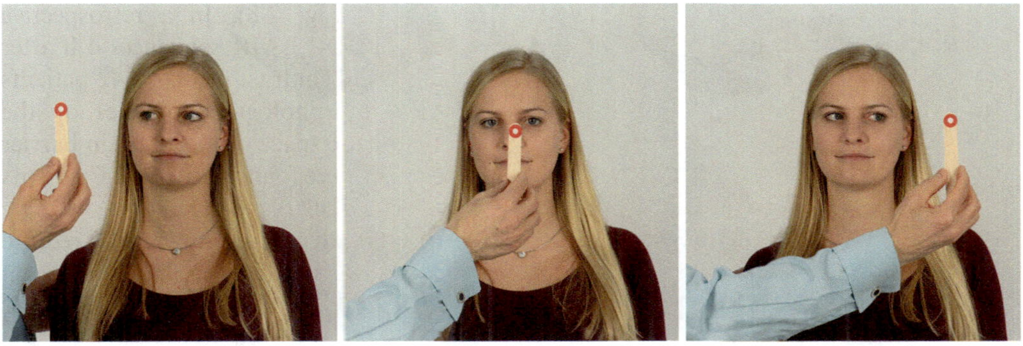

■ **Fig. 3.13** Clinical examination of smooth pursuit eye movements. It is important to note that the patient has to have a very good fixation point and the amplitudes of the horizontal and vertical smooth pursuit eye movement should not be too large, i.e., ±40° for horizontal and ± 20° for vertical eye movements. Further, one should start with a low angular velocity. For the examination of vertical eye movements, eyelids must always be lifted up; otherwise, it is not possible to perform a correct examination

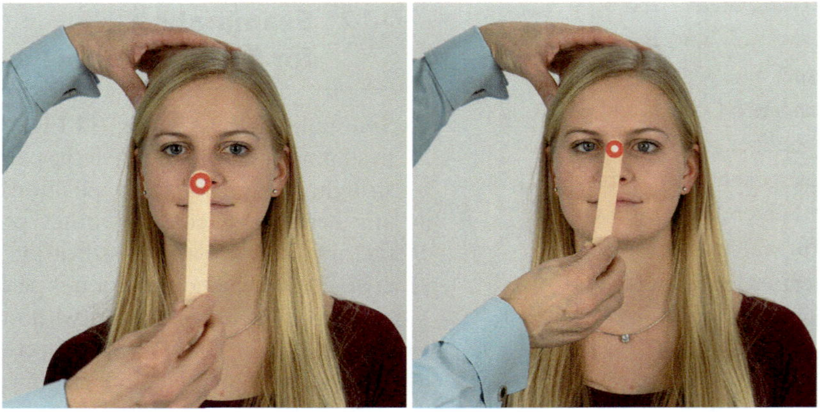

Fig. 3.14 Vergence test with convergence reaction. The vergence reaction is a combination of an adduction, myosis, and an accommodation, the latter is not directly visible to the observer

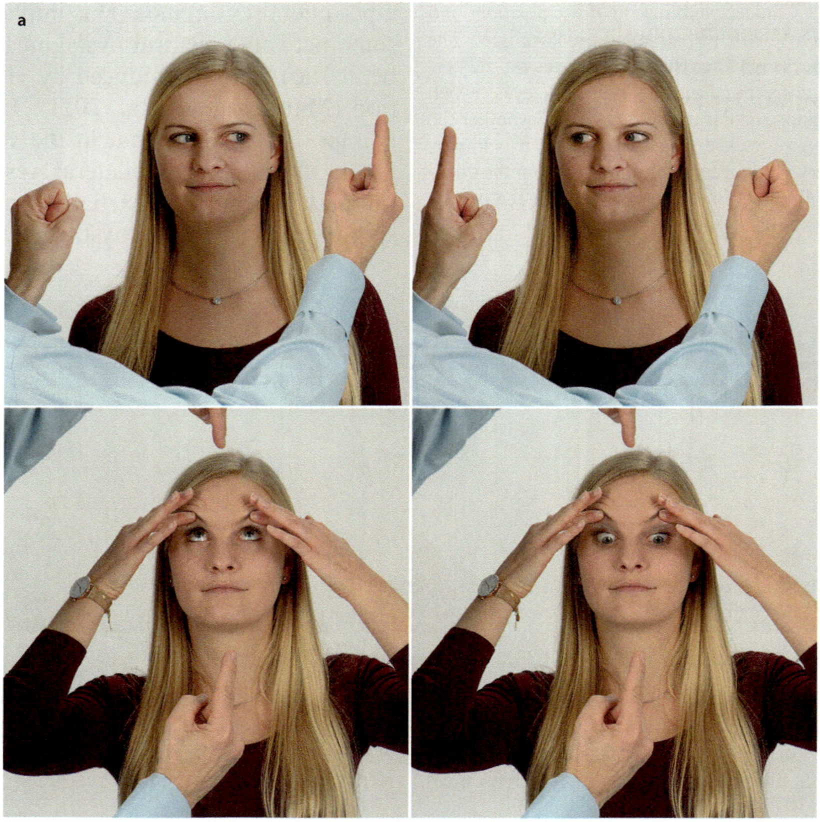

Fig. 3.15 **a**, **b** Clinical examination of horizontal and vertical saccades. A target could be **a** the tip of the examiner's finger, which moves up and down or **b** a so-called saccade stick, which allows a standardized examination. It is important that the patient has a very good target, that the amplitudes are not too large (0 ± 30° for horizontal and 0 ± 20° for vertical saccades) and that the eyelids are lifted up during examination of vertical saccades because otherwise it is not possible to examine vertical saccades properly because an impairment is often covered by blinking which drives saccades

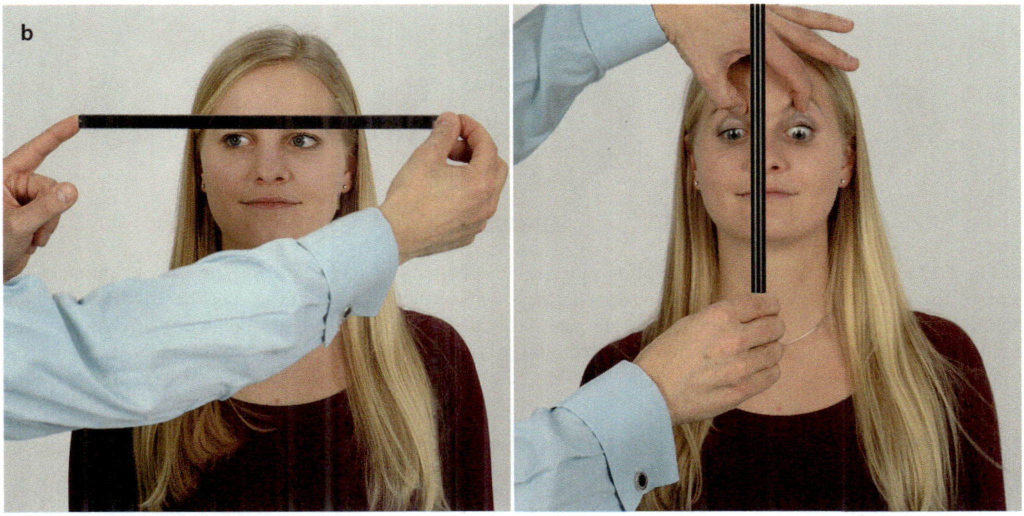

■ **Fig. 3.15** (continued)

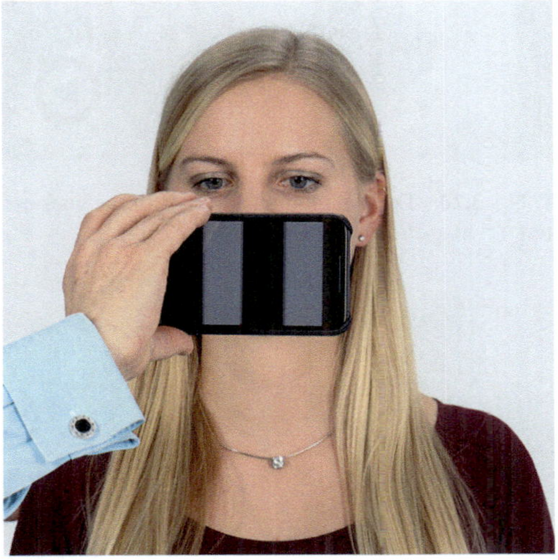

■ **Fig. 3.16** Examination of optokinetic nystagmus (OKN). This can also be done with a smartphone with a large screen and an app with horizontally and vertically moving stripes or figures in front of the patient's eyes. Full-field stimulation is important for the OKN

Spontaneous nystagmus is caused by a peripheral or central vestibular tone imbalance. Sensu stricto, the pathological phase is the slow phase. The direction (horizontal, vertical, torsional, or combined), however, is given according to the fast phase, which can be seen more easily by the examiner. In peripheral vestibular spontaneous nystagmus, the fast phase beats toward the relatively more active labyrinth. The classification and diagnosis of nystagmus primarily depend on the type, the direction, and provoking/modulating factors (Eggers et al. 2019):

1. **Type of nystagmus:**
   - Saw tooth with a fast and a slow phase, which is typical for a peripheral vestibular nystagmus, but can also occur in central or even cerebellar lesions.
   - Pendular, which is typical for a central fixation pendular nystagmus (■ Fig. 3.22) or, for instance, a central seesaw nystagmus.

2. **Direction of the fast phase:**
   - Horizontal, e.g., toward the right ear with a torsional component anticlockwise, which is typical for an acute vestibular lesion on the left side. Rule: The fast phase of a nystagmus beats toward the relatively more active labyrinth. In this case, the nystagmus is caused by a vestibular tone imbalance: The right labyrinth is more active, which leads to a slow drift toward the left and a fast correction

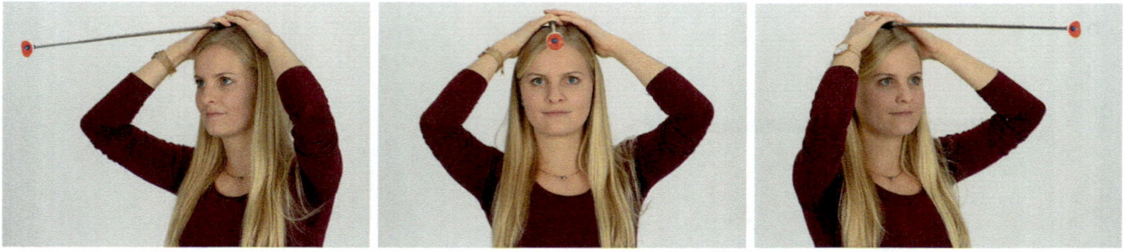

■ **Fig. 3.17** Clinical testing of visual fixation suppression of the VOR. Healthy individuals can suppress the VOR by fixation. The eyes remain on the target. A minimal shift of the image on the retina (so-called retinal slip) is the signal to suppress the VOR; the same signal is also important for the smooth pursuit. The observance of saccades during this examination indicates an impairment of the smooth pursuit system, typically found in cerebellar disorders involving the flocculus or paraflocculus or cerebellar pathways

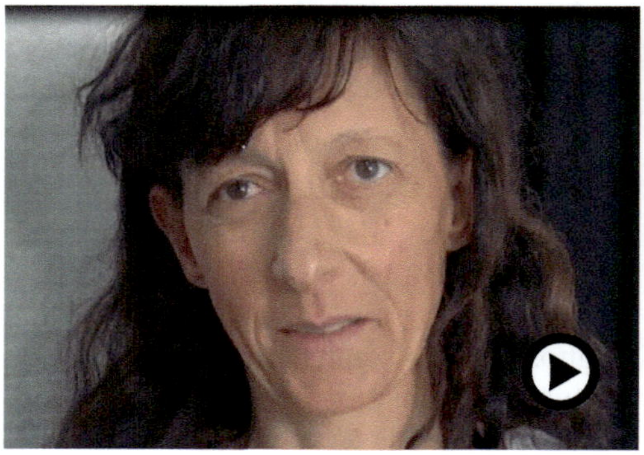

■ **Fig. 3.18** Trochlear nerve palsy on the left (► https://doi.org/10.1007/000-94f)

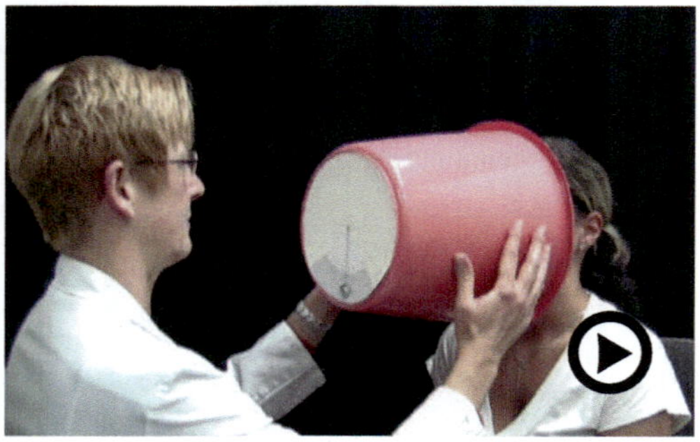

■ **Fig. 3.20** Determination of SVV with the bucket test (► https://doi.org/10.1007/000-92p)

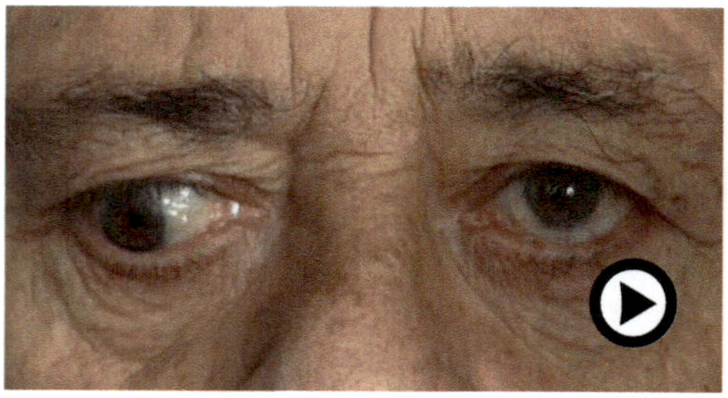

■ **Fig. 3.19** Skew cover test (► https://doi.org/10.1007/000-92n)

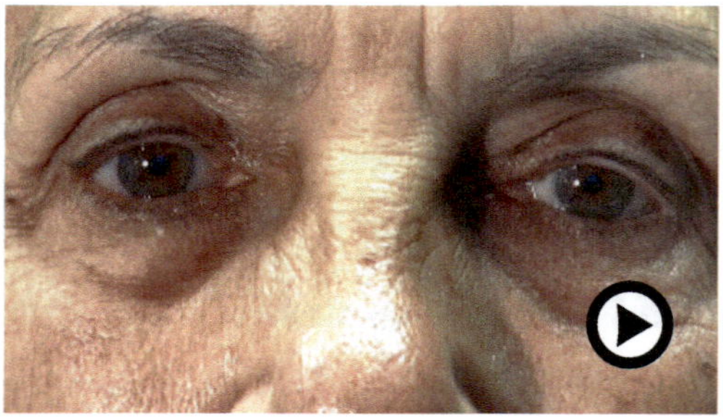

■ **Fig. 3.21** Peripheral vestibular spotaneous nystagmus (► https://doi.org/10.1007/000-92q)

saccade to the right. This is in parallel to the ipsiversive tendency to fall toward the less active side.

- Vertical downward or upward: downbeat and upbeat nystagmus (Figs. ■ 3.23 and ■ 3.24). It is important for the diagnosis of a downbeat nystagmus that the patient is examined when looking to the right or to the left as well as downward because in primary position the intensity of the nystagmus can be very low and the diagnosis is therefore often missed. If the patient looks to the right or to the left, there is often a more intense diagonally downwardly beating nystag-

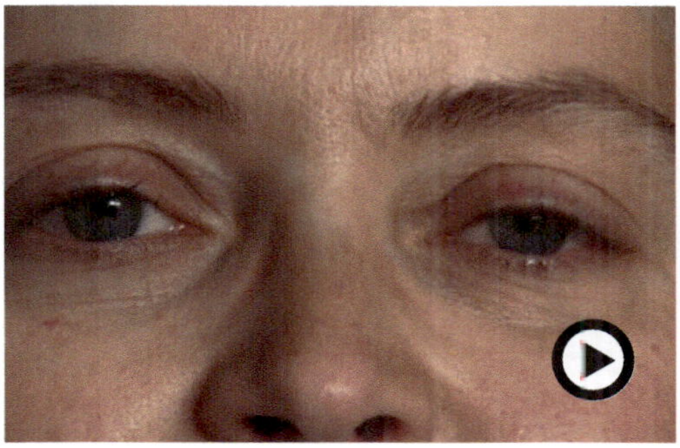

Fig. 3.22 Fixation pendular nystagmus (▶ https://doi.org/10.1007/000-92r)

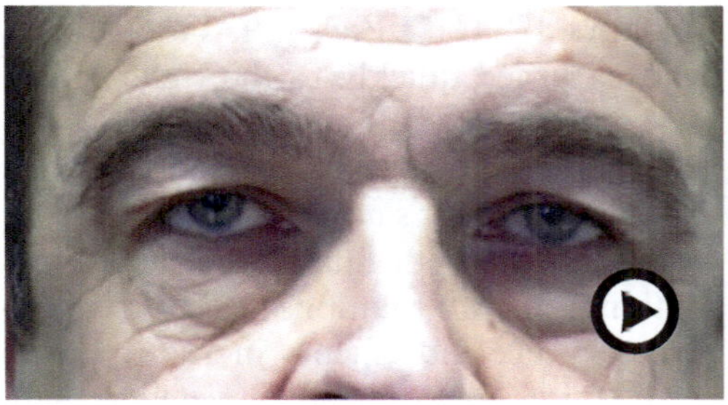

Fig. 3.23 Downbeat nystagmus (▶ https://doi.org/10.1007/000-92s)

mus, because downbeat nystagmus is often associated with a gaze-holding deficit.

- Purely torsional, for instance due to a lesion in the medulla oblongata or in the mesencephalon. Clinical rule: A purely vertical or a purely torsional nystagmus is a central nystagmus.

3. **Provoking or modulating factors:**
   - Reduction or suppression by visual fixation, i.e., when the patient is fixating a target, the intensity of the nystagmus is less, or it is completely suppressed. If the patient then puts on Frenzel's goggles or M-glasses, the intensity of the nystagmus increases. This is a typical sign of a spontaneous peripheral vestibular nystagmus (Fig. 3.25), as in acute unilateral vestibulopathy/vestibular neuritis. There is one caveat: As mentioned above often central types of spontaneous nystagmus, e.g., in a brainstem infarction, can also be reduced by visual fixation (Mantokoudis et al. 2021). Therefore, the following clinical rule applies: A nystagmus which is *not* reduced by visual fixation is *not* a peripheral nystagmus.
   - Using Frenzel's goggles or M-glasses, patients should also be examined during the head-shaking maneuver, during hyperventilation, and during maneuvers with changing pressure or applying loud sounds. The latter two to look for a syndrome of the third mobile windows (see below).

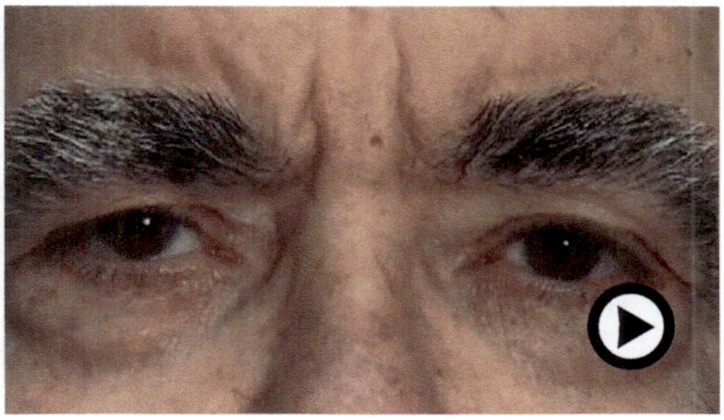

Fig. 3.24 Upbeat nystagmus (▶ https://doi.org/10.1007/000-92t)

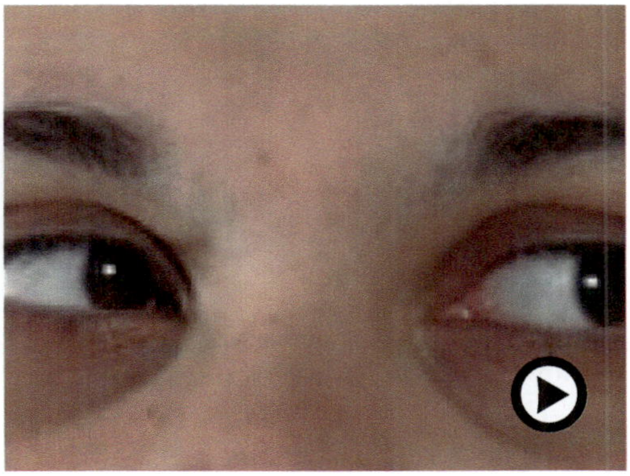

Fig. 3.25 Acute unilateral vestibulopathy/vestibular neuritis on the right side (▶ https://doi.org/10.1007/000-92v)

To look for a spontaneous nystagmus, one can alternatively examine the patient using an ophthalmoscope while the non-examined eye is covered. This is a very sensitive method for

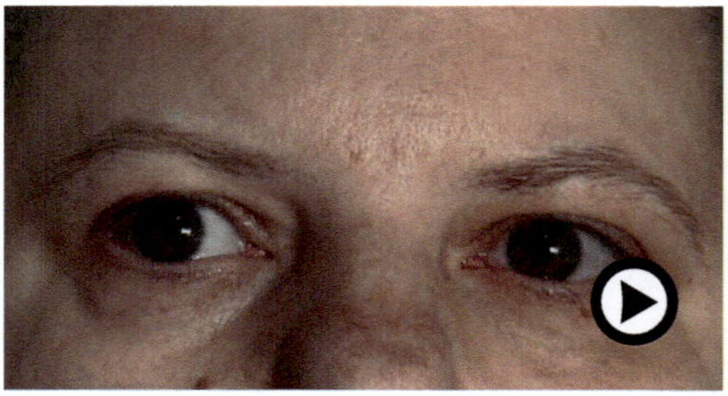

◼ **Fig. 3.26** Square-wave jerks (► https://doi.org/10.1007/000-92w)

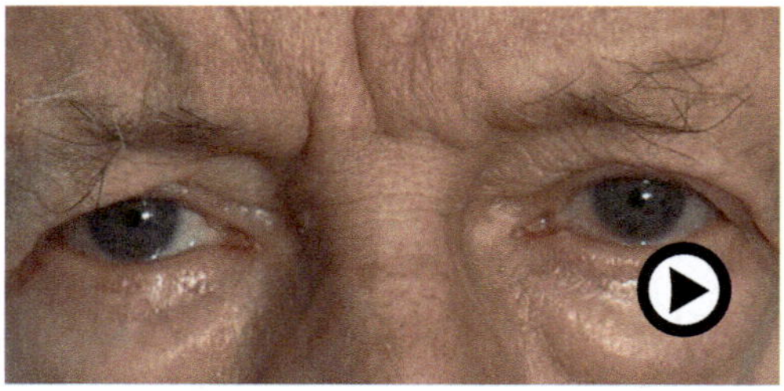

◼ **Fig. 3.27** Progressive supranuclear gaze palsy (► https://doi.org/10.1007/000-92x)

the diagnosis of a nystagmus, even with a low intensity or a low frequency, and for the diagnosis of square-wave jerks (◼ Fig. 3.26), i.e., small saccades with an amplitude of between 0.5° and 5°, which are, for instance, found in patients with tauopathies (◼ Fig. 3.27) or cerebellar diseases. When the patient is examined for the presence of a nystagmus using an ophthalmoscope, one carefully looks at the movements of the papilla or retinal vessels. Since the retina is behind the rotational axis of the eye, the direction of the observed retinal movements is opposite to the direction of a horizontal or vertical nystagmus, i.e., in a patient with a downbeat nystagmus, there is a quick upward movement of the papilla and the retinal vessels.

3.1.3 Head Impulse Test, Halmagyi-Curthoys Test

The head impulse test (HIT) allows the function of the VOR in the high-frequency range to be examined, to look for a unilateral or bilateral VOR deficit (Halmagyi and Curthoys 1988) (◼ Fig. 3.5). The patient's head is turned quickly to the right and to the left with an amplitude of about 20–30° and the patient is asked to fixate a target (e.g., the examiner's nose):

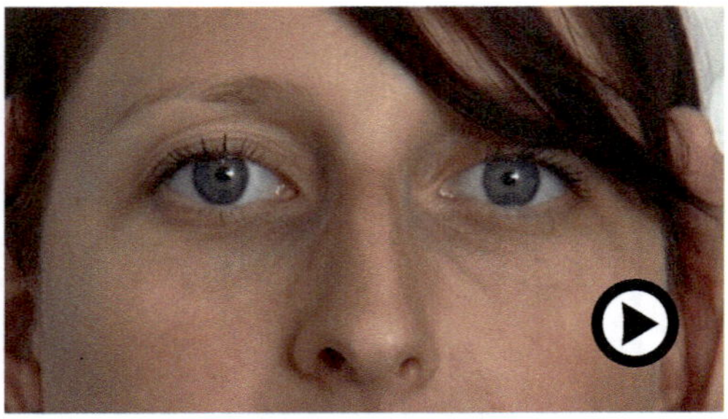

◼ **Fig. 3.28** Head impulse test, normal findings (► https://doi.org/10.1007/000-92y)

- In patients with intact vestibular function, the head rotations lead to compensatory eye movements in the opposite direction to the head movements with the same angular velocity (◼ Fig. 3.28). The image of the visual surroundings thereby stays stable on the retina and the patient does not need to perform a refixation saccade.
- In patients with a unilateral vestibular deficit (◼ Fig. 3.29) (◼ Fig. 3.5b shown for a deficit of the right horizontal semicircular canal), the eyes move with the head toward the right and the patient has to perform a refixation saccade to the left (◼ Fig. 3.5b), which is the clinical sign of a VOR deficit in the high-frequency range, in this case on the right.
- In bilateral vestibulopathy (◼ Fig. 3.30), there are refixation saccades on both sides, indicating a bilateral high-frequency VOR deficit.

One caveat: The head impulse test (video-HIT) (see below) is clearly superior to the bedside head impulse test: The latter has a sensitivity of only 65% for the diagnosis of a unilateral or a bilateral vestibulopathy (Yip et al. 2016). Therefore, nowadays, the video-

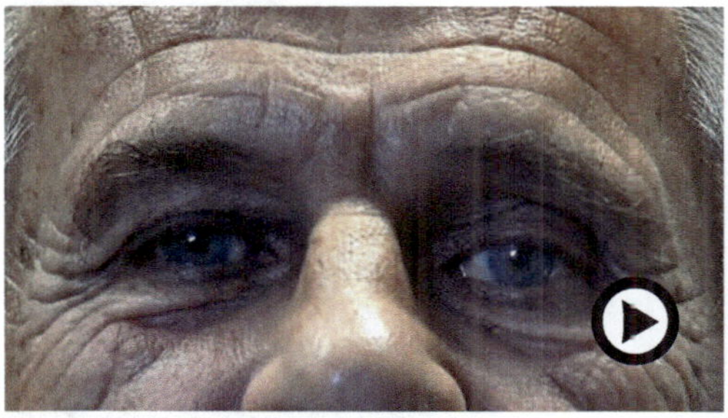

■ **Fig. 3.29** Left unilateral vestibulopathy (► https://doi.org/10.1007/000-92z)

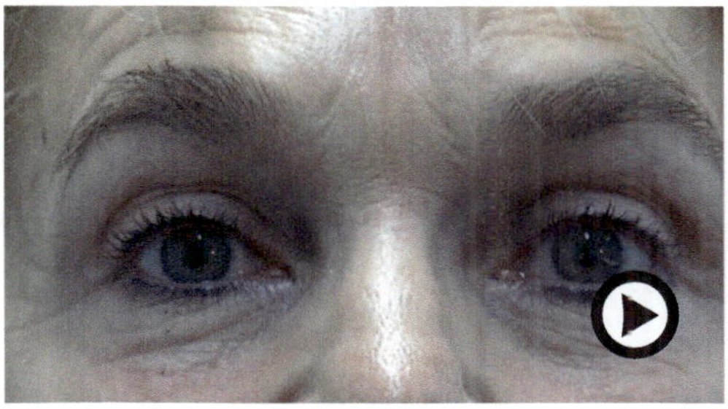

■ **Fig. 3.30** Bilateral vestibulopathy (► https://doi.org/10.1007/000-930)

HIT should be performed routinely as the gold standard.

3.1.4 Diagnostic Positioning Maneuvers to Look for BPPV of the Posterior, Horizontal or Anterior Canal or a Central Positional Nystagmus

3.1.4.1 Diagnosis of BPPV of the Posterior Canal

In addition to the Dix-Hallpike maneuver, nowadays the diagnostic Semont maneuver (■ Figs. 3.6a and ■ 3.31) (von Brevern et al. 2015) and the suggested so-called diagnostic SemontPLUS maneuver (■ Fig. 3.6g, h) are recommended, in particular because after the two latter maneuvers one can immediately continue with the therapeutic Semont maneuvers. For the diagnostic Semont maneuver, the head of the patient sitting in

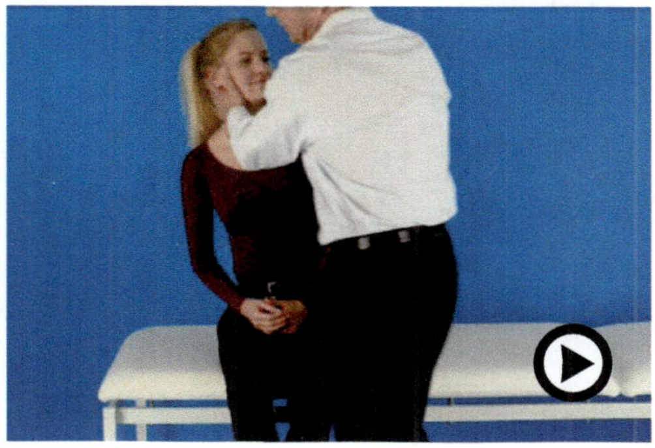

■ **Fig. 3.31** Diagnostic SemontPlus maneuver (► https://doi.org/10.1007/000-931)

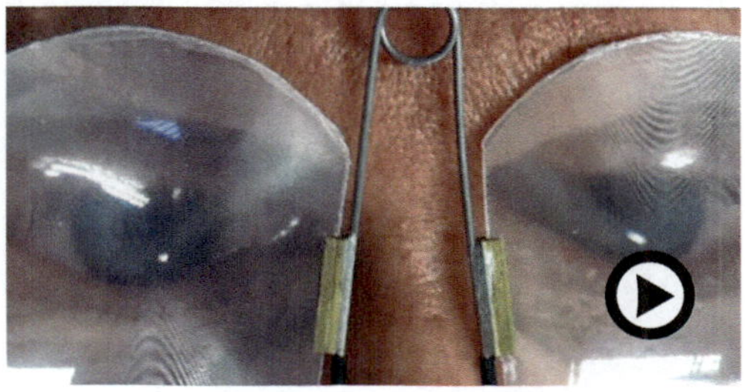

■ **Fig. 3.32** Nystagmus in right-sided posterior canal BPVV (► https://doi.org/10.1007/000-932)

an upright position is turned 45° to one side and then the patient is moved 90° toward the other side, while the examiner inspects the eye movements using Frenzel's goggles or M-glasses. For the diagnostic SemontPLUS maneuver, the patient is moved by at least 150°. In BPPV of a posterior canal, the nystagmus beats vertically toward the forehead and torsionally toward the undermost ear with a crescendo-decrescendo time course and a duration of less than 1 min (right posterior canal/left posterior canal) (■ Figs. 3.32 and 3.33). The pathophysiology is an ampullofugal excitation of the affected posterior canal due to a freely moving otoconia (■ Fig. 3.34) with a nystagmus in the plane of the affected posterior canal according to Ewald's first law.

If one does not know from the patient history which side is most likely affected, one should always begin with the right side

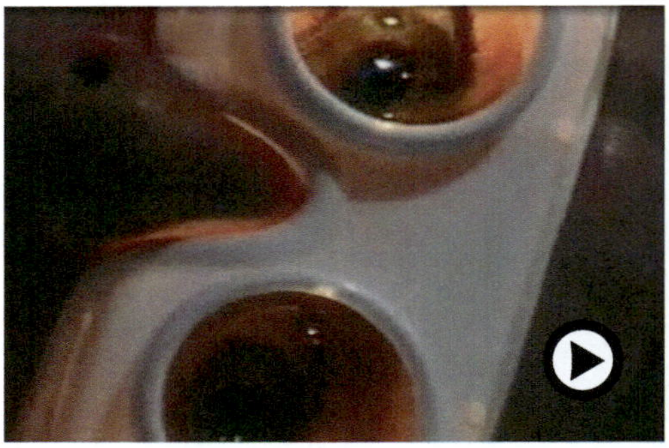

◘ **Fig. 3.33** Nystagmus in left-sided posterior canal BPVV (► https://doi.org/10.1007/000-933)

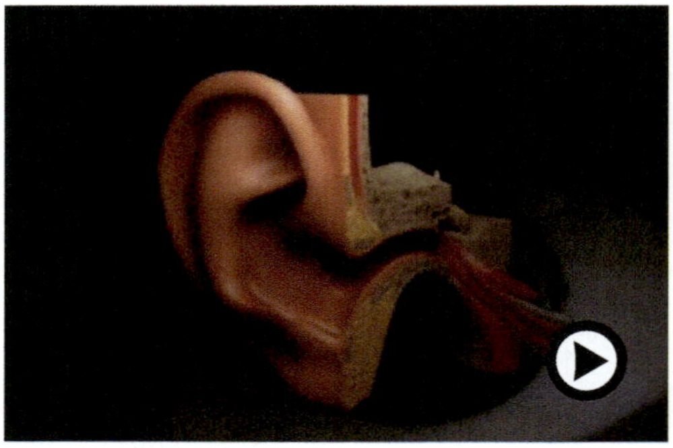

◘ **Fig. 3.34** Model of canalolithiasis (► https://doi.org/10.1007/000-934)

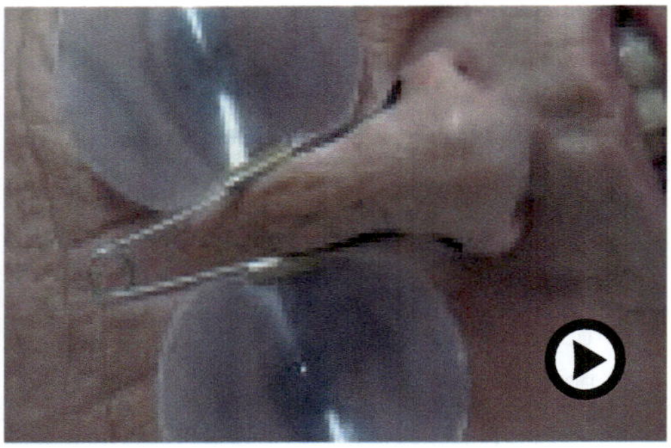

◘ **Fig. 3.35** Horizontal canal BPPV, canalolithiasis on the right side (► https://doi.org/10.1007/000-935)

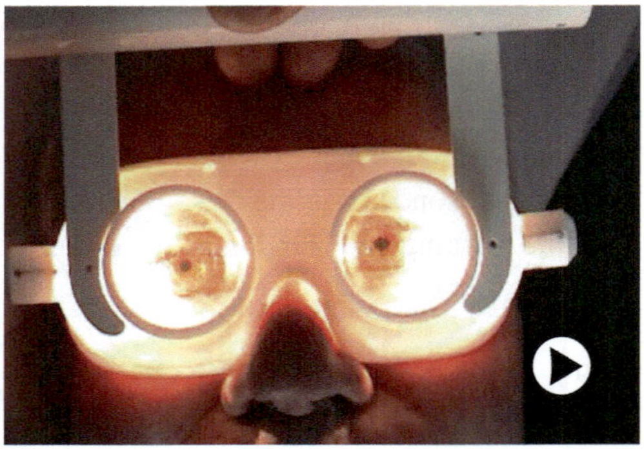

◘ **Fig. 3.36** Horizontal canal BPPV, cupulolithiasis on the left side (► https://doi.org/10.1007/000-936)

because a right-sided posterior canal is affected at least twice as often as a left-sided posterior canal because most people sleep on their right side. Further, with the diagnostic maneuvers for BPPV of a posterior semicircular canal, one does not overlook BPPV of a horizontal semicircular canal (see below).

3.1.4.2 Diagnosis of a BPPV of a Horizonal Semicircular Canal

The patient lies supine with the head tilted 25° upward (◘ Fig. 3.7) so that the horizontal canal is vertically oriented. Subsequently, the patient's head is turned 90° to the right, then back to the middle position, and then 90° to the left (supine roll test), while the patient's eye movements are examined with Frenzel's goggles or M-glasses:

- Canalolithiasis (freely moving otoconia within the affected semicircular canal): the nystagmus beats toward the undermost ear geotropically (◘ Fig. 3.35) in both head positions, i.e., with the head turned toward the right or the left ear, with a crescendo-decrescendo time course (Bhattacharyya et al. 2017, Bhandari et al. 2022). It is important to note that the affected side is the side with the higher intensity of the nystagmus.
- Cupulolithiasis (otoconia attached to the cupula): the nystagmus beats toward the uppermost ear, i.e., ageotropically (◘ Fig. 3.36), which can persist for a very long time because the otoconia are attached to the cupula, leading to a persistent deflection of the cupula. The affected side is the side with the lower intensity of the nystagmus.

3.1.4.3 Diagnosis of a BPPV of an Anterior Semicircular Canal

The positional test is the supine head-hanging test. Anterior canal BPPV is characterised by a vertical downwardly beating nystagmus with a torsional component towards the affected side. However, the torsional component depends on the eye position, is not always clear and is less intense than the vertical one. Therefore, determining the affected side can often be difficult, thus further complicating proper diagnosis and differential diagnosis to central positional nystagmus.

3.1.4.4 Central Positional Nystagmus

An important diagnostic criterion to differentiate a peripheral from a central positional nystagmus (CPN) is the direction of the nystagmus (Buttner et al. 1999). In peripheral positional vertigo, the direction of the nystagmus corresponds to the plane of the affected canal: vertical torsional in posterior canal BPPV, linear-horizontal in horizontal canal BPPV. In CPN, one finds a very similar direction of the nystagmus in different head positions because it is most often caused by an otolith dysfunction. Most often, one sees a downwardly beating central positional nystagmus (◘ Fig. 3.37) in all positions, i.e., right ear down, left ear down, or supine with the head overextended. Clinically it is important to note that CPN is often associated with other central, often cerebellar ocular motor or other neurological signs; typically, it is not improved by the therapeutic maneuvers for BPPV (Lemos and Strupp, 2022).

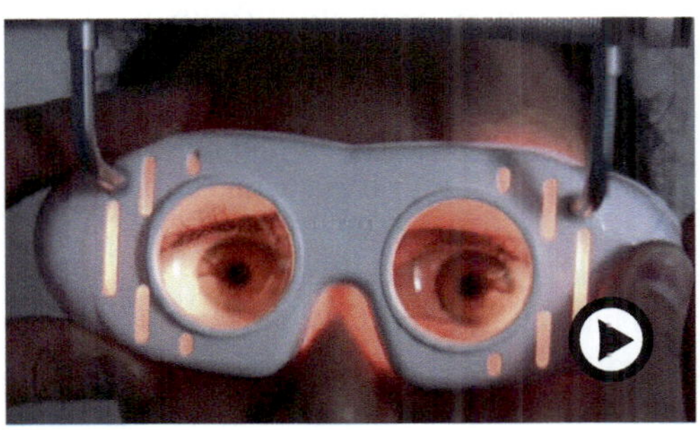

◘ **Fig. 3.37** Central positional nystagmus (▶ https://doi.org/10.1007/000-937)

3.1.5 Examination of Stance and Gait

3.1.5.1 Romberg Test

The Romberg test has different conditions—from easy to difficult: (1) legs wide apart, (2) both feet together, (3) one foot in front of the other (heel-to-toe: the tandem Romberg test), (4) standing on one leg (◘ Figs. 3.8 and ◘ 3.38). These conditions should be performed with eyes open and eyes closed. Healthy subjects can stand on one leg with the eyes closed for more than 5 s:

- If a subject sways with the eyes closed much more than with the eyes open, this will indicate a sensory deficit of the vestibular (uni- or bilateral vestibulopathy) and/or the somatosensory system (e.g., polyneuropathy).
- In acute unilateral vestibulopathy, there is typically a tendency to fall toward the affected side (◘ Table 3.1).
- Acute brainstem infarctions, in particular Wallenberg syndrome, lead to a strong lateropulsion. Lesions of the medullary brain-

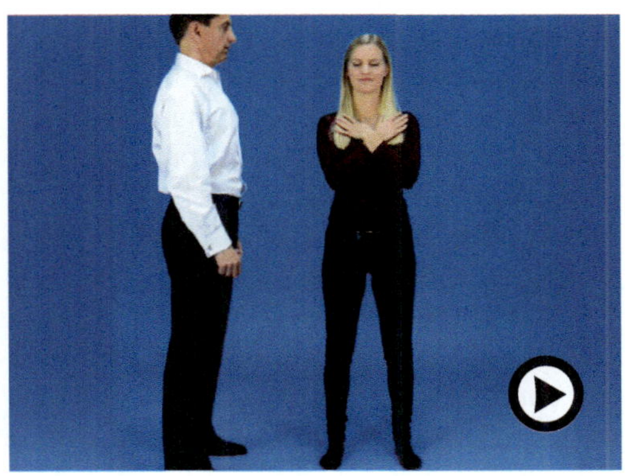

◘ **Fig. 3.38** Romberg Test (▶ https://doi.org/10.1007/000-938)

Table 3.1 Disturbances of posture and gait control in peripheral vestibular disorders (in alphabetical order)

Disease	Direction of deviation	Pathomechanism
Acute unilateral vestibulopathy/vestibular neuritis	Ipsiversive	Vestibular tone imbalance due to failure of the horizontal and anterior semicircular canal and utricle
Bilateral vestibulopathy	Different directions	Failure of vestibulospinal postural reflexes, exacerbated in the dark and on uneven ground
BPPV, e.g., of the posterior canal (during changes in head position)	Forward and ipsiversive	Ampullofugal stimulation of the posterior canal due to canalolithiasis that leads to endolymph flow
Menière's disease, during an attack, and Tumarkin's otolithic catastrophy	Lateral, ipsiversive, or contraversive, sudden falls in Tumarkin's otolithic catastrophy	Excitation and subsequent inhibition of the otoliths; sudden vestibulospinal tone failure in Tumarkin's otolithic catastrophy
Tullio phenomenon	Backward, contraversive, diagonal	Stimulation of the otoliths by sounds of certain frequencies, in the syndrome of the third mobile windows
Vestibular paroxysmia	Contraversive or in different directions	Neurovascular compression of the vestibulocochlear nerve and excitation (rarely inhibition) of the vestibular nerve

stem cause a lateropulsion toward the side of the lesion, whereas lesions of the pontomesencephalic brainstem cause a lateropulsion to the opposite side (Table 3.2).

- In downbeat and upbeat nystagmus syndrome, there is an increased forward and back (to-and-fro) sway with the eyes closed.

Patients with functional dizziness can sway in various directions with sometimes bizarre body movements without falls. Distraction by dual task (e.g., counting down from 100 or writing numbers on the patient's skin) often leads to a reduction of body sway in such conditions.

3.1.5.2 Clinical Gait Analysis

Gait should also be examined under different conditions (Schniepp et al. 2019): (1) walking with eyes open and closed with a self-selected gait velocity; (2) walking with eyes open and closed on an imaginary line (tandem gait); (3) walking with eyes open and closed during a dual task (e.g., counting down from 100). The following gait parameters are evaluated: velocity, step length, rhythm, gait variability, base of gait, posture, and asymmetry of walking and arm swing. Typical findings are found, for instance, in:

1. Sensory deficit (vestibular and/or somatosensory): reduced self-selected gait velocity, broad-based gait with worsening after closing the eyes
2. Cerebellar ataxia: high gait variability, broad-based gait, improvement of gait with higher gait velocities
3. Functional gait disorder: often bizarre gait patterns, high variability and asymmetries of walking and arm swing, improvement during distraction and when walking backward (dual task)
4. Hypokinetic-rigid syndrome: reduced gait velocity with reduced step length, rigor, often ventral flexion, reduced arm swing, typically asymmetrical in patients with Parkinson's disease

Table 3.2 Disturbance of posture and gait control in central vestibular disorders (in alphabetical order)

Disease/syndrome	Direction of deviation	Pathomechanism
Downbeat/upbeat nystagmus syndrome	Backward and forward	Vestibular tone imbalance in the pitch plane
Ocular tilt reaction (OTR)	Contraversive with mesencephalic lesions, ipsiversive with pontomedullary lesions, ipsi- or contraversive with unilateral cerebellar lesions (uvula or dentate nucleus)	Tone imbalance of the VOR in the roll plane with lesions of the vertical canals or otolith pathways
Paroxysmal ocular tilt reaction	Ipsiversive with mesencephalic excitation, contraversive with pontomedullary excitation or excitation of the vestibular nerve	Pathological excitation of the otolith or vertical canal pathways (VOR in the roll plane)
Thalamic astasia (often overlooked)	Contraversive or ipsiversive	Vestibular tone imbalance due to lesions of the posterolateral or centromedian thalamus
Vestibular epilepsy (rare)	Contraversive	Focal seizures due to epileptic discharges of the vestibular cortex
Wallenberg's syndrome: Lateropulsion	Ipsiversive, diagonal	Central vestibular tone imbalance (roll and yaw planes) with tilt of subjective vertical

3.1.6 Additional Clinical Vestibular Examinations

3.1.6.1 Head-Shaking Test

The patient shakes his/her head about 20 times to the right and to the left; subsequently, eye movements are observed using Frenzel's goggles or M-glasses. The head-shaking nystagmus (Fig. 3.39) is based on an asymmetrical charging of the velocity storage mechanism (Raphan et al. 1979). This can occur in peripheral and in central lesions. In a unilateral peripheral vestibular lesion, a head turn toward the healthy side causes a charging of the velocity storage mechanism, whereas a head turn in the opposite direction does not, which leads to asymmetrical charging. In such a situation, the fast phase of the nystagmus typically beats toward the healthy, more active labyrinth. In central and in particular cerebellar dysfunction, one may find a "cross-coupling," i.e., horizontal head shaking can lead to a vertical nystagmus (Fig. 3.40), or a spontaneous nystagmus can change direction after head shaking, which is also a central sign (Huh and Kim 2011; Choi et al. 2016), which, however, is not specific for a central lesion (Yang et al. 2020).

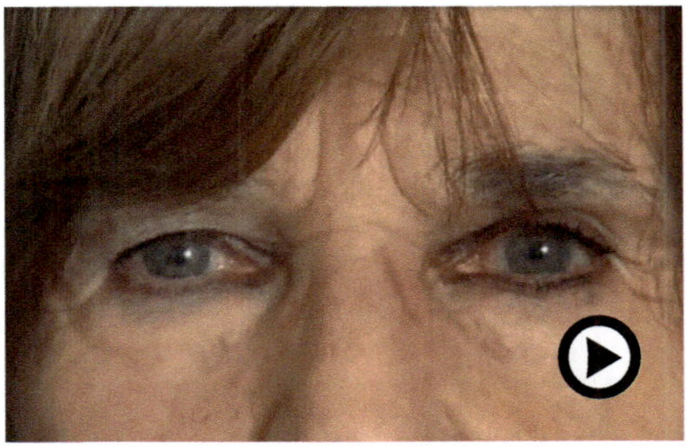

Fig. 3.39 Head-shaking nystagmus (▶ https://doi.org/10.1007/000-939)

3.1.6.2 Hyperventilation-Induced Nystagmus

The patient hyperventilates for 3 min, and subsequently, the patient's eyes are observed using Frenzel's goggles or M-glasses. Hyperventilation-induced nystagmus can be found in up to 70% of patients with vestibular paroxysmia (Hufner et al. 2008) and in patients with a vestibular schwannoma or central lesions (Eggers et al. 2019).

3.1.6.3 Examination for Signs of a Third Mobile Window

There are several tests to look for signs of the syndrome of a third mobile windows (► Chap. 12): changes of pressure in the middle ear using a Politzer balloon (◘ Fig. 3.9, which allows the application of positive and negative pressure), the tragal pressure test, pressing against the open and closed vocal cords or the closed nostrils (Valsalva maneuvers) (◘ Fig. 3.41), and the application of sounds with specific frequencies and sound levels (Tullio phenomenon). All of these tests can induce attacks of vertigo/dizziness or nystagmus in the plane of the affected canal. Since superior canal dehiscence syndrome is the most frequent subtype, this leads to a vertical torsional nystagmus in the plane of the anterior/superior canal (◘ Table 3.3).

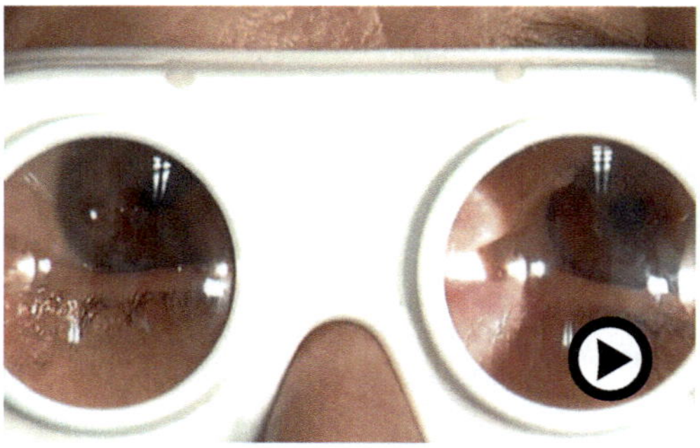

◘ **Fig. 3.40** Head-shaking nystagmus with cross coupling (► https://doi.org/10.1007/000-93a)

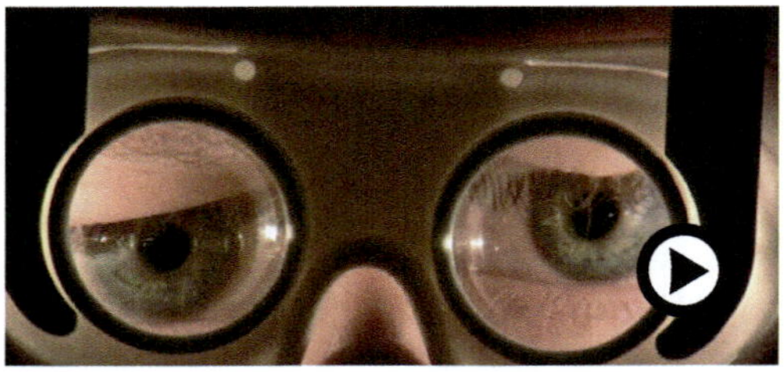

◘ **Fig. 3.41** Valsalva maneuver in a patient with left-sided superior canal dehiscence syndrome (► https://doi.org/10.1007/000-93b)

◘ **Table 3.3** Combined examination of the vestibular and ocular motor systems

Type of examination	Question	Possible findings
Body and head position	Head tilt or head torsion/body tilt	Head tilt, e.g., as a component of the ocular tilt reaction or in trochlear palsy
Position of the eyes when looking straight ahead (primary position)	Ocular misalignment	Skew deviation/vertical deviation or manifest strabismus (tropia)
Cover and uncover test and alternating cover test	Horizontal or vertical ocular misalignment: manifest or latent strabismus, or central vertical deviation	Ocular misalignment, eye muscle nerve or eye muscle paresis, skew deviation

■ Table 3.3 (continued)

Type of examination	Question	Possible findings
Looking straight ahead with and without Frenzel's goggles/M-glasses	Spontaneous nystagmus in primary position: suppressed or not suppressed by visual fixation	Peripheral vestibular spontaneous nystagmus vs. central fixation nystagmus
Vergence test and convergence reaction	Reduced or absent vergence reaction	Reduced or absent vergence reaction in lesions of the mesencephalon
Head-shaking test	Head-shaking nystagmus	Peripheral head-shaking nystagmus in a unilateral vestibular lesion or central head-shaking nystagmus; cross-coupling typical of a cerebellar lesion as well as direction-changing nystagmus
Smooth pursuit horizontally ±40° and vertically ±20°	Smooth or saccadic	Saccadic smooth pursuit, most often due to cerebellar dysfunction
Gaze-holding function: horizontal and vertical gaze to the endpoint (i.e., the point at which the patient is still able to fixate the target with both eyes)	Unsustained, sustained endpoint nystagmus or gaze-evoked nystagmus horizontally or vertically	Gaze-evoked nystagmus
Looking for rebound nystagmus: patient fixates a target for 30–60s in the endpoint position; then, the eyes jump back to the primary position	Rebound nystagmus	Rebound nystagmus indicates a cerebellar lesion most often affecting the flocculus
Saccades: spontaneous saccades and voluntary and reflexive saccades: ±20° horizontally and ± 20° vertically	Velocity, accuracy, conjugacy, and latency	Slowing of saccades, saccade dysmetria, i.e., hypo- or hypermetric, dysconjugate saccades in INO
Horizontal and vertical optokinetic nystagmus using the optodrum or e.g., the optodrum app	Normal or impaired optokinetic nystagmus, change of direction/phase	Reduced or absent optokinetic nystagmus, indicating a dysfunction of the smooth pursuit/saccadic system Change of direction or beating diagonally during monocular stimulation typical of infantile nystagmus nystagmus
Head-impulse test	Deficit of the VOR unilaterally or bilaterally	Refixation saccade unilaterally or bilaterally, indicating a VOR deficit in the high-frequency range
Visual fixation suppression of the VOR: combine oscillating turning of the head/body and a fixation point about 50 cm in front of the eyes with the same angular velocity	Impairment of visual fixation suppression of the VOR	Impaired visual fixation suppression of the VOR, most often indicating a floccular dysfunction

(continued)

Table 3.3 (continued)

Type of examination	Question	Possible findings
Measurement of the subjective visual vertical (SVV) using the bucket test	Deviation of the subjective visual verticality	Deviation of >2.5° indicating an acute peripheral or central unilateral vestibular lesion
Diagnostic positioning maneuver	BPPV of the posterior, horizontal or anterior semicircular canal and central positional nystagmus	Nystagmus: Torsional-vertical upward: posterior canal Linear-horizontal: horizontal canal Torsional vertical downward: anterior canal
Romberg test with the eyes open and closed under simple and difficult conditions with and without distraction (counting backward from 100 7s)	Sway and direction of sways Functional components	Increased sway with closed eyes: Indicates a sensory deficit of the vestibular and/or somatosensory system Reduction of sway during distraction: Indicates functional dizziness
Examination of gait with eyes open, eyes closed, heel-to-toe, and during dual task	Gait velocity, step length, rhythm, gait variability, base of gait, body position, and asymmetry of gait and arm swing	Reduced gait velocity, reduced step length, increased gait variability, impaired gait rhythm, broad base, reduced arm swing unilaterally or bilaterally

3.2 Examination of the Ocular Motor System

3.2.1 Examination in Primary Position and the Various Cover Tests

In primary position, one looks for ocular misalignments with the cover tests and for a nystagmus (see above and below). The cover tests allow diagnosis of a latent or manifest strabismus. The prerequisite for all cover tests is the presence of foveal fixation.

In the **one-eye cover test** (Fig. 3.42), the presence of a so-called heterotropia (i.e., manifest strabismus) can be observed in the uncovered eye; the latter moves when the other eye is covered. Heterotropia is defined as a misalignment of the visual axes, even during binocular fixation.

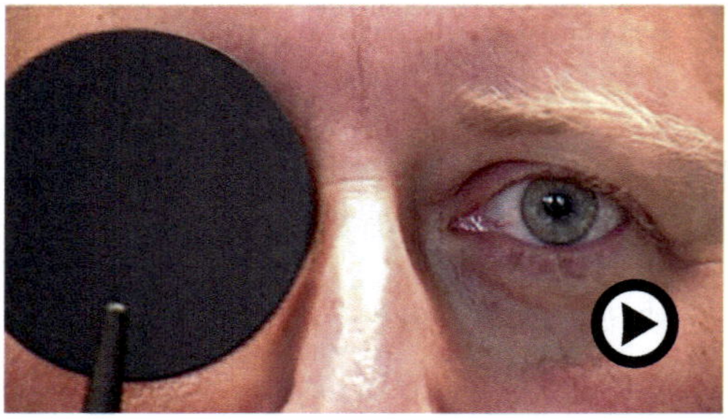

Fig. 3.42 One-eye cover test (▶ https://doi.org/10.1007/000-93c)

First, the patient is asked to fixate either a near target (at a distance of 30–40 cm) or one 5–6 m away. Then, the examiner covers one eye and looks for correction movements of the now uncovered eye. If the uncovered eye moves:

- From the inside outward, esotropia is present
- From the outside inward, exotropia
- From above downward, hypertropia
- From below upward, hypotropia

Then, the other eye is examined.

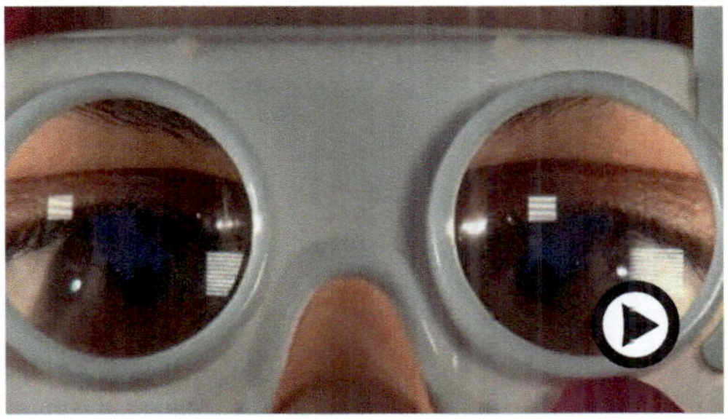

■ **Fig. 3.43** Peripheral vestibular spontaneous nystagmus (▶ https://doi.org/10.1007/000-93d)

The one-eye cover/uncover test (■ Figs. 3.2 and 3.43) is used to prove the presence of a heterophoria (i.e., latent strabismus). This is a misalignment of the eye axes when a target is fixated with one eye only. It is important to perform the above-mentioned cover part of the test before the cover/uncover part in order to exclude a heterotropia first of all. First one eye is covered for about 3 sec, then uncovered; the possible corrective movements of the previously covered eye are observed. If it moves:

- Outward, esophoria is present
- Inward, an exophoria
- Downward, a hyperphoria
- Upward, a hypophoria

Then, the other eye is examined.

The alternating cover test (■ Figs 3.10 and ■ 3.44) is useful for determining the maximal misalignment of the eye axes in both a tropia and a phoria. The alternating cover test is also helpful when establishing a vertical deviation/skew deviation (in the context of an OTR, see above), i.e., a vertical misalignment of the eyes that cannot be explained by an ocular muscle palsy or damage to a peripheral nerve. It is necessary to look for vertical corrective movements, when the cover is switched from one eye to the other. In contrast to trochlear nerve palsy or superior oblique muscle paresis, in skew deviation as a component of the OTR the vertical misalignment changes little or not at all during different directions of gaze. The only rare exception is the alternating skew deviation in cerebellar lesions.

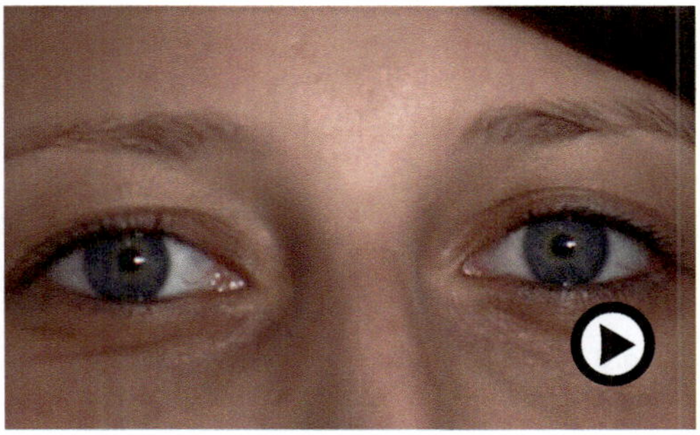

■ **Fig. 3.44** Nine different gaze positions, normal findings (▶ https://doi.org/10.1007/000-93e)

In the clinical examination of the eyes in **nine different positions** (■ Fig. 3.11, for more details, see below, ■ Fig. 3.44), it is necessary to look for misalignment of the axes of the eyes (see above), fixation disorders, peripheral vestibular spontaneous nystagmus and central fixation nystagmus, the range of eye movements and gaze-evoked nystagmus, i.e., disorders of the gaze-holding function. The examination can be performed with an object for fixation or a small rod-shaped flashlight.

3.2.2 Specific Examination for Nystagmus or Nystagmus-like Periodic Eye Movements

In the primary position, one should also look for periodic eye movements, in particular for spontaneous nystagmus (■ Fig. 3.4, see above: with and without Frenzel's goggles/M-glasses ■ Fig. 3.43) and nystagmus-like periodic eye movements, such as ocular flutter or opsoclonus (Eggers et al. 2019).

- **Spontaneous Nystagmus**
  - Horizontal-torsional peripheral vestibular spontaneous nystagmus (due to an acute unilateral vestibulopathy/vestibular neuritis) ■ Fig. 3.45).
  - Vertical nystagmus with the fast phase beating downwards or upwards, i.e., down-

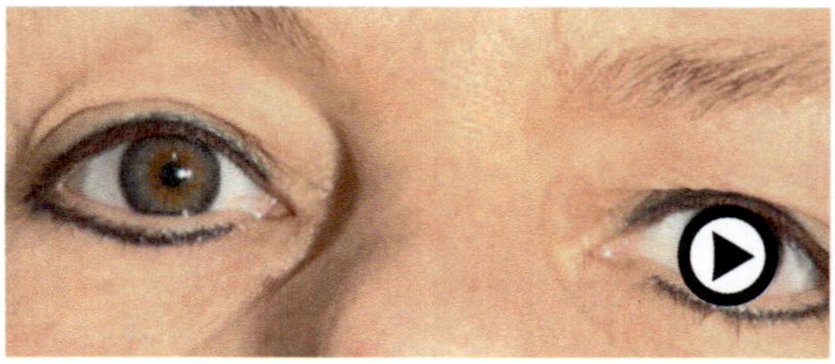

Fig. 3.45 Spontaneous horizontal torsional nystagmus (► https://doi.org/10.1007/000-93f)

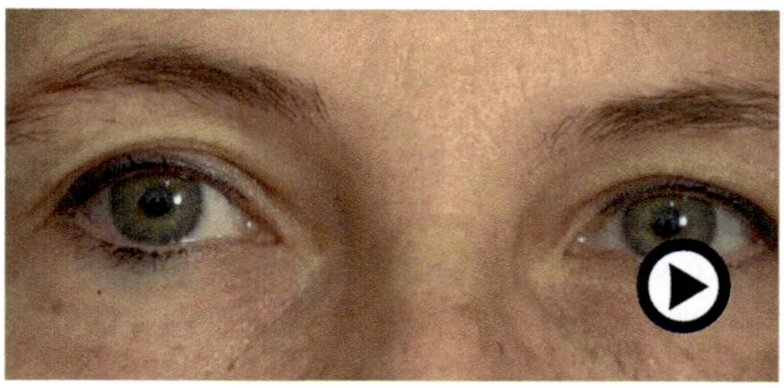

Fig. 3.46 Infantile nsytagmus (► https://doi.org/10.1007/000-93g)

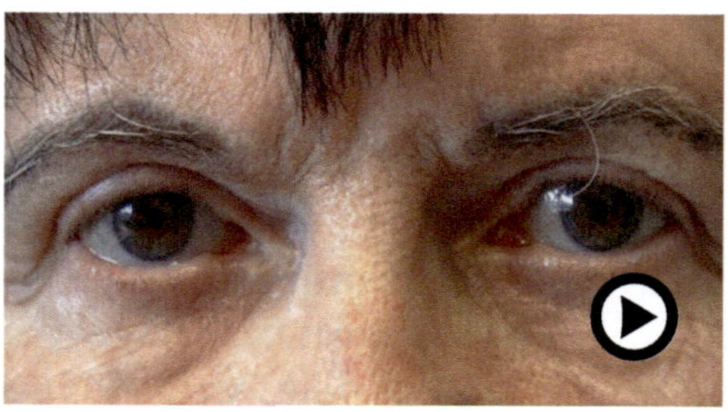

Fig. 3.47 Ocular flutter (► https://doi.org/10.1007/000-93h)

beat or downbeat nystagmus (Figs. 3.46 and 3.47).

- Purely torsional nystagmus, as in Wallenberg's syndrome or in mesencephalic lesions.
- Seesaw and hemi-seesaw nystagmus with one half cycle consisting of elevation and intorsion of one eye and synchronous depression and extorsion of the other eye; the vertical and torsional movements reverse during the next cycle, due to several types of brainstem lesions, bitemporal visual field defects, or congenital defects.

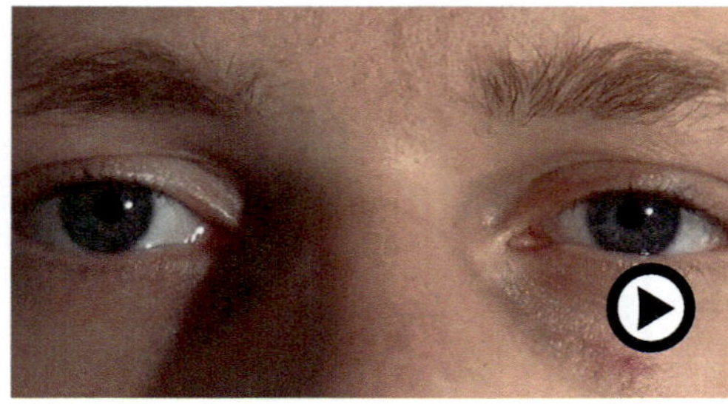

Fig. 3.48 Opsoclonus (► https://doi.org/10.1007/000-93j)

- Infantile nystagmus (Fig. 3.48), which is normally mainly horizontal with pathological waveform and varying frequency and amplitude, increases with fixation (fixational nystagmus); it normally does not cause oscillopsia despite a high intensity.

Nystagmus-Like Periodic Eye Movements

- **Saccadic intrusions and oscillations:** These are characterized by saccades, which drive the eyes away from the fixation point. Therefore, they are not a nystagmus sensu stricto.
  - Square-wave jerks (Fig. 3.26): Pairs of small horizontal conjugate saccades (most often <2°), which drive the eyes away from the fixation point and then, after a short interval of 200 ms to 400 ms, bring them back. This is often found in elderly subjects. In patients with cerebellar or brainstem lesions, they may occur continuously and then they are called square-wave oscillations. Macro square-wave jerks have an amplitude of >5° and a frequency of 2–3 Hz with an intersaccadic interval of 70–150 ms (Eggers et al. 2019).
  - Ocular flutter (Fig. 3.47): intermittent bursts of fast horizontal conjugate saccades with a frequency of 10–25 Hz without an intersaccadic interval, which often occur after a saccade.
  - Opsoclonus (Fig. 3.48): combined horizontal, vertical, and/or torsional

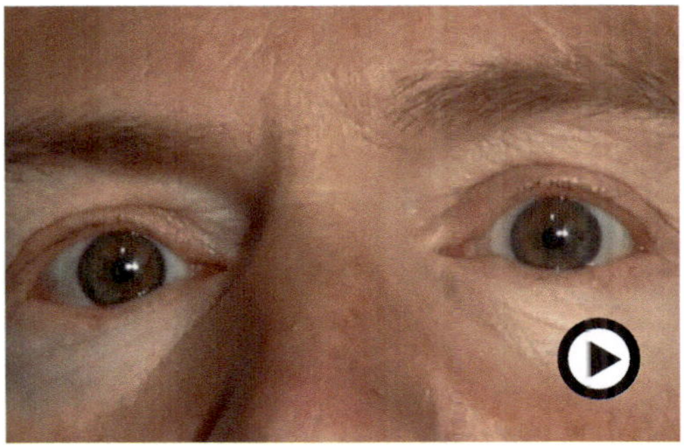

■ **Fig. 3.49** Convergence-retraction nystagmus (▶ https://doi.org/10.1007/000-93k)

saccadic oscillations with a large amplitude which are increased by smooth pursuit, convergence, and blinking; to the observer, they appear a little chaotic.

  - Ocular flutter and opsoclonus occur in various lesions of the brainstem and the cerebellum, e.g., in encephalitis, autoimmune/paraneoplastic syndromes, tumors, or intoxications. Pathophysiologically, they are caused by a disinhibition of burst neurons in the PPRF and/or riMLF.

- **Other nystagmus-like periodic eye movements:**
  - Convergence-retraction nystagmus (■ Fig. 3.49): combined vertical saccades, converging with retraction of the bulbi, which are typically induced by upward gaze. They are topographically very specific because they are found in lesions of the posterior commissure or bilateral lesions of the rostral interstitial nucleus of the medial longitudinal fascicle (riMLF).
  - Ocular bobbing: intermittent fast conjugate movements of the eyes at downward movement of the eyes with slow upward eye movements. They are most often caused by pontine lesions (compression and hemorrhage).
  - Superior oblique myokymia (■ Fig. 3.50): The leading symptom is monocular oscillopsia. Clinical examination reveals a monocular vertical torsional nystagmus in the plane of the superior oblique muscle due to an excitation of the trochlear nerve analogous to other neurovascular cross-compression syndromes.

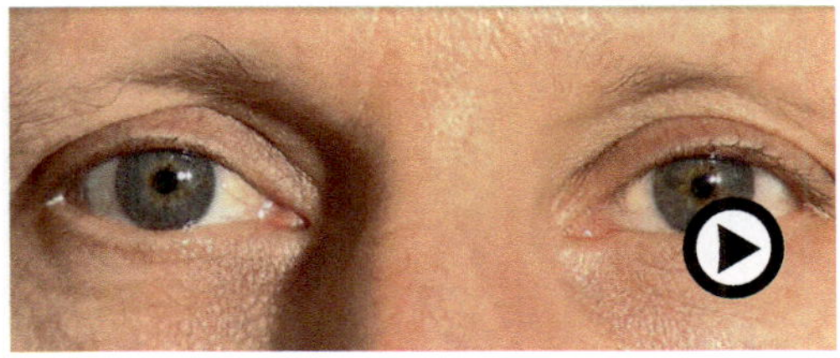

■ **Fig. 3.50** Superior oblique myokomia (▶ https://doi.org/10.1007/000-93m)

3.2.3 Examination of the Range of Eye Movements (Motility)

After examining for possible ocular misalignment (see cover tests above) and pathological eye movements in primary position (spontaneous nystagmus), the range of eye movements should be determined monocularly and binocularly in the eight end positions, i.e., determination of eye mobility (■ Fig. 3.11). One sees deficits, for instance, in eye muscle or eye muscle nerve or eye muscle nerve nuclei palsies (oculomotor, abducens, and trochlear nerve palsy, ■ Figs. 3.51, 3.52, and 3.53). A small rod-shaped flashlight has the advantage that one can precisely see the corneal reflex images and thereby easily determine ocular misalignments in the various positions. It is important to examine the corneal reflex images from the perspective of the flashlight and to advise the patient to fixate the flashlight precisely.

In addition to peripheral ocular motor paresis (eye muscle paresis), there are also central supranuclear gaze palsies, which normally affect both eyes, e.g., in progressive supranuclear palsy (■ Fig. 3.54), a tauopathy, or in Niemann-Pick type C (■ Fig. 3.55),

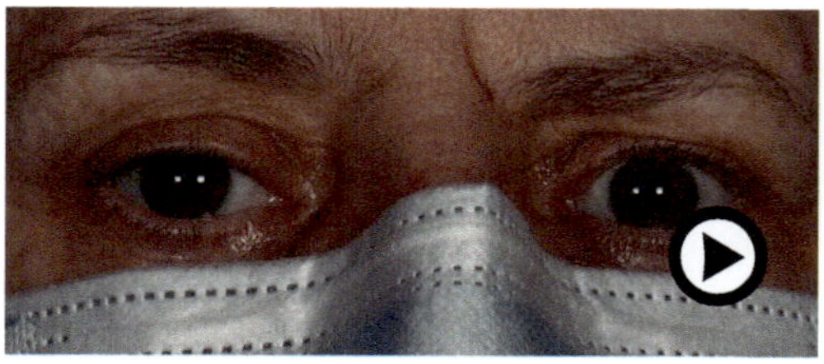

Fig. 3.51 Ocular motor nerve palsy on the right (► https://doi.org/10.1007/000-93n)

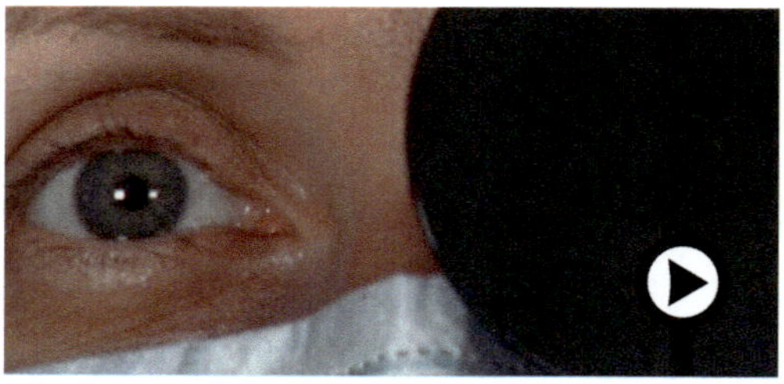

Fig. 3.52 Abducens nerve palsy on the right (► https://doi.org/10.1007/000-93p)

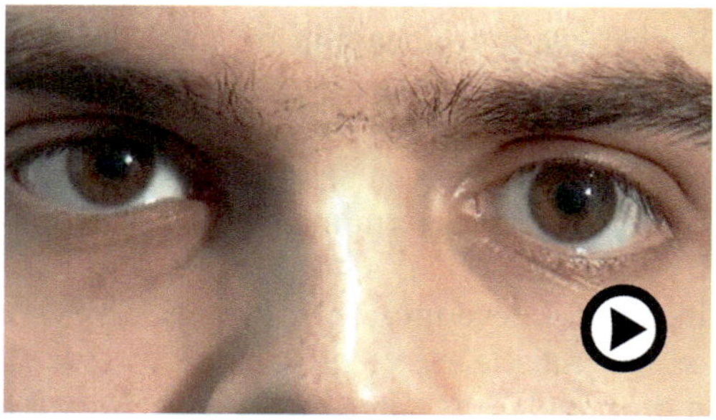

Fig. 3.53 Trochlear nerve palsy (► https://doi.org/10.1007/000-93q)

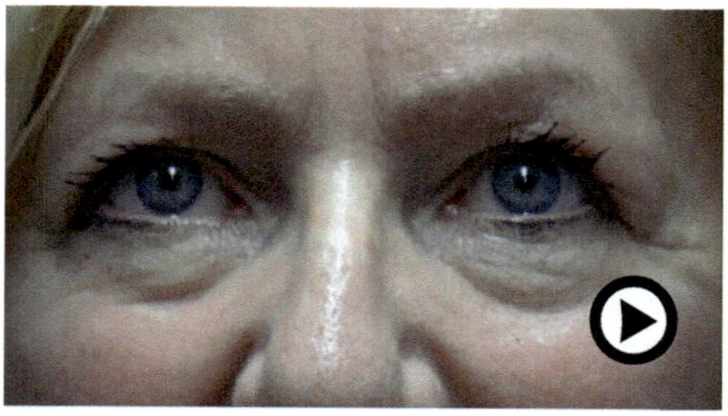

Fig. 3.54 Supranuclear gaze palsy (► https://doi.org/10.1007/000-93r)

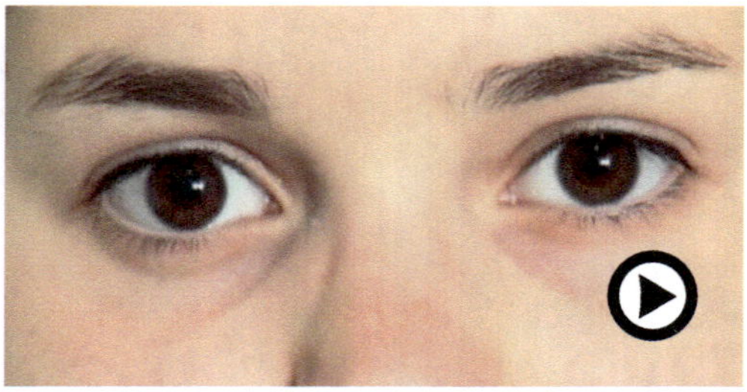

Fig. 3.55 Typical ocular motor findings in Niemann-Pick type C (► https://doi.org/10.1007/000-93s)

a lysosomal storage disease; in the latter, patients first have a saccade and then a gaze palsy (see below).

3.2.4 Examination for a Gaze-Holding Deficit

To examine gaze-holding function, the patient has to look to the right, to the left, up, and down. By definition, the endpoint is the point at which the patient is still able to fixate the target with both eyes (Figs. 3.12 and 3.56). Healthy subjects can have a transient endpoint nystagmus which lasts only a few seconds, i.e., a few nystagmus beats. The typical clinical sign of gaze-evoked nystagmus (Fig. 3.57) is that the fast phase always beats in the direction of the gaze, i.e., the direction changes depending on the gaze direction, so it is also a direction-changing nystagmus that occurs before the eccentric endpoint.

Pathophysiologically, gaze-evoked nystagmus is caused by a so-called *leaky neural integrator* of the gaze-holding system, which leads to a drift of the eyes from the eccentric position to the primary position with a compensatory gaze-evoked nystagmus with the fast phase beating in the direction of the fixation point. The relevant anatomical structures for the neural integrator are the cerebellar flocculus/paraflocculus, the vestibular nuclei, the interstitial nucleus of Cajal (INC) for vertical gaze-holding, and

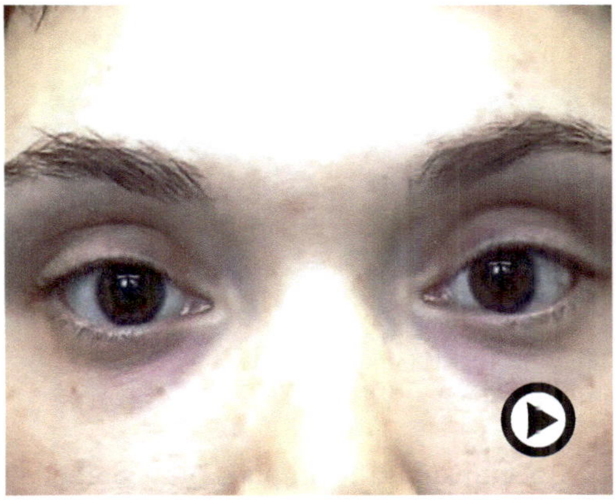

■ **Fig. 3.56** Smooth pursuit, normal findings (▶ https://doi.org/10.1007/000-93t)

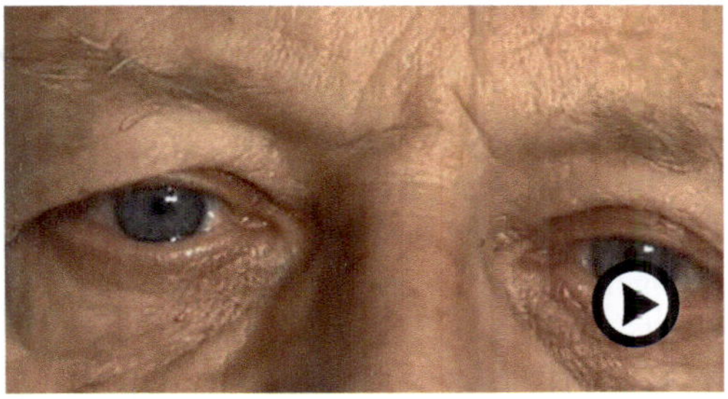

■ **Fig. 3.57** Gaze-evoked nystagmus (▶ https://doi.org/10.1007/000-93v)

the nucleus praepositus hypoglossi (NPH) for horizontal gaze-holding (see below). There are three types of gaze-holding deficit/gaze-evoked nystagmus:

- Physiological: unsustained/transient endpoint nystagmus (the endpoint is defined as the point at which the patient is still able to fixate the target with both eyes), duration <10 s
- Sustained endpoint nystagmus: as an isolated finding most often clinically not relevant; in combination with other central ocular motor disorders, most likely pathological
- Gaze-evoked nystagmus sensu stricto, i.e., more proximally than the endpoint: pathological, indicating a leaky integrator

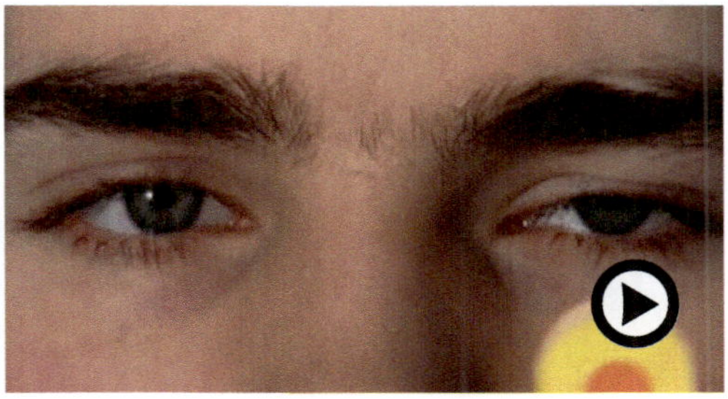

■ **Fig. 3.58** Gaze-evoked nystagmus in all directions (▶ https://doi.org/10.1007/000-93w)

Clinical Rules

- *Gaze-evoked nystagmus in all directions* occurs in cerebellar disorders (■ Fig. 3.58) (especially impaired function of the flocculus/paraflocculus), above all in neurodegenerative diseases affecting the cerebellum, but can also be caused by drugs (e.g., anticonvulsants, sedatives) or alcohol.
- A purely *horizontal gaze-evoked nystagmus* (■ Fig. 3.57) can indicate a structural lesion in the area of the brainstem (namely the NPH, more rarely the vestibular nuclei) or cerebellum (flocculus/paraflocculus), i.e., the neural integrator for horizontal gaze-holding function.
- A purely *vertical gaze-evoked nystagmus* is observed in midbrain lesions involving the INC, i.e., the neural integrator for vertical gaze-holding function.
- A *dissociated horizontal gaze-evoked nystagmus* (greater in the abducting than the adducting eye) in combination with an adduction deficit are the signs of an internuclear ophthalmoplegia (INO) due to a unilateral lesion of the medial longitudinal fascicle (MLF), which connects the abducens nucleus via interneurons with the contralateral oculomotor nucleus (the INO is on the same side as the adduction deficit).
- *Downbeat nystagmus* (DBN, ■ Fig. 3.59) usually increases when looking down and especially to the side

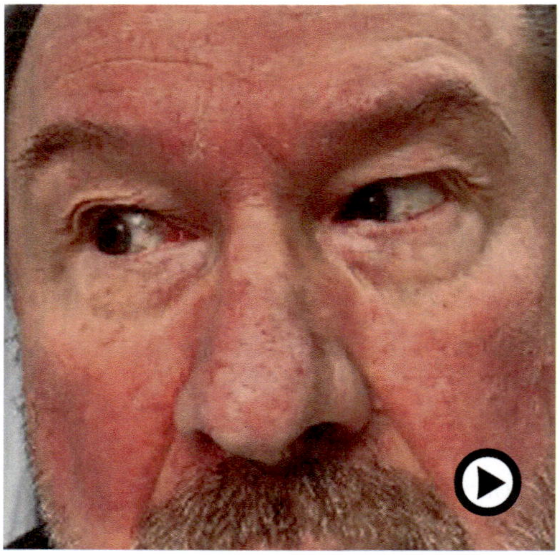

Fig. 3.59 Downbeat nystagmus (▶ https://doi.org/10.1007/000-93x)

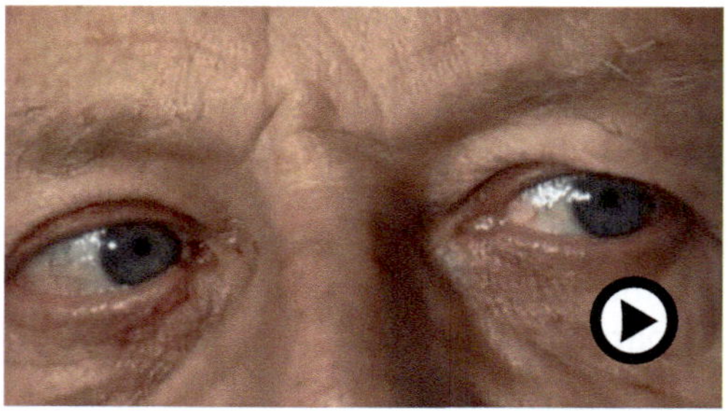

Fig. 3.60 Rebound_nystagmus (▶ https://doi.org/10.1007/000-93y)

because of an additional gaze-holding deficit. Therefore, one often finds a nystagmus beating diagonally downward in the sideward gaze in DBN. The cause of DBN is generally a bilaterally impaired function of the flocculus/paraflocculus.

- To examine for a *rebound nystagmus* (Figs. 3.60 and 3.61), the patient should gaze for 30–60s to one side and then return the eyes quickly to the primary position; this can cause a transient nystagmus to appear with the fast phases opposite to the direction of the previous eye position. Rebound nystagmus generally indicates damage to the flocculus/paraflocculus or cerebellar pathways and is thereby also helpful for the diagnosis of cerebellar dizziness (Feil et al. 2019).

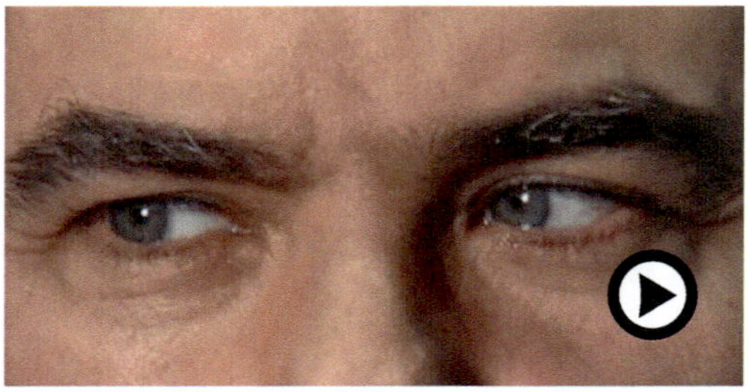

Fig. 3.61 Rebound nystagmus (▶ https://doi.org/10.1007/000-93z)

3.2.5 Clinical Examination of Smooth Pursuit Eye Movements

The generation of smooth pursuit eye movements (Fig. 3.56), which keep the image of an object stable on the fovea is a reflex driven by retinal slip. It involves diverse anatomical structures: the visual cortex, medial temporal area, medial superior temporal area (MST), frontal eye fields, dorsolateral pontine nuclei, cerebellum (flocculus), vestibular, and ocular motor nuclei. These eye movements are influenced by alertness, a number of drugs and also by age. Even healthy people exhibit a slightly saccadic smooth pursuit (Fig. 3.62) during vertical downward eye movements.

The patient is asked to track visually an object moving slowly in horizontal and vertical directions (10–20°/s) while keeping the head stationary (Fig. 3.13). Corrective (catch-up or back-up) saccades are looked for; they indicate a smooth pursuit gain (ratio of eye movement velocity and gaze target velocity) that is too low or too high:

- A saccadic smooth pursuit in all directions (Fig. 3.63) indicates an impaired function of the flocculus/ paraflocculus, e.g., in spinocerebellar ataxias, drug poi-

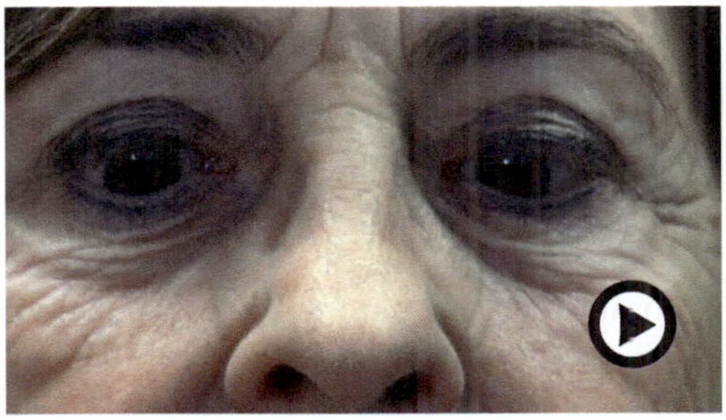

Fig. 3.62 Saccadic smooth pursuit, vertical downward (▶ https://doi.org/10.1007/000-940)

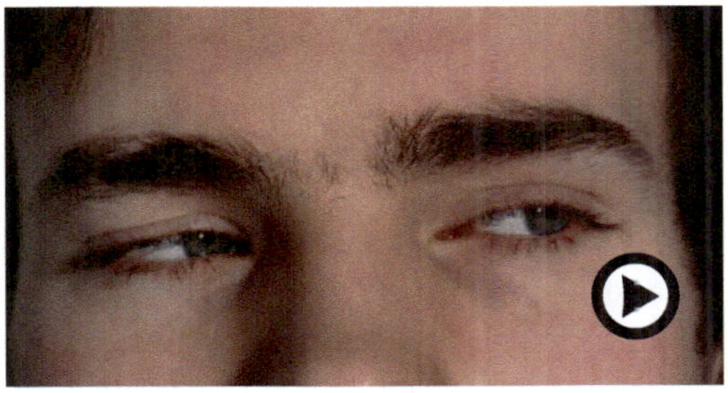

Fig. 3.63 Saccadic smooth pursuit in all directions (▶ https://doi.org/10.1007/000-941)

soning (anticonvulsants, sedatives, benzodiazepines), or alcohol.

- Marked asymmetries of smooth pursuit, however, indicate a structural lesion; e.g., if the smooth pursuit is saccadic to the left, this indicates a left-sided lesion of the flocculus/paraflocculus.
- A reversal of smooth pursuit eye movements is typical for infantile nystagmus.

3.2.6 Vergence Test and Convergence Reaction

To induce *vergence,* a target is moved from a distance of about 50 cm toward the patient's eyes or the patient looks back and forth between a distant and a near target (■ Fig. 3.14). Looking nearby causes vergence, accommodation, and miosis, i.e., the convergence reaction. Neurons important for the convergence reaction are in the area of the mesencephalic reticular formation and the oculomotor nucleus.

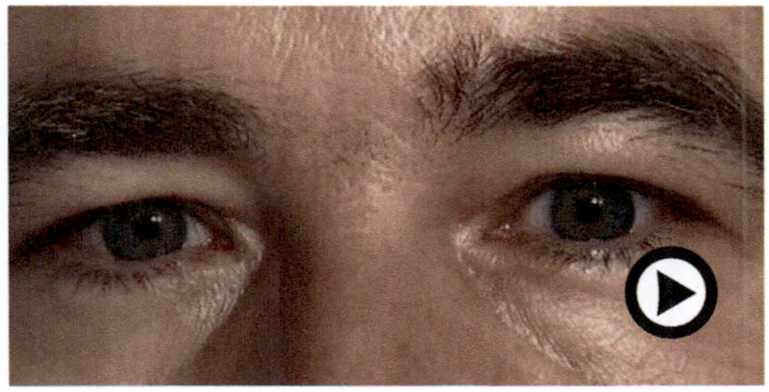

Fig. 3.64 Convergence-retraction nystagmus (▶ https://doi.org/10.1007/000-942)

This explains why the convergence reaction is disturbed in rostral midbrain lesions and tumors of the pineal region, aqueduct, and thalamus, and why abnormalities of vertical gaze are often associated with these defects. In certain neurodegenerative disorders such as progressive supranuclear palsy, convergence is also often impaired. Inborn defects of the convergence reaction also occur in some forms of strabismus.

Convergence-retraction nystagmus (■ Fig. 3.64) can be induced by having the patient look upward, having him/her make saccades vertically upward, or look at a moving optokinetic drum with its stripes going downward. Instead of vertical saccades, rapid, convergent eye movements result that are associated with retractions of the eyeball. The site of damage is the posterior commissure or in rare cases a bilateral disorder of the rostral interstitial nucleus of medial longitudinal fasciculus (riMLF).

A *spasm of the near reflex* is a voluntary convergence accompanied by pupillary constriction; the latter is an important clinical sign for the diagnosis. Occasionally, spasm of the near reflex is psychogenic. It can mimic bilateral abducens palsy.

3.2.7 Clinical Examination of Saccades

First, it is necessary to observe spontaneous saccades triggered by visual or auditory stimuli. Then, the patient is asked to glance back and forth between two horizontal or two vertical targets (◘ Figs. 3.15a, ◘ 3.56, and 3.65). The use of a so-called saccade stick is very useful for a standardized bedside examination (◘ Fig. 3.15b). The amplitudes for the horizontal saccades should be 0 ± 20° to 30° and those for the vertical saccades should be 0 ± 20°. When examining vertical saccades, it is essential to lift the upper eyelids; otherwise, saccade palsy can easily be overlooked.

The velocity, accuracy, and the conjugacy of the saccades should be noted:

- Normal individuals can immediately reach the target with a single fast movement or one small corrective saccade.
- Isolated *slowing* of *vertical saccades* (◘ Fig. 3.66) indicates a midbrain lesion in which the rostral interstitial nucleus of the medial longitudinal fascicle (riMLF) is involved, in fact in ischemic or neurodegenerative diseases, especially progressive supranuclear palsy/tauopathies (◘ Fig. 3.54), Niemann-Pick type C (◘ Fig. 3.55), or acutely in vascular lesions or encephalitis.
- Isolated *slowing* of *horizontal saccades* (◘ Fig. 3.67) is observed in pontine brainstem lesions due to a dysfunction of the burst neurons in the paramedian pontine reticular formation (PPRF); unilateral lesions lead to an ipsiversive slowing of horizontal saccades.
- *Slowing of saccades in all directions*—often accompanied by hypometric saccades (◘ Fig. 3.68)—occurs, for example, in neurodegenerative disorders or with intoxication (especially anticonvulsants, sedatives, benzodiazepines).
- *Hypermetric saccades* (◘ Fig. 3.69): the best test for this are saccades back from an eccentric position to the primary position. Hypermetric saccades can be identified by an overshooting and a corrective saccade back to the object. They indicate

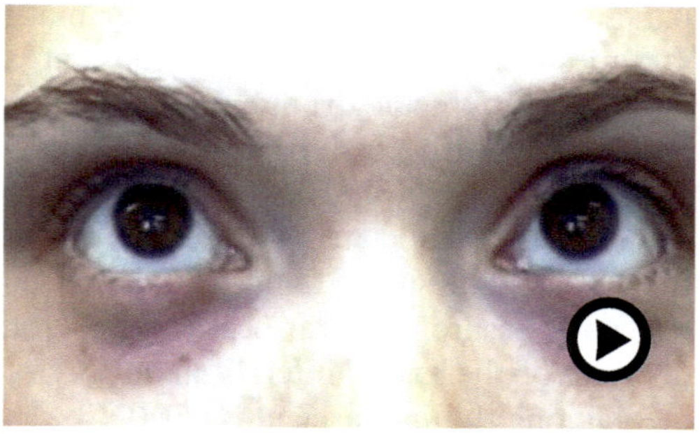

◘ **Fig. 3.65** Normal saccades vertical (▶ https://doi.org/10.1007/000-943)

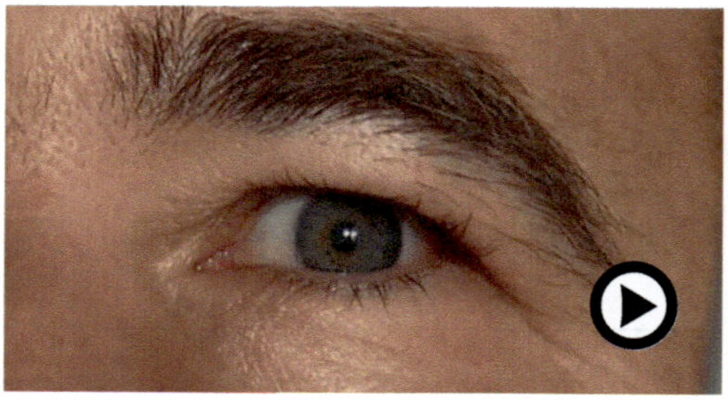

◘ **Fig. 3.66** Slowing of vertical saccades (▶ https://doi.org/10.1007/000-944)

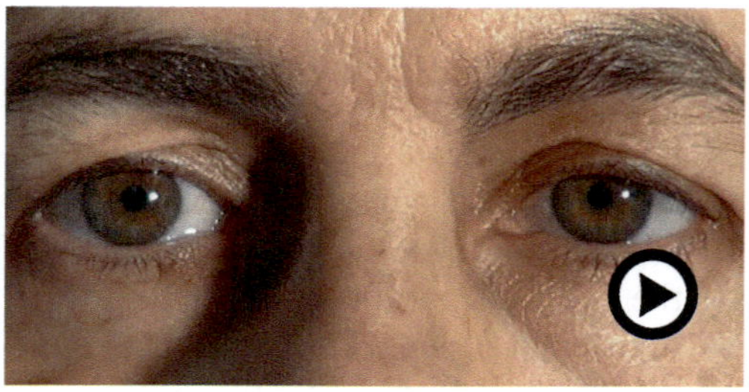

◘ **Fig. 3.67** Slowing of horizontal saccades (▶ https://doi.org/10.1007/000-945)

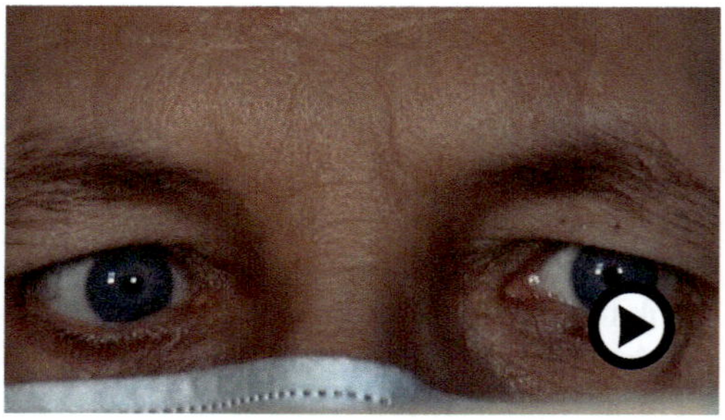

◘ **Fig. 3.68** Hypometric saccades (▶ https://doi.org/10.1007/000-946)

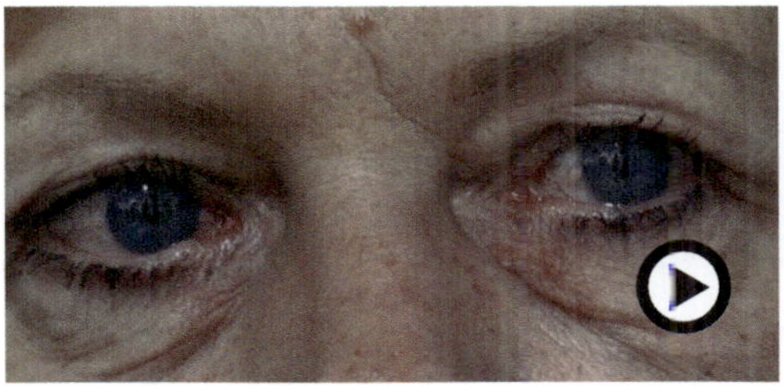

Fig. 3.69 Hypermetric saccades (▶ https://doi.org/10.1007/000-947)

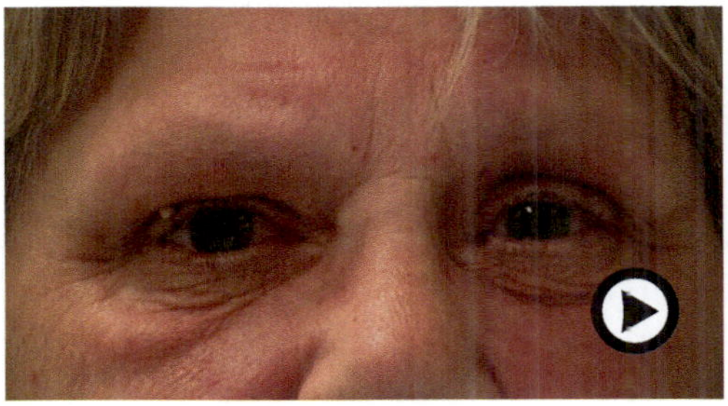

Fig. 3.70 Wallenberg's syndrome. Slowing of the adducting saccade (▶ https://doi.org/10.1007/000-948)

lesions of the cerebellum (namely the fastigial nucleus) or cerebellar pathways leading to a not precise signal to the riMLF and PPRF neurons.

- *Hypometric saccades*, (Fig. 3.68) which can be identified as staircase saccades because they are caught in flight, indicate a lesion of the dorsal cerebellar ocular motor vermis or its pathways.
- Patients with Wallenberg's syndrome (Fig. 3.70) make *hypermetric saccades toward the side of the lesion and hypometric saccades toward the opposite side* due to a dysfunction of the inferior cerebellar peduncle; defects of the superior cerebellar peduncle, conversely, lead to contralateral hypermetric saccades. In addition, when examining vertical saccades, there is an ipsipulsion of vertical saccades toward the side of the lesion.
- A *slowing of the adducting saccade* ipsilateral to a lesion of the MLF (Figs. 3.71 and 3.72) is pathognomonic for internuclear ophthalmoplegia (INO).

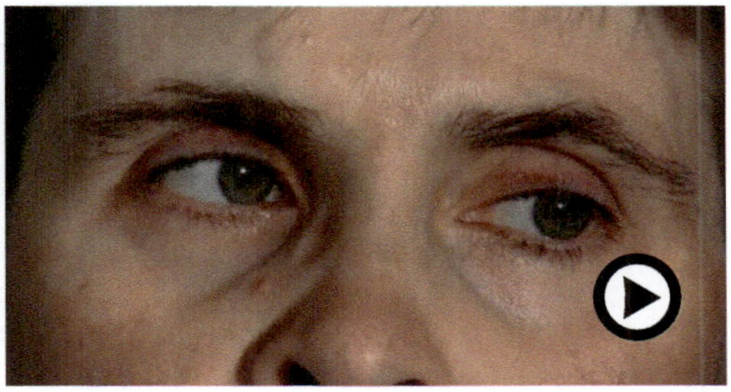

Fig. 3.71 Impairment of the adducting saccade on the left in internuclear ophthalmoplegia on the left side (▶ https://doi.org/10.1007/000-949)

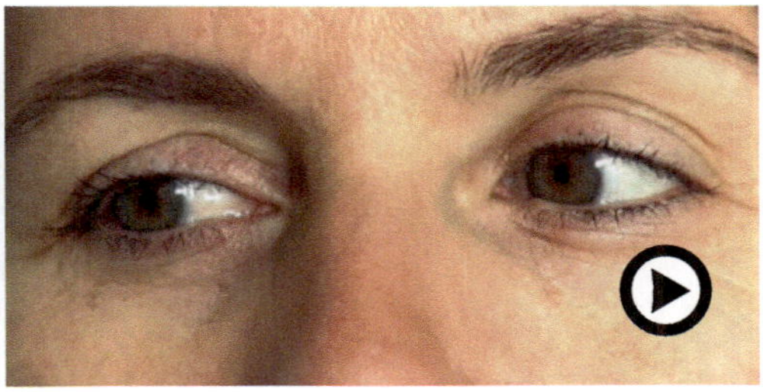

Fig. 3.72 Bilateral impairment of adduction in bilateral internuclear ophthalmoplegia (▶ https://doi.org/10.1007/000-94a)

- *Delayed initiation* of saccades is most often due to a supratentorial cortical dysfunction, affecting the frontal or parietal eye field (e.g., Balint's syndrome, multisystem atrophy); this, however, is difficult to identify during bedside examination and requires video-oculography to be properly diagnosed (see ▶ Chap. 4).
- In rare cases, patients with frontal cortical lesions may also suffer from *ocular motor apraxia*, i.e., they are not able to generate voluntary saccades. The best test to examine these patients is to ask them to perform saccades with the eyes closed, which avoids any reflexive saccades.

3.2.8 Examination of Optokinetic Nystagmus

The examination of eye movements with the optokinetic drum (Fig. 3.73) or a smartphone with a large screen and an app (e.g.,

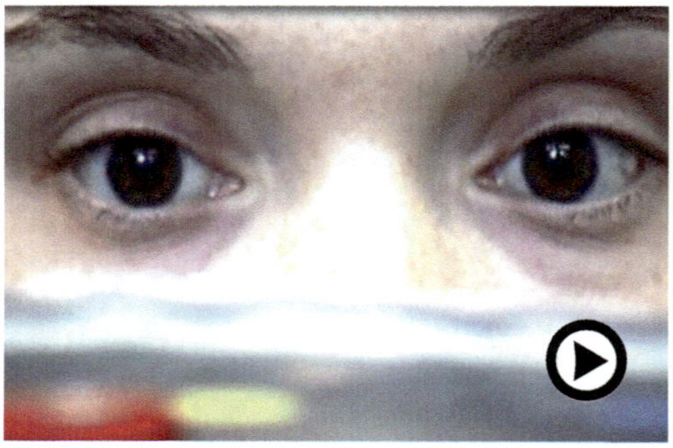

Fig. 3.73 Optokinetic nystagmus, normal findings (▶ https://doi.org/10.1007/000-94b)

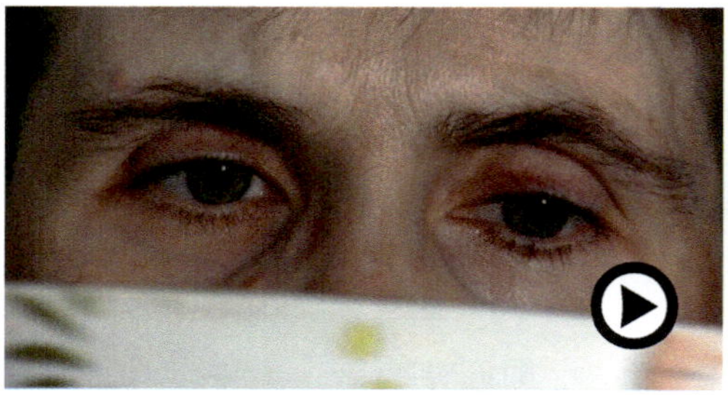

Fig. 3.74 Dissociation of the optokinetic nystagmus in left sided internuclear ophthalmoplegia (▶ https://doi.org/10.1007/000-94c)

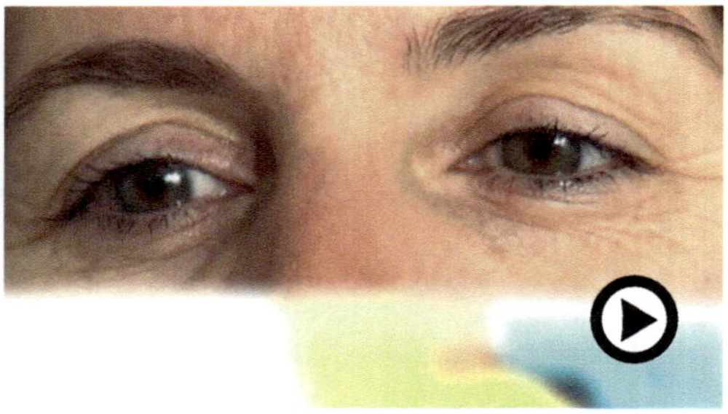

Fig. 3.75 Dissociation of the optokinetic nystagmus in bilateral internuclear ophthalmoplegia (▶ https://doi.org/10.1007/000-94d)

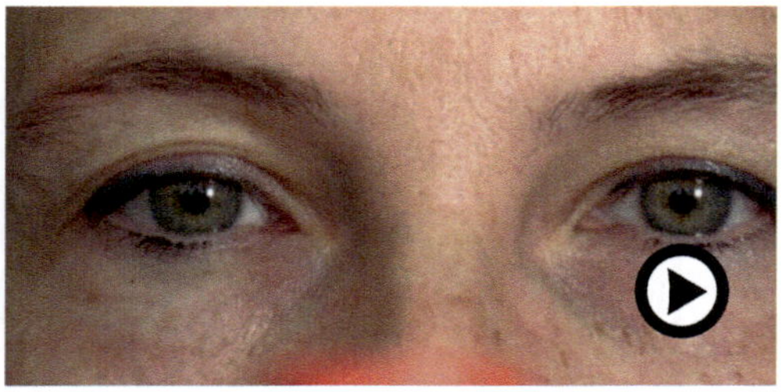

Fig. 3.76 Reversal of pursuit of the optokinetic nystagmus in infantile nystagmus (▶ https://doi.org/10.1007/000-94e)

OptoDrum Fig. 3.16) allows combined testing of smooth pursuit movements and saccades in horizontal and vertical directions. It is especially helpful with uncooperative or drowsy patients as well as children and patients with low visual acuity. It is also helpful in patients in whom functional blindness is assumed because OKN cannot easily be suppressed voluntarily (one caveat: patients with cortical blindness do have OKN). An intact horizontal and vertical optokinetic nystagmus speaks probably for intact function of the midbrain and the pons.

Look for:

- Asymmetries, e.g., between right and left (indicates a unilateral cortical or pontine lesion), vertical OKN worse than horizontal (indicative of a supranuclear gaze palsy due to a mesencephalic lesion)
- Dissociations (Figs. 3.74 and 3.75) of the two eyes (a sign of diminished adduction in INO) and
- Reversal of pursuit which is typically found in infantile nystagmus (Fig. 3.76)

3.2.9 Testing the Visual Fixation Suppression of the Vestibulo-Ocular Reflex

Before performing this test, the examiner must be sure that the VOR is intact (see above). The patient is then asked to fixate a target in front of his/her eyes while moving his/her head as sinusoidally and uniformly as possible with the same angular velocity as the target in front of the eyes, first horizontally and then vertically, back and forth at moderate speed (Figs. 3.17 and 3.77). The examiner should watch for corrective saccades, which indicate a disorder of the visual fixation suppression of the VOR. Impaired visual fixation suppression of the VOR (◘ Fig. 3.78)—which as a rule occurs with smooth pursuit abnormalities, as these two functions use the same nuclei and neural pathways—typically indicates lesions of the cerebellum (flocculus or paraflocculus) or of cerebellar pathways. Unilateral floccular lesions lead to an ipsilesional impairment of the suppression of the VOR. Drugs, especially anticonvulsants and sedatives, and alcohol can also impair visual fixation suppression of the VOR, because of their effects on the cerebellum. In general, this test is particularly important for the diagnosis of a cerebellar dysfunction leading to cerebellar dizziness (Feil et al. 2019).

An overview of the topographical and pathological anatomy of central ocular motor disorders can be found in ◘ Table 3.4 and ◘ Figs. 3.5, 3.79, and 3.80.

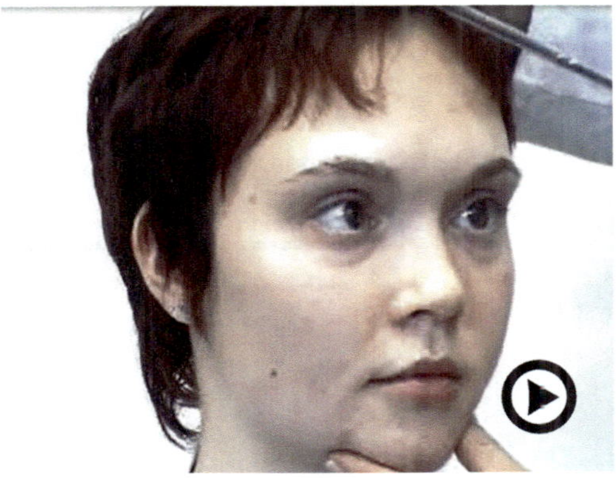

◘ **Fig. 3.77** Clinical testing of visual fixation suppression of the vestibulo-ocular reflex, normal findings (► https://doi.org/10.1007/000-92m)

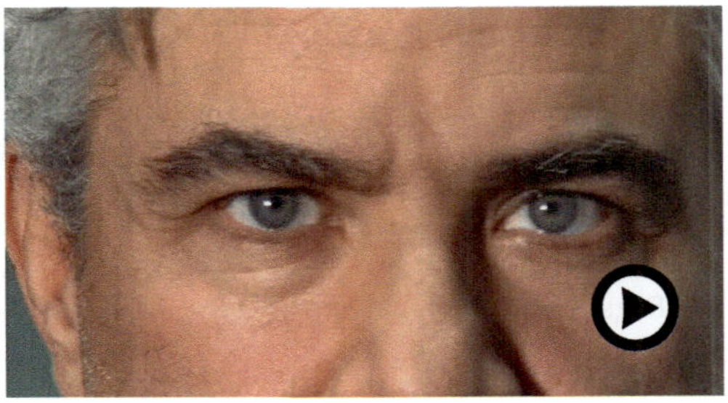

◘ **Fig. 3.78** Impaired visual fixation suppression of the vestibulo-ocular reflex (► https://doi.org/10.1007/000-94g)

◘ **Table 3.4** (A) Anatomy and pathological anatomy of structures relevant for ocular motor disorders and nystagmus, (B) Functional anatomy and pathological anatomy of the cerebellum in relation to ocular motor disorders and nystagmus

(A) Ocular motor dysfunctions and nystagmus and their pathological and topographical anatomy.	
Clinical findings: ocular motor disturbances and nystagmus	**Likely topographical anatomical location in brainstem and cerebellum**
Isolated vertical saccade palsy	Mesencephalon (rostral interstitial nucleus of the medial longitudinal fascicle, riMLF)
Isolated horizontal saccade palsy Isolated *unilateral* horizontal saccade palsy	Pons (paramedian pontine reticular formation, PPRF) Put that down by one line on the level of Isolated unilateral...
Hypermetric saccades	Cerebellar (fastigial nucleus) or cerebellar pathways
Hypometric saccades	Cerebellar (dorsal ocular motor vermis or pathways)
Isolated vertical gaze-evoked nystagmus	Mesencephalon (interstitial nucleus of Cajal, INC)

(continued)

Table 3.4 (continued)

Isolated horizontal gaze-evoked nystagmus	Ponto-medullary/cerebellar lesions (nucleus prepositus hypoglossi, vestibular nuclei, vestibulocerebellum)
Internuclear ophthalmoplegia	MLF lesion ipsilateral to the side of the impaired adduction
Downbeat nystagmus	Mainly cerebellum with bilateral floccular lesion, rarely bilateral lower brainstem
Upbeat nystagmus	Medulla oblongata or mesencephalon
Convergence-retraction nystagmus	Mesencephalon (posterior commissure or bilateral riMLF lesions)
(B) Functional and pathological anatomy of the cerebellum in relation to ocular motor disorders and nystagmus	
Site of the lesion	**Typical findings**
Flocculus/paraflocculus	Saccadic smooth pursuit, gaze-evoked nystagmus in all directions, downbeat nystagmus, rebound nystagmus, impaired visual fixation suppression of the VOR
Nodulus/uvula	Central positional nystagmus, Periodic alternating nystagmus
Fastigial nucleus Dorsal ocular motor vermis	Hypermetric saccades Hypometric saccades

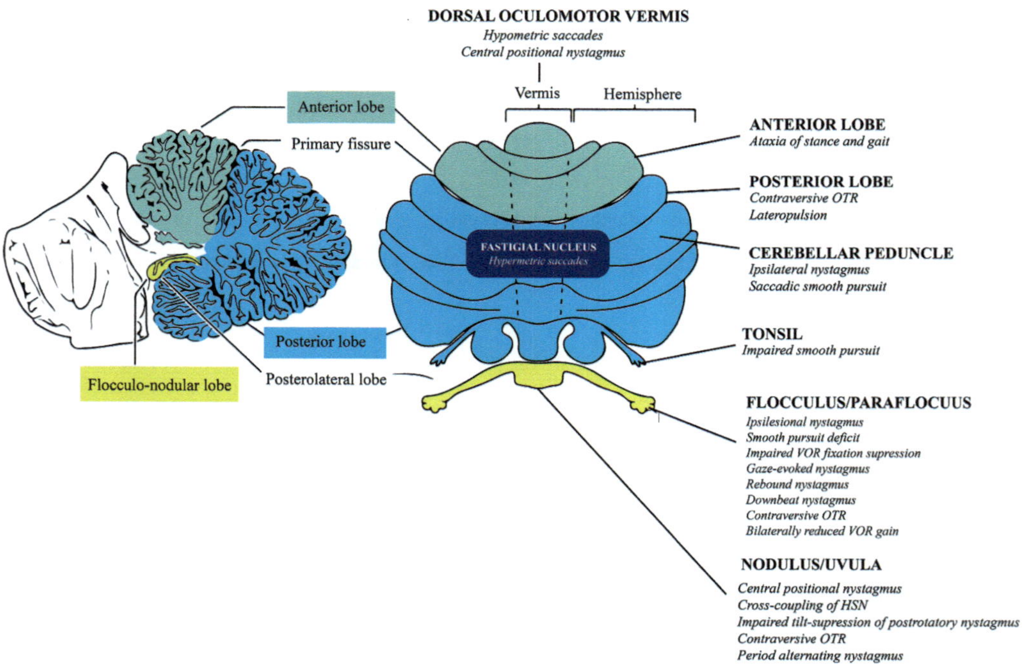

Fig. 3.79 Overview of the ocular motor centers in the area of the brainstem

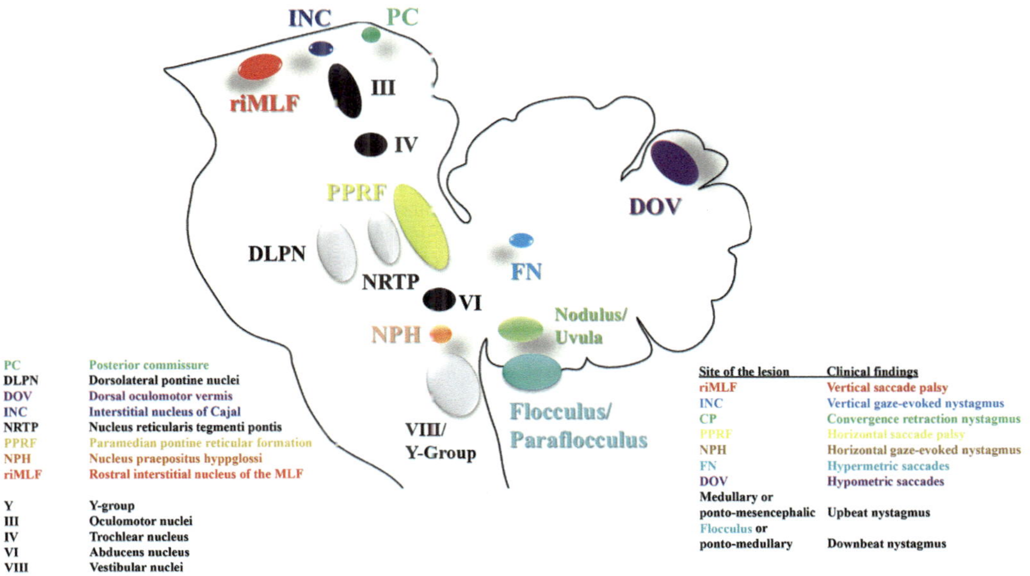

Fig. 3.80 Overview of the relevant ocular motor structures of the cerebellum

References

Bhandari A, Bhandari R, Kingma H, Strupp M (2022) Modified interpretations of the supine roll test in horizontal canal BPPV based on simulations: How the initial position of the debris in the canal and the sequence of testing affects the direction of the nystagmus and the diagnosis. Front Neurol 13:881156

Bhattacharyya N, Gubbels SP, Schwartz SR, Edlow JA, El-Kashlan H, Fife T, Holmberg JM, Mahoney K, Hollingsworth DB, Roberts R, Seidman MD, Steiner RW, Do BT, Voelker CC, Waguespack RW, Corrigan MD (2017) Clinical practice guideline: benign paroxysmal positional vertigo (update). Otolaryngol Head Neck Surg 156(3_suppl):S1–S47

Brandt T, Dieterich M (1993) Skew deviation with ocular torsion: a vestibular brainstem sign of topographic diagnostic value. Ann Neurol 33(5):528–534

Buttner U, Helmchen C, Brandt T (1999) Diagnostic criteria for central versus peripheral positioning nystagmus and vertigo: a review. Acta Otolaryngol 119(1):1–5

Choi JY, Jung I, Jung JM, Kwon DY, Park MH, Kim HJ, Kim JS (2016) Characteristics and mechanism of perverted head-shaking nystagmus in central lesions: video-oculography analysis. Clin Neurophysiol 127(9):2973–2978

Dieterich M, Brandt T (1992) Wallenberg's syndrome: lateropulsion, cyclorotation, and subjective visual vertical in thirty-six patients. Ann Neurol 31(4):399–408

Dieterich M, Brandt T (1993) Ocular torsion and tilt of subjective visual vertical are sensitive brainstem signs. Ann Neurol 33(3):292–299

Dieterich M, Brandt T (2019) Perception of verticality and vestibular disorders of balance and falls. Front Neurol 10:172

Eggers SDZ, Bisdorff A, von Brevern M, Zee DS, Kim JS, Perez-Fernandez N, Welgampola MS, Della Santina CC, Newman-Toker DE (2019) Classification of vestibular signs and examination techniques: nystagmus and nystagmus-like movements. J Vestib Res 29(2-3):57–87

Feil K, Strobl R, Schindler A, Krafczyk S, Goldschagg N, Frenzel C, Glaser M, Schoberl F, Zwergal A, Strupp M (2019) What is behind cerebellar vertigo and dizziness? Cerebellum 18(3):320–332

Halmagyi GM, Curthoys IS (1988) A clinical sign of canal paresis. Arch Neurol 45:737–739

Halmagyi GM, McGarvie LA, Strupp M (2020) Nystagmus goggles: how to use them, what you find and what it means. Pract Neurol 20:446–450

Hufner K, Barresi D, Glaser M, Linn J, Adrion C, Mansmann U, Brandt T, Strupp M (2008) Vestibular paroxysmia: diagnostic features and medical treatment. Neurology 71(13):1006–1014

Huh YE, Kim JS (2011) Patterns of spontaneous and head-shaking nystagmus in cerebellar infarction: imaging correlations. Brain 134(Pt 12):3662–3671

Lemos J, Strupp M (2022) Central positional nystagmus: an update. J Neurol 269:(4)1851–860

Mantokoudis G, Wyss T, Zamaro E, Korda A, Wagner F, Sauter TC, Kerkeni H, Kalla R, Morrison M, Caversaccio MD (2021) Stroke Prediction Based on the Spontaneous Nystagmus Suppression Test in Dizzy Patients: A Diagnostic Accuracy Study. Neurology 97:e42–e51

Korda A, Zamaro E, Wagner F, Morrison M, Caversaccio MD, Sauter TC, Schneider E, Mantokoudis G (2022) Acute vestibular syndrome: is skew deviation a central sign? J Neurol 269:1396–1403

Raphan T, Matsuo V, Cohen B (1979) Velocity storage in the vestibulo-ocular reflex arc (VOR). Exp Brain Res 35(2):229–248

Schniepp R, Mohwald K, Wuehr M (2019) Clinical and automated gait analysis in patients with vestibular, cerebellar, and functional gait disorders: perspectives and limitations. J Neurol 266(Suppl 1):118–122

Strupp M, Fischer C, Hanss L, Bayer O (2014) The takeaway Frenzel goggles: a Fresnel-based device. Neurology 83(14):1241–1245

von Brevern M, Bertholon P, Brandt T, Fife T, Imai T, Nuti D, Newman-Toker D (2015) Benign paroxysmal positional vertigo: diagnostic criteria. J Vestib Res 25(3-4):105–117

Westheimer G, Blair SM (1975) The ocular tilt reaction - brainstem ocular motor routine. Investig Ophthalmol 14:833–839

Yang TH, Lee J, Oh SY, Kang JJ, Kim JS, Dieterich M (2020) Clinical implications of head-shaking nystagmus in central and peripheral vestibular disorders: is perverted head-shaking nystagmus specific for central vestibular pathology? Eur J Neurol 27:1296–1303

Yip CW, Glaser M, Frenzel C, Bayer O, Strupp M (2016) Comparison of the bedside head-impulse test with the video head-impulse test in a clinical practice setting: a prospective study of 500 outpatients. Front Neurol 7:58

Zwergal A, Rettinger N, Frenzel C, Frisen L, Brandt T, Strupp M (2009) A bucket of static vestibular function. Neurology 72:1689–1692

Laboratory Examinations and Imaging

Contents

Supplementary Information The online version contains supplementary material available at [https://doi.org/10.1007/978-3-030-78260-3_4]. The videos can be accessed by scanning the related images with the SN More Media App.

M. Strupp et al., *Vertigo and Dizziness*, https://doi.org/10.1007/978-3-030-78260-3_4

After the patient history and the bedside examination of the vestibular, ocular motor, and cerebellar systems, laboratory examinations form the third pillar of clinical diagnostics. They are also most relevant for the quantification and documentation of vestibular deficits (Starkov et al. 2021), the course of the disease, and the effects of treatment (van de Berg et al. 2018). The high relevance of quantitative testing of function by means of the video head impulse test (video-HIT) and caloric testing for a precise diagnosis has also been highlighted in the diagnostic criteria of the Bárány Society, e.g., for the diagnosis of bilateral vestibulopathy (Strupp et al. 2017), presbyvestibulopathy (Agrawal et al. 2019) and acute unilateral vestibulopathy/vestibular neuritis (Strupp et al. 2022). In addition, the video-HIT can also contribute to the differentiation between an acute peripheral and an acute central vestibular syndrome (Saber Tehrani et al. 2018; Machner et al. 2021).

When it comes to quantitative testing of vestibular function, it is, however, still very problematic that there are no internationally accepted criteria for reference and pathological values for the different tests. They not only vary from laboratory to laboratory (Strupp et al. 2020), but even from technical assistant to technical assistant within the same clinic (Ertl et al. 2016).

The most important laboratory examinations are as follows:

- For the vestibular system:
  - Video head impulse test (video-HIT): Function of the angular VOR in the high-frequency range (for references, see Halmagyi et al. 2017).
  - Caloric testing: Function of the horizontal semicircular canal in the low-frequency range (for references, see Shepard and Jacobson 2016).
  - Rotatory chair examination: Function of the horizontal canals in the low- and middle-frequency range (to be applied in exceptional cases (for references, see Furman 2016)).
  - In clinical routine, the following order of these three examinations has proved to be useful: (1) Video-HIT, because this can be easily and reliably applied; (2) if this is normal, caloric testing, which may be associated with a lot of potential artifacts; (3) if both are normal and the patient history makes a peripheral vestibular deficit likely, rotatory chair testing can be indicated.
  - Vestibular-evoked myogenic potentials (VEMP) (Colebatch et al. 2016; Rosengren et al. 2019) to test the function of the otolith organs (Taylor and Welgampola 2019): The major indication for VEMP is the diagnosis of a syndrome of the third mobile windows, i.e., in particular superior canal dehiscence syndrome (Fife et al. 2017; Verrechia et al. 2019; Ward et al. 2021; Kim et al. 2022a):
    - Cervical VEMP (cVEMP): mainly saccular function
    - Ocular VEMP (oVEMP): mainly utricular function.
  - Subjective visual verticality (SVV): Function of graviceptive pathways, which arise from the otolith organs and the vertical semicircular canals; a deviation of the SVV toward one side indicates an ipsilateral peripheral vestibular lesion or a contralateral excitation (Zwergal et al. 2009a, b; Dieterich and Brandt 1993); in terms of topographic anatomic diagnosis lesions within the labyrinth/vestibular nerve and the lower brainstem lead to an ipsilateral deviation and upper brainstem lesions to a contralateral deviation of SVV.
- For the ocular motor system:
  - Video-oculography (VOG) (for references, see Larrazabal et al. 2019; Falls 2019); this, for instance, allows a quantification of the velocity and precision of saccades.

- For stance and gait:
  - Posturography (in selected cases) (for references, see Falls 2019).
- For gait:
  - Quantitative gait analysis (in selected cases) (for references, see Schniepp et al. 2019).

In ◘ Table 4.1 and ◘ Figs. 4.1, 4.2, 4.3, 4.4, 4.5, 4.6, 4.7, 4.8, 4.9, and 4.10, the clinically relevant neurootological and neuroophthalmological laboratory examinations with typical findings and their interpretation are summarized.

4.1 Laboratory Testing of Vestibular Function

4.1.1 Video Head Impulse Test (Video-HIT)

▪ Function of the Angular VOR in the High-Frequency Range

The simultaneous measurement of the head and eye angular velocity during fast head turns allows a quantification of the function of the angular VOR in the high-frequency range (Bartl et al. 2009; MacDougall et al.

◘ **Table 4.1** Laboratory examinations of the vestibular and ocular motor systems

Technique	Features	Advantages	Disadvantages
Vestibular system			
Video-HIT	Quantification of the function of the angular VOR in the high-frequency range	Non-invasive, can be performed quickly and easily, examination of the VOR function close to the optimal range of stimulation of the semicircular canals between 0.1 and 10 Hz	This test does not allow examination of a single semicircular canal, but only a pair of semicircular canals
Caloric testing	Quantification of the function of the horizontal semicircular canals in the low-frequency range	Non-invasive, simple to perform, allows the examination of single horizontal canals	Only the function of the horizontal canals can be quantified, time-consuming, there can be several artifacts; it may cause nausea or vomiting in patients
Rotatory chair examination	Quantification of the function of the horizontal semicircular canals in the lower- and middle-frequency range	Non-invasive	Expensive equipment, only possible to examine pairs of semicircular canals, not single canals (similar to video-HIT); indicated in selected cases when video-HIT and caloric testing are normal, although the patient history indicates a peripheral vestibular deficit. Nowadays, only rarely applied.

(continued)

Table 4.1 (continued)

Technique	Features	Advantages	Disadvantages
Cervical vestibular-evoked myogenic potentials (cVEMP)	Mainly examination of saccular function	Non-invasive, is well tolerated, quite easy to perform	Interpretation of the findings is heterogeneous; different normative and pathological values recommended; the function of the vertical canals is also partially tested
Ocular vestibular-evoked myogenic potentials (oVEMP)	Mainly examination of utricular function	Non-invasive, is well tolerated, easy to perform	Similar to cVEMP
Subjective visual verticality (SVV)	Examination of an acute vestibular tone imbalance of the graviceptive pathways from the otolith organs (mainly utricle) and vertical semicircular canals	Non-invasive, is well tolerated, easy to perform, e.g., with the bucket test	Will be normalized during central compensation despite a persisting deficit; thus, deviation indicates an acute or not compensated lesion
Ocular motor system			
Video-oculography (VOG)	Measurement range ± 40° horizontally and ± 20° vertically, resolution of 0.1–1°; allows the recording of nystagmus, smooth pursuit, saccades, gaze-holding function, optokinetic nystagmus, suppression of the VOR	Non-invasive, well tolerated, combined with caloric testing and the head impulse test to determine the function of the VOR; nowadays widely used	Only possible with open eyes, artifacts possible: 3D analysis more complicated and expensive
Magnetic-coil technique by lens	Measurement range horizontal ±40°, vertical ±40°, resolution of 0.02°	Best resolution of horizontal, vertical, and torsional movements (research); can be combined with head impulse test if angular head velocity is also measured	Semi-invasive, unpleasant, expensive, only with cooperative patients, maximum of 30 min, local anesthesia necessary

2009; Halmagyi et al. 2017) (Fig. 4.1). It is important to note that the testing is close to the functionally relevant stimulation range of the semicircular canals from 0.1 to 10 Hz. Further, with the video head impulse test pairs of semicircular canals and not isolated semicircular canals are examined, e.g., during a head turn to the right, there is an excitation of the right horizontal and an inhibition of the left horizontal canal. Since

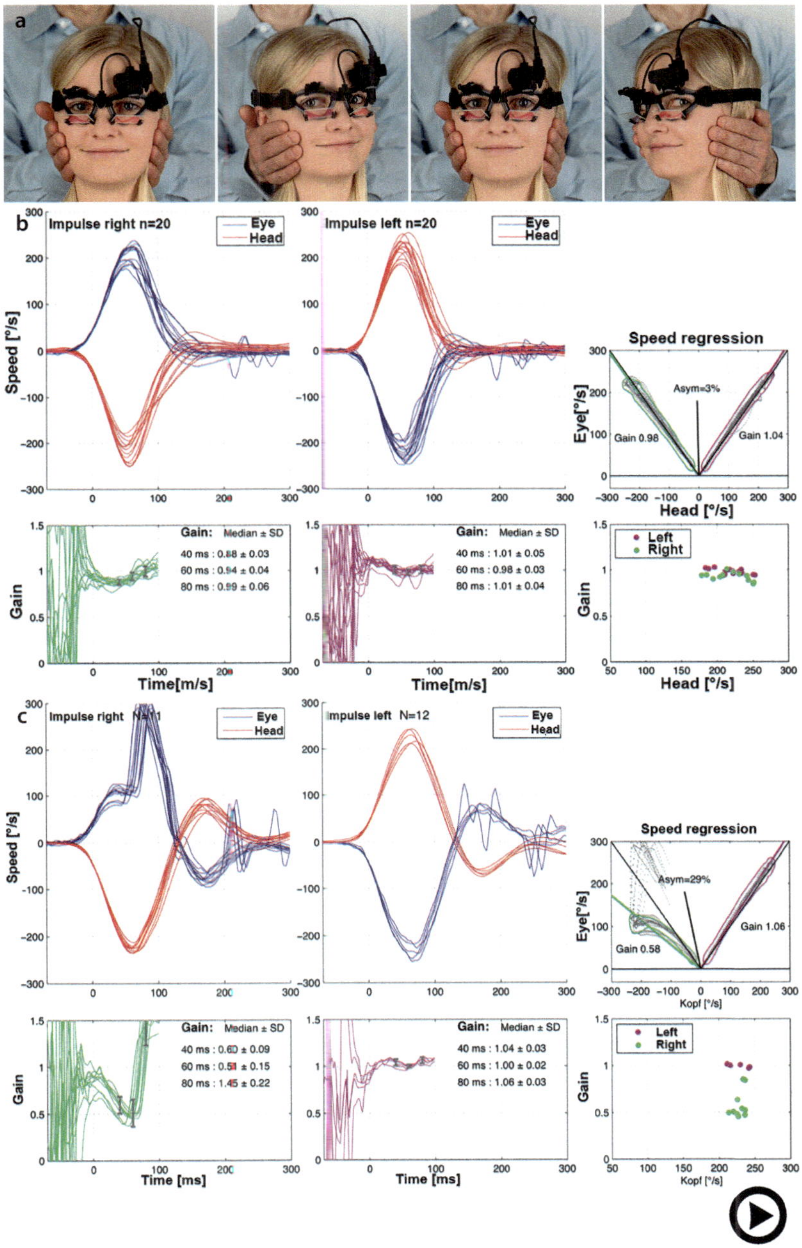

Fig. 4.1 **a–c** Head impulse test with video-oculography (video-HIT) to quantify the function of the angular VOR. **a** During fast head turns to the right and to the left, there is a simultaneous recording of the eye movements by a high-resolution infrared camera and the head movements by sensors in the mask. This allows measurement of the angular velocities after calibration. **b** In the system depicted, the quotient of the angular eye and head velocity at 60 ms is calculated: the VOR gain. The recording shows a normal VOR gain. **c** During quick head turns to the left, a normal VOR gain of 1.0 is found. During quick head turns to the right, the gain is reduced to 0.51. Already 70 ms after the initiation of the head turn to the right, the patient performs so-called refixation saccades, which are not recognized by the clinical examiner and are therefore called covert saccades. For clinical practice, this means: If only the bedside head impulse test is performed in such patients, the results could be false normal (► https://doi.org/10.1007/000-94p)

in almost all cases of a peripheral vestibular deficit the horizontal canal is affected, the examination of this canal by the video-HIT is clinically sufficient in most patients.

For the calculation of the VOR gain, different algorithms are used; e.g., the angular eye velocity is divided by the angular head velocity at 60 ms or the area under the curve of the eye angular velocity is divided by head angular velocity. Despite these different approaches to the analysis, the calculated values are practically identical (Lee et al. 2018; Murnane et al. 2014; Strupp et al. 2018). Depending on the position of the camera in front of the examined eye, there is a right-left difference for the VOR gain, which has not been well explained so far: For instance, if the camera is placed in front of the right eye, the gain to the right is around 5% higher than the gain to the left (Strupp et al. 2018).

The applied normative values/reference range of the video-HIT are mainly based on studies with a large number of healthy subjects, also for different age groups (e.g., McGarvie et al. 2015; Matino-Soler et al. 2015; Bachmann et al. 2018; Yang et al. 2016). A VOR gain above 0.8 is often classified as normal; a VOR gain below 0.7 on one side could be interpreted as a unilateral peripheral vestibular deficit (Strupp et al. 2022); a bilateral VOR gain of between 0.8 and 0.6 in combination with an appropriate patient history and bedside examination is compatible with a presbyvestibulopathy (Agrawal et al. 2019); and a bilaterally reduced VOR gain of below 0.6 indicates a bilateral vestibulopathy (Strupp et al. 2017).

4.1.2 Caloric Testing

▪ Function of the Horizontal Canal in the Low-Frequency Range

Caloric testing allows a quantification of the function of a single horizontal canal (in the low—unphysiological—frequency range of about 0.003 Hz) by irrigation of the external auditory canal with 30 °C cold and 44 °C warm water, while the eye movements induced are recorded. The peak slow phase velocity of the caloric-induced nystagmus is quantified by means of VOG (see below). An advantage of this technology is that each horizontal canal can be examined separately, in contrast to video-HIT and rotatory chair testing.

The irrigation with 44 °C warm water causes—by means of a combination of convective and non-convective mechanisms—an excitation of the hair cells of the horizontal canal with slow contraversive eye movements; 30 °C cool water causes an inhibition with slow phase ipsiversive eye movements (for references, see Shepard and Jacobson 2016) (◘ Fig. 4.2).

The parameter to quantify the function is the mean peak slow phase velocity of the calorically induced nystagmus (mPSPV). Since there is a huge interindividual variability of the caloric excitability, for the comparison of the function of both horizontal canals additionally the vestibular paresis formula of Jongkees is used (Jongkees et al. 1962): [((R 33° + R 44°) – (L 30° + L 44°)]/[(R 30° + R 44° + L 30° + L 44°))] × 100; for instance, R 30° decrease means mPSPV during caloric irrigation with 30°C cold water.

Although caloric irrigation was already described by Robert Bárány in 1907 (Barany 1907), there is so far no general consensus about normal reference values and pathological values for either the absolute or the relative values (Bruner and Norris 1971; Peterka et al. 1990; Mallinson and Longridge 2004; Shepard and Jacobson 2016; Van Der Stappen et al. 2000). For the absolute values for warm and cold water irrigation, most often mPSPV values <3° – 6°/s are assumed to be pathological for a unilateral peripheral deficit (Strupp et al. 2022). For bilateral vestibulopathy (BVP), according to the current diagnostic criteria, the sum of the mPSPV for warm and cold irrigation is assumed to be <6°/s on each side (Strupp et al. 2017).

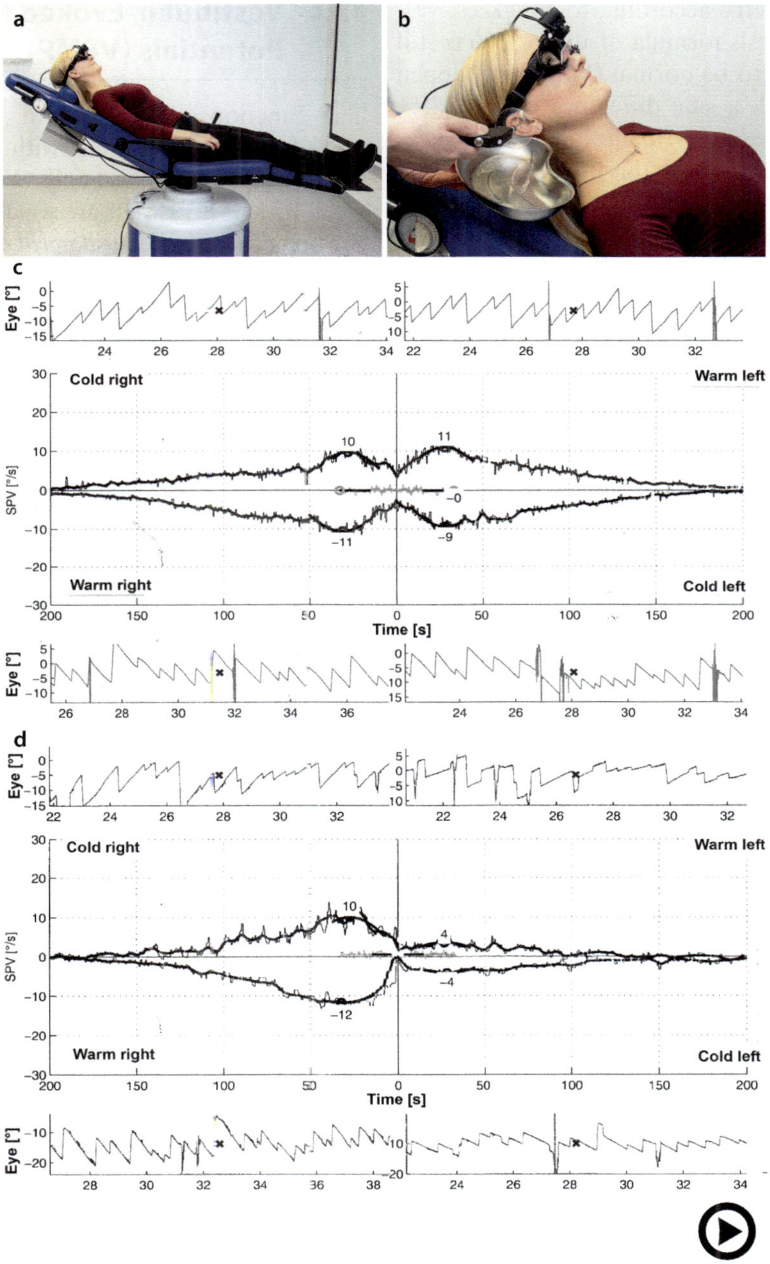

Fig. 4.2 a–d Caloric testing with recording of eye movements by video-oculography. By means of caloric testing, the excitability of the individual horizontal canals can be determined and thus whether or not they are functioning properly. **a** After excluding the possibility of a lesion of the eardrum, the head of the patient is tilted 30° upward so that the horizontal semicircular canals approach the vertical plane. This allows optimal caloric stimulation. **b** The external auditory canals on each side are separately irrigated under standard conditions with 30 °C cold and 44 °C warm water and the horizontal and vertical eye movements are recorded by means of video-oculography. **c** Caloric testing in a healthy individual. **d** Pathological finding: relative reduced caloric excitability on the left (according to Jongkees' vestibular paresis formula, side difference of 47%). (► https://doi.org/10.1007/000-94j)

An asymmetry according to Jongkees' vestibular paresis formula of up to 19% is still considered to be normal (Van Der Stappen et al. 2000), a side difference of >20–25% is considered to be pathological (Jongkees et al. 1962), although this has so far not been correlated with clinical deficits, functioning, or the quality of life of affected patients (Shepard and Jacobson 2016).

4.1.3 Rotatory Chair Testing

Using a rotatory chair and simultaneous measurement of eye movements by VOG, the function of the pairs of horizontal semicircular canals can—depending on the stimulation method—be quantified in the low- and middle-frequency range (Furman 2016; Maes et al. 2008). Sinusoidal stimulation is used to quantify the function in the low-frequency range of the VOR from 0.005 to 0.64 Hz. The so-called velocity step test (VST), e.g., constant rotation with 100°/s and subsequent deceleration with 200°/s, is used to quantify the function in a higher and more physiologically relevant range (Goulson et al. 2014). The reference values given in the literature for normal and pathological data vary greatly, however. Therefore, it is recommended that each laboratory generates its own normative/reference values (Wall et al. 1984). For the diagnosis of BVP, a reduced horizontal angular VOR gain ≤0.1 upon sinusoidal stimulation on a rotatory chair (0.1 Hz, Vmax=50°/sec) and a phase lead≥15 degrees (time constant≤6sec) is proposed (Strupp et al. 2017). In general, the clinical relevance of the rotatory chair examination has decreased considerably over the last years, in particular since VOR function can be reliably examined by the video-HIT, and is therefore only indicated in exceptional cases.

4.1.4 Vestibular-Evoked Myogenic Potentials (VEMP)

The function of the otolith organs can nowadays be measured with vestibular-evoked myogenic potentials (VEMP): cervical VEMP (cVEMP) are used to evaluate the function of the *ipsilateral* saccule and ocular VEMP (oVEMP) that of the *contralateral* utricle (◘ Fig. 4.3) (for references, see Rosengren et al. 2019). It has so far not been clarified whether these tests exclusively stimulate the otolith organs or also, in addition, the semicircular canals. VEMP use the sensitivity of the otolith organs to sound (air-conducted sound = ACS) and vibration (bone-conducted vibration = BCV). A prerequisite for the application of ACS stimuli is intact middle ear function; therefore, it is necessary to exclude a conduction hearing loss before applying the VEMP. On the other hand, sensorineural hearing loss does not cause any methodological problems because, in ACS-VEMP, the sensitivity of the otolith organs and not the cochlea to sounds is measured. In contrast to the ACS stimuli, BCV stimuli can be applied independent of middle ear function. Clinically and scientifically, VEMP are important laboratory tests, in particular if one considers that previously testing of the function of the otolith organs could only be done with considerable time and effort. However, the clinical relevance of VEMP needs to be evaluated further in basic and clinical studies (for references, see: Fife et al. 2017; Curthoys and Dlugaiczyk 2020).

Based on the clinical guidelines of the American Academy of Neurology, the most important indication for the use of cVEMP and oVEMP is their contribution to the diagnosis of the syndrome of the third mobile windows (▶ Chap. 12), in particular superior canal dehiscence syndrome (Fife et al. 2017; Verrechia et al. 2019; Ward et al. 2021; Kim et al. 2022a). As was shown in several studies

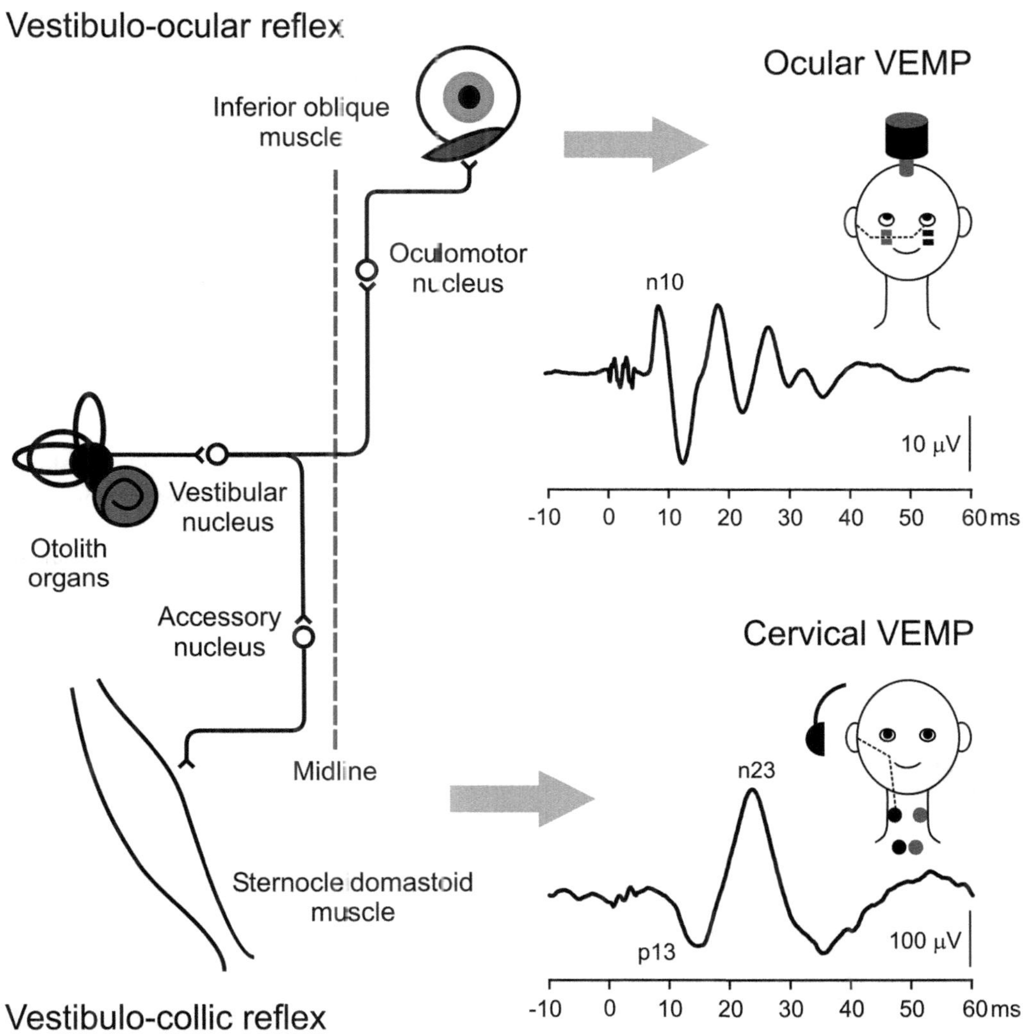

Fig. 4.3 Vestibular-evoked myogenic potentials (VEMP)): Cervical vestibular-evoked myogenic potentials (cVEMP) and ocular-vestibular-evoked potentials (oVEMP). Schematic drawing and recording of cVEMP and oVEMP. The stimulation for oVEMP (**upper part**) is usually by vibration, preferably with the so-called minishaker on the forehead and recording over the inferior oblique muscle while the subject is looking upward. In healthy subjects, there is a contralateral negative (n10) and positive (p15) wave. This test allows an evaluation of the function of the utricle, but probably semicircular canal function is also partially involved. It is a vestibulo-ocular reflex. cVEMP (**lower part**) allow mainly a measurement of the function of the saccule via the vestibulo-colic reflex (VCR) over the vestibular nerves, vestibular nuclei, interneurons, and motoneurons to the neck sternocleidomastoid muscle. It is a vestibulo-spinal reflex (kindly provided by Sally Rosengren, Sydney)

(for references, see Fife et al. 2017; Ward et al. 2021), the amplitudes of the oVEMP are increased and the threshold of the cVEMP is decreased in superior canal dehiscence syndrome. In clinical practice, oVEMP can be performed more easily than cVEMP and do not depend on a threshold. In addition, oVEMP are evidently more sensitive and specific than cVEMP for the diagnosis of superior canal dehiscence syndrome and other third mobile windows (Fife et al. 2017; Verrechia et al. 2019; Ward et al. 2021).

4.1.4.1 Cervical Vestibular-Evoked Myogenic Potentials (cVEMP)

The vestibulo-colic reflex (VCR) is used to test the reflex arc of the saccule, which extends over the vestibular nerves, vestibular nuclei, interneurons, and motor neurons to the neck musculature (namely the sternocleidomastoid muscles) (◘ Fig. 4.4) (for references, see Rosengren et al. 2019). The reflex can be induced by a loud monaural pure tone (e.g., 500-Hz, 2 ms duration, 130 dB pSPL = peak sound pressure level). One should take care that the patient does not experience a sound-induced trauma. The patient should lift his/her head while lying supine to increase the muscle tension of the sternocleidomastoid muscle. The inhibitory potential from the sternocleidomastoid muscle is recorded by a superficial EMG. In healthy subjects, there is first an ipsilateral positive, i.e., inhibitory, wave after about 13 ms (P13) and a subsequent negative excitatory wave after 23 ms (N23) (◘ Fig. 4.3). Criteria for the evaluation are the presence of P13 and N23 with amplitude and latency; the latter is less relevant. If there are no waves or there is a significant asymmetry between right and left, this is assumed to be pathological. Increased latencies were observed in certain neurological diseases, such as multiple sclerosis, and are evidently clinically less relevant (for references, see Fife et al. 2017; Curthoys and Dlugaiczyk 2020).

Clinically relevant pathological findings for cVEMP were described for the following diseases:

- Syndrome of the third mobile windows, in particular canal dehiscence syndrome: Typically, the threshold for cVEMP is reduced, i.e., even sounds with low decibel values can induce waves with increased amplitudes (Kim et al. 2022a). The currently recommended threshold measurement for cVEMP is done with a

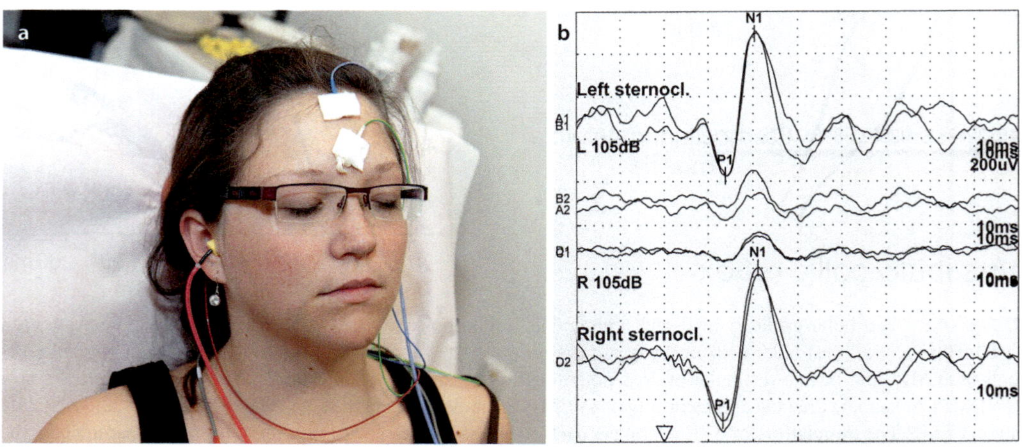

◘ **Fig. 4.4** a, b Cervical VEMP. **a** Depiction of the recording conditions. The prerequisite for the application of air-conducted sound stimuli (ACS) is intact middle ear function; intact sensorineural hearing function (cochlea and pathways) is not necessary, since cVEMP use the sound sensitivity of the saccule. The reflex is most often induced by a 500-Hz pure tone with a duration of 2 ms and up to 130 dB peak sound pressure level. The recording is done with a superficial EMG from both sternocleidomastoid muscles. It is important that the patient lifts his/her head by about 30° while lying supine to increase the muscle tension. **b** In healthy subjects, there is an initial ipsilateral positive wave (about 13 ms after the stimulus, P13), indicating an inhibition, and a subsequent negative wave (after about 23 ms, N23) (curves 1 and 3). Contralaterally, these amplitudes are normally not seen (curves 2 and 4). About 50–100 stimuli are necessary for the recording. Criteria for the evaluation of cVEMP are the presence of P13 and N23 waves and their amplitudes; the latency is less important. For cVEMP, threshold measurements are also used, in particular when superior canal dehiscence syndrome or an other syndrome of the third mobile windows are suspected stimulation frequency of 2000 Hz; this has a specificity of almost 100% and a sensitivity of 92% (Noij et al. 2019).

- Acute unilateral vestibulopathy/vestibular neuritis: In two thirds of the patients, cVEMP are normal, which can be explained by sparing of the inferior part of the vestibular nerve, which goes to the saccule and the posterior semicircular canal (for references, see Colebatch et al. 2016; Rosengren et al. 2019).
- Bilateral vestibulopathy: cVEMP are reduced or absent in only a small number of patients with bilateral vestibulopathy (Rosengren et al. 2018; Zingler et al. 2008). It is so far not known why otolith function is evidently more preserved than semicircular canal function in bilateral vestibulopathy.
- Menière's disease (MD): Patients with MD—but not with vestibular migraine (VM)—showed a higher asymmetry ratio for cVEMP than for oVEMP amplitudes (Dlugaiczyk et al. 2020). This is in line with a more common saccular than utricular dysfunction in MD and a more permanent loss of otolith function in MD versus VM.

4.1.4.2 Ocular-Vestibular-Evoked Potentials (oVEMP)

For oVEMP, the stimulation is performed by vibration (bone-conducted vibration), most often with a so-called minishaker in the middle of the forehead (Fz) and the recording is done from the inferior oblique muscle when the patient looks upward. The EMG signals of the inferior oblique muscle mainly arise from the contralateral utricle (for references, see (Rosengren et al. 2019)). In healthy subjects, there is a contralateral (excitatory) wave (N10) about 10 ms after the stimulus and a positive wave (P15) about 15 ms after the stimulus (◘ Fig. 4.5).

Technically, the recording of oVEMP is easier than that of cVEMP. Criteria for the evaluation of oVEMP are the presence or absence of N10 and P15 waves and their amplitude. Increased latencies were observed in neurological disorders, e.g., multiple sclerosis, with an involvement of the brainstem (Fife et al. 2017; Curthoys and Dlugaiczyk 2020). No waves or a significant asymmetry of the amplitudes is considered pathological, although there are so far no normative values (Strupp et al. 2020).

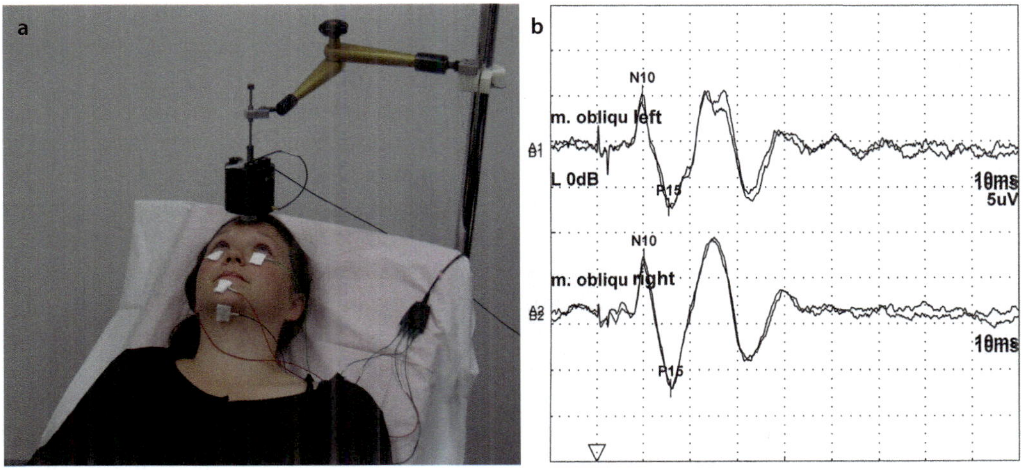

◘ **Fig. 4.5** **a**, **b** Ocular VEMP. **a** Depiction of the recording conditions: Stimulation with a minishaker (bone-conducted vibration) in the middle of the forehead at the hairline (Fz). The recording is performed over the inferior oblique muscles while the subject looks 30° upward. **b** In healthy subjects, about 10 ms after the stimulus there is a negative (i.e., excitatory) wave (N10) and after about 15 ms there is a positive (i.e., inhibitory) wave (P15). Criteria for the evaluation are the presence of these waves and their amplitudes; the latency is less important

The major indication for the use of oVEMP is for the diagnosis of syndrome of the third mobile windows (Fife et al. 2017): A peak-to-peak amplitude of the oVEMP of more than 16.7 μV (ACS, 500 Hz, 125 dB SPL) has a sensitivity of 100% and a specificity of 89% for superior canal dehiscence syndrome (Verrecchia et al. 2019).

cVEMP and oVEMP can be used to differentiate between a superior, the very rare inferior and the even rarer complete acute unilateral vestibulopathy/vestibular neuritis. In superior and complete unilateral vestibulopathy, oVEMP are typically reduced or absent (Oh et al. 2013; Curthoys et al. 2011), because the superior part of the vestibular nerves innervates the utricle. On the other hand, cVEMP, which mainly arise from the saccule, which is innervated by the inferior part of the vestibular nerve, are reduced or absent in inferior and complete acute unilateral vestibulopathy/vestibular neuritis (Chihara et al. 2012; Curthoys 2012; Manzari et al. 2013; Murofushi et al. 1996; Oh et al. 2013). However, cVEMP are normal in more than two thirds of patients with acute superior unilateral vestibulopathy (Oh et al. 2013; Curthoys 2012; Manzari et al. 2013).

4.2 Pure-Tone Audiogram and Acoustic-Evoked Potentials

ENT physicians test hearing by means of a pure-tone audiogram. In connection with the main symptom of vertigo, audiometry and other tests of the audiological system, e.g., acoustic-evoked potentials or oto-acoustic emissions, are of particular importance for diagnosing Menière's disease, vestibular schwannoma, Cogan's syndrome, and other diseases affecting the vestibulo-cochlear nerve and inner ear (► Box 2.2). For the diagnosis of Menière's disease, the following criteria in terms of hearing are recommended (Lopez-Escamez et al. 2015): Pure-tone audiogram impairment of hearing <2000 Hz of at least – 30 dB in two neighboring frequencies, associated with an attack of vertigo, mainly ±24 h. It has been shown to be helpful for the diagnosis of Menière's disease if patients use apps or portable iPad-based audiometry devices to perform their own hearing tests before, during, and after an attack (Tse et al. 2019).

Acoustic-evoked potentials, which were often used for the diagnosis of vestibular schwannoma in the past—which is now diagnosed by high-resolution contrast-enhanced MRI—and otoacoustic emissions are nowadays less important in patients with the leading symptom of vertigo and dizziness.

4.3 Laboratory Examinations of the Ocular Motor System

▪ Video-Oculography (VOG)

Video-oculography is a non-invasive, valid, and reliable method to record eye movements. Using one or two video cameras (i.e., monocular or binocular recording), which are integrated in a mask attached to the head, eye movements are filmed with a high resolution (◘ Fig. 4.6).

For the two-dimensional recording of eye movements, an image analysis, mainly of the movements of the pupil, is performed. This method allows quick and reliable recording of horizontal and vertical eye movements. In this way, different types of eye movements can be examined: spontaneous nystagmus with and without fixation, smooth pursuit, gaze-holding function, saccades, optokinetic nystagmus, and fixation suppression of the VOR. The three-dimensional recording of eye movements, i.e., including torsional eye movements, requires a more demanding analysis of the structure of the iris or the application of two additional markers on the sclera. Video-oculography can be combined with the head impulse test (video head impulse test, ◘ Fig. 4.1) and caloric irrigation (◘ Fig. 4.2).

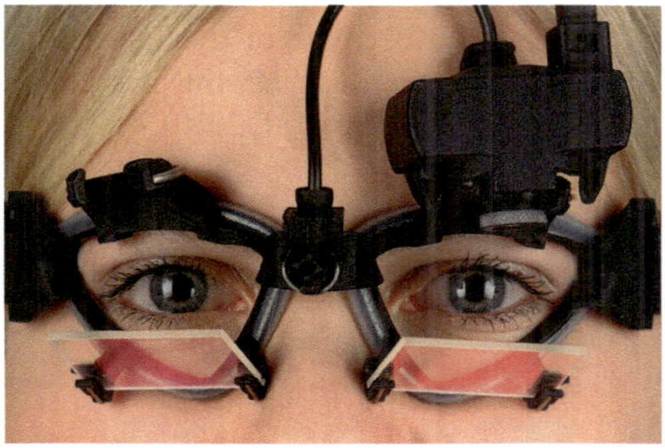

◘ **Fig. 4.6** Video-oculography (VOG) with a mask attached to the head and an integrated video camera. An infrared light is integrated into the mask and allows the recording of eye movements with a camera even in complete darkness, which is particularly important for the recording of spontaneous nystagmus. The recordings of eye movements can be seen online and the analysis occurs automatically or semi-automatically

4.4 Neuro-Orthoptic and Psychophysical Tests

Neuro-orthoptic and psychophysical tests have become increasingly relevant for topographic anatomical diagnosis, in particular to discriminate between peripheral and central vestibular or ocular motor lesions, as well as for a precise diagnosis in the brainstem and cerebellum. The following methods are used:

- Cover tests, in particular to detect vertical deviation (skew deviation) (see above).
- Psychophysical measurement of the subjective visual vertical (SVV), as depicted in ◘ Fig. 4.7, or with the simple bucket test (◘ Fig. 3.3) to detect an acute or subacute imbalance of the labyrinths or graviceptive pathways and to differentiate a monocular infranuclear lesion (e.g., third or fourth nerve) from a vestibular lesion (Dieterich and Brandt 1993, 2019). A deviation of the SVV under binocular as well as monocular

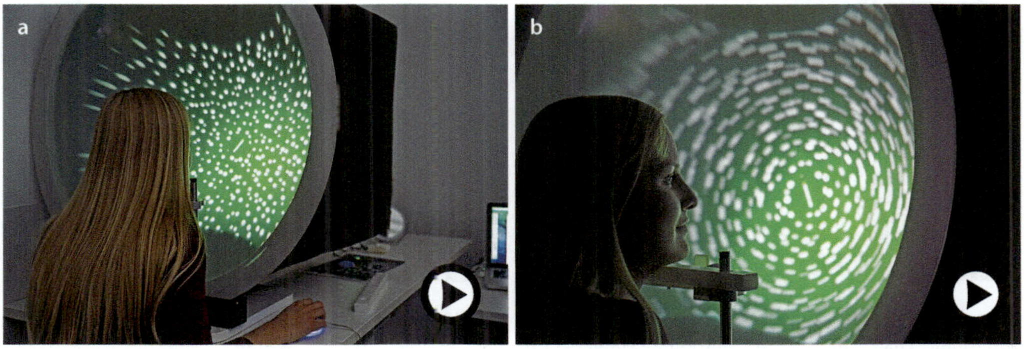

◘ **Fig. 4.7** **a, b** The subjective visual vertical (SVV). **a** For determination of the SVV, the patient sits upright in front of a hemispheric dome (60 cm in diameter) and looks into it. The dome extends beyond the limits of the patient's visual field with the result that the patient cannot orient himself spatially by fixed external structures. The hemispheric dome is illuminated with spots of light that can rotate. A short bar (14° of the visual field) is projected at the eye level of the subject. The patient is asked to turn it by means of a potentiometer from a random initial position until he has the subjective impression that the bar is "vertical." The deviation of the bar from the objective vertical axis is measured in degrees and recorded on a PC. The mean of ten measurements equals the SVV. Under these conditions, the normal range (mean ± 2 SDs) of the SVV is 0° ± 2.5° (▶ https://doi.org/10.1007/000-94k). **b** Measurements can be made under static and dynamic conditions. Under dynamic conditions, the spots either rotate to the right or to the left. In addition, the measurement can be made with both eyes or each eye individually. This is helpful when differentiating between central and peripheral ocular motor disorders (▶ https://doi.org/10.1007/000-94m)

viewing conditions indicates a vestibular lesion, whereas a third or fourth nerve palsy causes a deviation of the affected eye only.

- Scanning laser ophthalmoscope (SLO) for the quantification of eye torsion in the roll plane and to differentiate a monocular infranuclear lesion (e.g., third or fourth nerve) from a vestibular lesion (Dieterich and Brandt, 1993) (▣ Fig. 4.8). A torsion of both eyes (symmetric or asymmetric) indicates a vestibular imbalance.
- Measurement of dynamic visual acuity (DVA), including the VOR reading test, i.e., determination of visual acuity under static conditions and during head turns. If there is a decrease of dynamic visual acuity of more than 0.2, this indicates a VOR deficit (Vital et al. 2010).

4

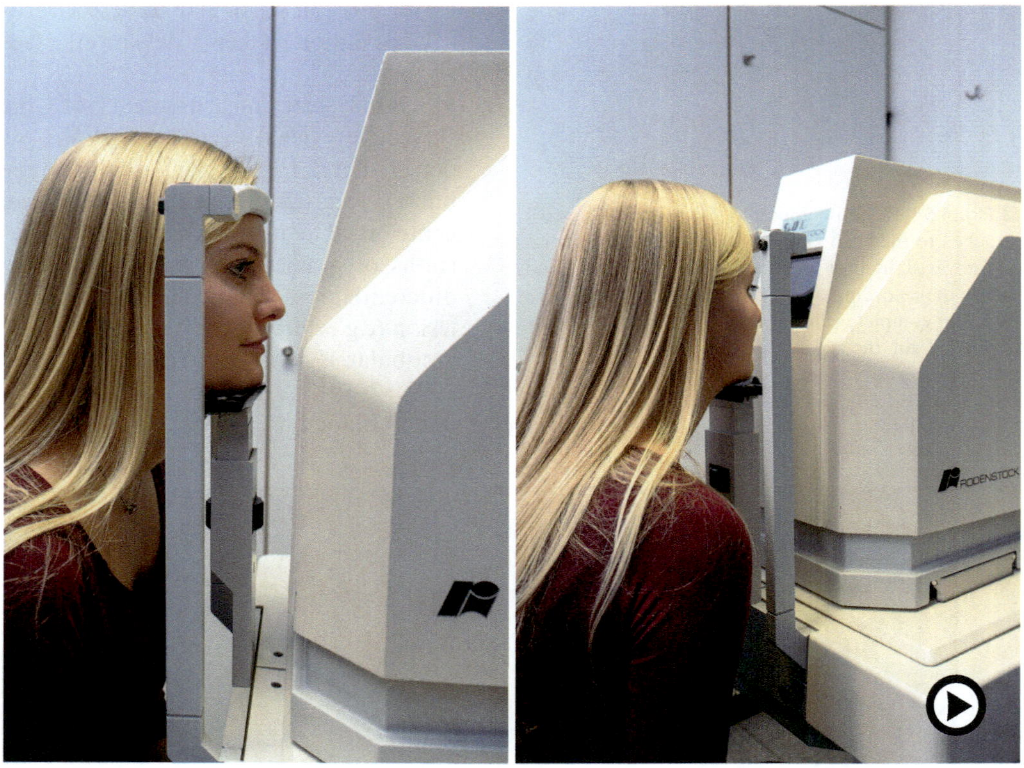

▣ **Fig. 4.8** Measurement of the eye position in the roll plane. The scanning laser ophthalmoscope (SLO) can be used to take photographs and videos of the fundus of the eye (examination is also possible with a fundus camera). The cyclorotation (rolling) of the eye or eye torsion can be measured in degrees on the fundus photographs as the angle between the horizontal and the so-called papillofoveal meridian. The patient sits upright, looks into the SLO, and fixates a dot. (With the SLO, it is not necessary to administer a mydriatic drug; however, this is necessary if the measurement is made with traditional fundus photography.) Both eyes of healthy controls exhibit a slightly excyclotropic position in the roll plane, i.e., counterclockwise rotation of the right eye and a clockwise rotation of the left eye (from the viewpoint of the examiner). The normal range (±2 SDs) is from −1 to 11.5°. Values outside this range are considered pathological (e.g., patients with a peripheral vestibular lesion show an ipsiversive torsion of both eyes, i.e., excyclotropia of the ipsilateral eye and incyclotropia of the contralateral eye) (▶ https://doi.org/10.1007/000-94n)

4.5 Posturography and Gait Analysis

▪ Posturography

Posturography (◘ Fig. 4.9) allows measurement of body sway under different conditions, e.g., with eyes open or closed, or while standing on firm ground or foam rubber. For many years, this method was considered sensitive but not specific. Now with the use of neuronal networks and automatic analysis of the sway patterns under the above-mentioned various conditions, it is possible to decide in many cases whether, for example, a peripheral vestibular deficit, a cerebellar syndrome, an orthostatic tremor, or functional dizziness is present (Krafczyk et al. 2006; Ahmadi et al. 2019). It is also useful for long-term studies to evaluate the course of the diseases (e.g. Feil et al. 2015) or to detect a secondary functional dizziness (by co-contraction of the leg muscles) following an acute vestibular syndrome (Brandt et al. 2012).

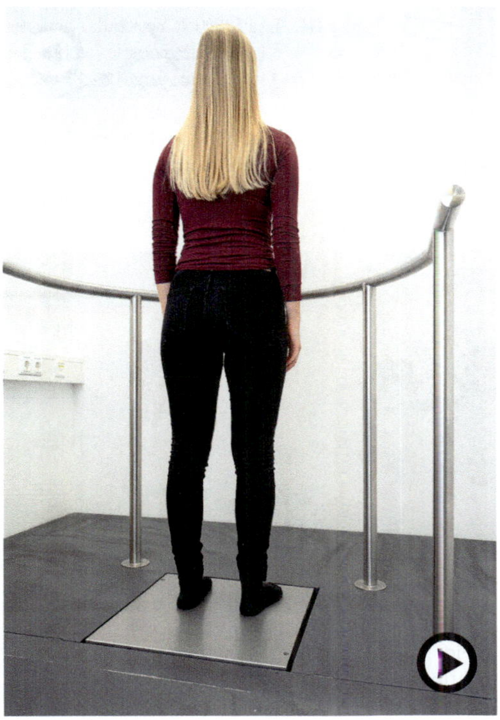

◘ Fig. 4.9 Posturography. Posturography (here the Kistler platform) allows the examination of control of stance and postural stability under different conditions: eyes open, eyes closed, Romberg and Tandem-Romberg, or standing on firm ground or on a compliant foam rubber padded platform The parameters to be measured are body sway to the right or left, forward or backward, upward or downward with a subsequent analysis of the so-called sway path values (SP, "sway path") and frequency (by a Fourier analysis). The SP is defined as the length of the path described by the center of foot pressure during a given time. Healthy subjects also exhibit body sway as a result of inherent physiological instability. Sway path is increased in patients with a vestibular deficit in particular with the eyes closed. In cerebellar disorders, one finds a typical 3-Hz sway and in orthostatic tremor a 14–16 Hz sway. Nowadays, an automated analysis with a neuronal network allows differentiation between sensory (namely vestibular) deficits, functional dizziness, cerebellar ataxia, and orthostatic tremor (► https://doi.org/10.1007/000-94h)

▪ Quantitative Gait Analysis

Quantitative gait analysis, e.g., with GAITrite (◘ Fig. 4.10), has been shown

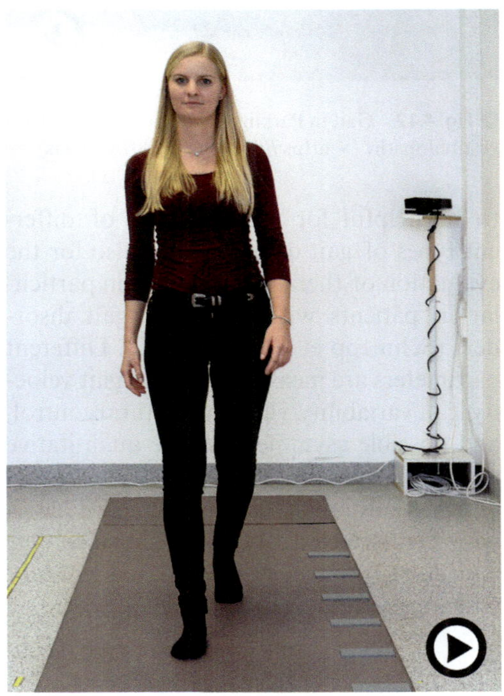

◘ Fig. 4.10 Quantitative gait analysis. Different parameters are measured and analyzed: gait velocity, gait variability, rhythm, asymmetries (all with eyes open and closed), and the effects of distraction (► https://doi.org/10.1007/000-94q)

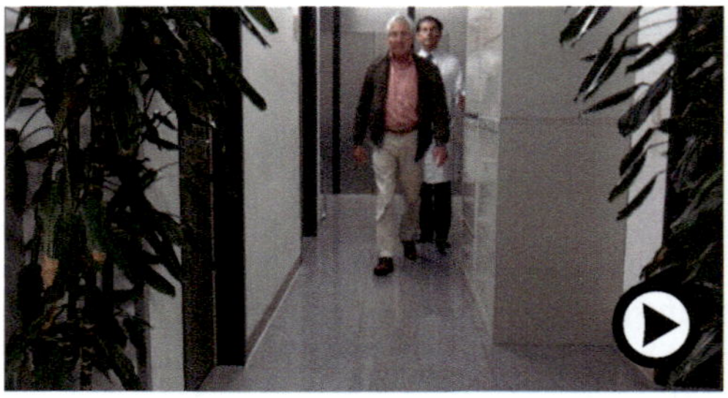

Fig. 4.11 Gait in bilateral vestibulopathy (▶ https://doi.org/10.1007/000-94r)

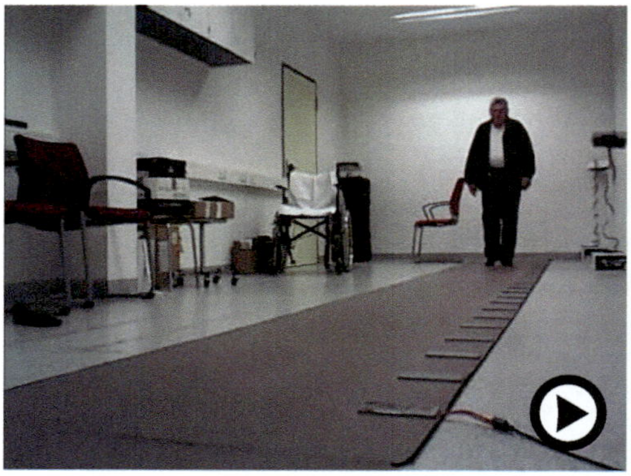

Fig. 4.12 Gait in Parkinson's disease plus bilateral vestibulopathy (▶ https://doi.org/10.1007/000-94s)

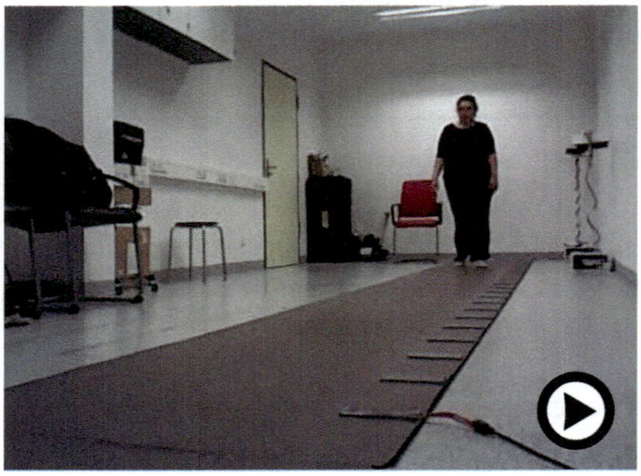

Fig. 4.13 Gait in cerebellar ataxia (▶ https://doi.org/10.1007/000-94t)

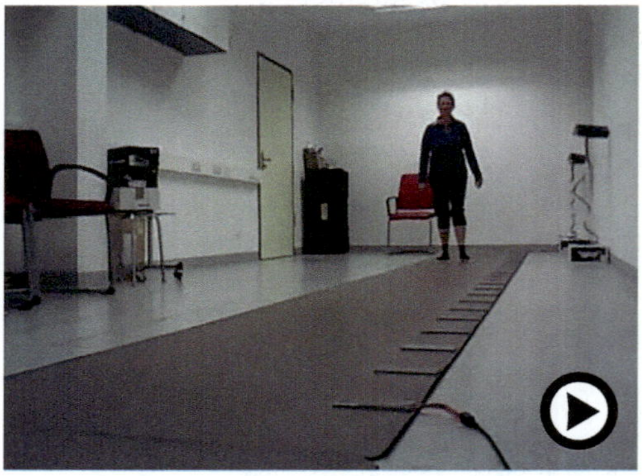

Fig. 4.14 Gait in functional gait disorder (▶ https://doi.org/10.1007/000-94v)

to be helpful for the diagnosis of different types of gait disorders and also for the evaluation of therapeutic effects, in particular in patients with cerebellar gait disorders (Schniepp et al. 2011, 2012). Different parameters are measured such as gait velocity, gait variability, rhythm, postural control, and possible asymmetries. The quantitative measurements are performed under different conditions with three gait velocities (slow, self-selected, and high gait velocities) and with eyes open, eyes closed, tandem gait, with and without distraction (dual task, e.g., counting backward). The analysis is semiautomatic and often allows a discrimination between the following possible causes: sensory deficits (vestibular, in particular bilateral vestibulopathy, (Figs. 4.11, 4.12, 4.13 and 4.14) proprioceptive, visual), cerebellar (Figs. 4.11, 4.12, 4.13 and 4.14), or other central and functional (Figs. 4.11, 4.12, 4.13 and 4.14) gait disorders (Tables 4.2 and 4.3).

Table 4.2 Disturbances of posture and gait control in peripheral vestibular disorders

Illness	Direction of deviation	Pathomechanism
Bilateral vestibulopathy	Different directions	Failure of vestibulospinal postural reflexes, exacerbated in the dark and on uneven ground
Acute unilateral vestibulopathy/ vestibular neuritis	Ipsiversive	Vestibular tone imbalance due to failure of the horizontal and anterior semicircular canal and utricle
Tumarkin's otolithic catastrophy	Lateral, ipsiversive, or contraversive (sudden falls)	Variations of endolymph pressure lead to an abnormal stimulation or inhibition of the otoliths and sudden vestibulospinal tone failure
Tullio phenomenon	Backward, contraversive, diagonal	Stimulation of the otoliths by sounds of certain frequencies, e.g., in cases of a syndrome of the third mobile windows
Vestibular paroxysmia	Contraversive or in different directions	Neurovascular compression of the vestibulocochlear nerve and excitation (rarely inhibition) of the vestibular nerve

Table 4.3 Disturbance of posture and gait control in central vestibular disorders

Illness	Direction of deviation	Pathomechanism
Downbeat nystagmus syndrome	Backward and forward	Vestibular tone imbalance in the pitch plane
Lateropulsion (Wallenberg's syndrome)	Ipsiversive, diagonal	Central vestibular tone imbalance (roll and yaw planes) with tilt of subjective vertical
Ocular tilt reaction (OTR)	Contraversive with mesencephalic lesions, ipsiversive with pontomedullary lesions, ipsi- or contraversive with unilateral cerebellar lesions (uvula or dentate nucleus)	Tone imbalance of the VOR in the roll plane with lesions of the vertical canals or otolith pathways
Paroxysmal ocular tilt reaction	Ipsiversive with mesencephalic excitation, contraversive with pontomedullary excitation or excitation of the vestibular nerve	Pathological excitation of the otolith or vertical canal pathways (VOR in the roll plane)
Thalamic astasia (often overlooked)	Contraversive or ipsiversive	Vestibular tone imbalance due to lesions of the posterolateral (rarely centromedian) thalamus
Vestibular epilepsy (rare)	Contraversive	Focal seizures due to epileptic discharges of the vestibular cortex

4.6 Additional Laboratory Examinations

To clarify the cause of disorders (differential diagnoses: ischemia, hemorrhage, tumor, inflammation, neurodegenerative disease, malformation, or fracture), additional imaging techniques are often necessary, e.g.,

- Cranial magnetic resonance imaging (MRI), namely with sections of the brainstem, cerebellopontine angle, cerebellum, and labyrinth
- High-resolution computed tomography, in particular of the bony labyrinth

If ischemia is suspected, Doppler/duplex sonography is also performed, particularly of the vertebral and basilar arteries, and further cardiovascular diagnostics are called for. If a central inflammatory origin is suspected, a spinal tap and visual and somatosensory-evoked potentials should also be performed.

4.6.1 Imaging of the Petrous Bone, the Cerebellopontine Angle, the Brainstem, and Cerebellum with Computed Tomography and Magnetic Resonance Imaging

In general, with high-resolution magnetic resonance imaging (MRI) and computed tomography (CT) of the petrous bone, it is now possible to reliably identify the following peripheral and central vestibular diseases:

- Masses in the cerebellopontine angle, internal auditory canal (e.g., vestibular schwannoma which requires T1 with and without gadolinium and T2 sequences) or middle ear (e.g., cholesteatoma).
- Post-traumatic forms of vertigo due to petrous bone fractures.
- "Vestibular pseudoneuritis" due to fascicular lesions of the vestibular nerve at the entry zone of the brainstem (e.g., MS plaques or ischemic lesions) and other acute central vestibular syndromes, most often due to ischemia of the brainstem or cerebellum. It is important to note that MRI is often normal within the first 48 hours after symptom onset (Saber Tehari et al. 2014) so that an MRI later is recommended to confirm the diagnosis of a central lesion (Kim et al. 2022b).

Imaging is also important for the diagnosis of:

- Inflammatory (e.g., labyrinthitis, Cogan's syndrome), hereditary (e.g., Mondini–Alexander dysplasia), or neoplastic (e.g., meningeosis carcinomatosa) inner ear diseases.
- Vestibular paroxysmia, looking for neurovascular cross-compression of the vestibular nerve; this, however, is also found in 45% of healthy subjects (Sivarasan et al. 2019). Therefore, imaging is mainly performed in these patients to exclude other pathologies, in particular vestibular schwannomas or brainstem lesions (see ► Chap. 11).
- Syndrome of the third mobile windows, in particular superior canal dehiscence syndrome (see ► Chap. 12).
- Acute unilateral vestibulopathy, e.g., in patients with herpes zoster with a contrast enhancement of the eighth cranial nerve.
- Superficial siderosis, which often also affects the vestibular nerve and may lead to bilateral vestibulopathy.

An endolymphatic hydrops can be indirectly visualized by transtympanic or intravenous application of gadolinium in high-resolution temporal bone MRI (see ► Chap. 10).

Note, for the diagnosis of an acute central vestibular syndrome: Even a normal high-resolution MRI including diffusion-weighted imaging can, in symptomatic patients, not exclude a brainstem or cerebellar lesion within the first 48 h: 50% of MRIs with lesions <10 mm are often false negative (Saber Tehrani et al. 2014, 2018). This underlines the importance of a detailed patient history and a systematic clinical neurological, neurootological, and neuroophthalmological examination, which are superior to imaging within the first 48 hours. It is important to note that in the acute phase of an acute vestibular syndrome, cranial CT is indicated as the first imaging technique, namely to exclude bleeding and tumors, as well CT angiography to look for stenosis or thrombosis in the vertebro-basilar system.

High-Resolution Computed Tomography of the Petrous Bone

Modern multi-slice CT machines allow spatially very high-resolution imaging of the petrous bone structures, in particular the bony labyrinth, the facial nerve canal, and the skull base. An examination in the spiral mode of operation (with 1-mm slice thickness, 1-mm table feed, 140 kV, 111 mA, and 0.75 s revolution) yields a local spatial resolution of 0.3 × 0.3 × 1 mm. The data are reconstructed for each side separately. Typically, transversal and coronal reconstructions are made; 3-D surface reconstructions are also possible. CT of the petrous bone is indicated when the bone is also to be assessed, e.g., to prove the presence of fractures, malformations (e.g., Mondini–Alexander dysplasia), and in particular SCDS as well as ossifications of the labyrinth in chronic illnesses (e.g., otosclerosis or Cogan's syndrome) and accompanying bone alterations in benign and malignant growth processes (e.g., cholesteatoma, cholesterol cysts, vestibular schwannoma, rhabdomyosarcoma, basalioma, or adenocarcinoma).

In particular in a syndrome of the third mobile windows, namely SCDS, a high-resolution thin-slice CT (≤ 0.6 mm) with 3D reconstruction parallel and perpendicular to the superior canal (◘ Fig. 12.4) is necessary (Mau et al. 2018; Ho 2019)—ideally with a so-called flat panel CT (Tunkel et al. 2019)—in particular in order not to get false pathological findings.

High-Resolution Magnetic Resonance Imaging of the Petrous Bone and the Cerebellopontine Angle

The MRI examination of the petrous bone and the cerebellopontine angle is performed in a circularly polarized head coil. This technique is clearly superior to CT as regards the imaging of non-osseous structures or lesions, e.g., tumors and inflammatory soft-tissue growths, especially in the petrous bone. The numerous anatomical structures confined in a very small space within the petrous bone make high demands on the MRI technology. The examination protocol should include the following (or similar) sequences:

- Transversal proton-weighted and T2-weighted fast spin-echo sequence with a double echo in a 3-mm-thick slice and an interslice distance of less than 0.8 mm for evaluating the brainstem and cerebellum.
- A transversal T1-weighted sequence (e.g., 2-D fast low angle shot, FLASH) with a 2-mm-thick slice and a spatial resolution of ca. 0.55 mm, before and, if applicable, after intravenous administration of an MRI contrast medium. After the contrast medium is applied, it is advisable to perform coronal imaging as well.
- A high-resolution, strongly T2-weighted sequence (e.g., 3-D constructive interference in steady state, CISS, or 3-D FIESTA, fast imaging employing steady-state acquisition) of ca. 0.5 mm spatial resolution and 0.6–0.8 mm slice thickness. This sequence is especially suitable for imaging the cerebral nerves and the fluid-filled inner ear structures. It is the method of choice for detecting a neurovascular cross-compression which is also found in about 45% of healthy individuals (Sivarasan et al. 2019). Since it is a 3-D sequence, multiple plane reconstructions can be made in all directions, especially also parallel to the course of each cerebral nerve. By using the maximum

intensity projection (MIP) procedure, it is possible to represent the signal-intense structures of the inner ear three dimensionally and in any orientation.

- If a pathological neurovascular cross-compression is suspected, another complementary examination with MR angiography (e.g., TOF, time of flight) is performed (Donahue et al. 2017). If the TOF-MRA is performed before and after intravenous administration of contrast medium, it is possible to identify and differentiate contacts with arteries and with veins.
- If an endolymphatic hydrops is suspected, delayed MR sequences for the improved imaging of the endolymphatic space 4 h after intravenous administration of a standard dose contrast agent can be added. The sequences consist of high-resolution heavily T2-weighted MR cisternography (MRC, free water weighted image) for an anatomical reference of the total lymph fluid, a hT2w-3D- FLAIR scan with a 16,000 ms TR, and a 2900 ms inversion time (positive perilymph image [PPI]), and a positive endolymph image (PEI) with the same TR, and a 2500 ms inversion time (Naganawa et al. 2017). Image processing to increase the contrast-to-noise ratio (Boegle et al. 2021) enables the assessment of the endolymphatic space (hypointense signal) in contrast to the perilymph space (hyperintense signal) and in relation to the total lymph fluid.

References

Agrawal Y, van de Berg R, Wuyts F, Walther L, Magnusson M, Oh E, Sharpe M, Strupp M (2019) Presbyvestibulopathy: diagnostic criteria consensus document of the classification committee of the Barany Society. J Vestib Res 29(4):161–170

Ahmadi SA, Vivar G, Frei J, Nowoshilow S, Bardins S, Brandt T, Krafczyk S (2019) Towards computerized diagnosis of neurological stance disorders: data mining and machine learning of posturography and sway. J Neurol 266(Suppl 1):108–117

Bachmann K, Sipos K, Lavender V, Hunter LL (2018) Video head impulse testing in a pediatric population: normative findings. J Am Acad Audiol 29(5):417–426

Barany R (1907) Physiologie und Pathologie des Bogengangsapparates beim Menschen. Franz Deuticke, Vienna

Bartl K, Lehnen N, Kohlbecher S, Schneider E (2009) Head impulse testing using video-oculography. Ann N Y Acad Sci 1164:331–333

Boegle R, Gerb J, Kierig E, Becker-Bense S, Ertl-Wagner B, Dieterich M, Kirsch V (2021) Intravenous Delayed Gadolinium-Enhanced MR Imaging of the Endolymphatic Space: A Methodological Comparative Study. Front Neurol 12:647296

Brandt T, Strupp M, Novozhilov S, Krafczyk S (2012) Artificial neural network posturography detects the transition of vestibular neuritis to phobic postural vertigo. J Neurol 259:182–184

Bruner A, Norris TW (1971) Age-related changes in caloric nystagmus. Acta Otolaryngol Suppl 282:1–24

Chihara Y, Iwasaki S, Murofushi T, Yagi M, Inoue A, Fujimoto C, Egami N, Ushio M, Karino S, Sugasawa K, Yamasoba T (2012) Clinical characteristics of inferior vestibular neuritis. Acta Otolaryngol 132(12):1288–1294

Colebatch JG, Rosengren SM, Welgampola MS (2016) Vestibular-evoked myogenic potentials. Handb Clin Neurol 137:133–155

Curthoys IS (2012) The interpretation of clinical tests of peripheral vestibular function. Laryngoscope 122(6):1342–1352

Curthoys IS, Dlugaiczyk J (2020) Physiology, clinical evidence and diagnostic relevance of sound-induced and vibration-induced vestibular stimulation. Curr Opin Neurol 33(1):126–135

Curthoys IS, Iwasaki S, Chihara Y, Ushio M, McGarvie LA, Burgess AM (2011) The ocular vestibular-evoked myogenic potential to air-conducted sound; probable superior vestibular nerve origin. Clin Neurophysiol 122(3):611–616

Donahue JH, Ornan DA, Mukherjee S (2017) Imaging of Vascular Compression Syndromes. Radiol Clin North Am 55:123–138

Dieterich M, Brandt T (1993) Ocular torsion and perceived vertical in oculomotor, trochlear and abducens nerve palsies. Brain 116:1095–1104

Dieterich M, Brandt T (2019) Perception of Verticality and Vestibular Disorders of Balance and Falls. Front Neurol 10:172

Dlugaiczyk J, Habs M, Dieterich M (2020) Vestibular evoked myogenic potentials in vestibular migraine and Menière's disease: cVEMPs make the difference. J Neurol 267:169–180

Ertl M, Boegle R, Kirsch V, Dieterich M (2016) On the impact of examiners on latencies and amplitudes in cervical and ocular vestibular-evoked myogenic

potentials evaluated over a large sample (N = 1,038). Eur Arch Otorhinolaryngol 273(2):317–323
Falls C (2019) Videonystagmography and Posturography. Adv Otorhinolaryngol 82:32–38
Feil K, Bottcher N, Guri F, Krafczyk S, Schoberl F, Zwergal A, Strupp M (2015) Long-term course of orthostatic tremor in serial posturographic measurement. Parkinsonism Relat Disord 21(8):905–910
Fife TD, Colebatch JG, Kerber KA, Brantberg K, Strupp M, Lee H, Walker MF, Ashman E, Fletcher J, Callaghan B, Gloss DS (2017) Practice guideline: cervical and ocular vestibular evoked myogenic potential testing: report of the guideline development, dissemination, and implementation Subcommittee of the American Academy of neurology. Neurology 89(22):2288–2296
Furman JM (2016) Rotational testing. Handb Clin Neurol 137:177–186
Goulson AM, McPherson JH, Shepard NT (2014) Background and introduction to whole-body rotational testing. In Jacobson GP, Shepard NT (eds) Balance function assessment and management. Plural Publishing Inc., San Diego, USA
Halmagyi GM, Chen L, MacDougall HG, Weber KP, McGarvie LA, Curthoys IS (2017) The video head impulse test. Front Neurol 8:258
Ho ML (2019) Third window lesions. Neuroimaging Clin N Am 29(1):57–92
Jongkees LB, Maas J, Philipszoon A (1962) Clinical electronystagmography: a detailed study of electronystagmography in 341 patients with vertigo. Pract Otorhinolaryngol Basel 24:65–93
Kim DH, Kim SW, Kim SH, Jung JH, Hwang SH (2022a) Usefulness of Cervical Vestibular-Evoked Myogenic Potentials for Diagnosing Patients With Superior Canal Dehiscence Syndrome: A Meta-Analysis. Otol Neurotol 43:146–152
Kim JS, Newman-Toker DE, Kerber KA, Jahn K, Bertholon P, Waterston J, Lee H, Bisdorff A, Strupp M (2022b) Vascular vertigo and dizziness: diagnostic criteria 32(3):205–22.
Krafczyk S, Tietze S, Swoboda W, Valkovic P, Brandt T (2006) Artificial neural network: a new diagnostic posturographic tool for disorders of stance. Clin Neurophysiol 117(8):1692–1698
Larrazabal AJ, Garcia Cena CE, Martinez CE (2019) Video-oculography eye tracking towards clinical applications: a review. Comput Biol Med 108 57–66
Lee SH, Yoo MH, Park JW, Kang BC, Yang CJ, Kang WS, Ahn JH, Chung JW, Park HJ (2018) Comparison of video head impulse test (vHIT) gains between two commercially available devices and by different gain analytical methods. Otol Neurotol 39(5):e297–e300
Lopez-Escamez JA, Carey J, Chung WH, Goebel JA, Magnusson M, Mandala M, Newman-Toker DE, Strupp M, Suzuki M, Trabalzini F, Bisdorff A (2015) Diagnostic criteria for Meniere's disease. J Vestib Res 25(1):1–7
MacDougall HG, Weber KP, McGarvie LA, Halmagyi GM, Curthoys IS (2009) The video head impulse test: diagnostic accuracy in peripheral vestibulopathy. Neurology 73(14):1134–1141
Machner B, Erber K, Choi JH, Trillenberg P, Sprenger A, Helmchen C (2021) Usability of the head impulse test in routine clinical practice in the emergency department to differentiate vestibular neuritis from stroke. Eur J Neurol 28:1737–1744
Maes L, Dhooge I, De VE, D'haenens W, Bockstael A, Keppler H, Philips B, Swinnen F, Vinck BM (2008) Normative data and test-retest reliability of the sinusoidal harmonic acceleration test, pseudorandom rotation test and velocity step test. J Vestib Res 18(4):197–208
Mallinson AI, Longridge NS (2004) Caloric response does not decline with age. J Vestib Res 14(5): 393–396
Manzari L, Burgess AM, MacDougall HG, Curthoys IS (2013) Vestibular function after vestibular neuritis. Int J Audiol 52(10):713–718
Matino-Soler E, Esteller-More E, Martin-Sanchez JC, Martinez-Sanchez JM, Perez-Fernandez N (2015) Normative data on angular vestibulo-ocular responses in the yaw axis measured using the video head impulse test. Otol Neurotol 36(3):466–471
Mau C, Kamal N, Badeti S, Reddy R, Ying YM, Jyung RW, Liu JK (2018) Superior semicircular canal dehiscence: diagnosis and management. J Clin Neurosci 48:58–65
McGarvie LA, MacDougall HG, Halmagyi GM, Burgess AM, Weber KP, Curthoys IS (2015) The video head impulse test (vHIT) of semicircular canal function – age-dependent normative values of VOR gain in healthy subjects. Front Neurol 6:154
Murnane O, Mabrey H, Pearson A, Byrd S, Akin F (2014) Normative data and test-retest reliability of the SYNAPSYS video head impulse test. J Am Acad Audiol 25(3):244–252
Murofushi T, Halmagyi GM, Yavor RA, Colebatch JG (1996) Absent vestibular evoked myogenic potentials in vestibular neurolabyrinthitis. An indicator of inferior vestibular nerve involvement? Arch Otolaryngol Head Neck Surg 122(8):845–848
Naganawa S, Kawai H, Taoka T, Sone M (2017) Improved HYDROPS: imaging of endolymphatic hydrops after intravenous administration of Gadolinium. Magn Reson Med Sci 16(4):357–361
Noij KS, Herrmann BS, Guinan JJ Jr, Rauch SD (2019) Toward optimizing cVEMP: 2,000-Hz tone bursts improve the detection of superior canal dehiscence. Audiol Neurootol 23(6):335–344
Oh SY, Kim JS, Yang TH, Shin BS, Jeong SK (2013) Cervical and ocular vestibular-evoked myogenic potentials in vestibular neuritis: comparison

between air- and bone-conducted stimulation. J Neurol 260(8):2102–2109

Peterka RJ, Black FO, Schoenhoff MB (1990) Age-related changes in human vestibulo-ocular reflexes: sinusoidal rotation and caloric tests. J Vestib Res 1(1):49–59

Rosengren SM, Colebatch JG, Young AS, Govender S, Welgampola MS (2019) Vestibular evoked myogenic potentials in practice: methods, pitfalls and clinical applications. Clin Neurophysiol Pract 4:47–68

Rosengren SM, Welgampola MS, Taylor RL (2018) Vestibular-evoked myogenic potentials in bilateral vestibulopathy. Front Neurol 9:252

Saber Tehrani AS, Kattah JC, Kerber KA, Gold DR, Zee DS, Urrutia VC, Newman-Toker DE (2018) Diagnosing stroke in acute dizziness and vertigo: pitfalls and pearls. Stroke 49(3):788–795

Saber Tehrani AS, Kattah JC, Mantokoudis G, Pula JH, Nair D, Blitz A, Ying S, Hanley DF, Zee DS, Newman-Toker DE (2014) Small strokes causing severe vertigo: frequency of false-negative MRIs and nonlacunar mechanisms. Neurology 83(2):169–173

Schniepp R, Mohwald K, Wuehr M (2019) Clinical and automated gait analysis in patients with vestibular, cerebellar, and functional gait disorders: perspectives and limitations. J Neurol 266(Suppl 1):118–122

Schniepp R, Wuehr M, Ackl N, Danek A, Brandt T, Strupp M, Jahn K (2011) 4-aminopyridine improves gait variability in cerebellar ataxia due to CACNA 1A mutation. J Neurol 258(9):1708–1711

Schniepp R, Wuehr M, Neuhaeusser M, Kamenova M, Dimitriadis K, Klopstock T, Strupp M, Brandt T, Jahn K (2012) Locomotion speed determines gait variability in cerebellar ataxia and vestibular failure. Mov Disord 27(1):125–131

Shepard NT, Jacobson GP (2016) The caloric irrigation test. Handb Clin Neurol 137:119–131

Sivarasan N, Touska P, Murdin L, Connor S (2019) MRI findings in vestibular paroxysmia – an observational study. J Vestib Res 29(2-3):137–145

Starkov D, Strupp M, Pleshkov M, Kingma H, van de Berg R (2021) Diagnosing vestibular hypofunction: an update. J Neurol 268:377–385

Strupp M, Bisdorff A, Furman J, Hornibrook J, Jahn K, Maire R, Newman-Toker D, Magnusson M (2022) Acute unilateral vestibulopathy/vestibular neuritis:diagnostic criteria 32(5):389–06.

Strupp M, Grimberg J, Teufel J, Laurell G, Kingma H, Grill E (2020) Worldwide survey on laboratory testing of vestibular function. Neurol Clin Pract 10:(5)379–387

Strupp M, Kichler A, McGarvie L, Kremmyda O (2018) The video head impulse test: a right-left imbalance. J Neurol 265(Suppl 1):40–43

Strupp M, Kim JS, Murofushi T, Straumann D, Jen JC, Rosengren SM, Della Santina CC, Kingma H (2017) Bilateral vestibulopathy: diagnostic criteria consensus document of the classification Committee of the Barany Society. J Vestib Res 27(4):177–189

Taylor RL, Welgampola MS (2019) Otolith function testing. Adv Otorhinolaryngol 82:47–55

Tse D, Ramsay T, Lelli DA (2019) Novel use of portable audiometry to track hearing fluctuations in Meniere's disease: a pilot study. Otol Neurotol 40(2):e130–e134

Tunkel AE, Carey JP, Pearl M (2019) Flat panel computed tomography in the diagnosis of superior semicircular canal dehiscence syndrome. Otol Neurotol 40(2):213–217

van de Berg R, Rosengren S, Kingma H (2018) Laboratory examinations for the vestibular system. Curr Opin Neurol 31(1):111–116

Van Der Stappen A, Wuyts FL, Van de Heyning PH (2000) Computerized electronystagmography: normative data revisited. Acta Otolaryngol 120(6):724–730

Verrechia L, Brantberg K, Tawfique Z, Maoli D (2019) Diagnostic accuracy of ocular vestibular evoked myogenic potentials for superior canal dehiscence syndrome in a large cohort of dizzy patients. Ear Heart 40(2):287–294

Vital D, Hegemann SC, Straumann D, Bergamin O, Bockisch CJ, Angehrn D, Schmitt KU, Probst R (2010) A new dynamic visual acuity test to assess peripheral vestibular function. Arch Otolaryngol Head Neck Surg 136(7):686–691

Wall C, Black FO, Hunt AE (1984) Effects of age, sex and stimulus parameters upon vestibulo- ocular responses to sinusoidal rotation. Acta Otolaryngol Stockh 98(3-4):270–278

Ward BK, van de Berg R, Van R, V, Bisdorff A, Hullar TE, Welgampola MS, Carey JP (2021) Superior semicircular canal dehiscence syndrome: Diagnostic criteria consensus document of the committee for the classification of vestibular disorders of the Barany Society. J Vestib Res 31:131–141

Yang CJ, Lee JY, Kang BC, Lee HS, Yoo MH, Park HJ (2016) Quantitative analysis of gains and catch-up saccades of video-head-impulse testing by age in normal subjects. Clin Otolaryngol 41(5):532–538

Zingler VC, Weintz E, Jahn K, Botzel K, Wagner J, Huppert D, Mike A, Brandt T, Strupp M (2008) Saccular function less affected than canal function in bilateral vestibulopathy. J Neurol 255(9):1332–1336

Zwergal A, Rettinger N, Frenzel C, Frisen L, Brandt T, Strupp M (2009a) A bucket of static vestibular function. Neurology 72:1689–1692

Zwergal A, Strupp M, Brandt T, Buttner-Ennever JA (2009b) Parallel ascending vestibular pathways: anatomical localization and functional specialization. Ann N Y Acad Sci 1164:51–59

General Principles of Therapy

Contents

M. Strupp et al., *Vertigo and Dizziness*, https://doi.org/10.1007/978-3-030-78260-3_5

The treatment of the various forms of vertigo and dizziness depends on the underlying disease. It consists of five principles:

1. Explaining the symptoms and signs, pathophysiology, etiology, and treatment options to the patient. This also includes which therapeutic measures can be applied, what the assumed success rate is, what the potential side effects are, and how long it takes until one can expect a therapeutic effect. This is also essential for the compliance, persistence and adherence of the patients with therapeutic measures. The patient should also be told to keep a diary in chronic relapsing diseases to quantify the response to the treatment. If necessary, there should be a timetable for follow-up consultations to monitor therapeutic effects and adjust treatment, which can include the use of other treatment options or a combination of various treatment options. In addition, the patient should be informed that many vestibular disorders have a good prognosis, e.g., recovery of peripheral vestibular function in acute unilateral vestibulopathy, central compensation of a peripheral vestibular tone imbalance, and spontaneous remissions in BPPV. On the other hand, patients should also be informed about recurrence rates, for instance, of 50% in BPPV and of the possibility of developing a secondary functional dizziness in particular in vestibular migraine.
2. Physical therapy (■ Table 5.1).
3. Drug therapy (■ Tables 5.2 and 5.3; overviews in Strupp and Zwergal 2020; Zwergal et al. 2019).
4. Psychotherapeutic measures.
5. Surgery: nowadays only very rarely (■ Table 5.4).

5.1 Physical Therapy

■ Vestibular Rehabilitation, Balance Training, and Gait Exercises

A specific form of balance training is performed to improve central vestibular compensation in cases of peripheral and central vestibular damage. It entails exercises for the vestibular, somatosensory, and ocular motor systems in order to promote substitution of the missing vestibular information by other systems and central vestibular compensation (overviews in Hall et al. 2022; Dunlap et al. 2019). Such a substitution was also demonstrated by fMRI: In patients with bilateral vestibulopathy, larger areas of the visual and multisensory cortex areas are activated during visual stimulation than in age-matched healthy controls (Dieterich et al. 2007).

The most important indications for vestibular rehabilitation are acute and chronic vestibular deficits and central vestibular syndromes, e.g., after brainstem or cerebellar infarction and cerebellar dizziness (Feil et al. 2019). The efficacy of vestibular rehabilitation is demonstrated, at least for acute unilateral vestibulopathy, by several randomized controlled trials (overviews in Dunlap et al. 2019; McDonnell and Hillier 2015; Hall et al. 2022). Specific exercises for the vestibular, ocular motor, and somatosensory systems are performed, first under the instruction of a physiotherapist, then by the patients independently. Ideally, the exercises should be performed daily. For instance, in acute unilateral vestibulopathy, active head turns with fixation of a visual target (Lehnen et al. 2018; Meldrum and Jahn 2019) increase the vestibular tone imbalance as the driving force of vestibular compensation and improve vestibular rehabilitation. This should be combined under dynamic conditions with gait exercises and prophylactic treatment of falls, if necessary. I acute unilateral vestibulopathy treatment should be performed at least three times per day for at least 20 min each session for about 8 weeks. The Nintendo Wii was demonstrated to be a simple and effective tool (Jahn et al. 2018). If patients are suffering from persisting peripheral vestibular deficits—as in bilateral vestibulopathy—the exercises should be performed daily for the rest of their lives. It is important to note that patients often experience an improvement only after 6–12 weeks.

The efficacy of vestibular rehabilitation depends on many factors, such as age, duration of the pre-existing symptoms, and comorbidities. In particular, musculoskeletal diseases, impairments of cognition, and additional psychiatric comorbidities, such as depression or anxiety, particularly fear of falls, reduce the efficacy of such measures (Whitney et al. 2020). These comorbidities and additional factors should be evaluated before the beginning of the treatment and should be considered when deciding on the frequency, duration, and type of treatment measures.

■ **Liberatory Maneuvers for BPPV**

The different liberatory maneuvers for the different types of BPPV (◘ Table 5.1, see ► Chap. 8) lead to a recovery in more than 95% of all cases within a few days, if they are properly performed (overview in Bhattacharyya et al. 2017).

◘ **Table 5.1** Physiotherapeutic strategies for vertigo and dizziness

Treatment strategy	Indications
Vestibular exercises, balance training, gait training	Improvement of the central vestibular compensation of a vestibular tone imbalance (e.g., acute unilateral vestibulopathy) Substitution, better strategies and reduction of risk of falls in persisting vestibular deficits and central lesions Habituation to prevent motion sickness (physical therapy)
Liberatory maneuvers, e.g., Semont/ SemontPlus or Epley Modified Roll-over, forced prolonged position e.g., head shaking Modified Yacovino	Benign paroxysmal positioning vertigo of the Posterior canal Horizontal canal Canalolithiasis Cuplulolithiasis Anterior canal

5.2 Pharmacotherapy: The Four Ds

For the pharmacotherapy of vestibular disorders, there are two approaches and options: first, an unspecific symptomatic treatment of vertigo, dizziness, and nausea at the beginning and, second, if possible, a specific causative therapy depending on the underlying etiology of the vestibular disease. The symptomatic treatment of acute vertigo and nausea by vestibular suppressants delays central vestibular compensation and should therefore be limited to a maximum of 1–3 days and the side effects of the drugs carefully considered. Depending on the disease, corticosteroids, betahistine, and sodium or potassium channel blockers can be used for the specific treatment, but we still need state-of-the-art randomized placebo-controlled trials to prove their efficacy (overview in Strupp and Zwergal 2020).

When applying drug therapy, "The four Ds" should be considered:

- Diagnosis: Is the diagnosis correct? This should be based on the current diagnostic criteria of the Bárány Society.
- Drug: Appropriate, effective, well tolerated?
- Dosage: What is the best dosage? This requires adjustments depending on effects and side effects.
- Duration: How long does it take until one can expect an effect? When does the dosage have to be adjusted? How long should the drug be given? When should another treatment session be initiated?

5.2.1 Symptomatic Therapy of Acute Vertigo, Nausea, and Vomiting

In the acute phase, antivertiginous drugs might be given, but only for a maximum of 1–3 days because they delay central compensation (overview in Soto et al. 2013; Chabbert 2016, ◘ Table 5.2). They act on various receptors, the most relevant of which are histamine, muscarine, dopamine, serotonin, and GABA, which can also explain the major side effects of each class of pharmacological agents:

- **H1R antagonists:** The so-called first-generation antihistamines evidently have a combined effect on the peripheral and the central vestibular system (see Soto et al. 2013; Chabbert 2016; Takumida et al. 2016). Typical examples are as follows:
  - Dimenhydrinate (combination of diphenhydramine, an inverse agonist of the H1 receptor (H1R) and 8-chlortheophylline (an adenosine-receptor antagonist to reduce drowsiness, the major side effect of diphenhydramine)) or
  - Promethazine (orally 25–50 mg); this is also a moderate muscarinergic receptor (MR) antagonist, and dopamine D2 receptor (D2R) antagonist, like neuroleptics; therefore, it can also lead to tardive dyskinesia.
- **H1R agonist and H3R inverse agonist, i.e., antagonist: betahistine:** Betahistine is the most frequently used drug worldwide for the treatment of vertigo (Agus et al. 2013). It is a weak H1R agonist and an inverse H3R agonist, i.e., a H3R antagonist. A Cochrane review and a meta-analysis concluded that it is probably effective in acute vertigo (Murdin et al. 2016).
- **Serotonin 5-HT3 receptor (5HT3R) antagonists:** Ondansetron (4–8 mg single dosage) or granisetron (single dosages

◘ **Table 5.2** Antivertiginous and antiemetic drugs (for a maximum of 1–3 days but not for long-term therapy)

Drug group	Dosage	Mode of action
Antihistamines		
Dimenhydrinate	Tablet (50 mg) every 4–6 h Suppository (150 mg) 1–2/d	Histamine (H_1) antagonist
Serotonin antagonists		
Ondansetron	Tablet 4–8 mg (up to 24 mg/d) or 4–8 mg i.v.	5 HT3-antagonist
Benzodiazepines		
Diazepam	Tablet (5 or 10 mg) every 4–6 h or injected solution of 10 mg i.m.	$GABA_A$ agonist
Clonazepam	Tablet (0.5 mg) every 4–6 h	
Anticholinergics		
Scopolamine	Transdermal 1.0 mg/72 h	Muscarine antagonist

1–2 mg) are effective in acute vertigo against nausea and vomiting and have few side effects.

- **GABAA agonists,** namely benzodiazepines, e.g., clonazepam (single dosage 0.5–1.0 mg) with GABA being the main inhibitory neurotransmitter of vestibular neurons which can lead to drowsiness and, in the long-term, drug addiction.
- **Anticholinergics, i.e., anti-muscarinergic drugs:** These drugs act on the peripheral and central vestibular system. Scopolamine, an unspecific inhibitor of the muscarine receptor (best applied as a transdermal patch, 1.0 mg), is used; it has typical anticholinergic side effects such as dry mouth or blurred vision. It can be used as an antiemetic but is rarely used to treat acute vertigo nowadays.
- **Dopamine D2 receptor (D2R) antagonists**, such as metoclopramide (10 mg tid) or domperidone (10–20 mg tid), act mainly on the chemoreceptor trigger zone in the brainstem; they also have a so-called gastroprokinetic effect (via muscarinergic receptors). The major side effects are movement disorders, mainly focal dystonia and akathisia. Therefore, they should be used very rarely.

The efficacy of symptomatic treatment with antihistamines, anticholinergics, $GABA_A$ agonists, D2R- and 5HT3R antagonists has been proven in many clinical trials (for references, see Soto et al. 2013; Chabbert 2016). Since most of these drugs (except betahistine) are sedatives, the respective substances most likely delay vestibular compensation. This is in line with animal studies: In an animal model of acute unilateral vestibulopathy, the potassium channel blocker, 4-aminopyridine, significantly reduced postural imbalance, but also delayed vestibular compensation (Beck et al. 2014) most likely by reducing the vestibular tone imbalance, which is evidently the driving force for vestibular compensation. Evidence from experiments on isolated amphibian preparations suggests that 4-aminopyridine increases the resting discharge of phasic vestibular afferent fibers through a block of voltage-dependent potassium conductances, thereby potentially reducing a bilateral imbalance between the two sides after a unilateral vestibular impairment (Bagus et al. 2019). All in all, antivertiginous drugs should not be given for longer than 1–3 days after symptom onset. The drug of choice also depends on the side effects and contraindications in individual patients.

Clinically, in the acute phase dimenhydrinate 50–100 mg is often given orally, rectally, or i.v. (recommended maximum dosage per day: 400 mg), or ondansetron 4–8 mg tablets are applied orally (up to 8 mg tid) or 4–8 mg i.v. (recommended maximum dosage per day 32 mg).

5.2.2 Improvement of Central Compensation, Enhancement of Central Vestibular Plasticity, and Adaption

A promising therapeutic strategy for acute unilateral vestibular disorders is the use of drugs to improve and accelerate central vestibular compensation. Drugs that enhance vestibular compensation and functional recovery have been extensively studied in various animal species. The most important and well-established compounds are betahistine, N-acetyl-L-leucine, and the Ginkgo biloba extract EGb 761 (for review, see Chabbert 2016). There are, however, so far no convincing randomized, placebo-controlled trials (RCTs).

Betahistine

Oral administration of betahistine at high daily doses of 50 mg/kg or 100 mg/kg accelerates the time course of recovery in cats after an acute unilateral vestibular lesion (Tighilet et al. 1995). Co-administration of a lower dose of betahistine (0.2 mg/kg/day) and selegiline (1 mg/kg/day) in this cat model increased the effect on postural recovery compared with betahistine monotherapy (Tighilet et al. 2018). Betahistine is considered to have multiple modes of action at the level of the peripheral and central vestibular networks: (1) increased blood flow in the vestibular system as an H3R antagonist (Bertlich et al. 2015, 2017); (2) increased histamine turnover and enhanced histamine release in the central nervous system (especially in the vestibular nuclei) via its property as an H3R inverse agonist; and (3) a potential inhibitory influence exerted at the level of the peripheral end organs and vestibular nerve afferent fibers through combined H3/H4 receptor effects (Lacour 2013). Beneficial effects of betahistine on the time course of vestibular compensation were also reported for humans (see Lacour 2013): In a randomized, double-blind, placebo-controlled study on patients, who underwent a vestibular neurectomy as a treatment for Menière's disease, betahistine reduced the time for recovery for most of the static postural, ocular motor, and perceptive symptoms, as well as for the patients' self-evaluation of stability, compared with placebo. Other animal studies demonstrated that the positive effect of betahistine on central compensation is based on the activation of the H1 receptor (Chen et al. 2019). In analogy to the animal studies on selegiline (Tighilet et al. 2018), one can conclude that high plasma concentrations are necessary, which can be achieved either by high oral dosages of at least 96 mg tid or probably by combination with selegiline. So far, however, there are no clinical trials.

Acetyl-leucine

Several studies in cats and rats have shown that *N-acetyl-DL-leucine* improves and accelerates postural compensation after unilateral labyrinthectomy relative to controls and that this effect is dose-dependent and driven by the L-isomer of the racemate (Gunther et al. 2015; Tighilet et al. 2015). N-acetyl-L-leucine also has an effect on cerebellar and thalamic networks during vestibular compensation (Gunther et al. 2015). In vitro electrophysiological recordings of neurons in the vestibular nuclei and vestibular-related networks in guinea pigs suggest that N-acetyl-DL-leucine may act by rebalancing the abnormal membrane potential in the vestibular nuclei (Vibert and Vidal 2001). One observational study described improvements of postural compensation in patients after vestibular neurotomy and labyrinthectomy (Ferber-Viart et al. 2009). Although N-acetyl-DL-leucine has been used in clinical practice to treat acute vertigo since 1957, a meta-analysis concludes that there is insufficient evidence for its efficacy (Vanderkam et al. 2019).

Gingko biloba extract

EGb 761 is a standardized extract of *Ginkgo biloba*, which contains flavonoids and terpene lactones (ginkgolides A, B, bilobalide) at defined doses (see Ude et al. 2013). Several studies have shown improvements of static and dynamic vestibular symptoms by EGb 761 after unilateral vestibular damage in rats, cats, and guinea pigs (Lacour et al. 1991; Maclennan et al. 1996; Lindner et al. 2019). In rats, oral administration of EGb 761 causes a dose-dependent improvement of the postural asymmetry and locomotor velocity via modulation of cerebral vestibular networks (vestibular nucleus, cerebellum, hippocampus) (Lindner et al. 2019). Experimental data suggest multiple effects of EGb 761 on neural plasticity, modulation of long-term potentiation, neuronal spine morphology and density, neurito- and neurogenesis mostly by terpene lactones (Muller et al. 2012).

5.2.3 Specific and Causative Pharmacotherapy

In addition to the above-mentioned symptomatic antivertiginous drugs, other agents with more specific modes of action are recommended for—if possible—causative therapy (Table 5.3) although there is often a lack of state-of-the art placebo-controlled RCTs. Examples are as follows:

- For peripheral vestibular syndromes: glucocorticoids to improve the recovery of peripheral vestibular function in acute unilateral vestibulopathy/vestibular neuritis (Strupp et al. 2004b; Sjogren et al. 2019); carbamazepine (Brandt et al. 2016), oxcarbazepine (Bayer et al. 2018), and lacosamide (Strupp et al. 2019) in vestibular paroxysmia; and betahistine as well as intraympanic gentamicin and glucocorticoids in Menière's disease (overview in: Naples et al. 2019) with, however, limited evidence (van Esch et al. 2022).
- For central vestibular syndromes, including cerebellar dizziness: 4-aminopyridine (sustained release form 2 × 10 mg/d) for the treatment of downbeat and upbeat nystagmus, episodic ataxia type 2 (EA 2), and cerebellar gait disorders (Strupp

Table 5.3 Drug therapy for various vestibular syndromes and for nystagmus according to different modes of action

Mode of action	Indication	Drug example and dosage
Anticonvulsants	Vestibular paroxysmia (neurovascular compression) Other (central) vestibular paroxysmias: paroxysmal brainstem or cerebellar attacks Myokymia of the superior oblique muscle Paroxysmal dysarthrophonia and ataxia Vestibular epilepsy	Lacosamide (100–400 mg/d) Oxcarbazepine (600–900 mg/d) Carbamazepine (400–800 mg/d)
	Vestibular migraine	For prophylaxis: Topiramate (50–150 mg/d)
Antivertiginous substances	For symptoms of nausea and vomiting in cases of Acute peripheral or central vestibular lesions Central "positional vomiting" Prophylaxis for nausea Vomiting due to liberatory maneuvers in BPPV Prevention of motion sickness	Dimenhydrinate (50 mg every 4–6 h) Ondansetron (4–8 mg every 8 h) Diazepam (5–10 mg every 4–6 h) For a maximum of 1–3 days but not for long-term therapy See also Table 5.3

(continued)

5

Table 5.3 (continued)

Mode of action	Indication	Drug example and dosage
Beta-receptor blocker	Vestibular migraine	For prophylaxis: Metoprolol SR (50–200 mg/d)
Betahistine: H1 agonist and H3 antagonist	Menière's disease, acute unilateral vestibulopathy/vestibular neuritis	Betahistine-dihydrochloride (>3 × 48–96 mg/d); can be probably combined with selegiline (5 mg/d) or rasagiline (1 mg/d) (currently being studied, caveat: contraindications); intranasal application under development.
Ototoxic antibiotics	Menière's disease Tumarkin's otolithic catastrophe (vestibular drop attacks)	Gentamicin (10–20 mg) intratympanally at intervals of 8–12 weeks
Chlorzoxazone	Downbeat nystagmus	Chlorzoxazone (1.5 g/d)
Corticosteroids	Acute unilateral vestibulopathy/vestibular neuritis	Methylprednisolone (100 mg/day, reduce dose every fourth day by 20 mg)
	Cogan's syndrome and other autoimmune inner ear diseases	Methylprednisolone (1000 mg/d i.v., reduce according to treatment effect)
Potassium channel blockers: 4-Aminopyridine	Downbeat nystagmus Upbeat nystagmus	4-Aminopyridine SR (2 × 10 mg/d)
Potassium channel blockers: 4-Aminopyridine	Episodic ataxia type 2	4-Aminopyridine SR (2 × 10 mg/d)
Carbonic anhydrase inhibitor: Acetazolamide		Acetazolamide (125–1000 mg/d)
Selective serotonin and noradrenaline reuptake inhibitors (SSRI, SSNRI)	Functional dizziness Vestibular migraine	Escitalopram (5–10 mg/d in the morning) Venlafaxine (37.5 – 75 mg/d)
Acetyl-DL-leucine	Certain types of ataxias, e.g., Niemann-Pick type C or gangliosidoses 2, currently being studied	Acetyl-DL-leucine (5 g/d)

et al. 2003, 2004a; Kalla et al. 2004; Glasauer et al. 2005; Muth et al. 2021; Schniepp et al. 2011, 2012; Strupp et al. 2011b, 2011a) (overview in Strupp et al. 2017); acetazolamide in EA 2 (Muth et al. 2021); or N-acetyl-leucine for certain patients with cerebellar dizziness (Strupp et al. 2013), in particular due to neurometabolic diseases such as Niemann-Pick type C or gangliosides type 2 (Tay-Sachs disease, Sandhoff disease) (Bremova et al. 2015; Bremova-Ertl et al. 2020, 2022; Kaya et al. 2020, 2021; Martakis K et al. 2022).

5.3 Psychological/Psychiatric and Behavioral Treatment

Functional dizziness is the most frequent type of vertigo in our dizziness outpatient unit, and as such, its treatment is of special importance. Treatment consists mainly of psychoeducation in combination with cognitive behavioral therapy involving desensitization by self-exposure to the precipitating situations and regular exercise. Often a combination with drugs, in particular, selective serotonin reuptake inhibitors (SSRIs) is necessary. These procedures should also be used in cases of secondary functional dizziness (see ▶ Chap. 15).

5.4 Surgical Treatment (◘ Table 5.4)

If vertigo or dizziness are caused by a vestibular schwannoma or a cavernoma of the brainstem, surgery or gamma knife—depending on the location, size, and course—will be the treatment options. Otherwise, surgery is necessary only in very rare cases.

◘ Table 5.4 Surgical treatment strategies for vertigo

"Canal plugging," "resurfacing," or "capping"	Syndrome of the third mobile windows
Surgical resection or gamma knife treatment	Tumours (e.g., vestibular schwannoma) Brainstem/cerebellar cavernomas
Surgical decompression	Arachnoid cysts of the posterior cranial fossa
Neurovascular decompression	Vestibular paroxysmia (last option)
Vestibular implant (under development)	Bilateral vestibulopathy

of vestibular paroxysmia when drug therapy was effective but not tolerated by the patient. Surgery should also be considered in cases of the syndrome of the third mobile windows with "canal plugging," "resurfacing," or "capping" (see ▶ Chap. 12). In the other forms of vertigo, surgery is of marginal importance compared with other treatments.

References

Agus S, Benecke H, Thum C, Strupp M (2013) Clinical and demographic features of vertigo: findings from the REVERT registry. Front Neurol 4:48

Bagus IG, Gordy C, Sanchez-Gonzalez R, Strupp M, Straka H (2019) Impact of 4-aminopyridine on vestibulo-ocular reflex performance. J Neurol 266:93–100

Bayer O, Bremova T, Strupp M, Hufner K (2018) A randomized double-blind, placebo-controlled, cross-over trial (Vestparoxy) of the treatment of vestibular paroxysmia with oxcarbazepine. J Neurol 265(2):291–298

Beck R, Gunther L, Xiong G, Potschka H, Boning G, Bartenstein P, Brandt T, Jahn K, Dieterich M, Strupp M, La FC, Zwergal A (2014) The mixed blessing of treating symptoms in acute vestibular failure–evidence from a 4-aminopyridine experiment. Exp Neurol 261:638–645

Bertlich M, Ihler F, Freytag S, Weiss BG, Strupp M, Canis M (2015) Histaminergic H-Heteroreceptors as a potential mediator of Betahistine-induced increase in Cochlear blood flow. Audiol Neurootol 20(5):283–293

Bertlich M, Ihler F, Weiss BG, Freytag S, Strupp M, Jakob M, Canis M (2017) Role of capillary pericytes and precapillary arterioles in the vascular mechanism of betahistine in a guinea pig inner ear model. Life Sci 187:17–21

Bhattacharyya N, Gubbels SP, Schwartz SR, Edlow JA, El-Kashlan H, Fife T, Holmberg JM, Mahoney K, Hollingsworth DB, Roberts R, Seidman MD, Steiner RW, Do BT, Voelker CC, Waguespack RW, Corrigan MD (2017) Clinical practice guideline: benign paroxysmal positional vertigo (update). Otolaryngol Head Neck Surg 156(3_suppl):S1–S47

Brandt T, Strupp M, Dieterich M (2016) Vestibular paroxysmia: a treatable neurovascular cross-compression syndrome. J Neurol 263(Suppl 1): 90–96

Bremova T, Malinova V, Amraoui Y, Mengel E, Reinke J, Kolnikova M, Strupp M (2015) Acetyl-dl-leucine in Niemann-Pick type C: a case series. Neurology 85(16):1368–1375

Bremova-Ertl T, Platt F, Strupp M (2020) Sandhoff-disease: improvement of gait by acetyl-DL-leucine – a case report. Neuropediatrics 51:450–452

Bremova-Ertl T, Claassen J, Foltan T, Gascon-Bayarri J, Gissen P, Hahn A, Hassan A, Hennig A, Jones SA, Kolnikova M, Martakis K, Raethjen J, Ramaswami U, Sharma R, Schneider SA (2022) Efficacy and safety of N-acetyl-L-leucine in Niemann-Pick disease type C. J Neurol 269:1651–1662

Chabbert C (2016) Principles of vestibular pharmacotherapy. Handb Clin Neurol 137:207–218

Chen ZP, Zhang XY, Peng SY, Yang ZQ, Wang YB, Zhang YX, Chen X, Wang JJ, Zhu JN (2019) Histamine H1 receptor contributes to vestibular compensation. J Neurosci 39(3):420–433

Dieterich M, Bauermann T, Best C, Stoeter P, Schlindwein P (2007) Evidence for cortical visual substitution of chronic bilateral vestibular failure (an fMRI study). Brain 130(Pt 8):2108–2116

Dunlap PM, Holmberg JM, Whitney SL (2019) Vestibular rehabilitation: advances in peripheral and central vestibular disorders. Curr Opin Neurol 32(1):137–144

Feil K, Strobl R, Schindler A, Krafczyk S, Goldschagg N, Frenzel C, Glaser M, Schoberl F, Zwergal A, Strupp M (2019) What is behind cerebellar vertigo and dizziness? Cerebellum 18(3):320–332

Ferber-Viart C, Dubreuil C, Vidal PP (2009) Effects of acetyl-DL-leucine in vestibular patients: a clinical study following neurotomy and labyrinthectomy. Audiol Neurootol 14(1):17–25

Glasauer S, Kalla R, Buttner U, Strupp M, Brandt T (2005) 4-aminopyridine restores visual ocular motor function in upbeat nystagmus. J Neurol Neurosurg Psychiatry 76(3):451–453

Gunther L, Beck R, Xiong G, Potschka H, Jahn K, Bartenstein P, Brandt T, Dutia M, Dieterich M, Strupp M, La FC, Zwergal A (2015) N-acetyl-L-leucine accelerates vestibular compensation after unilateral labyrinthectomy by action in the cerebellum and thalamus. PLoS One 10(3):e0120891

Hall CD, Herdman SJ, Whitney SL, Anson ER, Carender WJ, Hoppes CW, Cass SP, Christy JB, Cohen HS, Fife TD, Furman JM, Shepard NT, Clendaniel RA, Dishman JD, Goebel JA, Meldrum D, Ryan C, Wallace RL, Woodward NJ (2022) Vestibular Rehabilitation for Peripheral Vestibular Hypofunction: An Updated Clinical Practice Guideline From the Academy of Neurologic Physical Therapy of the American Physical Therapy Association. J Neurol Phys Ther. 46(2):118–77.

Jahn K, Saul AK, Elstner M, Sapa K, Kellerer S (2018) Vestibular rehabilitation therapy and Nintendo Wii balance board training both improve postural control in bilateral vestibulopathy. J Neurol 265(Suppl 1):70–73

Kalla R, Glasauer S, Schautzer F, Lehnen N, Buttner U, Strupp M, Brandt T (2004) 4-aminopyridine improves downbeat nystagmus, smooth pursuit, and VOR gain. Neurology 62(7):1228–1229

Kaya E, Smith DA, Smith C, Boland B, Strupp M, Platt FM (2020) Beneficial effects of acetyl-DL-leucine (ADLL) in a mouse model of Sandhoff disease. J Clin Med 9(4):1050

Kaya E, Smith DA, Smith C, Morris L, Bremova-Ertl T, Cortina-Borja M, Fineran P, Morten KJ, Poulton J, Boland B, Spencer J, Strupp M, Platt FM (2021) Acetyl-leucine slows disease progression in lysosomal storage disorders. Brain Commun 3:fcaa148

Lacour M (2013) Betahistine treatment in managing vertigo and improving vestibular compensation: clarification. J Vestib Res 23(3):139–151

Lacour M, Ez Zaher L, Raymond J (1991) Plasticity mechanisms in vestibular compensation in the cat are improved by an extract of Ginkgo biloba (EGb 761). Pharmacol Biochem Behav 40:367–379

Lehnen N, Kellerer S, Knorr AG, Schlick C, Jahn K, Schneider E, Heuberger M, Ramaioli C (2018) Head-movement-emphasized rehabilitation in bilateral vestibulopathy. Front Neurol 9:562

Lindner M, Gosewisch A, Eilles E, Branner C, Kramer A, Oos R, Wolf E, Ziegler S, Bartenstein P, Brandt T, Dieterich M, Zwergal A (2019) Ginkgo biloba extract EGb 761 improves vestibular compensation and modulates cerebral vestibular networks in the rat. Front Neurol 10:147

Maclennan K, Smith PF, Darlington CL (1996) The effects of ginkgolide B (BN52021) on guinea pig vestibular nucleus neurons in vitro: importance of controlling for effects of dimethyl sulphoxide (DMSO) vehicles. Neurosci Res 26(4):395–399

Martakis K, Claassen J, Gascon-Bayari J, Goldschagg N, Hahn A, Hassan A, Hennig A, Jones S, Kay R, Lau H, Perlman S, Sharma R, Schneider S, Bremova-Ertl T (2022) Efficacy and Safety of N-Acetyl-L-Leucine in Children and Adults With GM2 Gangliosidoses. Neurology. https://doi.org/10.1212/WNL.0000000000201660.

McDonnell MN, Hillier SL (2015) Vestibular rehabilitation for unilateral peripheral vestibular dysfunction. Cochrane Database Syst Rev (1):CD005397

Meldrum D, Jahn K (2019) Gaze stabilisation exercises in vestibular rehabilitation: review of the evidence and recent clinical advances. J Neurol 266(Suppl 1):11–18

Muller WE, Heiser J, Leuner K (2012) Effects of the standardized Ginkgo biloba extract EGb 761(R) on neuroplasticity. Int Psychogeriatr 24(Suppl 1):S21–S24

Murdin L, Hussain K, Schilder AG (2016) Betahistine for symptoms of vertigo. Cochrane Database Syst Rev (6):CD010696

Muth C, Teufel J, Schöls L, Synofzik M, Franke C, Timmann D, Mansmann U, Strupp M (2021)

Fampridine and Acetazolamide in EA2 and Related Familial EA: A Prospective Randomized Placebo-Controlled Trial. Neurol Clin Pract 11:e438–e446

Naples JG, Henry L, Brant JA, Eliades SJ, Ruckenstein MJ (2019) Intratympanic therapies in Meniere disease: evaluation of outcomes and early vertigo control. Laryngoscope 129(1):216–221

Schniepp R, Wuehr M, Ackl N, Danek A, Brandt T, Strupp M, Jahn K (2011) 4-aminopyridine improves gait variability in cerebellar ataxia due to CACNA 1A mutation. J Neurol 258(9):1708–1711

Schniepp R, Wuehr M, Neuhaeusser M, Benecke AK, Adrion C, Brandt T, Strupp M, Jahn K (2012) 4-Aminopyridine and cerebellar gait: a retrospective case series. J Neurol 259:2491

Sjogren J, Magnusson M, Tjernstrom F, Karlberg M (2019) Steroids for acute vestibular neuronitis-the earlier the treatment, the better the outcome? Otol Neurotol 40(3):372–374

Soto E, Vega R, Sesena E (2013) Neuropharmacological basis of vestibular system disorder treatment. J Vestib Res 23(3):119–137

Strupp M, Teufel J, Zwergal A, Schniepp R, Khodakhah K, Feil K (2017) Aminopyridines for the treatment of neurologic disorders. Neurol Clin Pract 7 65–76

Strupp M, Elger C, Goldschagg N (2019) Treatment of vestibular paroxysmia with lacosamide. Neurol Clin Pract 9(6):539–541

Strupp M, Kalla R, Claassen J, Adrion C, Mansmann U, Klopstock T, Freilinger T, Neugebauer H, Spiegel R, Dichgans M, Lehmann-Horn F, Jurkat-Rott K, Brandt T, Jen JC Jahn K (2011a) A randomized trial of 4-aminopyridine in EA2 and related familial episodic ataxias. Neurology 77(3):269–275

Strupp M, Kalla R, Dichgans M, Freilinger T, Glasauer S, Brandt T (2004a) Treatment of episodic ataxia type 2 with the potassium channel blocker 4-aminopyridine. Neurology 62(9):1623–1625

Strupp M, Schuler O, Krafczyk S, Jahn K, Schautzer F, Buttner U, Brandt T (2003) Treatment of downbeat nystagmus with 3,4-diaminopyridine: a placebo-controlled study. Neurology 61(2):165–170

Strupp M, Teufel J, Habs M, Feuerecker R, Muth C, van de Warrenburg BP, Klopstock T, Feil K (2013) Effects of acetyl-DL-leucine in patients with cerebellar ataxia: a case series. J Neurol 260(10): 2556–2561

Strupp M, Thurtell MJ, Shaikh AG, Brandt T, Zee DS, Leigh RJ (2011b) Pharmacotherapy of vestibular and ocular motor disorders, including nystagmus. J Neurol 258(7):1207–1222

Strupp M, Zingler VC, Arbusow V, Niklas D, Maag KP, Dieterich M, Bense S, Theil D, Jahn K, Brandt T (2004b) Methylprednisolone, valacyclovir, or the combination for vestibular neuritis. N Engl J Med 351(4):354–361

Strupp M, Zwergal A (2020) Pharmacotherapy of peripheral vestibular disorders. In: The senses. Academic Press/Elsevier, San Diego

Takumida M, Takumida H, Anniko M (2016) Localization of histamine (H1, H2, H3 and H4) receptors in mouse inner ear. Acta Otolaryngol 136(6):537–544

Tighilet B, Leonard J, Bernard-Demanze L, Lacour M (2015) Comparative analysis of pharmacological treatments with N-acetyl-dl-leucine (Tanganil) and its two isomers (N-acetyl-L-leucine and N-acetyl-D-leucine) on vestibular compensation: behavioral investigation in the cat. Eur J Pharmacol 769: 342–349

Tighilet B, Leonard J, Lacour M (1995) Betahistine dihydrochloride treatment facilitates vestibular compensation in the cat. J Vestib Res 5(1):53–66

Tighilet B, Leonard J, Watabe I, Bernard-Demanze L, Lacour M (2018) Betahistine treatment in a cat model of vestibular pathology: pharmacokinetic and pharmacodynamic approaches. Front Neurol 9:431

Ude C, Schubert-Zsilavecz M, Wurglics M (2013) Ginkgo biloba extracts: a review of the pharmacokinetics of the active ingredients. Clin Pharmacokinet 52(9):727–749

Vanderkam P, Blanchard C, Naudet F, Pouchain D, Vaillant RH, Perault-Pochat MC, Jaafari N, Boussageon R (2019) Efficacy of acetylleucine in vertigo and dizziness: a systematic review of randomised controlled trials. Eur J Clin Pharmacol 75:603

Van Esch BF, Zaag-Loonen H, Bruintjes T, Kuijpers T, van Benthem PPG (2022) Interventions for Meniere's disease: an umbrella systematic review. BMJ Evid Based Med 27:(4)235–45

Vibert N, Vidal PP (2001) In vitro effects of acetyl-DL-leucine (tanganil) on central vestibular neurons and vestibulo-ocular networks of the guinea-pig. Eur J Neurosci 13(4):735–748

Whitney SL, Sparto PJ, Furman JM (2020) Vestibular rehabilitation and factors that can affect outcome. Semin Neurol 40(1):165–172

Zwergal A, Strupp M, Brandt T (2019) Advances in pharmacotherapy of vestibular and ocular motor disorders. Exp Opin Pharmacother 20(10): 1267–1276

Peripheral Vestibular Syndromes

Contents

M. Strupp et al., *Vertigo and Dizziness*, https://doi.org/10.1007/978-3-030-78260-3_6

6.1 Introduction and Classification

Three forms of peripheral vestibular disorders, each with its typical symptoms and clinical signs, can be differentiated functionally, anatomically, and pathophysiologically (◘ Table 6.1):

1. Loss or severe impairment of function of the vestibular nerve and/or labyrinth: bilateral vestibulopathy (BVP) or a persisting severe unilateral peripheral vestibular deficit, characterized by postural imbalance and gait instablity.
2. Acute unilateral vestibulopathy leading to an acute vestibular tone imbalance manifesting as an acute peripheral vestibular syndrome.
3. Inadequate unilateral paroxysmal stimulation or rarely inhibition of the peripheral vestibular system, e.g., BPPV, Menière's disease, vestibular paroxysmia, or the syndrome of the third mobile window s, characterized by recurrent episodes of symptoms.

The lifetime prevalence of peripheral vestibular disorders is around 6.5% (Hulse et al. 2019).

6

◘ **Table 6.1** Three forms of peripheral vestibular disorders.

Type of disorder	Main symptoms	Examples and causes
Bilateral vestibulopathy or a persisting severe unilateral peripheral vestibular deficit	Postural imbalance and gait instability that increase in the dark and on unlevel ground (reduced or absent visual or somatosensory information) Oscillopsia during walking and head movements (loss of vestibulo-ocular reflexes) in some of the patients Disorders of spatial memory and navigation	Bilateral vestibulopathy due to Ototoxic substances (e.g., aminoglycosides) Bilateral Menière's disease Meningitis Neurodegeneration with or without additional cerebellar symptoms or signs Bilateral vestibular schwannoma (neurofibromatosis 2) Hemosiderosis
Acute/subacute unilateral vestibulopathy (labyrinth and/or vestibular nerve) with acute vestibular tone imbalance	Acute spinning vertigo (for days or a few weeks) Oscillopsia due to spontaneous nystagmus Tendency to fall in specific direction Nausea, vomiting	Acute unilateral vestibulopathy/vestibular neuritis, e.g., due to reactivation of a latent HSV 1 infection Labyrinthitis Trauma
Inadequate unilateral paroxysmal stimulation or rarely inhibition of the peripheral vestibular system	Attack or recurrent episodes of spinning vertigo or dizziness depending on cause, with or without triggers, of various durations and with various accompanying symptoms	Benign paroxysmal positional vertigo due to canalolithiasis or rarely cupulolithiais Menière's disease due to rupture of the endolymphatic membrane Vestibular paroxysmia due to neurovascular compression Syndrome of the third mobile windows, most often SCDS due to changes of pressure or sound

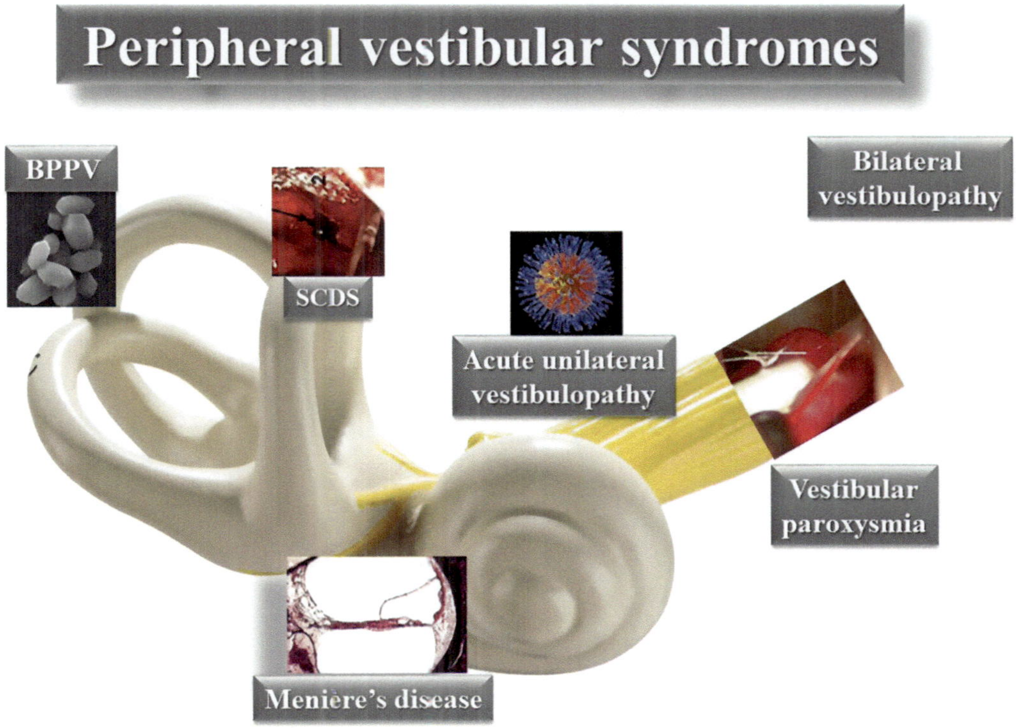

Fig. 6.1 Anatomy, pathophysiology, and etiology of the six most frequent peripheral vestibular syndromes

According to a study from South Korea the annual incidence of the three most frequent causes of peripheral vestibular was there for BPPV, acute unilateral vestibulopathy, vestibular neuritis, and Menière`s disease per 100,000 51.4, 22.7, and 12.4 in 2008 and 181.1, 62.9, and 50.5 in 2020, respectively. The incidence of each was significantly different by sex ($p < 0.001$), age ($p < 0.001$), and residence ($p < 0.001$), with the highest value in female, people aged 60 years or older, and people who resided in metropolitan cities (Jeong J et al. 2022).

In ► Chaps. 7, 8, 9, 10, 11, and 12, the six most frequent vestibular syndromes are presented based on the above-mentioned classification (overview in Fig. 6.1).

Reference

Hulse R, Biesdorf A, Hormann K, Stuck B, Erhart M, Hulse M, Wenzel A (2019) Peripheral vestibular disorders: an epidemiologic survey in 70 million individuals. Otol Neurotol 40(1):88–95

Jeong J, Youk TM, Choi HS (2022) Incidence of peripheral vestibular disorders based on population data of South Korea. J Vestib Res. https://doi.org/10.3233/VES-220085

Bilateral Vestibulopathy

Contents

Supplementary Information The online version contains supplementary material available at [https://doi.org/10.1007/978-3-030-78260-3_7]. The videos can be accessed by scanning the related images with the SN More Media App.

M. Strupp et al., *Vertigo and Dizziness*, https://doi.org/10.1007/978-3-030-78260-3_7

The leading symptoms of bilateral vestibulopathy (BVP) are unsteadiness, postural imbalance, impairment of gait, and, in some patients, movement-induced oscillopsia. Typically, the symptoms worsen in darkness and on uneven ground and patients have no symptoms while sitting or lying down under static conditions. The current diagnostic criteria for BVP and probable BVP according to the Classification Committee of the Bárány Society (Strupp et al. 2017) are as follows (▶ Box 7.1):

Box 7.1 Diagnostic Criteria for Bilateral and *Probable* Bilateral Vestibulopathy According to the Classification Committee of the Bárány Society (Strupp et al. 2017)

Bilateral vestibulopathy

1. Chronic vestibular syndrome with the following symptoms:
   (a) Unsteadiness when walking or standing plus at least one of 2 or 3
   (b) Movement-induced blurred vision or oscillopsia during walking or quick head/body movements and/or
   (c) Worsening of unsteadiness in darkness and/or on uneven ground
2. No symptoms while sitting or lying down under static conditions
3. Bilaterally reduced or absent angular VOR function documented by:
   - Bilaterally pathological horizontal angular VOR gain <0.6, measured by the video-HIT or scleral-coil technique and/or
   - Reduced caloric response (sum of bithermal max. peak SPV on each side <6°/s) and/or
   - Reduced horizontal angular VOR gain≤0.1 upon sinusoidal stimulation on a rotatory chair (0.1 Hz, Vmax=50°/sec) and a phase lead≥15 degrees (time constant≤6sec)
4. Not better accounted for by another disease

Probable bilateral vestibulopathy

1. Chronic vestibular syndrome with the following symptoms:
   (a) Unsteadiness when walking or standing plus at least one of 2 or 3
   (b) Movement-induced blurred vision or oscillopsia during walking or quick head/body movements and/or
   (c) Worsening of unsteadiness in darkness and/or on uneven ground
2. No symptoms while sitting or lying down under static conditions
3. Bilaterally pathological horizontal bedside head impulse test
4. Not better accounted for by another disease

The diagnosis of "bilateral vestibulopathy" requires quantitative testing of vestibular function by means of video-HIT and/or caloric testing, since the bedside head impulse test has a low sensitivity and specificity (Yip et al. 2016). Only the diagnosis of "*probable* BVP" can be made using bedside testing.

7.1 Epidemiology

BVP is evidently the most frequent cause of postural imbalance in the elderly requiring precise diagnosis. The prevalence in a US population was stated to be 28/100,000 (Ward et al. 2013); however, these data do not seem to be reliable because of the search criteria used (Neuhauser 2016). The relative frequency is 4–7% (Rinne et al. 1998; Zingler et al. 2007; Kim et al. 2011) (◘ Table 1.1). In our clinical experience, BVP is still often not diagnosed or is diagnosed too late.

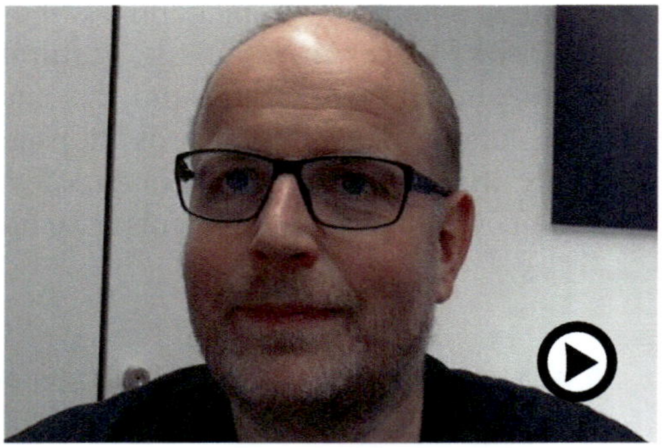

◘ **Fig. 7.1** Bilateral vestibulopathy: patient history (► https://doi.org/10.1007/000-950)

7.2 Diagnosis

The diagnosis is based on the patient history (leading symptoms: chronic postural imbalance and unsteadiness when walking, without symptoms under static conditions while sitting or lying down) in combination with a clinical and laboratory examination, the latter indicating a bilateral deficit of the vestibulo-ocular reflex based on the video-HIT, caloric testing and/or rarely examination using a rotatory chair (for reference, see Fujimoto et al. 2019, Starkov et al. 2020b).

7.2.1 Patient History

The typical symptoms (◘ Fig. 7.1) of BVP are:

- Postural imbalance, dizziness, and impaired gait and stance (worsening in darkness and/or on uneven ground). Therefore, patients have a higher risk of falling in darkness and on uneven ground (Fujimoto et al. 2013; Dobbels et al. 2020; Herssens et al. 2020).
- Typically, no symptoms while sitting or lying down under static conditions.
- Blurred vision while walking or during fast head movements (oscillopsia); however, blurred vision is reported only in 40–70% of the patients (Lucieer et al. 2018; Zingler et al. 2007) and often only if the patients are explicitly asked about it. In severe cases, the oscillopsia may even be pulse synchronous or induced by chewing.
- In particular at the beginning of the disease, recurrent attacks or episodes of spinning or non-spinning vertigo lasting for minutes to days. This is reported by 33–67% of the patients (Lucieer et al. 2018). Pathophysiologically, these are the periods in which vestibular function deteriorates unilaterally, leading to a transient vestibular tone imbalance: this is found in cases with so-called sequential BVP (Zingler et al. 2007).
- Impairment of spatial navigation and memory, as well as impaired spatial learning (Brandt et al. 2005; Kremmyda et al. 2016), but also reduced working memory and visual attention (Popp et al. 2017). These symptoms of a higher (cognitive) vestibular dysfunction (see ► Chap. 3) are often not noticed or spontaneously reported by the patient and therefore require specific testing.

7.2.2 Bedside Testing

The following three tests are important for the bedside testing of patients (Petersen et al. 2013):

- "Bedside head impulse test" (bHIT) (Halmagyi and Curthoys 1988); here one has to look for bilateral refixation saccades (Fig. 7.2). Since the bHIT has a sensitivity of only 65% for the diagnosis of BVP (Yip et al. 2016), only a diagnosis of *probable* BVP can be made using this test.

- Dynamic visual acuity (DVA): If this decreases by more than 0.2, it is evidence of an angular VOR deficit (Vital et al. 2010).
- Romberg test under four conditions and examination of gait: There is typically an increased sway after the eyes have been closed (Fig. 7.3) due to a deficit of vestibulo-spinal reflexes. An examination while standing on foam is evidently more sensitive (Sprenger et al. 2017). However, the Romberg test is not specific because patients with a somatosensory deficit show similar findings. Asymmetries of vestibular function can be recognized during walking with the eyes closed: There is a deviation of gait toward the more affected side (Fig. 7.4).

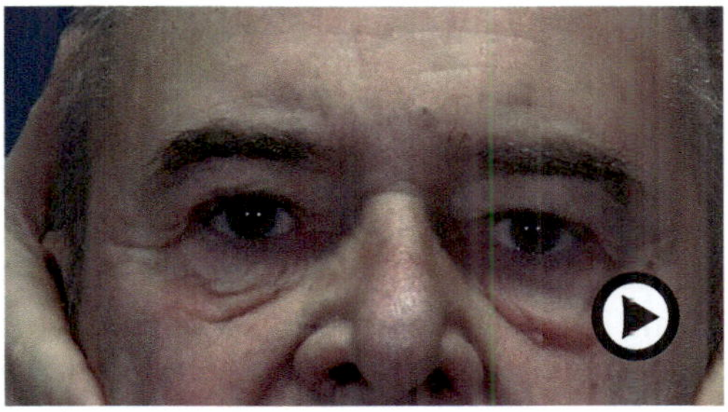

Fig. 7.2 Bilaterally pathological head impulse test (▶ https://doi.org/10.1007/000-94x)

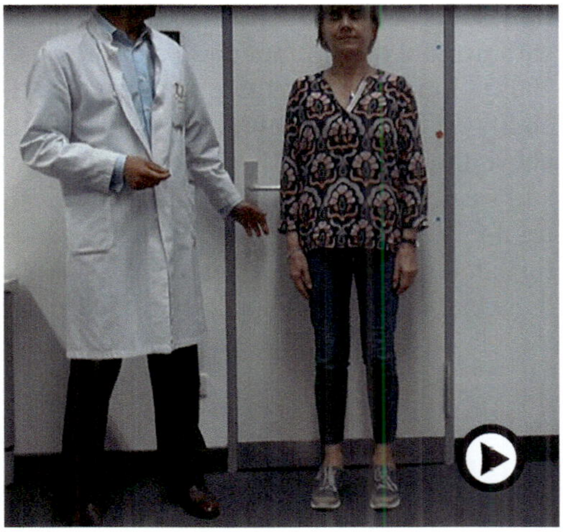

Fig. 7.3 Pathological Romberg test in bilateral vestibulopathy (▶ https://doi.org/10.1007/000-94y)

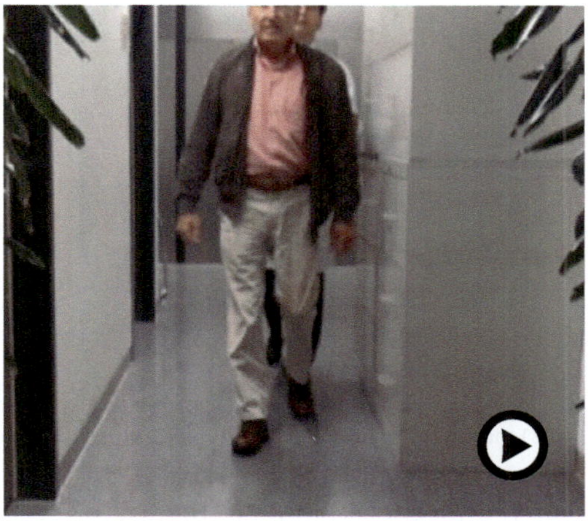

Fig. 7.4 Pathological gait in bilateral vestibulopathy (▶ https://doi.org/10.1007/000-94z)

7.2.3 Laboratory Testing

According to the above criteria, the precise diagnosis of BVP requires (Strupp et al. 2017) quantitative proof of bilaterally significantly reduced function of the VOR (Fujimoto et al. 2019; Starkov et al. 2020b). This can be measured by:

- The video-HIT (Halmagyi et al. 2017) in the high-frequency range; however, there are evident differences between the three major systems currently used, which should be taken into consideration for the diagnosis (van Dooren et al. 2020).
- Caloric irrigation with testing of the VOR in the low-frequency range (approximately 0.003 Hz). An advantage of this technique is that, in contrast to the video-HIT and the rotatory chair, each labyrinth can be examined separately.
- The rotatory chair in the middle-frequency range (0.1 Hz) (rarely necessary).

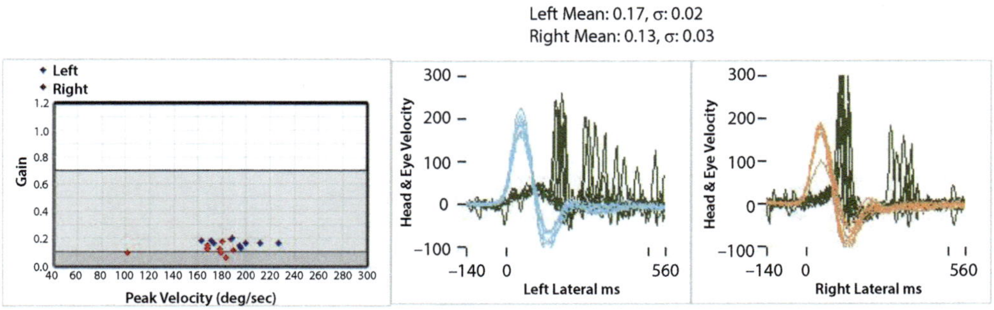

Fig. 7.5 Video head impulse test. Bilaterally significantly reduced VOR gain (left: 0.17; right: 0.13; normal >0.8) indicating bilateral vestibulopathy with a VOR deficit in the high-frequency range

For the diagnosis of BVP, the following is required (Strupp et al. 2017):

- VOR gain of <0.6 with an angular velocity of the head during stimulation of 150–300°/s (Fig. 7.5); for the diagnosis of presbyvestibulopathy (Agrawal et al. 2019), a VOR gain of between 0.6 and 0.8 is required; see differential diagnosis and/or
- Bilaterally reduced or absent caloric response (Fig. 7.6): sum of bithermal max. peak SPV on each side <6°/s; in particular in patients with bilateral Menière's disease, caloric irrigation is important because they often have a pseudo-normal video-HIT and/or
- Reduced horizontal angular VOR gain≤0.1 upon sinusoidal stimulation on a rotatory chair (0.1Hz, Vmax=50°/sec) and a phase lead≥15 degrees (time constant≤6sec) (Goulson et al. 2014)

Since in BVP the function of the horizontal semicircular canal is virtually always reduced (Tarnutzer et al. 2016, 2018), it is sufficient to test the function of this canal in the vast majority of cases.

7.2.4 Complementary Laboratory Testing

7.2.4.1 Cervical and Ocular Vestibular-Evoked Myogenic Potentials (c/oVEMP)

In BVP, the c/oVEMP are often normal for reasons we do not yet understand (Rosengren et al. 2018). Some case series show that the amplitude of the VEMP can be reduced (Fujimoto et al. 2009; Agrawal et al. 2013; Brantberg and Lofqvist 2007; Zingler et al. 2008a). The impairment of the function of the utricle correlates with that of the horizontal semicircular canals (Agrawal et al. 2013), which is to be expected for anatomical reasons. In addition, there is a very rare subgroup with bilateral sacculopathy with normal canal function (Fujimoto et al. 2009). Furthermore, there is a high variability of the VEMP amplitudes in subjects above the age of 60 (Colebatch et al. 2016) and we do not yet have good normative values for VEMPs (Strupp et al. 2020), which further limits the use of c/oVEMP in the diagnosis of BVP. All in all, VEMP can only

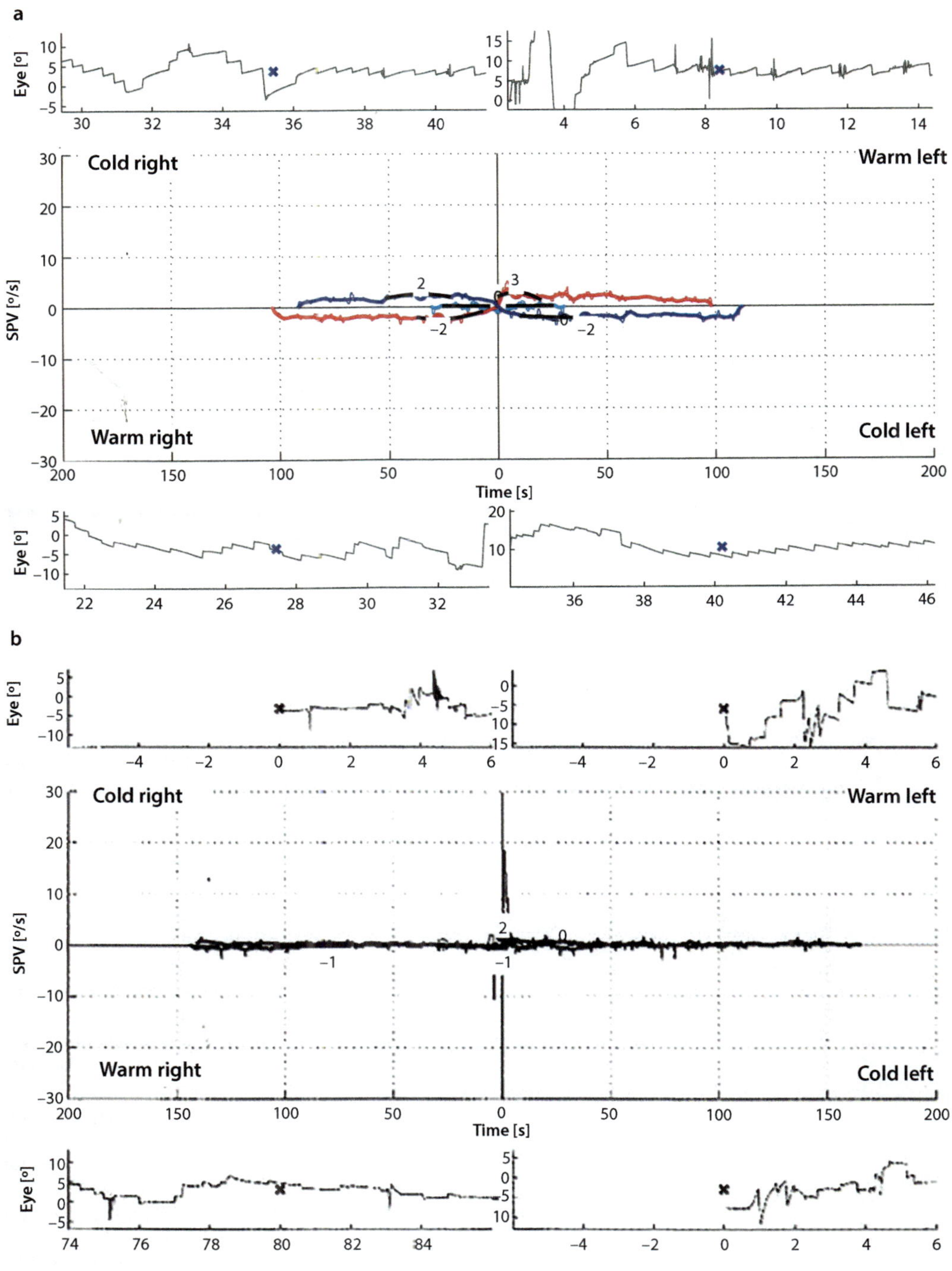

Fig. 7.6 **a**, **b** Caloric testing with warm and cold water in two patients with bilateral vestibulopathy. **a** Bilaterally reduced caloric response (sum of the maximum peak slow phase velocity on each side <6°/s). **b** Bilaterally no caloric response. Both patients have a VOR deficit in the low-frequency range

be complementary tests and are therefore not yet part of the diagnostic criteria.

7.2.5 Imaging

A contrast MRI should be performed in all patients with BVP, in particular to look for bilateral vestibular schwannoma (◘ Fig. 7.7) or, for example, a superficial siderosis (◘ Fig. 7.8). In a retrospective analysis of 3D-FLAIR sequences 4 h after administering contrast media to 42 patients with BV, morphologic anomalies of the endolymphatic space or blood-brain barrier impairment were found in 59.6% of patients (Eliezer et al. 2020).

Patients with post-traumatic BVP require a CCT, in particular to look for temporal bone fractures. A CCT is also helpful for

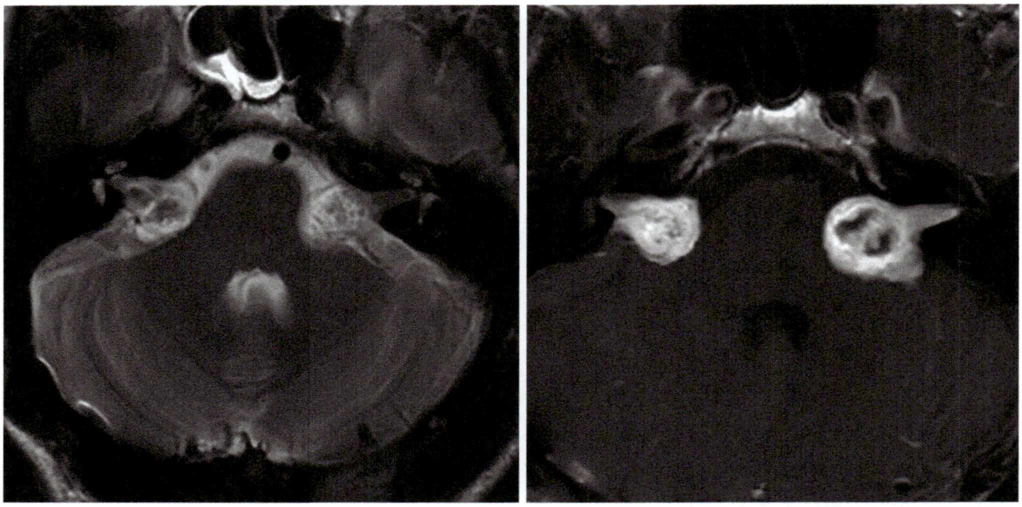

◘ **Fig. 7.7** Bilateral vestibular schwannoma with significant contrast enhancement on the right

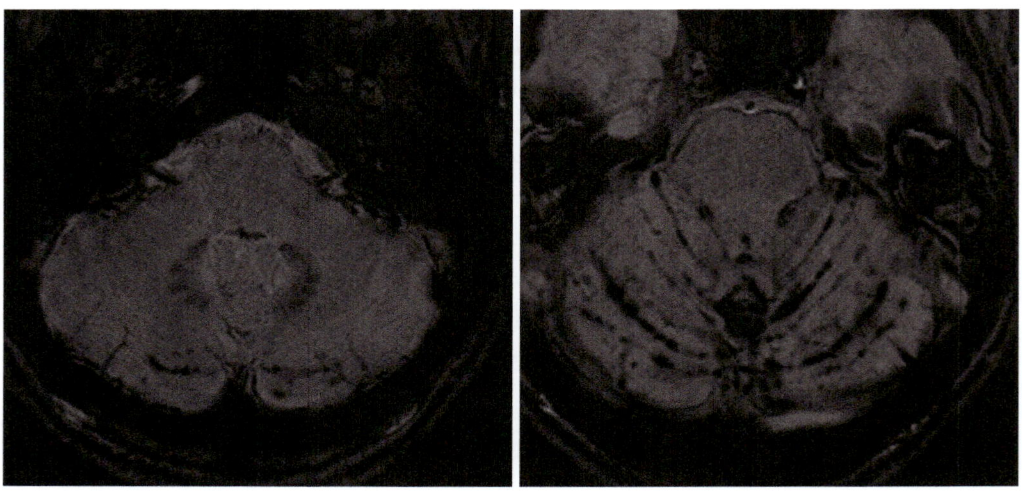

◘ **Fig. 7.8** MRI of the brain showing superficial siderosis (black layer) around the eighth cranial nerve (left) and on the surface of the cerebellum (right). In these cases, BVP is often associated with cerebellar ataxia

the diagnosis of congenital inner ear abnormalities in children with BVP (► Chap. 16).

7.3 Summary of Laboratory Testing and Clinically Relevant Points

For a precise diagnosis of BVP, quantitative testing of vestibular function is necessary, nowadays initially using video-HIT. If the VOR gain in the video-HIT is <0.6, the diagnosis of BVP can—in combination with an appropriate patient history – be made. If the VOR gain bilaterally is >0.6, caloric testing is required. Finally, in all patients with BVP, at least one contrast-enhanced MRI should be performed, in particular to look for a bilateral vestibular schwannoma.

7.4 Pathophysiology

The leading symptoms of BVP can be explained by the deficits of the vestibulo-ocular and vestibulo-spinal reflexes:

- **Unsteadiness of posture and gait,** increased in the dark and on uneven ground: Due to the redundant sensorimotor control of posture, the visual system can basically substitute for any defective regulation of postural control in light. The somatosensory system also contributes to the maintenance of balance, above all via the muscle spindle afferents and the mechanoreceptors of the joints and skin. If the contribution of the visual system (in darkness or due to visual disorders) is reduced, gait imbalance increases until the patient experiences a tendency to fall. This is further intensified if the patient walks in the dark over uneven or springy ground. Thus, a sensory polyneuropathy also reduces the somatosensory contribution to posture control and thereby exacerbates the symptoms of BVP. In a study with quantitative gait analysis, two significant predictive factors for falls in patients with BVP were established: a coexisting polyneuropathy (odds ratio: 3.6) and increased gait variability, in particular with low walking speed (odds ratio: 1.3) (Schniepp et al. 2017). The influence of proprioceptive, visual, vestibular and cognitive factors on posture was evaluated by posturography in patients with BVP (Sprenger et al. 2017). The best predictor of an impairment of function was standing on foam. This underlines how important proprioceptive input is, which correlates with the above-mentioned study on the risk of falls.
- **Oscillopsia and blurred vision** (◘ Fig. 7.9): During rapid head movements, the impaired VOR cannot maintain the target of gaze on the fovea, and thus, there is an involuntary movement of the image on the retina, which is experienced as an illusory movement that reduces the visual acuity. This symptom is found in only 40–70% of patients with BVP (Lucieer et al. 2018; Zingler et al. 2007); the patients often only mention it if they are explicitly asked about it. Conversely, when head movements are slow, the smooth pursuit system is able to sufficiently stabilize the gaze in space, and no illusory movement or blurriness occurs.

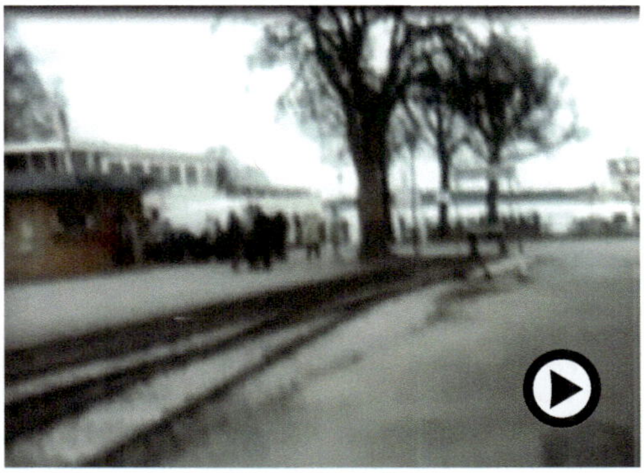

◘ **Fig. 7.9** Oscillopsia induced by walking in bilateral vestibulopathy (► https://doi.org/10.1007/000-94w)

- **Deficits of spatial memory, navigation, and other cognitive functions and morphological changes:** An intact vestibular function is important for spatial orientation, spatial memory, and navigation (Smith 1997). In patients with BVP, there are significant deficits of spatial orientation, navigation, and memory (Brandt et al. 2005); there is also a significant atrophy of the hippocampus (Brandt et al. 2005). Even patients with a partial bilateral BVP have a functional impairment of spatial learning, as well as an atrophy of the gray matter of the hippocampus (Gottlich et al. 2016) and the posterior parahippocampus (Kremmyda et al. 2016). In contrast, in patients with unilateral vestibulopathy the deficits are less pronounced. There are contrary results on spatial memory and hippocampus atrophy in unilateral deficits: Some did not find any changes (Hufner et al. 2007), whereas others demonstrated visuospatially impaired memory (Popp et al. 2017) and an atrophy of the posterior hippocampus in chronic deficits after 2.5 years (zu Eulenburg P. et al. 2010). Three months after vestibular neuritis, a bilateral increase of hippocampal volume was even reported (Hong et al. 2014).

7.5 Etiology

The etiology of BVP (◘ Table 7.1) remains unclear in 30–50% despite extensive diagnostics (Lucieer et al. 2016; Zingler et al. 2007). These patients can be assumed to have a neurodegenerative illness (see below) or the transition from a presbyvestibulopathy to a BVP. Two large case series have been published on the etiology of BVP. For example, in a retrospective study with 255 patients,

◘ **Table 7.1** Causes and underlying disease leading to bilateral vestibulopathy

Relatively frequent	Underlying cause
Idiopathic (>30–50%)	
Ototoxicity	Gentamicin and other antibiotics
	Anticancer chemotherapy
	Loop diuretics Amiodarone
	Aspirin
Bilateral Menière's disease	Endolymphatic hydrops
Meningitis or labyrinthitis	e.g., Streptococci, Neisseria meningitis, Mycobacterium tuberculosis
Combination with cerebellar disorders	Cerebellar ataxia and/or cerebellar ocular motor disorders, in particular downbeat nystagmus (frequent) CANVAS (cerebellar ataxia, neuropathy, and vestibular areflexia syndrome) Spinocerebellar ataxias Multiple system atrophy

■ **Table 7.1** (continued)

Relatively frequent	Underlying cause
Tumors	Neurofibromatosis type 2 (Bilateral vestibular schwannomas)
	Lymphomas
	Meningeosis carcinomatosa
	Infiltration of the skull base
Autoimmune disorders	Cogan's syndrome
	Neurosarcoidosis
	Behçet's disease
	Cerebral vasculitis
	Systemic lupus erythematosus
	Polychondritis
	Rheumatoid arthritis
	Polyarteritis nodosa
	Wegener's granulomatosis/ANCA-associated small vessel associated vasculitis and others
	Giant cell arteritis/large vascular vasculitis
	Antiphospholipid syndrome
	Hereditary sensory and autonomic neuropathy
Vitamin deficiencies	B1, B6, B12 deficiency
Bilateral sequential vestibular neuritis	Herpes simplex virus type I, varizella zoster
Other causes	
Congenital malformation	Usher's syndrome and other rare hereditary conditions
Other causes	Bilateral labyrinthine concussion Bilateral petrous bone fracture
	Paget's disease
	Macroglobulinemia
	Vertebrobasilar dolichoectasia Superficial siderosis

five frequent causes were found (Zingler et al. 2007): ototoxic aminoglycosides (13%), bilateral Menière's disease (7%), meningitis (5%), association with cerebellar disorders (4%, see below), and systemic autoimmune diseases (3%).

Patients with BVP frequently have a cerebellar syndrome and/or downbeat nystagmus syndrome and vice versa (Migliaccio et al. 2004; Zingler et al. 2007; Wagner et al. 2008). In these cases, one assumes a combined neurodegenerative disease which affects the peripheral and central vestibular and cerebellar systems. A variant, which is associated with ataxia and a ganglionopathy of the cranial and peripheral nerves, is the "Cerebellar Ataxia with Neuropathy and Vestibular Areflexia Syndrome" (CANVAS) (◘ Figs. 7.10, 7.11, and 7.12) (Szmulewicz et al. 2011; Kirchner et al. 2011; Pothier et al. 2011; Yacovino et al. 2019). In most cases, this is caused by certain mutations (autosomal recessive homozygote pentamer repeat disease) (Cortese et al. 2019; Rafehi et al. 2019), which are also associated with late-onset ataxias and not specific.

Other rare causes are bilateral vestibular schwannoma (◘ Fig. 7.7, neurofibromatosis type II), a superficial siderosis (◘ Fig. 7.8), and autoimmunological inner ear diseases such as Cogan syndrome (◘ Fig. 7.13) (for review, see Durtette et al. 2017). The latter is characterized by the combination of acute/subacute onset of spinning vertigo/non-spinning vertigo, reduced hearing, tinnitus, and eye pain with red eyes. If Cogan syndrome is not immediately treated, it often leads to BVP and bilateral hearing loss. In patients with Cogan syndrome, MRI typically shows bleedings and contrast enhance-

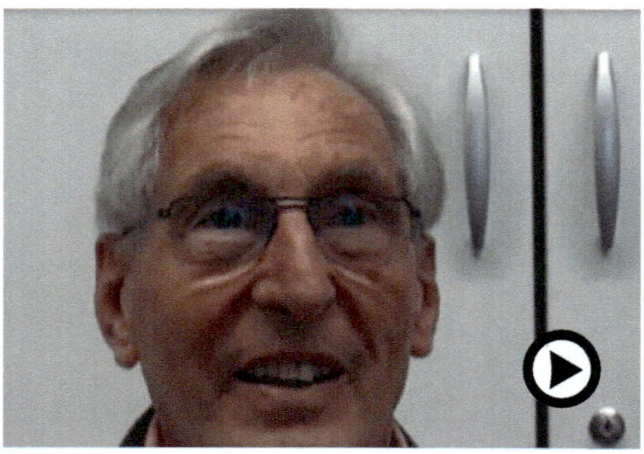

◘ **Fig. 7.10** Patient history in cerebellar ataxia, neuropathy and vestibular areflexia (CANVAS) (▶ https://doi.org/10.1007/000-951)

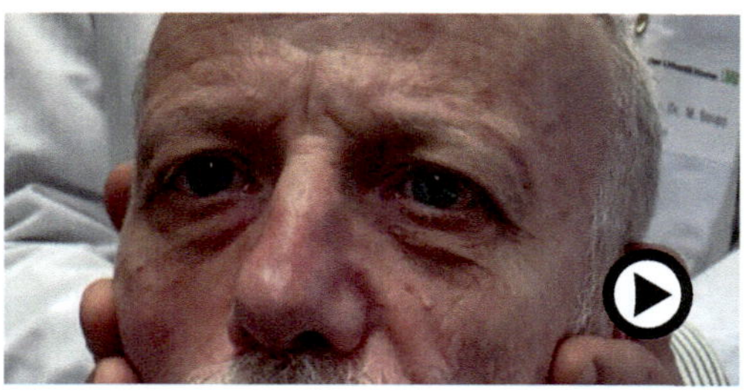

◘ **Fig. 7.11** Bilaterally pathological head impulse test in cerebellar ataxia, neuropathy and vestibular areflexia (CANVAS) (▶ https://doi.org/10.1007/000-952)

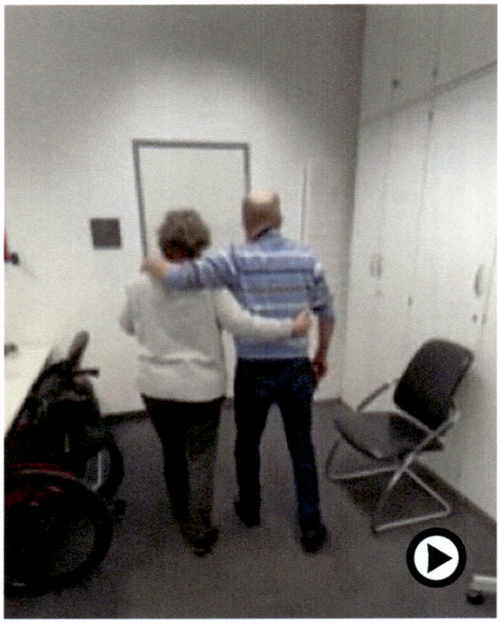

◘ **Fig. 7.12** Impaired walking in cerebellar ataxia, neuropathy and vestibular areflexia (CANVAS) (▶ https://doi.org/10.1007/000-953)

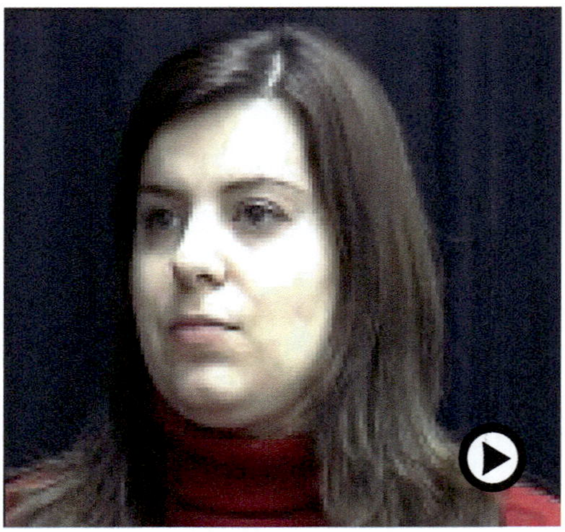

◘ **Fig. 7.13** Cogan-Sydrome: patient history (▶ https://doi.org/10.1007/000-954)

ment in the labyrinth and/or the cochlea. Finally, in a case series, the antiarrhythmic drug amiodarone was identified as an ototoxic substance: 15 of 126 patients (12%) with BVP had an exposition to this drug (Gurkov et al. 2018).

Depending on the etiology of the BVP, not all parts of the labyrinth, i.e., the semicircular canals and otolith organs, are equally impaired. In a retrospective study on 109 patients with BVP caused by aminoglycosides, Menière's disease, infectious inner ear diseases, CANVAS, and other causes, as well as idiopathic cases ($n = 47$), the functional deficits of all three semicircular canals were measured by video-HIT (Tarnutzer et al. 2016). The anterior semicircular canal was less frequently impaired ($n = 86/218$) than the horizontal semicircular canal ($n = 186/218$) or the posterior semicircular canal ($n = 194/218$). This was particularly the case in patients with BVP due to aminoglycosides and Menière's disease and in idiopathic cases. The impairment of the function of the six semicircular canals and four otolith organs also depends on the etiology of the BVP (Tarnutzer et al. 2018). A mean of 6.8 of 10 sensors was impaired. A significantly higher number was found in cases due to aminoglycosides (8.1) or inner ear infections (8.7) than in Menière's disease (5.5).

As mentioned above, an MRI study (3D-FLAIR, 4 h after contrast enhancement, 42 patients with BVP) showed morphological changes in almost 60%: A bilateral vestibular atelectasis was found in 21 of the 42 patients (50%) and a contrast enhancement of the labyrinth in 5 of the 42 patients (Eliezer et al. 2020). Therefore, a high-resolution MRI of the inner ear can contribute to the diagnosis of the underlying etiology.

7.6 Differential Diagnosis and Clinical Problems

The evaluation of the differential diagnosis should focus on two aspects:

- Differentiation from other vestibular and non-vestibular diseases that are also associated with postural imbalance, unsteadiness, and/or oscillopsia (▶ Box 2.1, 2.4 and 2.5)
- Evaluation of the possible underlying etiologies (see ◻ Table 7.1)

Important differential diagnoses:

Disorders with similar symptoms (in alphabetical order):

- Cerebellar ataxias without BVP.
- Cerebellar dizziness (Feil et al. 2019), typically with cerebellar ocular motor disorders in all patients, e.g., saccadic smooth pursuit, gaze-holding deficit, or downbeat nystagmus.
- Downbeat nystagmus syndrome, in particular in those patients without additional signs and symptoms of ataxia.
- Extrapyramidal diseases, such as Parkinson's disease, multiple system atrophy, or tauopathies, in particular progressive supranuclear palsy, which are often initially associated with postural imbalance, gait disorders, and falls.
- Functional dizziness.
- Intoxication, e.g., benzodiazepine or chronic alcohol abuse.
- Normal pressure hydrocephalus or subcortical vascular encephalopathy, in particular if impairment of gait and cognition are the leading symptoms.
- Orthostatic dizziness (Kim et al. 2019).
- Persisting unilateral peripheral vestibular deficit.

- Reduced visual acuity, also due to nystagmus, if oscillopsia is the leading symptom as in fixation pendular nystagmus.
- Syndrome of the third mobile windows (most often superior canal dehiscence syndrome), which can be associated with pressure- or sound-induced oscillopsia.

7.7 Combined Central and Peripheral Vestibular Deficits

There is increasing evidence of a combined impairment of the function of the peripheral and central vestibular systems (Chen and Halmagyi 2018): For instance, acute lesions of the cerebellar flocculus can lead to an isolated functional deficit of both horizontal canals, whereas lesions of the vestibular nuclei are associated with an impairment of the function of both horizontal and posterior semicircular canals.

In a case series of 14 patients with Wernicke encephalopathy, an impairment of the function of both horizontal canals was found in virtually all patients (Lee et al. 2018); this is most likely caused by the neurons of the median vestibular nuclei being extremely sensitive to the thiamine deficiency.

In Gaucher's disease, there is typically an impairment of the function of all semicircular canals with only minimal refixation saccades (Chen and Halmagyi 2018).

Infarctions in the AICA territory often lead to combined peripheral and central symptoms as well as VOR deficits and hearing impairment: ipsilaterally, one finds a deficit of all semicircular canals in combination with a contralateral deficit of the horizontal semicircular canal or a bilaterally isolated deficit of both horizontal canals (Chen and Halmagyi 2018).

7.8 Course of the Disease

A follow-up study of more than 80 patients with BVP over about 5 years showed that, in more than 80% of the patients, there is no significant improvement of vestibular function, which was independent of the etiology, time course of symptoms, sex, and age at the manifestation of the disease (Zingler et al. 2008b).

7.9 Treatment: Therapeutic Principles, Aims, and Pragmatic Therapy

The therapy of BVP is based on five principles:

1. Explanation of the signs and symptoms and the etiology to the patient
2. Primary prophylaxis, i.e., restrictive use of ototoxic substances (in particular, aminoglycosides, amiodarone, certain diuretics)
3. Therapy of the underlying disease, e.g., meningitis, Menière's disease
4. Physiotherapy with lifelong, daily vestibular exercises
5. New therapeutic measures, such as noisy galvanic stimulation, vibrotactile measures such as the balance belt, and—in the foreseeable future—the vestibular implant

7.9.1 Pragmatic Therapy

7.9.1.1 Informing and Educating the Patient

It is important to inform the patients carefully about the type, mechanism of symptoms and signs, and the benign course of their illness in most cases with no further deterioration of function during the course of the disease (Zingler et al. 2008b). It is our experience that the diagnosis of a BVP is still established much too late, despite many visits to the physician, a fact that only intensifies the complaints of the patients. It is important to note that the disease has a pronounced negative impact on physical and social functioning, leading to deterioration of quality of life (Guinand et al. 2012; Lucieer et al. 2018; Lucieer et al. 2020). Frequently, these subjective complaints are reduced by simply informing the patient about the disease. Finally, in terms of treatment with vestibular exercises, it is important to inform the patient that a benefit often occurs only after 6 to 12 weeks of treatment, which is relevant for the patient's compliance, adherence, and persistence to therapy.

7.9.2 Primary Prevention

Primary prevention is most important for the group of patients with ototoxic labyrinthine damage, above all that due to aminoglycosides. Aminoglycoside therapy should be used only if strictly indicated and then only in a once-daily dose. Plasma levels have to be monitored. Patients with renal insufficiency, advanced age, or familial susceptibility to aminoglycoside ototoxicity are at particular risk. Ototoxic antibiotics should not be combined with other ototoxic substances, such as loop diuretics, as this can have a potentiating effect on inner ear damage. Further, amiodarone was also identified as a relevant ototoxic drug (Gurkov et al. 2018). Careful follow-ups of the vestibular and hearing function are necessary during treatment. However, the physician must remain vigilant, as the ototoxic effects of gentamicin have a delayed onset, often appearing only after days or weeks (Magnusson and Padoan 1991).

7.9.3 Causative Treatment

Recovery of vestibular function is possible in post-meningitis cases due to a serous non-suppurative labyrinthitis and in individual cases of autoimmunologically induced forms of inner ear disease, which are diagnosed too infrequently. Although controlled prospective studies are lacking, immune treatment is theoretically expedient, if there are clinical signs of a systemic autoimmune disease or if antibodies against inner ear structures are detected (Schuler et al. 2003; Deutschlander et al. 2005). Initially, corticosteroids can be tried (e.g., prednisolone in doses of 80 mg/day, tapered over ca. 3–4 weeks). In Cogan's syndrome, initially high doses of steroids (1 g i.v. daily for 5 days) have to be given with subsequent dose reduction (for an overview, see Durtette et al. 2017); if the response is inadequate or relapses occur, additional but temporary administration of azathioprine or cyclophosphamide is recommended. In addition, treatment of the causative underlying disease (◘ Table 7.1) is important and in individual cases also successful.

7.9.4 Lifelong, Daily Vestibular Exercises for Stance and Gait and to Prevent Falls

Physical therapy with vestibular exercises should be performed daily and lifelong and has a high level of acceptance among patients. Primarily, it partially substitutes vestibular function with visual and somatosensory function. The substitution was also demonstrated by functional imaging: For instance, during visual stimulation, larger areas of the visual and multisensory cortex were activated in patients with BVP than in healthy controls (Dieterich et al. 2007). The efficacy of vestibular exercises is well proven by several clinical studies (for an overview, see Hall et al. 2022; Dunlap et al. 2019; Sulway and Whitney 2019; Whitney et al. 2020). It is important to inform the patient that it often takes more than 6 to 12 weeks before the patient notices a functional benefit; otherwise, patients may stop the vestibular exercises too early.

Physical therapy, in particular with head movements in all three planes (VOR exercises), can even increase dynamic visual acuity in individual patients due to an improvement of VOR function and saccadic compensatory processes (Lehnen et al. 2018). A more recent approach is so-called increased VOR adaptation, which, in a single case, caused a significant increase of the VOR gain (Gimmon et al. 2019). In addition to vestibular exercises, prevention of falls is particularly relevant in the elderly (for an overview, see Dunlap et al. 2019).

7.10 New Procedures, Measures, and Perspectives

Electrical stimulation of the labyrinth (for a review, see Sluydts et al. 2020) offers many potential treatment options. One option is so-called noisy vestibular stimulation, which increases the basic noise level and the perception of vestibular information (Wuehr et al. 2017). This improves dynamic gait stability (Wuehr et al. 2016), increases spontaneously selected gait velocity (Iwasaki et al. 2018), and reduces the threshold for the contribution of vestibular information to balance control (Schniepp et al. 2018), which seems to be a basic mode of action of noisy vestibular stimulation.

So-called vibrotactile measures, such as the balance belt which gives feedback to the patient about body sway, are now easy to apply and evidently effective in improving stance and gait: 31 of 39 patients reported a benefit (Kingma et al. 2019).

Finally, the vestibular implant (VI) is a promising approach which allows the vestibular deficit to be substituted (Guyot and Perez 2019; Boutabla et al. 2020, Chow et al. 2021). Although several patients have already been implanted, this measure is still in a mainly preclinical phase (Perez et al. 2017). In three patients, it was demonstrated that the function of the VOR could be substituted (Guinand et al. 2017) and the dynamic visual acuity increased (Starkov et al. 2020a). In patients with residual VOR function, there was a positive, but also a negative interaction with the VI (van de Berg et al. 2017a). The VI can also be used to improve otolith function (Fornos et al. 2019; Ramos et al. 2020). The translabyrinthine operative approach seems to be best because this allows hearing to be preserved (van de Berg et al. 2017b); fluoroscopy can improve the precision of the implantation of the electrodes in the semicircular canal (Stultiens et al. 2020). The diagnostic criteria and prerequisites for potential candidates for the VI have been elaborated (van de Berg et al. 2020).

References

Agrawal Y, Bremova T, Kremmyda O, Strupp M (2013) Semicircular canal, saccular and utricular function in patients with bilateral vestibulopathy: analysis based on etiology. J Neurol 260(3):876–883

Agrawal Y, van de Berg R, Wuyts F, Walther L, Magnusson M, Oh E, Sharpe M, Strupp M (2019) Presbyvestibulopathy: diagnostic criteria consensus document of the classification committee of the Barany Society. J Vestib Res 29(4):161–170

Boutabla A, Cavuscens S, Ranieri M, Cretallaz C, Kingma H, van de Berg R, Guinand N, Perez FA (2020) Simultaneous activation of multiple vestibular pathways upon electrical stimulation of semicircular canal afferents. J Neurol 267:273

Brandt T, Schautzer F, Hamilton D, Brüning R, Markowitsch HJ, Kalla R, Darlington CL, Smith PF, Strupp M (2005) Vestibular loss causes hippocampal atrophy and impaired spatial memory in humans. Brain 128:2732–2741

Brantberg K, Lofqvist L (2007) Preserved vestibular evoked myogenic potentials (VEMP) in some patients with walking-induced oscillopsia due to bilateral vestibulopathy. J Vestib Res 17(1):33–38

Chen L, Halmagyi GM (2018) Central lesions with selective Semicircular Canal involvement mimicking bilateral Vestibulopathy. Front Neurol 9:264

Chow MR, Ayiotis AI, Schoo DP, Gimmon Y, Lane KE, Morris BJ, Rahman MA, Valentin NS, Boutros PJ, Bowditch SP, Ward BK, Sun DQ, TreviÃ±o GC, Schubert MC, Carey JP, Della Santina CC (2021) Posture, Gait, Quality of Life, and Hearing with a Vestibular Implant. N Engl J Med 384:(6)521–532

Colebatch JG, Rosengren SM, Welgampola MS (2016) Vestibular-evoked myogenic potentials. Handb Clin Neurol 137:133–155

Cortese A, Simone R, Sullivan R, Vandrovcova J, Tariq H, Yau WY, Humphrey J, Jaunmuktane Z, Sivakumar P, Polke J, Ilyas M, Tribollet E, Tomaselli PJ, Devigili G, Callegari I, Versino M, Salpietro V, Efthymiou S, Kaski D, Wood NW, Andrade NS, Buglo E, Rebelo A, Rossor AM, Bronstein A, Fratta P, Marques WJ, Zuchner S, Reilly MM, Houlden H (2019) Biallelic expansion of an intronic repeat in RFC1 is a common cause of late-onset ataxia. Nat Genet 51(4):649–658

Deutschlander A, Glaser M, Strupp M, Dieterich M, Brandt T (2005) Steroid treatment in bilateral vestibulopathy with inner ear antibodies. Acta Otolaryngol (Stockh) 125:848–851

Dieterich M, Bauermann T, Best C, Stoeter P, Schlindwein P (2007) Evidence for cortical visual substitution of chronic bilateral vestibular failure (an fMRI study). Brain 130(Pt 8):2108–2116

Dobbels B, Lucieer F, Mertens G, Gilles A, Moyaert J, Van de Heyning P, Guinand N, Perez FA, Herssens N, Hallemans A, Vereeck L, Vanderveken O, Van RV, van de Berg R (2020) Prospective cohort study on the predictors of fall risk in 119 patients with bilateral vestibulopathy. PLoS One 15(3):e0228768

Dunlap PM, Holmberg JM, Whitney SL (2019) Vestibular rehabilitation: advances in peripheral and central vestibular disorders. Curr Opin Neurol 32(1):137–144

Durtette C, Hachulla E, Resche-Rigon M, Papo T, Zenone T, Lioger B, Deligny C, Lambert M, Landron C, Pouchot J, Kahn JE, Lavigne C, De WB, Dhote R, Gondran G, Pertuiset E, Quemeneur T, Hamidou M, Seve P, Le GT, Grasland A, Hatron PY, Fain O, Mekinian A (2017) Cogan syndrome: characteristics, outcome and treatment in a French nationwide retrospective study and literature review. Autoimmun Rev 16(12):1219–1223

Eliezer M, Hautefort C, Van NC, Duquesne U, Guichard JP, Herman P, Kania R, Houdart E, Attye A, Toupet M (2020) Electrophysiological and inner ear MRI findings in patients with bilateral vestibulopathy. Eur Arch Otorhinolaryngol 277:1305

Feil K, Strobl R, Schindler A, Krafczyk S, Goldschagg N, Frenzel C, Glaser M, Schoberl F, Zwergal A, Strupp M (2019) What Is Behind Cerebellar Vertigo and Dizziness? Cerebellum 18(3):320–332

Fornos AP, van de Berg R, Armand S, Cavuscens S, Ranieri M, Cretallaz C, Kingma H, Guyot JP, Guinand N (2019) Cervical myogenic potentials and controlled postural responses elicited by a prototype vestibular implant. J Neurol 266(Suppl 1):33–41

Fujimoto C, Murofushi T, Chihara Y, Suzuki M, Yamasoba T, Iwasaki S (2009) Novel subtype of idiopathic bilateral vestibulopathy: bilateral absence of vestibular evoked myogenic potentials in the presence of normal caloric responses. J Neurol 256(9):1488–1492

Fujimoto C, Murofushi T, Chihara Y, Ushio M, Suzuki M, Yamaguchi T, Yamasoba T, Iwasaki S (2013) Effect of severity of vestibular dysfunction on postural instability in idiopathic bilateral vestibulopathy. Acta Otolaryngol 133(5):454–461

Fujimoto C, Yagi M, Murofushi T (2019) Recent advances in idiopathic bilateral vestibulopathy: a literature review. Orphanet J Rare Dis 14(1):202

Gimmon Y, Migliaccio AA, Kim KJ, Schubert MC (2019) VOR adaptation training and retention in a patient with profound bilateral vestibular hypofunction. Laryngoscope 129(11):2568–2573

Gottlich M, Jandl NM, Sprenger A, Wojak JF, Munte TF, Kramer UM, Helmchen C (2016) Hippocampal gray matter volume in bilateral vestibular failure. Hum Brain Mapp 37(5):1998–2006

Goulson AM, McPherson JH, Shepard NT (2014) Background and introduction to whole-body rotational testing. In: Jacobson GP, Shepard NT (eds) Balance unction assessment and management. Plural Publishing Inc.

Guinand N, Boselie F, Guyot JP, Kingma H (2012) Quality of life of patients with bilateral vestibulopathy. Ann Otol Rhinol Laryngol 121(7):471–477

Guinand N, van de Berg R, Cavuscens S, Ranieri M, Schneider E, Lucieer F, Kingma H, Guyot JP, Perez FA (2017) The video head impulse test to assess the efficacy of vestibular implants in humans. Front Neurol 8:600

Gürkov R, Manzari L, Blodow A, Wenzel A, Pavlovic D, Luis L (2018) Amiodarone-associated bilateral vestibulopathy. Eur Arch Otorhinolaryngol 275(3):823–825

Guyot JP, Perez FA (2019) Milestones in the development of a vestibular implant. Curr Opin Neurol 32(1):145–153

Hall CD, Herdman SJ, Whitney SL, Anson ER, Carender WJ, Hoppes CW, Cass SP, Christy JB,

Cohen HS, Fife TD, Furman JM, Shepard NT, Clendaniel RA, Dishman JD, Goebel JA, Meldrum D, Ryan C, Wallace RL, Woodward NJ (2022) Vestibular Rehabilitation for Peripheral Vestibular Hypofunction: An Updated Clinical Practice Guideline From the Academy of Neurologic Physical Therapy of the American Physical Therapy Association. J Neurol Phys Ther 46:(2)118–177

Halmagyi GM, Curthoys IS (1988) A clinical sign of canal paresis. Arch Neurol 45:737–739

Halmagyi GM, Chen L, MacDougall HG, Weber KP, McGarvie LA, Curthoys IS (2017) The video head impulse test. Front Neurol 8:258

Herssens N, Verbecque E, McCrum C, Meijer K, van de Berg R, Saeys W, Vereeck L, Van RV, Hallemans A (2020) A systematic review on balance performance in patients with bilateral vestibulopathy. Phys Ther 100(9):1582–1594

Hong SK, Kim JH, Kim HJ, Lee HJ (2014) Changes in the gray matter volume during compensation after vestibular neuritis: a longitudinal VBM study. Restor Neurol Neurosci 32(5):663–673

Hufner K, Hamilton DA, Kalla R, Stephan T, Glasauer S, Ma J, Bruning R, Markowitsch HJ, Labudda K, Schichor C, Strupp M, Brandt T (2007) Spatial memory and hippocampal volume in humans with unilateral vestibular deafferentation. Hippocampus 17(6):471–485

Iwasaki S, Fujimoto C, Egami N, Kinoshita M, Togo F, Yamamoto Y, Yamasoba T (2018) Noisy vestibular stimulation increases gait speed in normals and in bilateral vestibulopathy. Brain Stimul 11(4): 709–715

Kim S, Oh YM, Koo JW, Kim JS (2011) Bilateral vestibulopathy: clinical characteristics and diagnostic criteria. Otol Neurotol 32(5):812–817

Kim HA, Bisdorff A, Bronstein AM, Lempert T, Rossi-Izquierdo M, Staab JP, Strupp M, Kim JS (2019) Hemodynamic orthostatic dizziness/vertigo: diagnostic criteria. J Vestib Res 29(2–3):45–56

Kingma H, Felipe L, Gerards MC, Gerits P, Guinand N, Perez-Fornos A, Demkin V, van de Berg R (2019) Vibrotactile feedback improves balance and mobility in patients with severe bilateral vestibular loss. J Neurol 266(Suppl 1):19–26

Kirchner H, Kremmyda O, Hufner K, Stephan T, Zingler V, Brandt T, Jahn K, Strupp M (2011) Clinical, electrophysiological, and MRI findings in patients with cerebellar ataxia and a bilaterally pathological head-impulse test. Ann N Y Acad Sci 1233(1):127–138

Kremmyda O, Hufner K, Flanagin VL, Hamilton DA, Linn J, Strupp M, Jahn K, Brandt T (2016) Beyond dizziness: virtual navigation, spatial anxiety and hippocampal volume in bilateral vestibulopathy. Front Hum Neurosci 10:139

Lee SH, Kim SH, Kim JM, Tarnutzer AA (2018) Vestibular dysfunction in Wernicke's encephalopathy: predominant impairment of the horizontal semicircular canals. Front Neurol 9:141

Lehnen N, Kellerer S, Knorr AG, Schlick C, Jahn K, Schneider E, Heuberger M, Ramaioli C (2018) Head-movement-emphasized rehabilitation in bilateral vestibulopathy. Front Neurol 9:562

Lucieer F, Vonk P, Guinand N, Stokroos R, Kingma H, van de Berg R (2016) Bilateral vestibular hypofunction: insights in etiologies, clinical subtypes, and diagnostics. Front Neurol 7:26

Lucieer F, Duijn S, Van RV, Perez FA, Guinand N, Guyot JP, Kingma H, van de Berg R (2018) Full Spectrum of reported symptoms of bilateral vestibulopathy needs further investigation-a systematic review. Front Neurol 9:352

Lucieer FMP, Van HR, van SL DS, Perez-Fornos A, Guinand N, Van RV KH, Joore M, van de Berg R (2020) Bilateral vestibulopathy: beyond imbalance and oscillopsia. J Neurol 267:241

Magnusson M, Padoan S (1991) Delayed onset of ototoxic effects of gentamicin in treatment of Meniere's disease. Rationale for extremely low dose therapy. Acta Otolaryngol (Stockh) 111:671–676

Migliaccio AA, Halmagyi GM, McGarvie LA, Cremer PD (2004) Cerebellar ataxia with bilateral vestibulopathy: description of a syndrome and its characteristic clinical sign. Brain 127(Pt 2):280–293

Neuhauser HK (2016) The epidemiology of dizziness and vertigo. Handb Clin Neurol 137:67–82

Perez FA, Cavuscens S, Ranieri M, van de Berg R, Stokroos R, Kingma H, Guyot JP, Guinand N (2017) The vestibular implant: a probe in orbit around the human balance system. J Vestib Res 27(1):51–61

Petersen JA, Straumann D, Weber KP (2013) Clinical diagnosis of bilateral vestibular loss: three simple bedside tests. Ther Adv Neurol Disord 6(1):41–45

Popp P, Wulff M, Finke K, Ruhl M, Brandt T, Dieterich M (2017) Cognitive deficits in patients with a chronic vestibular failure. J Neurol 264(3):554–563

Pothier DD, Rutka JA, Ranalli PJ (2011) Double impairment: clinical identification of 33 cases of cerebellar ataxia with bilateral vestibulopathy. Otolaryngol Head Neck Surg 146:804–808

Rafehi H, Szmulewicz DJ, Bennett MF, Sobreira NLM, Pope K, Smith KR, Gillies G, Diakumis P, Dolzhenko E, Eberle MA, Barcina MG, Breen DP, Chancellor AM, Cremer PD, Delatycki MB, Fogel BL, Hackett A, Halmagyi GM, Kapetanovic S, Lang A, Mossman S, Mu W, Patrikios P, Perlman SL, Rosemergy I, Storey E, Watson SRD, Wilson MA, Zee DS, Valle D, Amor DJ, Bahlo M, Lockhart PJ (2019) Bioinformatics-based identification of expanded repeats: a non-reference intronic pentamer expansion in RFC1 causes CANVAS. Am J Hum Genet 105(1):151–165

Ramos MA, de MA R, Rodriguez MI, Borkoski BS, Falcon Gonzalez JC (2020) Chronic electrical stimulation of the otolith organ: preliminary results in humans with bilateral vestibulopathy and sensorineural hearing loss. Audiol Neurootol 25(1–2): 79–90

Rinne T, Bronstein AM, Rudge P, Gresty MA, Luxon LM (1998) Bilateral loss of vestibular function: clinical findings in 53 patients. J Neurol 245(6–7):314–321

Rosengren SM, Welgampola MS, Taylor RL (2018) Vestibular-evoked myogenic potentials in bilateral vestibulopathy. Front Neurol 9:252

Schniepp R, Schlick C, Schenkel F, Pradhan C, Jahn K, Brandt T, Wuehr M (2017) Clinical and neurophysiological risk factors for falls in patients with bilateral vestibulopathy. J Neurol 264(2):277–283

Schniepp R, Boerner JC, Decker J, Jahn K, Brandt T, Wuehr M (2018) Noisy vestibular stimulation improves vestibulospinal function in patients with bilateral vestibulopathy. J Neurol 265(Suppl 1): 57–62

Schuler O, Strupp M, Arbusow V, Brandt T (2003) A case of possible autoimmune bilateral vestibulopathy treated with steroids. J Neurol Neurosurg Psychiatry 74(6):825

Sluydts M, Curthoys I, Vanspauwen R, Papsin BC, Cushing SL, Ramos A, de MA R, Borkoski BS, Barbara M, Manrique M, Zarowski A (2020) Electrical vestibular stimulation in humans: a narrative review. Audiol Neurootol 25(1–2):6–24

Smith PF (1997) Vestibular-hippocampal interactions. Hippocampus 7(5):465–471

Sprenger A, Wojak JF, Jandl NM, Helmchen C (2017) Postural control in bilateral vestibular failure: its relation to visual, proprioceptive, vestibular, and cognitive input. Front Neurol 8:444

Starkov D, Guinand N, Lucieer F, Ranieri M, Cavuscens S, Pleshkov M, Guyot JP, Kingma H, Ramat S, Perez-Fornos A, van de Berg R (2020a) Restoring the high-frequency dynamic visual acuity with a vestibular implant prototype in humans. Audiol Neurootol 25(1–2):91–95

Starkov D, Strupp M, Pleshkov M, Kingma H, van de Berg R (2020b) Diagnosing vestibular hypofunction: an update. J Neurol 268:377

Strupp M, Kim JS, Murofushi T, Straumann D, Jen JC, Rosengren SM, Della Santina CC, Kingma H (2017) Bilateral vestibulopathy: diagnostic criteria consensus document of the classification Committee of the Barany Society. J Vestib Res 27(4):177–189

Strupp, M., J. Grimberg, J. Teufel, G. Laurell, H. Kingma, and E. Grill (2020). Worldwide survey on laboratory testing of vestibular function. Neurol Clin Pract 10:(5)379–387

Stultiens JJA, Postma AA, Guinand N, Perez FA, Kingma H, van de Berg R (2020) Vestibular implantation and the feasibility of fluoroscopy-guided electrode insertion. Otolaryngol Clin N Am 53(1):115–126

Sulway S, Whitney SL (2019) Advances in vestibular rehabilitation. Adv Otorhinolaryngol 82:164–169

Szmulewicz DJ, Waterston JA, Halmagyi GM, Mossman S, Chancellor AM, Mclean CA, Storey E (2011) Sensory neuropathy as part of the cerebellar ataxia neuropathy vestibular areflexia syndrome. Neurology 76(22):1903–1910

Tarnutzer AA, Bockisch CJ, Buffone E, Weiler S, Bachmann LM, Weber KP (2016) Disease-specific sparing of the anterior semicircular canals in bilateral vestibulopathy. Clin Neurophysiol 127(8):2791–2801

Tarnutzer AA, Bockisch CJ, Buffone E, Weber KP (2018) Hierarchical cluster analysis of semicircular canal and otolith deficits in bilateral vestibulopathy. Front Neurol 9:244

van de Berg R, Guinand N, Ranieri M, Cavuscens S, Khoa Nguyen TA, Guyot JP, Lucieer F, Starkov D, Kingma H, van HM P-FA (2017a) The vestibular implant input interacts with residual natural function. Front Neurol 8:644

van de Berg R, Lucieer F, Guinand N, van TJ GE, Guyot JP, Kingma H, van HM TY, van OJ P-FA, Stokroos R (2017b) The vestibular implant: hearing preservation during Intralabyrinthine electrode insertion-a case report. Front Neurol 8:137

van de Berg R, Ramos A, Van Rompaey V, Bisdorff A, Perez-Fornos A, Rubinstein JT, Phillips JO, Strupp M, Della Santina CC, Guinand N (2020) The vestibular implant: opinion statement on implantation criteria for research. J Vestib Res 30(3):213–223

van Dooren TS, Starkov D, Lucieer FMP, Vermorken B, Janssen AML, Guinand N, Perez-Fornos A, Van Rompaey V, Kingma H, van de Berg R (2020) Comparison of three video head impulse test systems for the diagnosis of bilateral vestibulopathy. J Neurol 267:(Suppl 1):256–264

Vital D, Hegemann SC, Straumann D, Bergamin O, Bockisch CJ, Angehrn D, Schmitt KU, Probst R (2010) A new dynamic visual acuity test to assess peripheral vestibular function. Arch Otolaryngol Head Neck Surg 136(7):686–691

Wagner JN, Glaser M, Brandt T, Strupp M (2008) Downbeat nystagmus: aetiology and comorbidity in 117 patients. J Neurol Neurosurg Psychiatry 79(6):672–677

Ward BK, Agrawal Y, Hoffman HJ, Carey JP, Della Santina CC (2013) Prevalence and impact of bilateral vestibular hypofunction: results from the 2008

US National Health Interview Survey. JAMA Otolaryngol Head Neck Surg 139(8):803–810
Whitney SL, Sparto PJ, Furman JM (2020) Vestibular rehabilitation and factors that can affect outcome. Semin Neurol 40(1):165–172
Wuehr M, Nusser E, Decker J, Krafczyk S, Straube A, Brandt T, Jahn K, Schniepp R (2016) Noisy vestibular stimulation improves dynamic walking stability in bilateral vestibulopathy. Neurology 86(23):2196–2202
Wuehr M, Decker J, Schniepp R (2017) Noisy galvanic vestibular stimulation: an emerging treatment option for bilateral vestibulopathy. J Neurol 264(Suppl 1):81–86
Yacovino DA, Zanotti E, Hain TC (2019) Is cerebellar ataxia, neuropathy, and vestibular Areflexia syndrome (CANVAS) a vestibular ganglionopathy? J Int Adv Otol 15(2):304–308
Yip CW, Glaser M, Frenzel C, Bayer O, Strupp M (2016) Comparison of the bedside head-impulse test with the video head-impulse test in a clinical practice setting: a prospective study of 500 outpatients. Front Neurol 7:58
Zingler VC, Cnyrim C, Jahn K, Weintz E, Fernbacher J, Frenzel C, Brandt T, Strupp M (2007) Causative factors and epidemiology of bilateral vestibulopathy in 255 patients. Ann Neurol 61(6):524–532
Zingler VC, Weintz E, Jahn K, Bötzel K, Wagner J, Huppert D, Mike A, Brandt T, Strupp M (2008a) Saccular function less affected than canal function in bilateral vestibulopathy. J Neurol 255: 1332–1336
Zingler VC, Weintz E, Jahn K, Mike A, Huppert D, Rettinger N, Brandt T, Strupp M (2008b) Follow-up of vestibular function in bilateral vestibulopathy. J Neurol Neurosurg Psychiatry 79:284–288
zu Eulenburg P, Stoeter P, Dieterich M (2010) Voxel-based morphometry depicts central compensation after vestibular neuritis. Ann Neurol 68(2): 241–249

Acute Unilateral Vestibulopathy/Vestibular Neuritis

Contents

Supplementary Information The online version contains supplementary material available at [https://doi.org/10.1007/978-3-030-78260-3_8]. The videos can be accessed by scanning the related images with the SN More Media App.

M. Strupp et al., *Vertigo and Dizziness*, https://doi.org/10.1007/978-3-030-78260-3_8

(Synonyms used: vestibular neuronitis, acute vestibular loss, acute vestibular failure)

The neutral term "acute unilateral vestibulopathy" (AUVP) (Strupp and Magnusson 2015) as well as "vestibular neuritis" are used in the International Classification of Vestibular Disorders (► Box 8.1 and 8.2, Strupp et al. 2022) since the etiology of this disease has not yet been proven but is assumed to be viral in most cases. The leading symptoms of AUVP are an acute or rarely subacute onset of spinning vertigo, oscillopsia, a tendency to fall to the affected side, nausea, or vomiting. Clinical examination reveals a spontaneous peripheral vestibular nystagmus and a pathological head impulse test. The diagnostic criteria of AUVP/vestibular neuritis and for the probable AUVP/vestibular neuritis are as follows (► Box 8.1, Strupp et al. 2022):

Box 8.1 Diagnostic criteria for Acute Unilateral Vestibulopathy/Vestibular Neuritis

Each of the following criteria have to be fulfilled:

A. Acute or subacute onset of sustained spinning or non-spinning vertigo (i.e., an acute vestibular syndrome) of moderate to severe intensity with symptoms lasting for at least 24 hours.
B. Spontaneous peripheral vestibular nystagmus with a trajectory appropriate to the semicircular canal afferents involved, generally horizontal-torsional, direction-fixed, and enhanced by removal of visual fixation.
C. Unambiguous evidence of reduced VOR function on the side opposite the direction of the fast phase of the spontaneous nystagmus.
D. No evidence for acute central neurological, ontological or audiological symptoms.
E. No acute central neurological signs, namely no central ocular motor or central vestibular signs, in particular no pronounced skew deviation, no gaze-evoked nystagmus, and no acute audiologic or otological signs.
F. Not better accounted for by another disease or disorder.

Box 8.2 Diagnostic criteria for "Probable Acute Unilateral Vestibulopathy"

Each of the following criteria have to be fulfilled:

A. Acute or subacute onset of sustained spinning or non-spinning vertigo (i.e., an acute vestibular syndrome) of moderate to severe intensity with symptoms lasting for at least 24 hours.
B. Spontaneous peripheral vestibular nystagmus with a trajectory appropriate to the semicircular canal afferents involved, generally horizontal-torsional, direction-fixed, and enhanced by removal of visual fixation.
C. No clear evidence of reduced VOR function by bedside examination on the side opposite the direction of the fast phase of the spontaneous nystagmus.
D. No evidence for acute central neurological, ontological or audiological symptoms.
E. No acute central neurological signs, namely no central ocular motor or central vestibular signs, in particular no pronounced skew deviation, no gaze-evoked nystagmus, and no acute audiologic or otological signs.
F. Not better accounted for by another disease or disorder.

8.1 Epidemiology

An annual incidence of 3.5–15.5 per 100,000 persons was reported (Sekitani et al. 1993; Adamec et al. 2015); however, since the diagnostic criteria are not uniform, there are so far no valid state-of-the-art epidemiological studies (Neuhauser 2016). Two studies found no evidence for seasonal differences (Adamec et al. 2015; Koors et al. 2013). In a large cohort of more than 39000 patients who had a standardized evaluation, AUVP was the sixth most common cause of vertigo/dizziness and the third most common cause of peripheral vestibular disorders (BPPV ranks first, Menière's disease second). This ranking is also true for children (Gioacchini et al. 2014; Jahn et al. 2015). The usual age of onset is between 30 and 60 years (Depondt 1973; Adamec et al. 2015), with age distribution plateaus between 40 and 50 years (Sekitani et al. 1993; Adamec et al. 2015). There is no significant gender difference. The reported recurrence rate varies between 1.9% (Huppert et al. 2006) and 10.7% (Kim et al. 2011).

8.2 Diagnosis

8.2.1 Patient History

The **leading symptoms** of AUVP (◘ Fig. 8.1) are as follows:

- Acute or rarely subacute onset of sustained spinning or non-spinning vertigo, with symptoms untreated lasting at least 24 h. There are no antecedent signs or triggers, except for occasional spells of vertigo a few days before in some patients (Lee et al. 2009a). The vestibular symptoms typically worsen during head and body movements, so patients intuitively try to avoid any movements.
- Apparent movement of the visual surroundings (oscillopsia) due to the spontaneous nystagmus; patients often only report this when specifically asked about it.
- Postural imbalance with a tendency to fall in the direction of the slow phase of nystagmus (i.e., toward the side of the affected ear).
- Nausea and often vomiting.

To make the diagnosis—since there is no proving test—the absence of coinciding acute hearing loss, tinnitus, ear pain, or neurological symptoms, in particular from the brainstem and cerebellum, is required. Other events such as a recent trauma must also be excluded. Patients often have to be explicitly asked about symptoms.

8.2.2 Bedside Examination

For bedside examination of the patient, the following six tests are of particular interest (◘ Fig. 8.1):

- *Examination for spontaneous nystagmus* without and with Frenzel's goggles or M-glasses (◘ Fig. 8.2) (for references, see (Halmagyi et al. 2020)): There is a horizontal-torsional nystagmus with the fast phase beating toward the suspected non-affected ear (fast phase toward the more active labyrinth) with a torsional (beating counterclockwise-left or clockwise-right from the patient's point of view) and small upward component in AUVP. A peripheral vestibular spontaneous nystagmus is typically reduced in amplitude by fixation due to fixation suppression of the VOR. However, the strongly nauseated patient may not be able to cooperate adequately during the acute presentation of symptoms and in the very acute phase patients are often not able to significantly suppress the nystagmus. The intensity of spontaneous nystagmus is enhanced with Frenzel's goggles or M-glasses as well as by eye closure (that can be observed as seen or palpated through closed eyelids). Important to note: A nystagmus which is not reduced in intensity by visual fixation

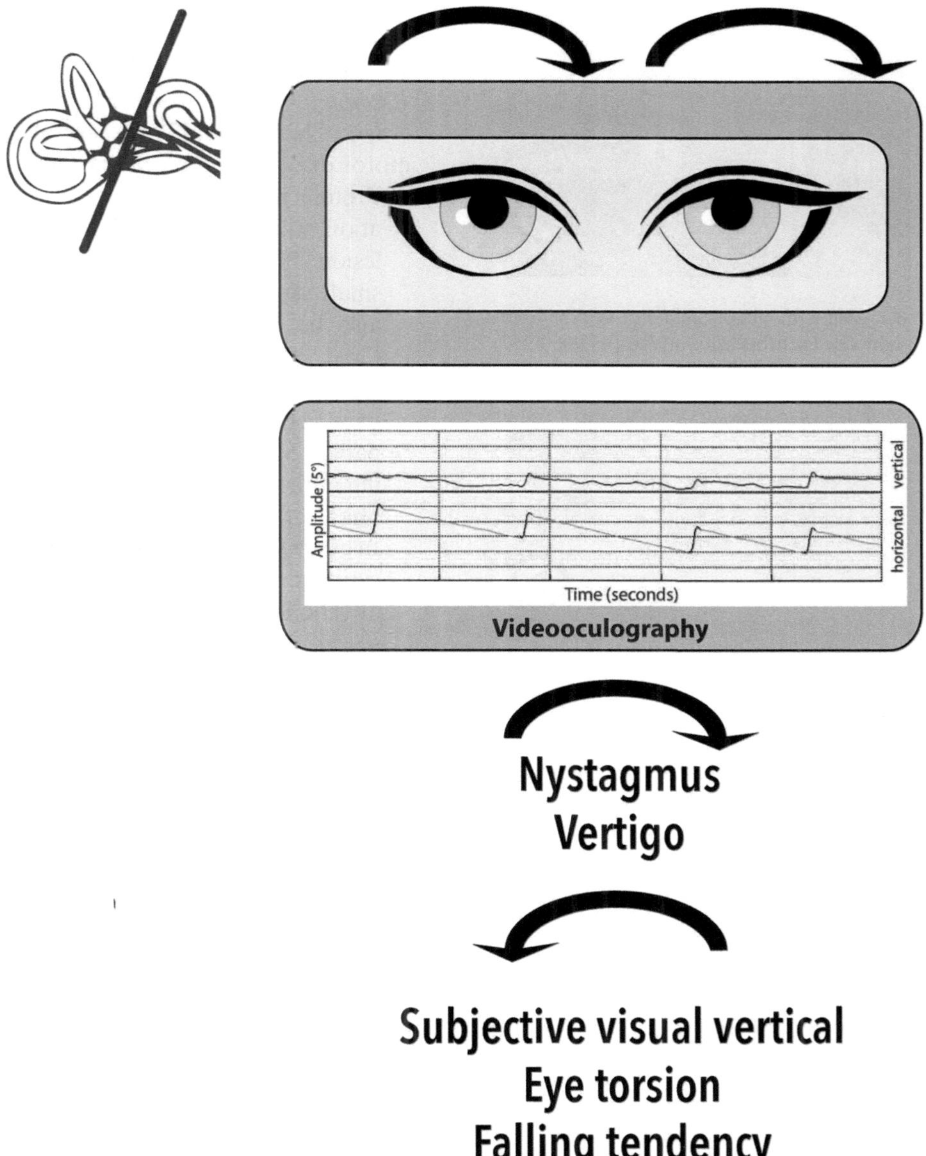

Fig. 8.1 Symptoms and signs of acute unilateral vestibulopathy (AUVP)/vestibular neuritis. Spinning or non-spinning vertigo toward the non-affected side, tendency to fall toward the affected side, and deviation of subjective visual vertical toward the affected side. Horizontal-torsional nystagmus with the fast phase beating toward the non-affected side with a torsional (beating counterclockwise-left or clockwise-right from the patient's point of view) and small upward component; it is reduced or suppressed by visual fixation

is not a peripheral vestibular spontaneous nystagmus; this implies that there are also central types, e.g., in brainstem infarction, which can be reduced by fixation (Mantokoudis et al. 2021b). According to Alexander's law, amplitude and slow-phase velocity are increased with gaze shifts toward the direction of the fast phase and decreased with gaze shifts toward the direction of the slow phase

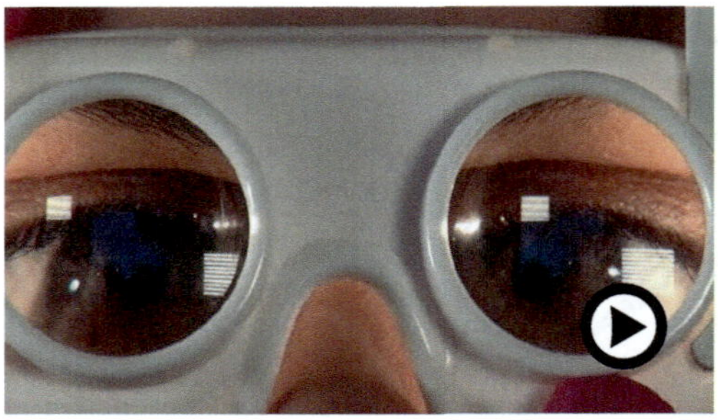

Fig. 8.2 Signs of acute unilateral vestibulopathy on the right side (▶ https://doi.org/10.1007/000-957)

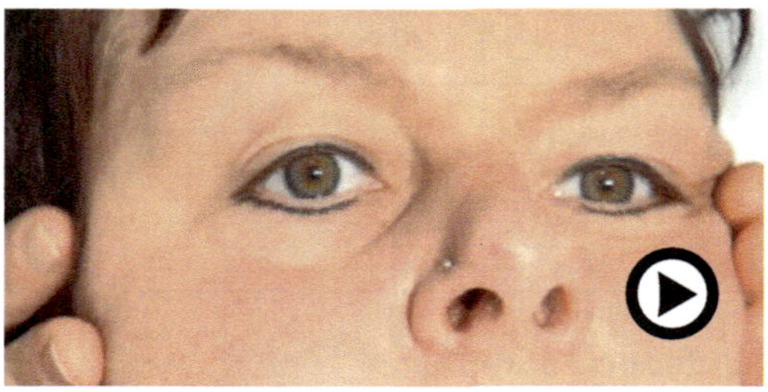

Fig. 8.3 Head impulse test in acute unilateral vestibulopathy on the left side (▶ https://doi.org/10.1007/000-956)

of the nystagmus. These are the typical characteristics of spontaneous peripheral vestibular nystagmus (for references, see Eggers et al. 2019; Strupp et al. 2021).

- *Head impulse test:* Pathological with a refixation saccade when the head is turned toward the suspected affected side (Fig. 8.3). If the result of the bedside HIT is unclear, a video-HIT and/or caloric testing are necessary; if available the video-HIT is strongly prefered also in the emergency room because it further increases the diagnostic accuracy (Machner et al. 2021a, 2021b). A normal HIT has a high negative predictive value.
- *Measurement of subjective visual vertical:* There is a mono- and binocular pathological deviation toward the affected ear (Bohmer and Rickenmann 1995, for references, see Dieterich and Brandt 2019) as one component of the *incomplete* ocular tilt reaction (see below) in AUVP.
- *Romberg Test:* Postural imbalance on the Romberg test, increased with the eyes closed, typically shows falling toward slow phase of nystagmus, i.e., the affected ear (Brandt and Dieterich 1993b).
- *Examination for central ocular motor disorders:* There should be no central ocular motor disorders, in particular *no*:
  - Prominent skew deviation/vertical deviation which would indicate a central lesion (Brandt and Dieterich 1993a). A small skew deviation of up to 3° can also be found in AUVP (Green and Gold, 2021; Korda et al. 2022).
  - Gaze-evoked nystagmus. To look for a gaze-holding deficit in AUVP, the patient has to be examined while looking in the opposite direction to the fast phase of the spontaneous nystagmus. In case of gaze-evoked nystagmus, indicating a central deficit, there will be a direction-changing nystagmus. This is a so-called Bruns' nystagmus which is found in about 30% of patients with an acute central vestibular syndrome (Mantokoudis et al. 2021a).
  - Pure vertical, pure horizontal, or pure torsional nystagmus.
- *Examination of hearing*: Hearing loss can be screened by using the finger rub test. The type of the hearing loss can be suspected by using the Rinne and Weber tests. An otoscopy has to be performed if indicated. There should be no evidence for acute hearing loss or, e.g., for herpes zoster when examining the ear by otoscopy.

8.2.3 Laboratory Tests

Since the bedside HIT is not very reliable to diagnose a vestibular deficit (Yip et al. 2016), laboratory tests are necessary to quantify the function of the VOR with:

- *Video head impulse test* (video-HIT) (Bartl et al. 2009; MacDougall et al. 2009; Halmagyi et al. 2017) to examine whether there is a VOR deficit in the high-frequency range (deficit: the gain should be less than <0.7

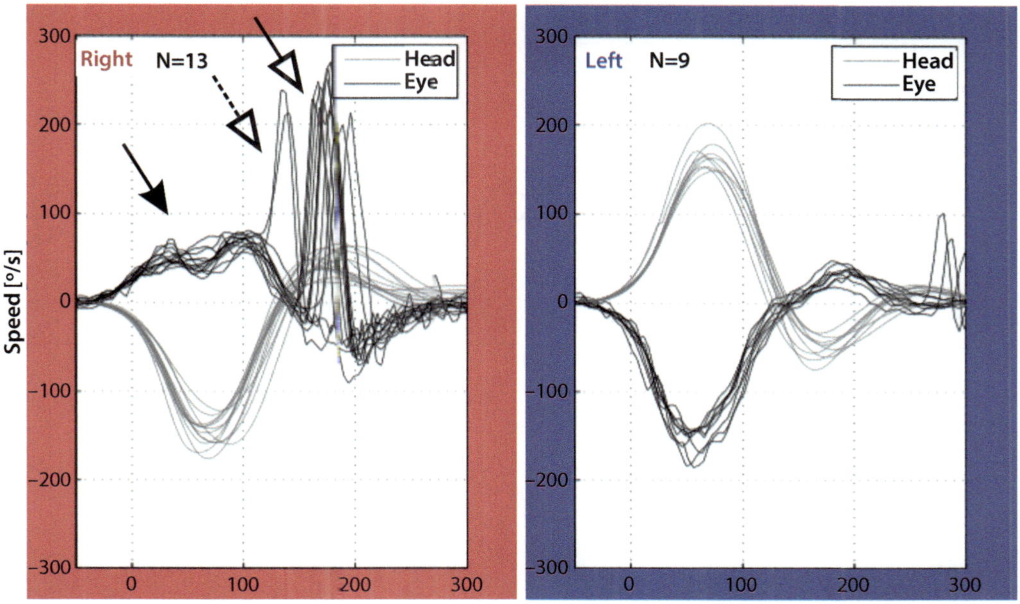

Fig. 8.4 Horizontal video head impulse test of a patient with right-sided vestibulopathy. The angular velocity of the eye and head movements is measured in °/s over a period of 300 ms, the integral of the area under curve is measured and the VOR gain calculated on this basis. In this patient, the VOR gain on the right side is about 0.3 (black arrow) and refixation saccades can be seen (white arrows)

and the side difference > 0.3) (Fig. 8.4); this also is helpful to differentiate between a peripheral and central vestibular lesion because a normal video-HIT is not compatible with AUVP (Chen et al. 2014; Mantokoudis et al. 2015; Saber Tehrani et al. 2018). The video-HIT is strongly recommended because of its high value for the diagnosis of AUVP (Manzari et al 2021) and because the video-HIT can be also used in the emergency department for quantitative testing and for discrimination between peripheral and central lesions (Chen et al. 2014, Mantokoudis 2015, Machner 2021a, b); if the video-HIT is normal, caloric testing is indicated.

- *Caloric testing* which should show a hypo- or unresponsiveness of the tested and affected horizontal canal (it tests the VOR in the low-frequency range of about 0.003 Hz). Since there is a large interindividual variability of the nystagmus induced by caloric irrigation and a small intraindividual variability of the response of the right and the left labyrinths, "Jongkees' formula for vestibular paresis" (Jongkees et al. 1962): (((R30° + R44°) – (L30° + L44°))/(R30° + R44° + L30° + L44°)) × 100 should be used to determine its presence. In this formula, for instance, R30° is the mean peak slow-phase velocity during caloric irrigation with 30 °C water. Vestibular paresis is usually defined as >25% asymmetry between the two sides (Honrubia 1994) or an absolute value for the sum of the mean peak slow phase velocity of the irrigation with warm and cold water <6°/s (Fig. 8.5). An advantage of caloric testing is that allows the separate examination of each labyrinth, in contrast to the video-HIT and rotational testing.

It is important to note that in rare "inferior vestibular neuritis," which affects the posterior canal only (see below), caloric testing and the video-HIT for the horizontal canal are typically normal.

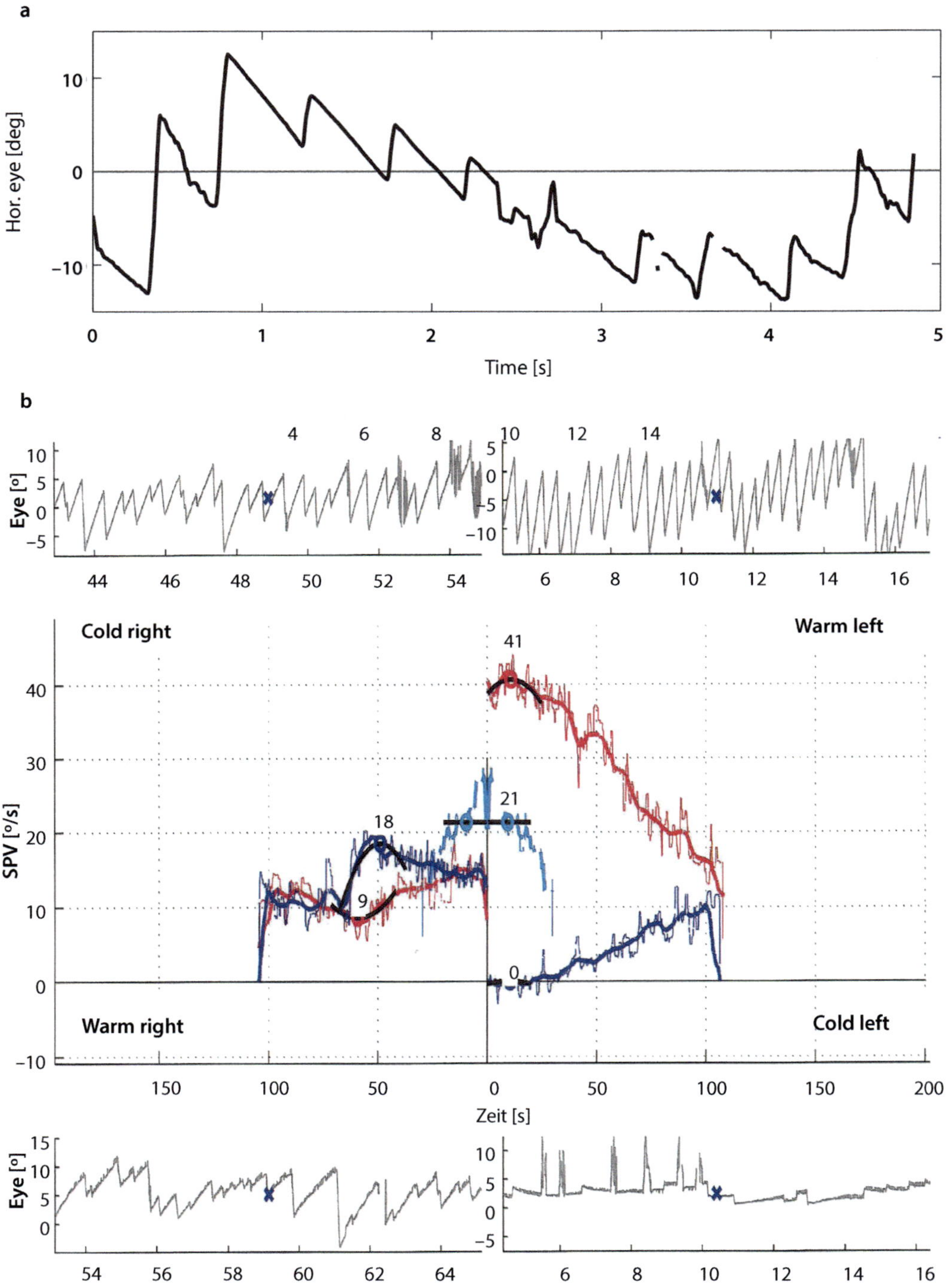

Fig. 8.5 **a**, **b** Caloric testing in a patient with an acute right-sided vestibulopathy. **a** The mean slow-phase velocity of the spontaneous nystagmus is about 21°/s (which eplains the shift of the baseline in **b**) with the fast phase beating toward the more active labyrinth; **b** caloric-induced nystagmus shows a significant hypofunction on the right side: 45% side difference according to the vestibular paresis formula of Jongkees (Jongkees et al. 1962)

8.3 Complementary Laboratory Examinations

8.3.1 Cervical and Ocular VEMP (c/oVEMP)

In contrast to video-HIT and caloric testing, VEMP are much less relevant for the diagnosis of AUVP (for references, see (Fife et al. 2017)). c/oVEMP help to differentiate between superior AUVP, which is the most frequent form, very rare inferior AUVP, and even rarer complete AUVP, which affects the superior and the inferior vestibular nerve and thus all semicircular canals and both otolith organs. oVEMP (Rosengren et al. 2019), which mainly evaluate the function of the utricle, are typically reduced or absent in superior and complete AUVP (Oh et al. 2013; Curthoys et al. 2011), since the pars superior of the vestibular nerve innervates the utricle (see below). cVEMP, which mainly evaluate the function of the saccule, that is mainly innervated by the inferior vestibular nerve, are reduced or absent in inferior and complete AUVP (Chihara et al. 2012; Curthoys 2012; Manzari et al. 2013; Murofushi et al. 1996; Oh et al. 2013).

8.3.2 Imaging

If the patient history and/or the clinical examination provide evidence of an acute central vestibular syndrome (ACVS), immediate imaging is indicated. CT can be used to rule out a hemorrhage; CT angiography allows the diagnosis of vertebral or basilar artery stenosis. It should be noted that even diffusion-weighted MRI in small brainstem or cerebellar lesions <10 mm is normal within the first 48 h after symptom onset in 50% of patients (Saber Tehrani et al. 2018). This strongly further supports the relevance of a systematic patient history and the clinical bedside examination of the vestibular and ocular motor systems to look for central signs, which permit a differentiation between AUVP and ACVS with a sensitivity and a specificity of about 90% (Cnyrim et al. 2008; Kattah et al. 2009; Saber Tehrani et al. 2018).

Imaging studies can also demonstrate that there might be a contrast enhancement of the vestibular nerve, in particular the superior vestibular nerve, 1–4 h after gadolinium injection (Byun et al. 2018; Eliezer et al. 2019; Venkatasamy et al. 2019); so far, this has no major clinical relevance. Finally, high-resolution MRI examinations ≥6 months after symptom onset in patients with a persisting peripheral deficit demonstrated an atrophy of the vestibular nerve in 5 of the 10 patients examined, in particular of the superior vestibular nerve (Freund et al. 2020).

8.3.3 Audiogram and Otoscopy

If there is evidence from the patient history and/or the clinical examination of an impairment of hearing, for instance, in the finger rub and/or Rinne and Weber test, an audiogram is indicated, in particular since patients with an attack of Menière's disease and patients with an AICA infarction show an impairment of hearing. If a patient complains of ear pain, otoscopy is indicated, namely to look for herpes zoster or otitis media.

8.4 Differential Diagnosis and Clinical Problems

It should be noted that the diagnosis of AUVP is a diagnosis of exclusion. The most important differential diagnoses are as follows:

- Acute central vestibular syndrome due to a lesion, most often an infarction, in the brainstem or the cerebellum.
- Combined acute central and peripheral lesions, for instance due to an AICA

infarction which can affect the labyrinth, cerebellum, and/or brainstem (Lee et al. 2009b).
- Other central vestibular syndromes, e.g., first attack of vestibular migraine.
- Other inner ear diseases, e.g., first attack of Menière's disease.

8.4.1 Acute Central Vestibular Syndrome (ACVS)

An ACVS which can mimic AUVP (vestibular pseudoneuritis) can occur due to:
1. A lesion in the root entry zone of the vestibular nerve in the lateral medulla (e.g., in multiple sclerosis (◘ Fig. 8.6)) or small lacunar strokes (Thömke and Hopf 1999), causing a fascicular nerve lesion.
2. A small lacunar infarction of the vestibular nuclei (◘ Fig. 8.7) (Kim and Lee 2010) or, e.g., the dorsolateral pons affecting the cerebellar peduncle (Chang and Wu 2010).
3. A small cerebellar infarction, e.g., of the flocculus which can even lead to a pathological HIT (Park et al. 2013) (for details, see ► Chap. 13).

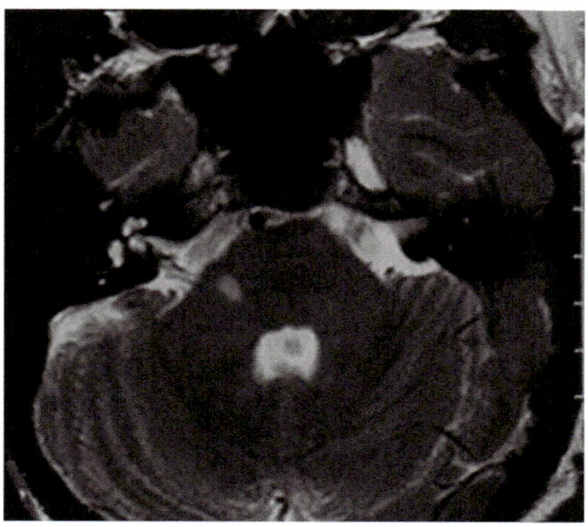

◘ **Fig. 8.6** Fascicular lesion of the right vestibular nerve, i.e., between the entry of the eighth nerve in the brainstem and the vestibular nuclei, in a patient with multiple sclerosis and the clinical features of an acute central vestibular syndrome

A sensitive and specific instrument to differentiate between AUVP and an ACVS is the combination of the patient history, with particular consideration of the ABDC² score (for references, see (Diener and Frank 2015)), and the clinical examination, in particular the HINTS and the HINTS plus (which includes testing of hearing) protocol (Cnyrim et al. 2008; Kattah et al. 2009; Saber Tehrani et al. 2018) to look for central signs (for references, see (Zwergal and Dieterich 2020; Kerber 2020; Gurley and Edlow 2019)).

Patient history The following aspects of the patient history would support a central origin:
- Cardiovascular risk factors, such as arterial hypertension, diabetes, nicotine consumption, atrial fibrillation, history of stroke or myocardial infarction
- Age > 60 years
- First attack of vertigo/dizziness
- Spontaneous occurence (i.e. no BPPV)
- Central additional symptoms, such as double vision, hemiparesis, hemi hypesthesia, or hemiataxia

▪ Bedside examination

The following five clinical signs (HINTS and HINTS plus) support a ***central*** origin (Cnyrim et al. 2008; Kattah et al. 2009; Saber Tehrani et al. 2018):
- Prominent vertical deviation/skew deviation (> 3°) (◘ Fig. 8.8): This is a sign of a central lesion, but only has a very low sensitivity because it is found in only 30% of patients with an acute brainstem or cerebellar lesion (Brandt and Dieterich 1993a). Small deviations can also be found in patients with AUVP (Green and Gold 2021; Korda et al. 2022), probably due to an impairment of utricular pathways.
- Type of spontaneous nystagmus: A spontaneous nystagmus that is not reduced or suppressed by visual fixation is not a

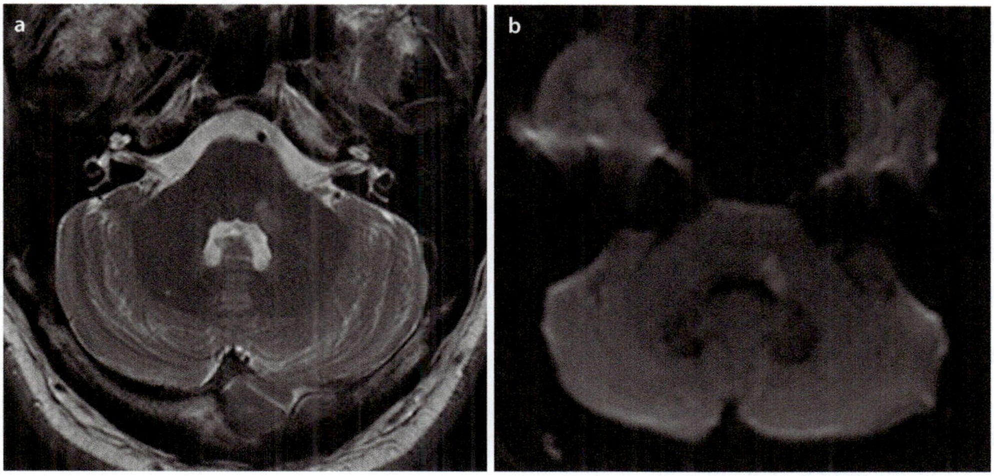

◘ **Fig. 8.7** **a, b** Acute ischemic lesion in the left vestibular nuclei region with a clinical picture of an acute central vestibular syndrome: **left** T2-weighted, **right** diffusion-weighted sequence

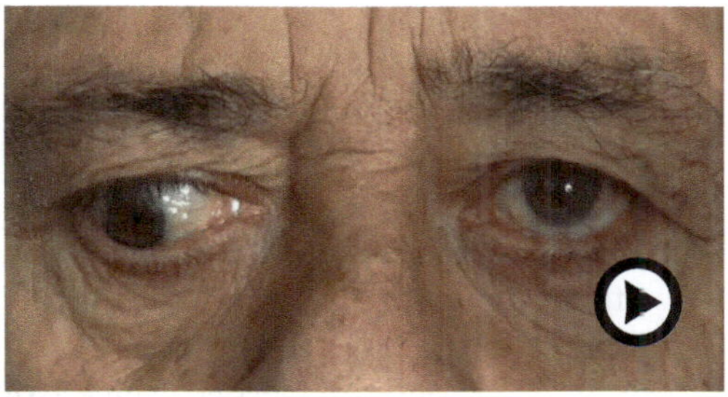

◘ **Fig. 8.8** Acute central vestibular syndrome with a skew deviation (▶ https://doi.org/10.1007/000-955)

peripheral vestibular spontaneous nystagmus (for references, see (Halmagyi et al. 2020)). It is important to note that that there are also central types of spontaneous nystagmus, e.g., in brainstem infarction, which can be reduced by fixation (Mantokoudis 2021b). A pure vertical nystagmus and a pure torsional nystagmus indicate a central lesion. A pure horizontal nystagmus also indicates a central lesion; however, it is also found in horizontal canal BPPV.

- A horizontal gaze-evoked nystagmus in the opposite direction to the fast phase of the spontaneous nystagmus i.e. a so-called Bruns' nystagmus (according to Alexander's law, the intensity of a spontaneous nystagmus increases when looking in the direction of the fast phase and therefore it is not helpful as a clinical sign to diagnose gaze-evoked nystagmus) or a vertical gaze-evoked nystagmus.
- A normal head impulse test in acute vestibular syndrome with nystagmus is not compatible with a peripheral lesion. It is important to note that the head impulse test can also be pathological in central lesions, in particular in a fascicular or nuclear lesion (◘ Figs. 8.5 and 8.6) or in floccular lesions (Park et al. 2013).
- Head-shaking nystagmus: If horizontal head-shaking leads to a change in the direction of the nystagmus or to a vertical nystagmus (cross-coupling) (◘ Fig. 8.9) (Choi et al. 2016a; Huh and Kim 2011), this is compatible with a central lesion, but it is not very specific (Yang et al. 2020).

Isolated clinical signs, such as prominent skew deviation, a normal HIT or a Bruns' nystagmus are specific, but not very sensitive (Cnyrim et al. 2008; Kattah et al. 2009; Newman-Toker et al. 2008). The combination of these clinical signs has a sensitivity and specificity of 80–95% (Cnyrim et al. 2008; New-

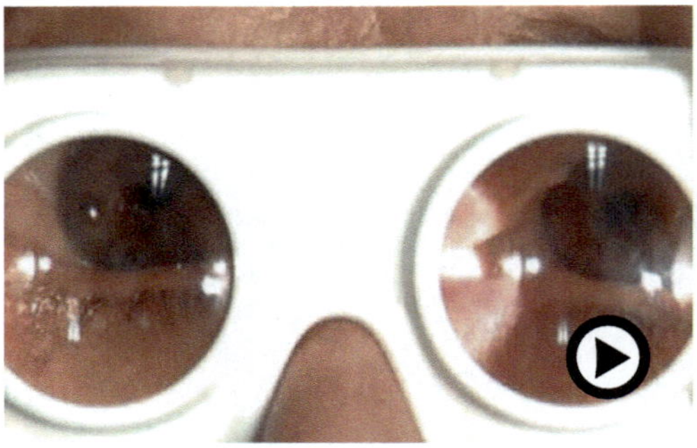

Fig. 8.9 Head shaking test with cross-coupling in a central lesion (▶ https://doi.org/10.1007/000-958)

man-Toker et al. 2008; Kattah et al. 2009; Chen et al. 2011). A meta-analysis (5 studies, 617 patients) concluded that the findings also depend on who is performing the examination (Ohle et al. 2020): Neurologists who used HINTS had a sensitivity of 96.7% and a specificity of 94.8%. Physicians, including neurologists, working in an ENT department had a sensitivity of 83% and a specificity of only 44%. This highlights the importance of combining the patient history, the $ABCD^2$ score, and HINTS.

Finally, the video-HIT also contributes to the differential diagnosis: a bilaterally normal or a bilaterally reduced or even increased VOR gain and crossed vertical refixation saccades are central signs (Choi et al. 2018a).

- **Cerebellar infarctions**

Infarctions in the territory of the posterior inferior cerebellar artery (PICA), the anterior inferior cerebellar artery (AICA) and rarely the superior cerebellar artery (SCA) can also manifest as ACVS. This is particularly true for PICA infarctions (Duncan et al. 1975; Huang and Yu 1985; Magnusson and Norrving 1991), which can lead to a vestibular pseudoneuritis. Cerebellar infarctions can also cause an incomplete ocular tilt reaction (OTR) (Mossman and Halmagyi 2000), in particular if the dentate nucleus (Baier et al. 2008), the flocculus (Park et al. 2013), the nodulus (Lee et al. 2019), the tonsil, uvula, and middle cerebellar peduncle (Baier et al. 2008) are affected.

Infarctions in the AICA territory, which supplies the cerebellum, brainstem, and inner ear, can manifest as ACVS with strong lateropulsion and hearing impairment in combination with central symptoms and signs (Lee et al. 2002; Lee et al. 2006): pseudolabyrinthitis (Choi et al. 2016b). It should be noted that they are often associated with acute severe unilateral hearing loss due to an infarction in the territory of the labyrinthine artery, which supplies the cochlea, the semicircular canals, and the otolith organs.

For clinical practice, it has been shown that the combination of the patient history, including the $ABCD^2$ score, and a systematic examination of the vestibular and the ocular motor systems with a particular focus on central signs allows a differentiation between an acute peripheral and an acute central vestibular syndrome (see ▶ Chap. 13).

Vestibular migraine The leading symptom of vestibular migraine (see ▶ Chap. 14; current diagnostic criteria (Lempert et al. 2012)) is also an acute onset of vertigo which can last for up to 72 h and which can also be associated with peripheral vestibular spontaneous nystagmus (von Brevern M. et al. 2005). Therefore, the differential diagnosis can be difficult, in particular in a first attack of vestibular migraine. Helpful criteria are a history of migraine, typical migrainous symptoms with the attack of vertigo, and a normal HIT during an attack.

8.4.2 Other Peripheral Vestibular Disorders

There is a broad spectrum of other peripheral vestibular disorders that can lead to similar symptoms and signs. Important differential diagnoses are Menière's disease that can begin monosymptomatically (see ▶ Chap. 10) or longer-lasting attacks in

Table 8.1 Peripheral vestibular syndromes as differential diagnoses for AUVP

Diagnosis	Clinical characteristics
Cogan's syndrome	Double triad: Vertigo, bilateral hearing loss/tinnitus, eye pain/"red eyes" Bilateral, often asymmetric peripheral vestibular deficits, bilateral hypoacusis, interstitial keratitis Symptoms or deficits often rapidly progress Mostly in young women; relatively rare, but requires immediate immunosuppressive therapy
Herpes zoster oticus (Ramsay-Hunt syndrome)	Initially burning ear pain and blisters, vertigo, hearing disorders, and facial paresis Can lead to complete AUVP, including a vertical deviation/skew deviation (Arbusow et al. 1998) Often contrast enhancement of the affected cranial nerves on MRI
Cupulolithiasis and canalithiasis of a horizontal canal	Clinical examination reveals horizontal spontaneous nystagmus which changes direction during the lean-and-bow test (Choi et al. 2018b) and during the diagnostic positioning maneuvers, which is helpful for the differential diagnosis. See also ► Chap. 9 and the current diagnostic criteria (von Brevern et al. 2015).
Serous or purulent labyrinthitis	Associated with ear pain, reduced hearing, and/or tinnitus. The course of the disease can be acute, subacute, or slowly progressive. Otoscopy is necessary.
Menière's disease	Can begin mono- or oligosymptomatically. Then, the differential diagnosis is difficult and can only be made during the course of the disease. See also ► Chap. 10 and the current diagnostic criteria (Lopez-Escamez et al. 2015).
Vestibular paroxysmia	In single cases, the oligosymptomatic attacks may last for hours and be associated with peripheral vestibular spontaneous nystagmus. Therefore, the diagnosis can only be made during the course of the disease. See also ► Chap. 11 and the current diagnostic criteria (Strupp et al. 2016).
Vestibular schwannoma	Often a slowly progressive course of the disease and associated with impairment of hearing and/or tinnitus. Nowadays, often diagnosed in patients who have impairment of hearing by means of contrast-enhanced MRI. Symptoms often occur only in the later stage of the disease. In rare cases, it may also be associated with attacks of vertigo.

vestibular paroxysmia, both of which can be associated with spontaneous nystagmus (see ► Chap. 11). The short duration of the episodes and the quick recovery of patients can be helpful for the differentiation. In addition, patients with Menière's disease develop other ear symptoms and signs during the course of the disease.

Cupulolithiasis and canalithiasis of a horizontal semicircular canal (see ► Chap. 9) also leads to spinning vertigo and horizontal nystagmus. Symptoms and signs in horizontal canal BPPV, however, occur in attacks that depend on head position and there is a change in the direction of the horizontal nystagmus during the lean-and-bow test and during the positioning maneuvers (Choi et al. 2018b).

Important inflammatory inner ear diseases that are associated with an acute peripheral vestibular syndrome are zoster oticus and labyrinthitis. Zoster oticus is usually associated with efflorescence and often with lesions of other cranial nerves, i.e., the facial nerve, and, like labyrinthitis, it is also associated with ear pain. In these patients, otoscopy is indicated. In Table 8.1, the most relevant peripheral vestibular diseases as differential diagnoses are summarized with their clinical features.

8.5 Diagnosis: The Essentials for Clinical Practice

The diagnosis of AUVP is a diagnosis of exclusion. It requires very careful taking of the patient history, with a particular focus on the $ABCD^2$ score and potential central symptoms, a systematic neurological and neuro-otological examination, ideally including video-HIT, a neurophthalmological examination, in particular to look for a prominent vertical deviation gaze-holding deficits and other central ocular motor disorders, and testing of hearing.

8.6 Pathophysiology and Pathological Anatomy

Static deficits, e.g., spinning vertigo, spontaneous peripheral vestibular nystagmus Normal vestibular end organs generate an equal resting-firing frequency of the axons, which is the same on both sides. This continuous excitation (resting discharge rate in monkey ≈100 Hz (Goldberg and Fernandez 1971); 18,000 vestibular afferents for each labyrinth (Bergstrom 1973), i.e., 1.8 million action potentials per second) is transmitted to the vestibular nuclei via the vestibular nerves. Pathological processes affecting an end organ or vestibular nerve alter its firing frequency, thereby creating a vestibular tone imbalance. This causes spontaneous nystagmus with the slow phase (which is the pathological component of the nystagmus) of the eye movements toward the impaired labyrinth. This imbalance is also the cause of the other manifestations on different levels, i.e., perceptual (spinning vertigo, ipsilateral displacement of the subjective vertical (for references, see (Dieterich and Brandt 2019)), ocular motor (ipsilateral ocular torsion in addition to spontaneous nystagmus), postural (ipsilateral gait deviation or falling), and vegetative (nausea). The static deficits are compensated over weeks (for ref. see (Lacour et al. 2016)).

Dynamic deficits Dynamic deficits of the VOR can be demonstrated by HIT, video-HIT, caloric irrigation, and rotational testing. If the peripheral vestibular deficit persists, the dynamic deficits do not recover because they cannot be compensated.

Superior vestibular nerve, inferior vestibular nerve, or total vestibular nerve lesion The 3-D features of the spontaneous nystagmus and the dynamic deficit of the VOR of the horizontal, anterior, and posterior semicircular canals were measured in patients with vestibular neuritis by means of the scleral coil technique and analyzed by a vector analysis previously in 1996 (Fetter and Dichgans 1996b). These measurements supported the earlier view (Büchele and Brandt 1988) that AUVP is—in most cases—a partial rather than a total unilateral vestibular lesion (see below): It most often affects the superior division of the vestibular nerve only (innervating the horizontal and anterior semicircular canals, the maculae of the utricle, and the antero-superior part of the sacculus), which has its own path and ganglion (Lorente de Nó 1933; Sando et al. 1972), whereas the inferior vestibular nerve (innervating the posterior semicircular canal and the postero-inferior part of the sacculus) is most often spared, leading to "superior vestibular neuritis." These findings were further supported by (a) measurements of the function of individual semicircular canals with the head impulse test and the scleral coil technique (Bohmer et al. 1997; Fetter and Dichgans 1996a; Aw et al. 2001) and (b) VEMP studies with the cVEMP being most often normal and the oVEMP reduced or absent (Chihara et al. 2012; Curthoys 2012; Manzari et al. 2013; Murofushi et al. 1996; Oh et al. 2013). The sparing of the inferior vestibular nerve has twofold implications: first, with respect to clinical findings, because it explains why patients with AUVP can suffer from "post-infectious" BPPV of the posterior canal; second, with respect to the pathophysiology and etiology, because a theory on that has to

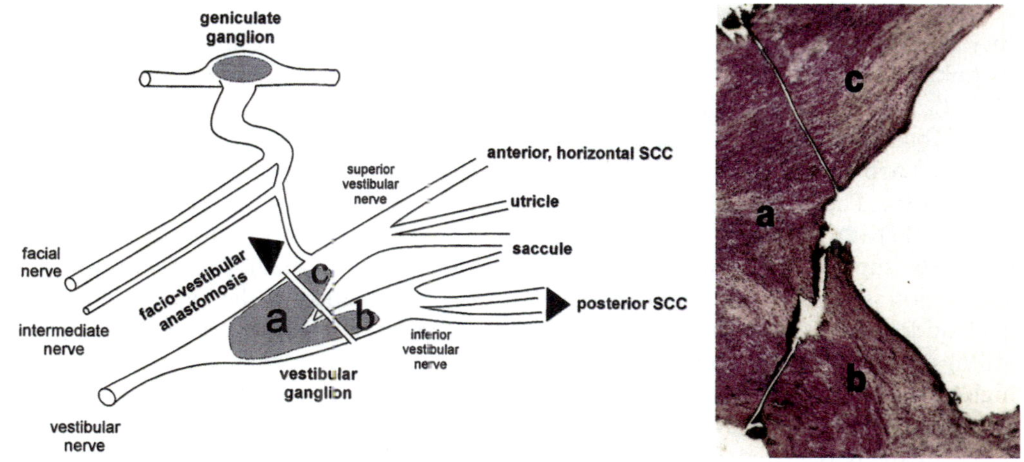

Fig. 8.10 *Left:* schematic drawing of the vestibular and facial nerves, the facio-vestibular anastomosis, the geniculate ganglion, and different sections of the vestibular ganglion (*a* stem, *b* inferior portion, *c* superior portion). *Right*: longitudinal cross-section of a human vestibular ganglion, in which the individual portions are separated. The presence of herpes simplex virus-1 DNA was confirmed by polymerase chain reaction in approximately 60% of the examined human vestibular ganglia. Moreover, the double innervation of the posterior canal, which may lead to the preservation of its function during vestibular neuritis, is visible (Arbusow et al. 1999). 1 ganglion geniculi, 2 vestibular ganglion, 3 facial nerve, 4 vestibular nerve, 5 intermediate nerve, 6 faciovestibular anastomoses, 7 superior vestibular nerve, 8 inferior vestibular nerve, 9 anterior, horizontal semicircular canal, 10 utricle, 11 saccule, 12 posterior semicircular canal

explain this fact. There are at least three possible explanations for the sparing of the inferior vestibular nerve: first, the longer and smaller bony canal through which the superior vestibular nerve runs (Goebel et al. 2001; Gianoli et al. 2005), which innervates the posterior semicircular canal; second, the double redundant innervation of the posterior canal with two nerves: the posterior ampullary and the accessory posterior ampullary nerve (Montandon et al. 1970; Arbusow et al. 1999; Arbusow et al. 2003; Büki and Ward 2021); and third, anastomoses between the facial nerve and the superior vestibular nerve through which reactivated herpes virus may spread (Arbusow et al. 1999; Büki and Ward 2021) (Fig. 8.10).

Using 3-D eye movement recordings and c/oVEMP, the first cases of rare **"inferior vestibular neuritis"** were described in 1996/1997 (Bohmer et al. 1997; Murofushi et al. 1996). The direction of the spontaneous nystagmus corresponds to the plane of the posterior canal, i.e., it is contraversively torsional with a downward component (the opposite direction to that which is found in posterior canal BPPV) (Kim and Kim 2012). It is often misdiagnosed as "central."

If the superior and the inferior vestibular nerve (**"total vestibular neuritis"**) are affected, horizontal nystagmus with torsional nystagmus is found with theoretically no vertical component because both vertical canals are affected. This also occurs in zoster oticus which can even lead to a complete OTR including a prominent skew deviation (Arbusow et al. 1998).

8.7 Etiology

A viral etiology of AUVP is—in analogy to Bell's palsy and some types of acute hearing loss—likely but so far not proven (Schuknecht and Kitamura 1981; Nadol, Jr. 1995; Baloh et al. 1996; Gacek and Gacek 2002; Baloh 2003; Le et al. 2019). There are several lines of evidence for such an etiology:

an autoptic study which showed inflammatory degenerations of the vestibular nerve (Schuknecht 1993), the demonstration of HSV-1, the latency-associated transcripts in vestibular ganglia, and activated CD8+ T cells (Arbusow et al. 1999, 2000a, b, 2003, 2010; Theil et al. 2001; Himmelein et al. 2017) (◘ Fig. 8.7). This hypothesis is further supported by two genome-wide association studies, which showed single nucleotide variants in the host factor for HSV1 replication (Rujescu et al. 2018) and high-risk allele for herpes labialis severity at the so-called IFNL3/4 locus (Rujescu et al. 2020). It is assumed that as a result of inter-current factors, HSV-1 replicates and induces an inflammation and edema and, thereby, secondary cell damage of the vestibular ganglion cells and axons in the bony canals, which may also explain the therapeutic effect of steroids (see below) in the very acute phase. Since—as mentioned above—the canal of the superior vestibular nerve is seven times longer and has more speculae (Gianoli et al. 2005) and the posterior semicircular canal is innervated by an additional anastomosis (Montandon et al. 1970; Arbusow et al. 2003), this may explain why the posterior canal is often but not always spared (◘ Fig. 8.10).

However, despite these findings, an inflammatory or even viral etiology has not so far been proved. The term "acute unilateral vestibulopathy" is preferred to "vestibular neuritis"; however, both can be synonymously used as in the International Classification of Vestibular Disorders (▶ Box 8.1 and 8.2).

8.8 Course of the Disease

The first phase of manifest loss of function is generally characterized by a severe feeling of illness, nausea, and vomiting. These symptoms are joined by vertigo, dizziness, and a tendency to fall to the ipsilateral side. The complaints resolve slowly over 1–2 weeks. As a rule, the patient is generally symptom-free within 3–5 weeks when at rest, i.e., under static conditions. In a retrospective study on 64 patients, different factors that could have an effect on the length of the hospital stay were investigated. The only correlation found was with the intensity of the spontaneous nystagmus at admission (Kim et al. 2020). Recovery is the result of a combination of the following:

- Central compensation of the peripheral vestibular tone imbalance, a multimodal process with different time courses, which occurs on different levels of the brainstem and cerebellum up to the cortex (for references, see Lacour et al. 2016, Zwergal et al. 2014)
- Substitution of the functional loss by the contralateral unaffected vestibular system as well as by somatosensory (e.g., neck proprioception (Strupp et al. 1998a)) and visual input (Eulenburg zu et al. 2010)
- Restoration of peripheral vestibular function (generally incomplete)

In the course of the illness, the peripheral vestibular function does not spontaneously recover in most patients (Brandt et al. 2010). A study with 60 patients showed that after 1 month 90% and after 6 months 80% of the patients still had a relevant deficit of peripheral vestibular function. In only 42% did a normalization occur in the further course (Okinaka et al. 1993). Lesion mapping was used to correlate the number of affected semicircular canals with the course of the disease in 50 patients with AUVP. The horizontal canal was affected in 97%, the anterior canal in 83%, the posterior canal in 46%, the utriculus in 73% and the sacculus in 44%. All five were affected in 32% and only the end organs of the superior vestibular nerve were affected in 22%. The more end organs were affected, the worse the course of the disease was (Navari and Casani 2020). Even in cases in which the peripheral deficit is complete, “static” symptoms (without head movement), such as spontaneous nystagmus, vertigo, and a tendency to fall, resolve. The remaining deficit, however, is still manifest in the form of a “dynamic” dysfunction: retinal slip of images of the visual scene with oscillopsia during rapid, high-frequency head movements, and walking and running because of the insufficiency of the VOR. Even if the caloric test normalizes in these patients, the head impulse test on the affected side is pathological in 30% (Schmid-Priscoveanu et al. 2001). A low VOR gain and many refixation saccades correlate with a poorer prognosis (Cerchiai et al. 2018); these patients require very intensive vestibular exercises (see below). The extent of the recovery of peripheral vestibular function is significantly better if only the superior vestibular nerve is affected rather than total AUVP (Hwang et al. 2019). In another study, the least symptoms and the shortest illness duration and intensity of the nystagmus were found in the inferior form (Lee et al. 2019). Visuo-vestibular psychological and personality traits are important for the long-term prognosis after AUVP (Bronstein and Dieterich 2019).

The long-term recurrence rate of vestibular neuritis is between 2% and 11% (Huppert et al. 2006; Kim et al. 2011).

8.9 Therapy: Principles, Aims, and Pragmatic Treatment

Based on the pathophysiology and assumed etiology of AUVP, treatment consists of four principles: (1) causative, i.e., theoretically anti-inflammatory and antiviral therapy; (2) symptomatic pharmacotherapy of vertigo, nausea, and vomiting; (3) vestibular exercises to improve central vestibular compensation, enhance central vestibular plasticity, adaption, and substitution; and (4) pharmacotherapy to improve central compensation.

8.9.1 Causative Treatment

In a randomized placebo-controlled four-arm trial, it was shown by caloric irrigation that a monotherapy with corticosteroids (methylprednisolone 100 mg per day, tapered every fourth day by 20 mg) significantly improved the recovery of peripheral vestibular function in AUVP after 12 months (Strupp et al. 2004). A virostatic agent, valacyclovir, led to neither a benefit nor an additional benefit when it was combined with methylprednisolone. The effects of steroids were supported by an observational study (Karlberg and Magnusson 2011). In a retrospective analysis, a positive effect of corticosteroids on spontaneous nystagmus, recovery of function, and quality of life was also found (Batuecas-Caletrio et al. 2015). In a single-blinded trial, it was demonstrated that vestibular exercises are equally effective as a treatment with corticosteroids in clinical, caloric, and otolith recovery (Goudakos et al. 2014); corticosteroid therapy seems to enhance earlier complete AUVP resolution during the first 6 months, with, however, no added benefit in the long-term prognosis after 12 months. These findings are supported by a more recent three-arm trial in 60 patients (Ismail et al. 2019). It was also demonstrated that the efficacy of corticosteroids significantly depended on the delay between the onset of symptoms and treatment: All 9 patients treated within 24 h after symptom onset had a normal caloric response after 3 months, while only 58% of those 14 patients treated between 25 and 72 h did (Sjogren et al. 2019).

A Cochrane review (Fishman et al. 2011) and a meta-analysis (Goudakos et al. 2010) made no general treatment recommendation for corticosteroids, mainly because there is only one randomized controlled trial; they may improve only the caloric extent and recovery of canal paresis (Goudakos et al. 2010) and their effects on life quality have still not been investigated sufficiently. A meta-analysis of six studies demonstrated that corticosteroids lead to a significant improvement of the caloric excitability after one month (95% CI, −16.33 – −0.32), but not after 12 months (Leong et al. 2021). The authors conclude that corticosteroids only have a positive effect in the acute phase. Another meta-analysis also concluded that corticosteroids improve the recovery (and particularly the long-term recovery) of peripheral vestibular function (Kim et al. 2022). All in all, we point out that further randomized placebo-controlled trials are necessary to evaluate the effects of corticosteroids in terms of recovery of vestibular function in the low- and high-frequency range, balance, functioning, and quality of life.

8.9.2 Symptomatic Therapy of Acute Vertigo, Nausea, and Vomiting

Various drugs have been recommended to acutely attenuate vertigo, nausea, and vomiting in vestibular disorders (for references, see Soto et al. 2013, Chabbert 2016, Strupp and Zwergal 2020). These agents are also often used for the symptomatic treatment of the acute phase, e.g., in Menière's disease or vestibular migraine. In addition, AUVP in humans and acute unilateral surgical or chemical vestibular lesions in animals are ideal models to evaluate the efficacy and mode of action of these drugs for symptomatic therapy and effects on central vestibular compensation (see below). The most relevant receptors involved are histamine, serotonin, GABA, dopamine, and muscarine, which can explain the major side effects of each class of pharmacological agents:

- H1R antagonists: The so-called first-generation antihistamines evidently have a combined effect on the peripheral and the central vestibular system (for references, see Soto et al. 2013, Chabbert 2016, Takumida et al. 2016). Examples are:
  - Dimenhydrinate (combination of diphenhydramine, an antagonist of the H_1-receptor (H1R), and 8-chlorthoeophylline (an adenosine-receptor antagonist to reduce drowsiness, the major side effect of diphenhydramine)).
  - Promethazine, which is also a moderate muscarinergic receptor (MR) antagonist, and dopamine D_2 receptor (D2R) antagonist, like neuroleptics; therefore, it can also lead to tardive dyskinesia.
- Serotonin 5-HT_3 receptor (5HT3R) antagonists, such as ondansetron or granisetron.
- $GABA_A$ agonists, namely benzodiazepines, with GABA being the main inhibitory neurotransmitter of vestibular neurons, which can lead to drowsiness and, in the long-term, drug addiction.
- H1R agonist and H3R inverse agonist, i.e., antagonist: betahistine. The most frequently used drug worldwide for the treatment of acute vertigo is betahistine (Agus et al. 2013). It is a weak H_1-agonist and H_3-inverse agonist, which attenuates the symptoms and also improves vestibular compensation in animal models (see below), but requires a sufficiently high plasma concentration (Tighilet et al. 2018). A Cochrane review and meta-analysis suggest that it is probably effective in acute vertigo (Murdin et al. 2016; Nauta 2014). More recently, it was shown that its effects can also be explained by an activation of central H1R leading to an activation of the vestibular system (Chen et al. 2019).
- Dopamine D_2 receptor (D2R) antagonists, such as metoclopramide (10 mg tid) or domperidone (10–20 mg tid), acting mainly on the chemoreceptor trigger zone in the brainstem; they have also a so-called gastroprokinetic effect (via muscarinergic receptors); the major side effects are movement disorders, mainly focal dystonia and akathisia.
- H4R antagonists: They act on the peripheral vestibular system, reduce the vestibular tone imbalance, and are effective in animal models (Kiss and Keseru 2014; Wersinger et al. 2013; Desmadryl et al. 2012; Venail et al. 2018).

- Anticholinergics act on the peripheral and central vestibular system. Scopolamine, an unspecific inhibitor of the muscarinergic receptors (best applied as a transdermal patch), has been the widely used; it has typical anticholinergic side effects such as dry mouth or blurred vision

The efficacy of symptomatic treatment with antihistamines, anticholinergics, $GABA_A$ agonists, D2R, and 5HT3R antagonists has been proven in many clinical trials (for references, see Soto et al. 2013; Chabbert 2016). Since most of these drugs (except betahistine) are sedatives, they most likely delay vestibular compensation. In an animal model of AUVP, the potassium channel blocker 4-aminopyridine significantly reduced postural imbalance, but on the other hand delayed vestibular compensation (Beck et al. 2014) most likely by reducing the vestibular tone imbalance, which is evidently the driving force for vestibular compensation.

Overall, symptomatic treatment with drugs that potentially delay central compensation should not be given for longer than 3 days after symptom onset. The drug of choice also depends on the side effects and contraindications in the individual patient.

8.9.3 Vestibular Exercises to Improve Central Compensation

So far, the most important principle of therapy is to promote central compensation by means of physical therapy (for references, see Hall et al. 2022, Sulway and Whitney 2019, Tjernstrom et al. 2016, Crane and Schubert 2018). Central compensation is not a uniform process. It involves various neural and structural mechanisms that operate in different locations (vestibulo-spinal or vestibulo-ocular structures) within different time courses, have various limited possibilities, and cause incomplete results, especially as regards head oscillations at high frequencies (Brandt et al. 1997). The central counter-regulation (compensation) of a unilateral labyrinthine lesion is enhanced and accelerated if movement stimuli trigger inadequate and incongruent afferent signals that provoke a sensory mismatch. The efficacy of balance training (for references, see Crane and Schubert 2018) has been demonstrated in animal studies and in several patient studies in AUVP (e.g., Strupp et al. 1998b; Tokle et al. 2020). These results are supported by a Cochrane review (McDonnell and Hillier 2015). Horizontal head turns are particularly important (Lehnen et al. 2018) to increase the vestibular tone imbalance and thus trigger vestibular compensation. The head turns can be done by the patients when they are still bedbound and thus do not involve the risk of falls.

Vestibular exercises, first recommended by Cawthorne and Cawthorne (1944), and later modified according to current knowledge of vestibular function (for references, see Hall et al. 2022, Whitney et al. 2020, Dunlap et al. 2019, Sulway and Whitney 2019):

- Active head movements to recalibrate the VOR voluntary eye movements and fixation to improve impaired gaze stabilization.
- Balance training, goal-directed movements, and gait exercises to improve the vestibulospinal regulation of posture and goal-directed motion.
- Voluntary eye movements and fixation to improve impaired gaze stabilization.

8.9.4 Pharmacotherapy for the Improvement of Central Compensation, Enhancement of Central Vestibular Plasticity, and Adaption

A theoretically promising therapeutic strategy for AUVP is the use of drugs to improve and accelerate central vestibular compensation.

However, there is so far no state-of-the-art placebo-controlled trial that shows any benefit in patients. Agents that enhance vestibular compensation have been extensively studied in various animal models and small prospective and placebo-controlled clinical studies. Compounds are betahistine, N-acetyl-DL-leucine, and the Ginkgo biloba extract EGb 761 (for review, see Chabbert 2016).

Betahistine Oral administration of betahistine at high daily doses of 50 mg/kg or 100 mg/kg accelerated the time-course of recovery in cats after unilateral vestibular damage (Tighilet et al. 1995). Co-administration of a lower betahistine dose (0.2 mg/kg/day) and selegiline (1 mg/kg/day) in this cat model increased the effect on postural recovery compared with betahistine monotherapy (Tighilet et al. 2018). Betahistine is considered to have multiple modes of action on the peripheral and central vestibular networks: (1) increased blood flow in the vestibular system as an H3R antagonist (Bertlich et al. 2015; Bertlich et al. 2017); (2) an increased histamine turnover and enhanced histamine release in the central nervous system (especially in the vestibular nuclei) via its property as an H3R inverse agonist; (3) a possibly inhibitory influence exerted at the level of the peripheral end organs and primary vestibular neurons through combined H3/H4 receptor effects (Lacour 2013). Beneficial effects of betahistine on vestibular compensation were also reported in humans, however, so far none in state-of-the art and sufficiently powered placebo-controlled trials (Redon et al. 2011; Lacour 2013).

Acetyl-DL-leucine Several studies in cats and rats have shown that N-acetyl-DL-leucine improves and accelerates postural compensation after unilateral labyrinthectomy relative to controls and that this effect is dose-dependent and driven by the L-isomer of the racemate (Gunther et al. 2015; Tighilet et al. 2015). N-acetyl-L-leucine also has an effect on cerebellar and thalamic networks during vestibular compensation (Gunther et al. 2015). In vitro electrophysiological recordings of neurons in the vestibular nuclei and vestibular-related networks in a guinea-pig model suggest that N-acetyl-DL-leucine may act by rebalancing the abnormal membrane potential in the vestibular nuclei (Vibert and Vidal 2001). One observational study described improvement of postural compensation in patients after vestibular neurotomy and labyrinthectomy (Ferber-Viart et al. 2009). Although N-acetyl-DL-leucine has been used in clinical practice to treat acute vertigo since 1957, a meta-analysis concludes that there is insufficient evidence for its efficacy (Vanderkam et al. 2019).

Gingko biloba extract EGb 761 is a standardized extract of *Ginkgo biloba*, which contains flavonoids and terpene lactones (ginkgolides A, B, bilobalide) at defined doses (for references, see Ude et al. 2013). Several studies have shown improvement of static and dynamic vestibular symptoms by EGb 761 after a unilateral vestibular lesion in rats, cats, and guinea pigs (Lacour et al. 1991; Maclennan et al. 1996; Lindner et al. 2019). In the rat model, oral administration of EGb 761 induced a dose-dependent improvement of postural asymmetry and locomotor velocity by means of a modulation of cerebral vestibular networks (vestibular nucleus, cerebellum, hippocampus) (Lindner et al. 2019). Experimental data suggest multiple effects of EGb 761 on neural plasticity, modulation of long-term potentiation, neuronal spine morphology and density, and neurogenesis mostly by terpene lactones (Muller et al. 2012).

8.9.5 Pragmatic Therapy

As explained above, the treatment of AUVP is based on the following therapeutic principles: (1) causal therapy, (2) symptomatic therapy, and (3) improvement of central vestibular compensation by vestibular exercises.

1. **Causal Therapy:** Although not proven, in clinical practice, currently 2 weeks of treatment with corticosteroids can be considered (e.g., methylprednisolone, 100 mg/day within 3 days after symptom onset (Strupp et al. 2004); taper off by 20 mg every fourth day) and—most importantly—they should be given as soon as possible after symptom onset (Sjogren et al. 2019).
2. **Symptomatic Therapy:** For the treatment of vertigo, nausea, and vomiting, we recommend the following drugs:
   - Dimenhydrinate (orally 50–100 mg or iv. or rectally (maximal daily dosage 400 mg)
   - Ondansetron (orally 4–8 mg up to 8 mg four times per day or i.v. 4 mg – 8 mg (maximal daily dosage 32)
   - Lorazepam (orally 0.5–1 mg up to 4 mg/d) (see also Table 5.2).

3. **Physiotherapy:** A gradual program of physical exercises initially under the supervision of a physiotherapist should be performed as soon as possible after symptom onset and if tolerated by the patient. We recommend about 15 min three times a day over a period of about 4 weeks. At the beginning, while the patients are still lying or sitting in bed, they should perform quick head turns to the right and left with fixation of a target in a sitting position because they increase vestibular tone imbalance without the risk of falls. Subsequently, vestibular exercises should be performed to improve stance and gait during combined head and body movements, which the patients should then continue to perform on their own. It should be noted that the degree of difficulty of these vestibular exercises with and without visual fixation should be slowly increased beyond normal levels.

Finally, we recommend a follow-up examination after 1, 6, and 12 months to evaluate the efficacy of the above measures and, if necessary, to intensify vestibular exercises and to document the potential recovery of peripheral vestibular function, which is important for the patient to know. Further, it is important to inform the patient that about 15% of those with AUVP develop post-infectious BPPV, which can explain a secondary deterioration. In addition, the patient should be informed about the risk of secondary functional dizziness and the recurrence rate, which is 2–11%.

References

Adamec I, Krbot SM, Handzic J, Habek M (2015) Incidence, seasonality and comorbidity in vestibular neuritis. Neurol Sci 36(1):91–95

Agus S, Benecke H, Thum C, Strupp M (2013) Clinical and demographic features of vertigo: findings from the REVERT registry. Front Neurol 4:48

Arbusow V, Dieterich M, Strupp M, Dreher V, Jäger L, Brandt T (1998) Herpes zoster neuritis involving superior and inferior parts of the vestibular nerve causes ocular tilt reaction. Neuro-Ophthalmology 19:17–22

Arbusow V, Schulz P, Strupp M, Dieterich M, von Reinhardstoettner A, Rauch E, Brandt T (1999) Distribution of herpes simplex virus type 1 in human geniculate and vestibular ganglia: implications for vestibular neuritis. Ann Neurol 46(3): 416–419

Arbusow V, Strupp M, Wasicky R, Horn AK, Schulz P, Brandt T (2000a) Detection of herpes simplex virus type 1 in human vestibular nuclei. Neurology 55(6):880–882

Arbusow V, Theil D, Strupp M, Mascolo A, Brandt T (2000b) HSV-1 not only in human vestibular ganglia but also in the vestibular labyrinth. Audiol Neurootol 6(5):259–262

Arbusow V, Theil D, Schulz P, Strupp M, Dieterich M, Rauch E, Brandt T (2003) Distribution of HSV-1 in human geniculate and vestibular ganglia: implications for vestibular neuritis. Ann N Y Acad Sci 1004:409–413

Arbusow V, Derfuss T, Held K, Himmelein S, Strupp M, Gurkov R, Brandt T, Theil D (2010) Latency of herpes simplex virus type-1 in human geniculate and vestibular ganglia is associated with infiltration of CD8+ T cells. J Med Virol 82(11):1917–1920

Aw ST, Fetter M, Cremer PD, Karlberg M, Halmagyi GM (2001) Individual semicircular canal function in superior and inferior vestibular neuritis. Neurology 57(5):768–774

Baier B, Bense S, Dieterich M (2008) Are signs of ocular tilt reaction in patients with cerebellar lesions mediated by the dentate nucleus? Brain 131(Pt 6):1445–1454

Baloh RW (2003) Clinical practice. Vestibular neuritis. N Engl J Med 348(11):1027–1032

Baloh RW, Ishyama A, Wackym PA, Honrubia V (1996) Vestibular neuritis: clinical-pathologic correlation. Otolaryngol Head Neck Surg 114(4):586–592

Bartl K, Lehnen N, Kohlbecher S, Schneider E (2009) Head impulse testing using video-oculography. Ann N Y Acad Sci 1164:331–333

Batuecas-Caletrio A, Yanez-Gonzalez R, Sanchez-Blanco C, Perez PB, Gonzalez-Sanchez E, Sanchez LA, Kaski D (2015) Glucocorticoids improve acute dizziness symptoms following acute unilateral vestibulopathy. J Neurol 262(11):2578–2582

Beck R, Gunther L, Xiong G, Potschka H, Boning G, Bartenstein P, Brandt T, Jahn K, Dieterich M, Strupp M, la FC, Zwergal A (2014) The mixed blessing of treating symptoms in acute vestibular failure--evidence from a 4-aminopyridine experiment. Exp Neurol 261:638–645

Bergstrom B (1973) Morphology of the vestibular nerve. I Anatomical studies of the vestibular nerve in man. Acta Otolaryngol Stockh 76(2):162–172

Bertlich M, Ihler F, Freytag S, Weiss BG, Strupp M, Canis M (2015) Histaminergic H-Heteroreceptors as a potential mediator of Betahistine-induced increase in Cochlear blood flow. Audiol Neurootol 20(5):283–293

Bertlich M, Ihler F, Weiss BG, Freytag S, Strupp M, Jakob M, Canis M (2017) Role of capillary pericytes and precapillary arterioles in the vascular mechanism of betahistine in a Guinea pig inner ear model. Life Sci 187:17

Bohmer A, Rickenmann J (1995) The subjective visual vertical as a clinical parameter of vestibular function in peripheral vestibular diseases. J Vestib Res 5(1):35–45

Bohmer A, Straumann D, Fetter M (1997) Three-dimensional analysis of spontaneous nystagmus in peripheral vestibular lesions. Ann Otol Rhinol Laryngol 106(1):61–68

Brandt T, Dieterich M (1993a) Skew deviation with ocular torsion: a vestibular brainstem sign of topographic diagnostic value. Ann Neurol 33(5):528–534

Brandt T, Dieterich M (1993b) Vestibular falls. J Vestib Res 3:3–14

Brandt T, Huppert T, Hufner K, Zingler VC, Dieterich M, Strupp M (2010) Long-term course and relapses of vestibular and balance disorders. Restor Neurol Neurosci 28:69–82

Brandt T, Strupp M, Arbusow V, Dieringer N (1997) Plasticity of the vestibular system: central compensation and sensory substitution for vestibular deficits. Adv Neurol 73:297–309

Bronstein AM, Dieterich M (2019) Long-term clinical outcome in vestibular neuritis. Curr Opin Neurol 32(1):174–180

Büchele W, Brandt T (1988) Vestibular neuritis - a horizontal semicircular canal paresis? Adv Otorhinolaryngol 42:157–161

Büki B, Ward BK (2021) Length of the narrow bony channels may not be the sole cause of differential involvement of the nerves in vestibular neuritis. Otol Neurotol 42:e918–e924

Byun H, Chung JH, Lee SH, Park CW, Park DW, Kim TY (2018) Clinical value of 4-hour delayed gadolinium-enhanced 3D FLAIR MR images in acute vestibular neuritis. Laryngoscope 128(8): 1946–1951

Cawthorne T, Cawthorn D (1944) The physiological basis for head exercises. J Chart Soc Physiother 106–107

Cerchiai N, Navari E, Sellari-Franceschini S, Re C, Casani AP (2018) Predicting the outcome after acute unilateral Vestibulopathy: analysis of Vestibulo-ocular reflex gain and catch-up saccades. Otolaryngol Head Neck Surg 158(3):527–533

Chabbert C (2016) Principles of vestibular pharmacotherapy. Handb Clin Neurol 137:207–218

Chang TP, Wu YC (2010) A tiny infarct on the dorsolateral pons mimicking vestibular neuritis. Laryngoscope 120(11):2336–2338

Chen L, Lee W, Chambers BR, Dewey HM (2011) Diagnostic accuracy of acute vestibular syndrome at the bedside in a stroke unit. J Neurol 258(5): 855–861

Chen L, Todd M, Halmagyi GM, Aw S (2014) Head impulse gain and saccade analysis in pontine-cerebellar stroke and vestibular neuritis. Neurology 83(17):1513–1522

Chen ZP, Zhang XY, Peng SY, Yang ZQ, Wang YB, Zhang YX, Chen X, Wang JJ, Zhu JN (2019) Histamine H1 receptor contributes to vestibular compensation. J Neurosci 39(3):420–433

Chihara Y, Iwasaki S, Murofushi T, Yagi M, Inoue A, Fujimoto C, Egami N, Ushio M, Karino S, Sugasawa K, Yamasoba T (2012) Clinical characteristics of inferior vestibular neuritis. Acta Otolaryngol 132(12):1288–1294

Choi JY, Jung I, Jung JM, Kwon DY, Park MH, Kim HJ, Kim JS (2016a) Characteristics and mechanism of perverted head-shaking nystagmus in central lesions: video-oculography analysis. Clin Neurophysiol 127(9):2973–2978

Choi KD, Lee H, Kim JS (2016b) Ischemic syndromes causing dizziness and vertigo. Handb Clin Neurol 137:317–340

Choi JY, Kim HJ, Kim JS (2018a) Recent advances in head impulse test findings in central vestibular disorders. Neurology 90(13):602–612

Choi S, Choi HR, Nahm H, Han K, Shin JE, Kim CH (2018b) Utility of the bow and lean test in predicting subtype of benign paroxysmal positional vertigo. Laryngoscope 128:2600–2604

Cnyrim CD, Newman-Toker D, Karch C, Brandt T, Strupp M (2008) Bedside differentiation of vestibular neuritis from central "vestibular pseudoneuritis". J Neurol Neurosurg Psychiatry 79(4):458–460

Crane BT, Schubert MC (2018) An adaptive vestibular rehabilitation technique. Laryngoscope 128(3):713–718

Curthoys IS (2012) The interpretation of clinical tests of peripheral vestibular function. Laryngoscope 122(6):1342–1352

Curthoys IS, Iwasaki S, Chihara Y, Ushio M, McGarvie LA, Burgess AM (2011) The ocular vestibular-evoked myogenic potential to air-conducted sound; probable superior vestibular nerve origin. Clin Neurophysiol 122(3):611–616

Depondt M (1973) Vestibular neuronitis. Vestibular paralysis with special characteristics. Acta Otorhinolaryngol Belg 27(3):323–359

Desmadryl G, Gaboyard-Niay S, Brugeaud A, Travo C, Broussy A, Saleur A, Dyhrfjeld-Johnsen J, Wersinger E, Chabbert C (2012) Histamine H4 receptor antagonists as potent modulators of mammalian vestibular primary neuron excitability. Br J Pharmacol 167(4):905–916

Diener HC, Frank B (2015) Stroke: stroke prevention--time to say goodbye to the ABCD2 score? Nat Rev Neurol 11(10):552–553

Dieterich M, Brandt T (2019) Perception of verticality and vestibular disorders of balance and falls. Front Neurol 10:172

Duncan GW, Parker SW, Fisher CM (1975) Acute cerebellar infarction in the PICA territory. Arch Neurol 32(6):364–368

Dunlap PM, Holmberg JM, Whitney SL (2019) Vestibular rehabilitation: advances in peripheral and central vestibular disorders. Curr Opin Neurol 32(1):137–144

Eggers SDZ, Bisdorff A, von BM, Zee DS, Kim JS, Perez-Fernandez N, Welgampola MS, Della Santina CC, Newman-Toker DE (2019) Classification of vestibular signs and examination techniques: nystagmus and nystagmus-like movements. J Vestib Res 29(2–3):57–87

Eliezer M, Maquet C, Horion J, Gillibert A, Toupet M, Bolognini B, Magne N, Kahn L, Hautefort C, Attye A (2019) Detection of intralabyrinthine abnormalities using post-contrast delayed 3D-FLAIR MRI sequences in patients with acute vestibular syndrome. Eur Radiol 29(6):2760–2769

Eulenburg zu P, Stoeter P, Dieterich M (2010) Voxel-based morphometry depicts central compensation after vestibular neuritis. Ann Neurol 68:241–249

Ferber-Viart C, Dubreuil C, Vidal PP (2009) Effects of acetyl-DL-leucine in vestibular patients: a clinical study following neurotomy and labyrinthectomy. Audiol Neurootol 14(1):17–25

Fetter M, Dichgans J (1996a) Three-dimensional human VOR in acute vestibular lesions. Ann N Y Acad Sci 781:619–621

Fetter M, Dichgans J (1996b) Vestibular neuritis spares the inferior division of the vestibular nerve. Brain 119:755–763

Fife TD, Colebatch JG, Kerber KA, Brantberg K, Strupp M, Lee H, Walker MF, Ashman E, Fletcher J, Callaghan B, Gloss DS (2017) Practice guideline: cervical and ocular vestibular evoked myogenic potential testing: report of the guideline development, dissemination, and implementation Subcommittee of the American Academy of neurology. Neurology 89(22):2288–2296

Fishman JM, Burgess C, Waddell A (2011) Corticosteroids for the treatment of idiopathic acute vestibular dysfunction (vestibular neuritis). Cochrane Database Syst Rev 5:CD008607

Freund W, Weber F, Schneider D, Mayer U, Scheithauer M, Beer M (2020) Vestibular nerve atrophy after vestibular neuritis – results from a prospective high-resolution MRI study. Rofo 192:854–861

Gacek RR, Gacek MR (2002) The three faces of vestibular ganglionitis. Ann Otol Rhinol Laryngol 111(2):103–114

Gianoli G, Goebel J, Mowry S, Poomipannit P (2005) Anatomic differences in the lateral vestibular nerve channels and their implications in vestibular neuritis. Otol Neurotol 26(3):489–494

Gioacchini FM, Alicandri-Ciufelli M, Kaleci S, Magliulo G, Re M (2014) Prevalence and diagnosis of vestibular disorders in children: a review. Int J Pediatr Otorhinolaryngol 78(5):718–724

Goebel JA, O'Mara W, Gianoli G (2001) Anatomic considerations in vestibular neuritis. Otol Neurotol 22:512–518

Goldberg JM, Fernandez C (1971) Physiology of peripheral neurons innervating semicircular canals of the squirrel monkey. I Resting discharge and response to constant angular accelerations. J Neurophysiol 34(4):635–660

Goudakos JK, Markou KD, Franco-Vidal V, Vital V, Tsaligopoulos M, Darrouzet V (2010) Corticosteroids in the treatment of vestibular neuritis: a systematic review and meta-analysis. Otol Neurotol 31(2):183–189

Goudakos JK, Markou KD, Psillas G, Vital V, Tsaligopoulos M (2014) Corticosteroids and vestibular exercises in vestibular neuritis. Single-blind randomized clinical trial. JAMA Otolaryngol Head Neck Surg 140(5):434–440

Green KE, Gold DR (2021) HINTS Examination in acute vestibular neuritis: do not look too hard for the skew. J Neuroophthalmol 41:e672–e678

Gunther L, Beck R, Xiong G, Potschka H, Jahn K, Bartenstein P, Brandt T, Dutia M, Dieterich M, Strupp M, la FC, Zwergal A (2015) N-acetyl-L-leucine accelerates vestibular compensation after unilateral labyrinthectomy by action in the cerebellum and thalamus. PLoS One 10(3):e0120891

Gurley KL, Edlow JA (2019) Acute Dizziness. Semin Neurol 39(1):27–40

Hall CD, Herdman SJ, Whitney SL, Anson ER, Carender WJ, Hoppes CW, Cass SP, Christy JB, Cohen HS, Fife TD, Furman JM, Shepard NT, Clendaniel RA, Dishman JD, Goebel JA, Meldrum D, Ryan C, Wallace RL, Woodward NJ (2022) Vestibular rehabilitation for P peripheral vestibular hypofunction: an updated clinical practice guideline from the academy of neurologic physical therapy of the American Physical Therapy Association. J Neurol Phys Ther 46:(2)118–177

Halmagyi GM, Chen L, MacDougall HG, Weber KP, McGarvie LA, Curthoys IS (2017) The video head impulse test. Front Neurol 8:258

Halmagyi GM, McGarvie LA, Strupp M (2020) Nystagmus goggles: how to use them, what you find and what it means. Pract Neurol 20:446–450

Himmelein S, Lindemann A, Sinicina I, Horn AKE, Brandt T, Strupp M, Hufner K (2017) Differential involvement during latent herpes simplex virus 1 infection of the superior and inferior divisions of the vestibular ganglia: implications for vestibular neuritis. J Virol 91(14):e00331-17

Honrubia V (1994) Quantitative vestibular function tests and the clinical examination. In: Herdman SJ (ed) Vestibular rehabilitation. F.A. Davis, Philadelphia, pp 113–164

Huang CY, Yu YL (1985) Small cerebellar strokes may mimic labyrinthine lesions. J Neurol Neurosurg Psychiatry 48(3):263–265

Huh YE, Kim JS (2011) Patterns of spontaneous and head-shaking nystagmus in cerebellar infarction: imaging correlations. Brain 134(Pt 12):3662–3671

Huppert D, Strupp M, Theil D, Glaser M, Brandt T (2006) Low recurrence rate of vestibular neuritis: a long-term follow-up. Neurology 67(10):1870–1871

Hwang K, Kim BG, Lee JD, Lee ES, Lee TK, Sung KB (2019) The extent of vestibular impairment is important in recovery of canal paresis of patients with vestibular neuritis. Auris Nasus Larynx 46(1):24–26

Ismail EI, Morgan AE, Abdel Rahman AM (2019) Corticosteroids versus vestibular rehabilitation in long-term outcomes in vestibular neuritis. J Vestib Res 28:417–424

Jahn K, Langhagen T, Heinen F (2015) Vertigo and dizziness in children. Curr Opin Neurol 28(1):78–82

Jongkees LB, Maas J, Philipszoon A (1962) Clinical electronystagmography: a detailed study of electronystagmography in 341 patients with vertigo. Pract Otorhinolaryngol Basel 24:65–93

Karlberg ML, Magnusson M (2011) Treatment of acute vestibular neuronitis with glucocorticoids. Otol Neurotol 32(7):1140–1143

Kattah JC, Talkad AV, Wang DZ, Hsieh YH, Newman-Toker DE (2009) HINTS to diagnose stroke in the acute vestibular syndrome: three-step bedside oculomotor examination more sensitive than early MRI diffusion-weighted imaging. Stroke 40(11):3504–3510

Kerber KA (2020) Acute Vestibular Syndrome. Semin Neurol 40(1):59–66

Kim G, Seo JH, Lee SJ, Lee DH (2022) Therapeutic effect of steroids on vestibular neuritis: systematic review and meta-analysis. Clin Otolaryngol 47:34–43

Kim JS, Kim HJ (2012) Inferior vestibular neuritis. J Neurol 259(8):1553–1560

Kim HA, Lee H (2010) Isolated vestibular nucleus infarction mimicking acute peripheral vestibulopathy. Stroke 41(7):1558–1560

Kim SJ, Lee HY, Lee MY, Choi JY (2020) Initial degree of spontaneous nystagmus affects the length of hospitalization of patients with vestibular neuritis. Otol Neurotol 41(6):836–842

Kim YH, Kim KS, Kim KJ, Choi H, Choi JS, Hwang IK (2011) Recurrence of vertigo in patients with vestibular neuritis. Acta Otolaryngol 131(11):1172–1177

Kiss R, Keseru GM (2014) Novel histamine H4 receptor ligands and their potential therapeutic applications: an update. Expert Opin Ther Pat 24(11):1185–1197

Koors PD, Thacker LR, Coelho DH (2013) Investigation of seasonal variability of vestibular neuronitis. J Laryngol Otol 127(10):968–971

Korda A, Zamaro E, Wagner F, Morrison M, Caversaccio MD, Sauter TC, Schneider E, Mantokoudis G (2022) Acute vestibular syndrome: is skew deviation a central sign? J Neurol 269:1396–1403

Lacour M (2013) Betahistine treatment in managing vertigo and improving vestibular compensation: clarification. J Vestib Res 23(3):139–151

Lacour M, Ez Zaher L, Raymond J (1991) Plasticity mechanisms in vestibular compensation in the cat are improved by an extract of Ginkgo biloba (EGb 761). Pharmacol Biochem Behav 40:367–379

Lacour M, Helmchen C, Vidal PP (2016) Vestibular compensation: the neuro-otologist's best friend. J Neurol 263(Suppl 1):S54–S64

Le TN, Westerberg BD, Lea J (2019) Vestibular neuritis: recent advances in etiology, diagnostic evaluation, and treatment. Adv Otorhinolaryngol 82:87–92

8

Lee H, Sohn SI, Jung DK, Cho YW, Lim JG, Yi SD, Lee SR, Sohn CH, Baloh RW (2002) Sudden deafness and anterior inferior cerebellar artery infarction. Stroke 33(12):2807–2812
Lee H, Sohn SI, Cho YW, Lee SR, Ahn BH, Park BR, Baloh RW (2006) Cerebellar infarction presenting isolated vertigo: frequency and vascular topographical patterns. Neurology 67(7):1178–1183
Lee H, Kim BK, Park HJ, Koo JW, Kim JS (2009a) Prodromal dizziness in vestibular neuritis: frequency and clinical implication. J Neurol Neurosurg Psychiatry 80(3):355–356
Lee H, Kim JS, Chung EJ, Yi HA, Chung IS, Lee SR, Shin JY (2009b) Infarction in the territory of anterior inferior cerebellar artery: spectrum of audiovestibular loss. Stroke 40(12):3745–3751
Lee J, Song K, Yu IK, Lee HY (2019) A case of isolated nodular infarction mimicking vestibular neuritis on the contralateral side. J Audiol Otol 23(3):167–172
Lee JY, Park JS, Kim MB (2019) Clinical characteristics of acute vestibular neuritis according to involvement site. Otol Neurotol 40(6):797–805
Lehnen N, Kellerer S, Knorr AG, Schlick C, Jahn K, Schneider E, Heuberger M, Ramaioli C (2018) Head-movement-emphasized rehabilitation in bilateral vestibulopathy. Front Neurol 9:562
Lempert T, Olesen J, Furman J, Waterston J, Seemungal B, Carey J, Bisdorff A, Versino M, Evers S, Newman-Toker D (2012) Vestibular migraine: diagnostic criteria. J Vestib Res 22(4):167–172
Leong KJ, Lau T, Stewart V, Canetti EFD (2021) Systematic review and meta-analysis: effectiveness of corticosteroids in treating adults with acute vestibular neuritis. Otolaryngol Head Neck Surg 165:255–266
Lindner M, Gosewisch A, Eilles E, Branner C, Kramer A, Oos R, Wolf E, Ziegler S, Bartenstein P, Brandt T, Dieterich M, Zwergal A (2019) Ginkgo biloba extract EGb 761 improves vestibular compensation and modulates cerebral vestibular networks in the rat. Front Neurol 10:147
Lopez-Escamez JA, Carey J, Chung WH, Goebel JA, Magnusson M, Mandala M, Newman-Toker DE, Strupp M, Suzuki M, Trabalzini F, Bisdorff A (2015) Diagnostic criteria for Meniere's disease. J Vestib Res 25(1):1–7
Lorente de Nó R (1933) Vestibulo-ocular reflex arc. Arch Neurol Psychiatr 30:245–291
MacDougall HG, Weber KP, McGarvie LA, Halmagyi GM, Curthoys IS (2009) The video head impulse test: diagnostic accuracy in peripheral vestibulopathy. Neurology 73(14):1134–1141
Machner B, Erber K, Choi JH, Sprenger A, Helmchen C, Trillenberg P (2021a) A Simple gain-based evaluation of the video head impulse test reliably detects normal vestibulo-ocular reflex indicative of stroke in patients with acute vestibular syndrome. Front Neurol 12:741859
Machner B, Erber K, Choi JH, Trillenberg P, Sprenger A, Helmchen C (2021b) Usability of the head impulse test in routine clinical practice in the emergency department to differentiate vestibular neuritis from stroke. Eur J Neurol 28:1737–1744
Maclennan K, Smith PF, Darlington CL (1996) The effects of ginkgolide B (BN52021) on Guinea pig vestibular nucleus neurons in vitro: importance of controlling for effects of dimethylsulphoxide (DMSO) vehicles. Neurosci Res 26(4):395–399
Magnusson M, Norrving B (1991) Cerebellar infarctions as the cause of 'vestibular neuritis'. Acta Otolaryngol (Stockh) Suppl 481:258–259
Mantokoudis G, Saber Tehrani AS, Wozniak A, Eibenberger K, Kattah JC, Guede CI, Zee DS, Newman-Toker DE (2012) VOR gain by head impulse video-oculography differentiates acute vestibular neuritis from stroke. Otol Neurotol 36:457–465
Mantokoudis G, Korda A, Zee DS, Zamaro E, Sauter TC, Wagner F, Caversaccio MD (2021a) Bruns' nystagmus revisited: a sign of stroke in patients with the acute vestibular syndrome. Eur J Neurol 28:2971–2979
Mantokoudis G, Wyss T, Zamaro E, Korda A, Wagner F, Sauter TC, Kerkeni H, Kalla R, Morrison M, Caversaccio MD (2021b) Stroke prediction based on the spontaneous nystagmus suppression test in dizzy patients: a diagnostic accuracy study. Neurology 97:e42–e51
Mantokoudis G, Tehrani AS, Wozniak A, Eibenberger K, Kattah JC, Guede CI, Zee DS, Newman-Toker DE (2015) VOR gain by head impulse video-oculography differentiates acute vestibular neuritis from stroke. Otol Neurotol 36:457-465
Manzari L, Burgess AM, MacDougall HG, Curthoys IS (2013) Vestibular function after vestibular neuritis. Int J Audiol 52(10):713–718
Manzari L, Princi AA, De AS, Tramontano M (2021) Clinical value of the video head impulse test in patients with vestibular neuritis: a systematic review. Eur Arch Otorhinolaryngol 278: 4155–4167
McDonnell MN, Hillier SL (2015) Vestibular rehabilitation for unilateral peripheral vestibular dysfunction. Cochrane Database Syst Rev 1:CD005397
Montandon P, Gacek RR, Kimura RS (1970) Crista neglecta in the cat and human. Ann Otol Rhinol Laryngol 79:105–112
Mossman S, Halmagyi GM (2000) Partial ocular tilt reaction due to unilateral cerebellar lesion. Neurology 49(2):491–493

Muller WE, Heiser J, Leuner K (2012) Effects of the standardized Ginkgo biloba extract EGb 761(R) on neuroplasticity. Int Psychogeriatr 24(Suppl 1):S21–S24

Murdin L, Hussain K, Schilder AG (2016) Betahistine for symptoms of vertigo. Cochrane Database Syst Rev 6:CD010696

Murofushi T, Halmagyi GM, Yavor RA, Colebatch JG (1996) Absent vestibular evoked myogenic potentials in vestibular neurolabyrinthitis. An indicator of inferior vestibular nerve involvement? Arch Otolaryngol Head Neck Surg 122(8):845–848

Nadol JB Jr (1995) Vestibular neuritis. Otolaryngol Head Neck Surg 112(1):162–172

Navari E, Casani AP (2020) Lesion patterns and possible implications for recovery in acute unilateral vestibulopathy. Otol Neurotol 41(2):e250–e255

Nauta JJ (2014) Meta-analysis of clinical studies with betahistine in Meniere's disease and vestibular vertigo. Eur Arch Otorhinolaryngol 271(5):887–897

Neuhauser HK (2016) The epidemiology of dizziness and vertigo. Handb Clin Neurol 137:67–82

Newman-Toker DE, Kattah JC, Alvernia JE, Wang DZ (2008) Normal head impulse test differentiates acute cerebellar strokes from vestibular neuritis. Neurology 70(24 Pt 2):2378–2385

Oh SY, Kim JS, Yang TH, Shin BS, Jeong SK (2013) Cervical and ocular vestibular-evoked myogenic potentials in vestibular neuritis: comparison between air- and bone-conducted stimulation. J Neurol 260(8):2102–2109

Ohle R, Montpellier RA, Marchadier V, Wharton A, McIsaac S, Anderson M, Savage D (2020) Can emergency physicians accurately rule out a central cause of vertigo using the HINTS exam? A systematic review and meta-analysis. Acad Emerg Med 27:887–896

Okinaka Y, Sekitani T, Okazaki H, Miura M, Tahara T (1993) Progress of caloric response of vestibular neuronitis. Acta Otolaryngol (Stockh) Suppl 503:18–22

Park HK, Kim JS, Strupp M, Zee DS (2013) Isolated floccular infarction: impaired vestibular responses to horizontal head impulse. J Neurol 260(6):1576–1582

Redon C, Lopez C, Bernard-Demanze L, Dumitrescu M, Magnan J, Lacour M, Borel L (2011) Betahistine treatment improves the recovery of static symptoms in patients with unilateral vestibular loss. J Clin Pharmacol 51(4):538–548

Rosengren SM, Colebatch JG, Young AS, Govender S, Welgampola MS (2019) Vestibular evoked myogenic potentials in practice: methods, pitfalls and clinical applications. Clin Neurophysiol Pract 4:47–68

Rujescu D, Hartmann AM, Giegling I, Konte B, Herrling M, Himmelein S, Strupp M (2018) Genome-wide association study in vestibular neuritis: involvement of the host factor for HSV-1 replication. Front Neurol 9:591

Rujescu D, Herrling M, Hartmann AM, Maul S, Giegling I, Konte B, Strupp M (2020) High-risk allele for herpes labialis severity at the IFNL3/4 locus is associated with vestibular neuritis. Front Neurol 11:570638

Saber Tehrani AS, Kattah JC, Kerber KA, Gold DR, Zee DS, Urrutia VC, Newman-Toker DE (2018) Diagnosing stroke in acute dizziness and vertigo: pitfalls and pearls. Stroke 49(3):788–795

Sando I, Black FO, Hemenway WG (1972) Spatial distribution of vestibular nerve in internal auditory canal. Ann Otol 81:305–319

Schmid-Priscoveanu A, Bohmer A, Obzina H, Straumann D (2001) Caloric and search-coil head-impulse testing in patients after vestibular neuritis. J Assoc Res Otolaryngol 2:72–78

Schuknecht HF (1993) Pathology of the ear., 2 ed. Lea & Febinger, Philadelphia

Schuknecht HF, Kitamura K (1981) Vestibular neuritis. Ann Otol 90(Suppl. 78):1–19

Sekitani T, Imate Y, Noguchi T, Inokuma T (1993) Vestibular neuronitis: epidemiological survey by questionnaire in Japan. Acta Otolaryngol (Stockh) Suppl 503:9–12

Sjogren J, Magnusson M, Tjernstrom F, Karlberg M (2019) Steroids for acute vestibular Neuronitis-the earlier the treatment, the better the outcome? Otol Neurotol 40:372–374

Soto E, Vega R, Sesena E (2013) Neuropharmacological basis of vestibular system disorder treatment. J Vestib Res 23(3):119–137

Strupp M, Magnusson M (2015) Acute Unilateral Vestibulopathy. Neurol Clin 33(3):669–685

Strupp M, Zwergal A (2020) Pharmacotherapy of peripheral vestibular disorders. In: The senses. Academic Press/Elsevier, San Diego

Strupp M, Arbusow V, Dieterich M, Sautier W, Brandt T (1998a) Perceptual and oculomotor effects of neck muscle vibration in vestibular neuritis. Ipsilateral somatosensory substitution of vestibular function. Brain 121(Pt 4):677–685

Strupp M, Arbusow V, Maag KP, Gall C, Brandt T (1998b) Vestibular exercises improve central vestibulospinal compensation after vestibular neuritis. Neurology 51(3):838–844

Strupp M, Bisdorff A, Furman J, Hornibrook J, Jahn K, Maire R, Newman-Toker D, Magnusson M (2022) Acute unilateral vestibulopathy/vestibular neuritis:diagnostic criteria. J Vest Res 32:(5)389–406

Strupp M, Straumann D, Helmchen C (2021) Nystagmus: diagnosis, topographic anatomical localization and therapy. Klin Monbl Augenheilkd 238(11):1186–1195

8

Strupp M, Zingler VC, Arbusow V, Niklas D, Maag KP, Dieterich M, Bense S, Theil D, Jahn K, Brandt T (2004) Methylprednisolone, valacyclovir, or the combination for vestibular neuritis. N Engl J Med 351(4):354–361

Strupp M, Lopez-Escamez JA, Kim JS, Straumann D, Jen JC, Carey J, Bisdorff A, Brandt T (2016) Vestibular paroxysmia: diagnostic criteria. J Vestib Res 26:409–415

Sulway S, Whitney SL (2019) Advances in vestibular rehabilitation. Adv Otorhinolaryngol 82:164–169

Takumida M, Takumida H, Anniko M (2016) Localization of histamine (H1, H2, H3 and H4) receptors in mouse inner ear. Acta Otolaryngol 136(6):537–544

Theil D, Arbusow V, Derfuss T, Strupp M, Pfeiffer M, Mascolo A, Brandt T (2001) Prevalence of HSV-1 LAT in human trigeminal, geniculate, and vestibular ganglia and its implication for cranial nerve syndromes. Brain Pathol 11(4):408–413

Thömke F, Hopf HC (1999) Pontine lesions mimicking acute peripheral vestibulopathy. J Neurol Neurosurg Psychiatry 66:340–349

Tighilet B, Leonard J, Lacour M (1995) Betahistine dihydrochloride treatment facilitates vestibular compensation in the cat. J Vestib Res 5(1):53–66

Tighilet B, Leonard J, Bernard-Demanze L, Lacour M (2015) Comparative analysis of pharmacological treatments with N-acetyl-dl-leucine (Tanganil) and its two isomers (N-acetyl-L-leucine and N-acetyl-D-leucine) on vestibular compensation: behavioral investigation in the cat. Eur J Pharmacol 769: 342–349

Tighilet B, Leonard J, Watabe I, Bernard-Demanze L, Lacour M (2018) Betahistine treatment in a cat model of vestibular pathology: pharmacokinetic and pharmacodynamic approaches. Front Neurol 9:431

Tjernstrom F, Zur O, Jahn K (2016) Current concepts and future approaches to vestibular rehabilitation. J Neurol 263(Suppl 1):S65–S70

Tokle G, Morkved S, Brathen G, Goplen FK, Salvesen O, Arnesen H, Holmeslet B, Nordahl SHG, Wilhelmsen KT (2020) Efficacy of vestibular rehabilitation following acute vestibular neuritis: a randomized controlled trial. Otol Neurotol 41(1):78–85

Ude C, Schubert-Zsilavecz M, Wurglics M (2013) Ginkgo biloba extracts: a review of the pharmacokinetics of the active ingredients. Clin Pharmacokinet 52(9):727–749

Vanderkam P, Blanchard C, Naudet F, Pouchain D, Vaillant RH, Perault-Pochat MC, Jaafari N, Boussageon R (2019) Efficacy of acetylleucine in vertigo and dizziness: a systematic review of randomised controlled trials. Eur J Clin Pharmacol 75(5):603–607

Venail F, Attali P, Wersinger E, Gomeni R, Poli S, Schmerber S (2018) Safety, tolerability, pharmacokinetics and pharmacokinetic-pharmacodynamic modelling of the novel H4 receptor inhibitor SENS-111 using a modified caloric test in healthy subjects. Br J Clin Pharmacol 84(12):2836–2848

Venkatasamy A, Huynh TT, Wohlhuter N, Vuong H, Rohmer D, Charpiot A, Meyer N, Veillon F (2019) Superior vestibular neuritis: improved detection using FLAIR sequence with delayed enhancement (1 h). Eur Arch Otorhinolaryngol 276(12):3309–3316

Vibert N, Vidal PP (2001) In vitro effects of acetyl-DL-leucine (tanganil) on central vestibular neurons and vestibulo-ocular networks of the guinea-pig. Eur J Neurosci 13(4):735–748

von Brevern M, Bertholon P, Brandt T, Fife T, Imai T, Nuti D, Newman-Toker D (2015) Benign paroxysmal positional vertigo: Diagnostic criteria. J Vestib Res 25(3–4):105–117

von Brevern M, Zeise D, Neuhauser H, Clarke AH, Lempert T (2005) Acute migrainous vertigo: clinical and oculographic findings. Brain 128(Pt 2): 365–374

Wersinger E, Gaboyard-Niay S, Travo C, Soto E, Baez A, Vega R, Brugeaud A, Chabbert C (2013) Symptomatic treatment of vestibular deficits: therapeutic potential of histamine H4 receptors. J Vestib Res 23(3):153–159

Whitney SL, Sparto PJ, Furman JM (2020) Vestibular rehabilitation and factors that can affect outcome. Semin Neurol 40(1):165–172

Yang TH, Lee J, Oh SY, Kang JJ, Kim JS, Dieterich M (2020) Clinical implications of head-shaking nystagmus in central and peripheral vestibular disorders: is perverted head-shaking nystagmus specific for central vestibular pathology? Eur J Neurol 27:1296–1303

Yip CW, Glaser M, Frenzel C, Bayer O, Strupp M (2016) Comparison of the bedside head-impulse test with the video head-impulse test in a clinical practice setting: a prospective study of 500 outpatients. Front Neurol 7:58

Zwergal A, Dieterich M (2020) Vertigo and dizziness in the emergency room. Curr Opin Neurol 33(1): 117–125

Zwergal A, Schlichtiger J, Xiong G, Beck R, Gunther L, Schniepp R, Schoberl F, Jahn K, Brandt T, Strupp M, Bartenstein P, Dieterich M, Dutia MB, la FC (2014) Sequential [F]FDG microPET whole-brain imaging of central vestibular compensation: a model of deafferentation-induced brain plasticity. Brain Struct Funct 221:159–170

Benign Paroxysmal Positional Vertigo

Contents

Supplementary Information The online version contains supplementary material available at [https://doi.org/10.1007/978-3-030-78260-3_9]. The videos can be accessed by scanning the related images with the SN More Media App.

M. Strupp et al., *Vertigo and Dizziness*, https://doi.org/10.1007/978-3-030-78260-3_9

Benign paroxysmal positional vertigo (BPPV)—the second most frequent vestibular disorder—is characterized by brief recurrent episodes of spinning vertigo, lasting seconds, induced by changes in head position relative to gravity, with a positional nystagmus. It is caused by otoconia that most often move freely in the affected semicircular canal leading to a deviation of the cupula by changes of head position. This pathophysiology explains why the attack of spinning vertigo and nystagmus is more correctly described by a positional than a positioning vertigo. It is the position of the head relative to gravity and not the movement itself that elicits the symptoms. This is similar to central positional vertigo/nystagmus syndromes in which the position of otoliths relative to gravity is causative (Choi and Kim 2019).

In 85–95%, the posterior semicircular canal is affected, in 10–15% the horizontal canal and very rarely the anterior canal. The affected side, canal and the mechanism can be identified with the diagnostic positional maneuvers. 95% of the cases are idiopathic. The treatment of choice is a side-, canal-, and mechanism-specific liberatory maneuver, with which practically all patients can be successfully treated. However, the cumulative recurrence rate is high (50%).

9.1 Epidemiology

BPPV is the most frequent peripheral vestibular disorder (for the relative frequency, see ◘ Fig. 1.3 and ◘ Table 1.1), despite being largely underdiagnosed (Neuhauser 2016). The reported prevalence is between 10 and 140/100,000 and the lifetime prevalence is at least 2.4% (von Brevern et al. 2007; van der Zaag-Loonen et al. 2015). In a population of subjects over 75, a very high prevalence of 9–11% was found (Oghalai et al. 2000; Kollen et al. 2012). BPPV can occur from childhood—where it is rare (Choi et al. 2020) but also the most frequent peripheral vestibular disorder (Hulse et al. 2019)—to old age. Idiopathic BPPV is a typical disorder of the elderly with a peak in the 5th to 7th decades (Neuhauser 2016). In idiopathic BPPV, women are affected at as twice as often as men (e.g., Katsarkas, 1999). 40% of geriatric patients who report vertigo suffer from BPPV (Ekvall et al. 2005). Screening techniques for BPPV either with tailored questionnaires (Lindell et al. 2018; Kim et al. 2020) or "smart" devices (Feil et al. 2018) have increased the accuracy of epidemiological estimates of its prevalence.

9.2 Posterior Canal BPPV

The diagnostic criteria for canalolithiasis of the posterior semicircular canal BPPV (pcBPPV) are as follows (von Brevern et al. 2015):

Box 9.1 Diagnostic Criteria of the Bárány-Society for Canalolithiasis of pcBPPV (von Brevern et al. 2015)

1. Recurrent attacks of positional vertigo or positional dizziness, provoked by lying down or turning over in the supine position.
2. Duration of attacks <1 min.
3. Positional nystagmus elicited after a latency of one or a few seconds by the Dix-Hallpike maneuver or side-lying maneuver (diagnostic Semont maneuver). The nystagmus is a combination of torsional nystagmus with the upper pole of the eyes beating toward the lower ear and vertical nystagmus beating upward (toward the forehead) typically lasting <1 min.
4. Not attributable to another disorder.

9.2.1 Diagnosis

9.2.1.1 Patient History

The leading symptom (Fig. 9.1) of pcBPPV is recurrent attacks of spinning vertigo, lasting seconds, which are induced by changes of head position relative to gravity (▶ Box 9.1). They can be associated with nausea, vomiting, or oscillopsia. Typical triggers include lying down or sitting up in bed, rolling over in bed, and bending over or extending the head backwards in order to look up or do something above the head. If BPPV is elicited while the patient is upright, there is a risk of falling. Attacks of vertigo are variable: They frequently occur in the morning, because over night the otoconia form an agglomerate which has a higher impact on endolymphatic flow than single crystals (Obrist et al. 2010) and repeated changes in position cause a transient lessening of the attacks. The complaints are often so typical ("my every morning vertigo") that a diagnosis can often be made solely on the basis of the patient history; occasionally even the affected ear can be identified ("spinning vertigo only occurs when lying down on my right side"). Questionnaires can contribute to the diagnosis (Lindell et al. 2018; Kim et al. 2020).

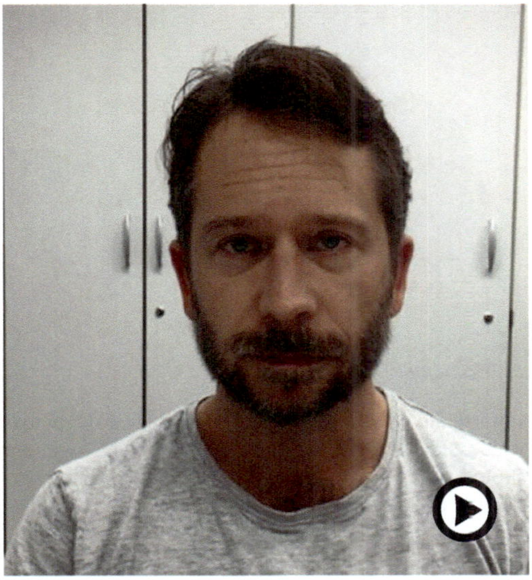

Fig. 9.1 Benign paroxysmal positioning vertigo (BPPV): patient history (▶ https://doi.org/10.1007/000-95f)

In addition to the episodes of spinning vertigo, about half of the patients (von Brevern et al. 2007) report—most often when specifically asked about it—postural imbalance and gait disorder. This is caused by so-called post-repositioning otolith dizziness, which can be explained by a partial repositioning of the otoconia back to the utricle (see below).

9.2.1.2 Bedside Examination

Diagnostic Semont-maneuver. As illustrated in Figs. 9.2, 9.3, 9.4 and 9.5, the head of the patient sitting in an upright position is turned 45° to one side. Subsequently, the patient's body is moved 90° or 150° ("diagnostic SemontPLUS maneuver," (Fig. 9.6) as already recommended earlier (Brandt et al. 1994)), at a medium velocity, toward the other side. In this position, one looks for nystagmus, using Frenzel goggles or M-glasses, for 1 min and asks the patient whether he/she experiences spinning vertigo. If there is posterior canal BPPV, one will see, after a short latency of a few seconds, a vertical-torsional positional nystagmus with a crescendo-decrescendo time course and a duration of less than 1 min. The fast phase of the nystagmus beats upward (toward the forehead) and the torsional component (upper pole of the eyes) beats toward the undermost ear (Figs. 9.4 and 9.5). The direction of the nystagmus depends on the direction of gaze: It is primarily torsional when the patient looks toward the undermost ear and vertical (to the forehead) when the patient eye position is parallel to the affected posterior canal. The nystagmus is caused by an (ampullofugal) excitation of the posterior canal of the undermost ear.

Dix-Hallpike maneuver (Dix and Hallpike 1952). The patient's head is turned 45° to one side; then, the patient is moved from an upright to a supine position with the head overextended by 20°; examination of eye movements as described above. Subsequently, the other side is examined.

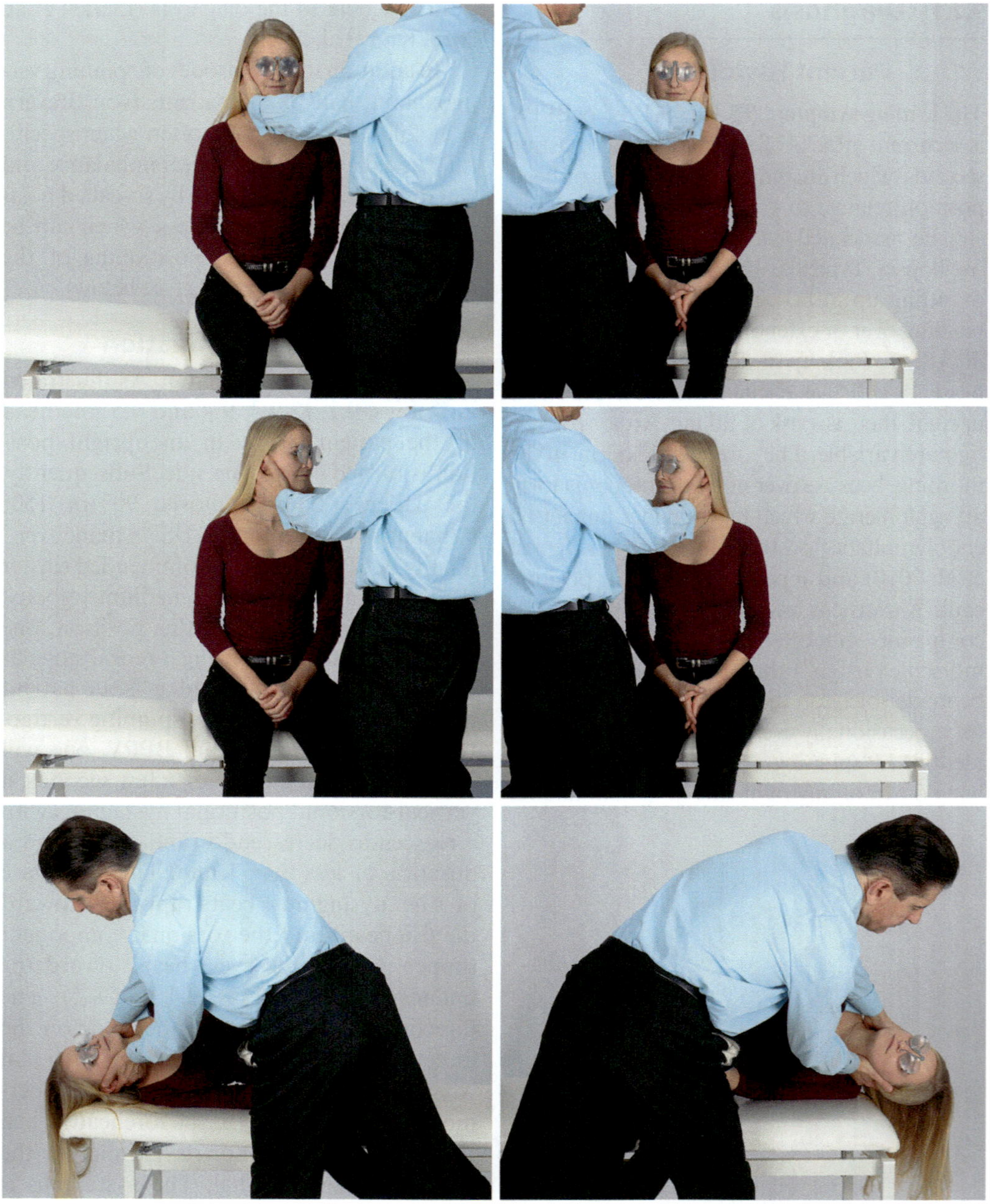

9

Fig. 9.2 Diagnostic Semont maneuver. On the left, for the right posterior canal and, on the right, for the left posterior canal. The patient's head is turned 45° to one side; then, the patient's body is moved toward the other side. If one is not able to conclude which side is affected from the patient history, one should start with the right side, because it is more frequently affected than the left side

If one is able to deduce the probable affected side from the patient history, one should begin with the examination of this side. If the affected side is not known, one should start by examining the right posterior canal because it is more frequently affected

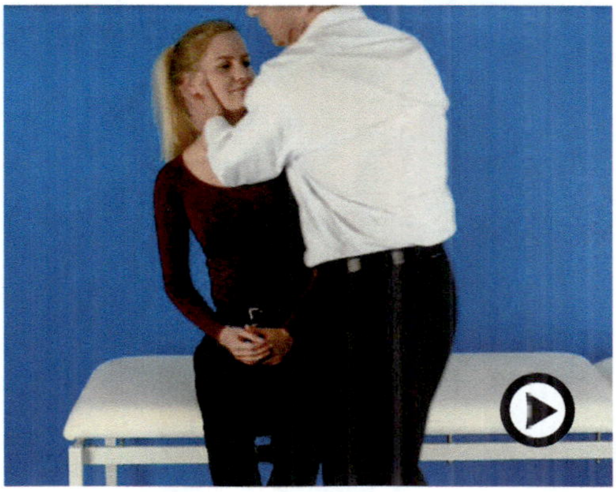

Fig. 9.3 Diagnostic SemontPLUS maneuver (▶ https://doi.org/10.1007/000-95a)

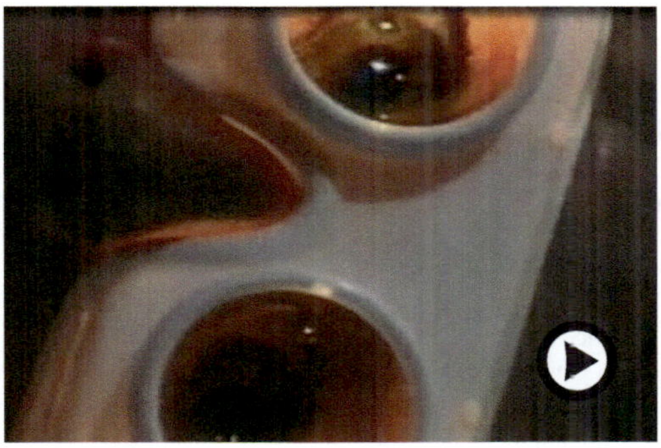

Fig. 9.4 Vertical torsional positional nystagmus in left-sided posterior canal BPPV (▶ https://doi.org/10.1007/000-95b)

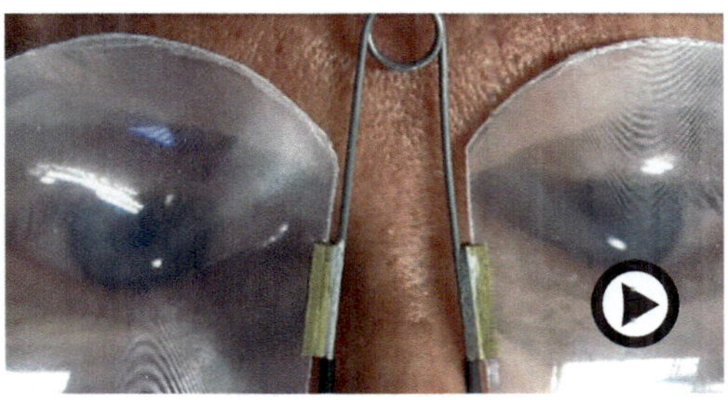

Fig. 9.5 Vertical torsional positional nystagmus in right-sided posterior canal BPPV (▶ https://doi.org/10.1007/000-95c)

than the left posterior canal (Lopez-Escamez et al. 2002); it is assumed that this is because most people sleep on their right side.

If one is not able to induce vertigo or nystagmus during the examination, we recommend that patients perform the diagnostic maneuvers every morning for 10 days according to written instructions. The accuracy of the diagnosis can be further increased by the patient using a smartphone to video his/her eye movements during the diagnostic positioning maneuvers (Shah et al. 2019, Strupp et al. 2023), by screening technologies with a special questionnaire and by smart devices (Feil et al. 2018).

9.2.1.3 Laboratory Examination

As already described by Dix and Hallpike in 1952 in a series of 100 patients (Dix and Hallpike 1952), BPPV is a relatively benign, non-destructive disease, which does not per se lead to vestibular deficits. Therefore, if the diagnosis is certain, additional laboratory examinations are normally not necessary (von Brevern et al. 2015; Bhattacharyya et al. 2017). If the patient history is not typical or the clinical findings are not unambiguous, laboratory examinations and imaging studies play an important role in looking for other causes (particularly central positional vertigo/nystagmus). Laboratory examinations are also indicated if there is evidence of other prior diseases, such as acute unilateral vestibulopathy or Menière's disease, which are both associated with a higher risk of BPPV (see below).

9.2.2 Differential Diagnoses and Clinical Problems

The most relevant differential diagnoses for pcBPPV are summarized in Table 9.1. They can be categorized as follows:

1. Peripheral vestibular disorders, with recurrent episodes of vertigo, namely
   - rare horizontal canal BPPV (hcBPPV, ▶ Sect. 9.3) and very rare anterior canal BPPV (acBPPV,

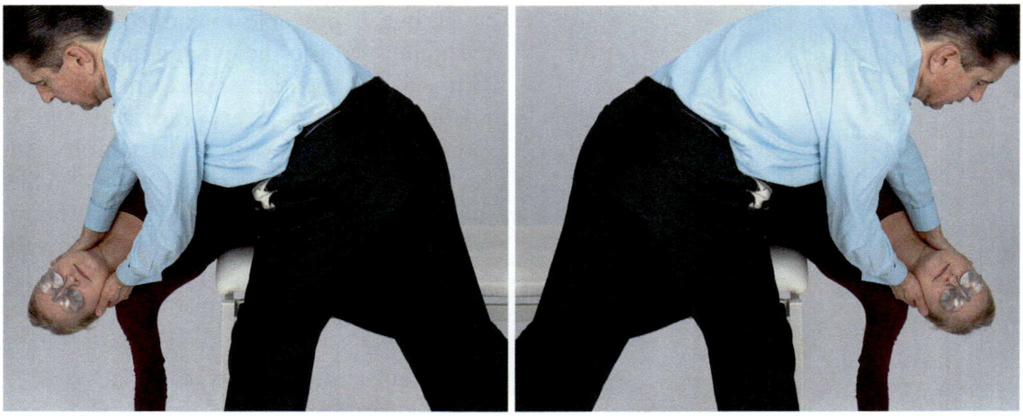

Fig. 9.6 Diagnostic SemontPLUS maneuver. The difference to the regular Semont maneuver is that the patient's head is overextended by 60°, which should theoretically increase the sensitivity of the diagnostic maneuver

Table 9.1 Differential diagnoses for pcBPPV with the leading symptom of recurrent short episodes of vertigo, and diseases or conditions associated with a higher risk of BPPV

Peripheral vestibular disorders	Central disorders	Other diseases	Diseases or conditions which are associated with a higher risk of BPPV
Horizontal canal BPPV Anterior canal BPPV Multiple canals affected Bilateral BPPV Syndrome of the third mobile windows Vestibular paroxysmia	Central positional vertigo/nystagmus Vestibular migraine TIA Vertebral artery compression/occlusion syndrome Paroxysmal brainstem attacks	Orthostatic dizziness Metabolic disorders, such as hypoglycemia Panic attacks Drug-induced	Head trauma Long bedrest Reduced physical activity Age After acute unilateral vestibulopathy Menière's disease Vestibular migraine Reduced hearing

▶ Sect. 9.4); the diagnosis can be made by observing the direction of the positional vertigo, which corresponds to the affected canal.

- BPPV which affects two or three semicircular canals. In such cases, it is recommended to wait a few days and then repeat the examination of the patient, because there is a high rate of spontaneous remission in hcBPPV and acBPPV.
- bilateral BPPV, which is relatively more frequent after head trauma: about 10% of post-traumatic BPPV are bilateral (Katsarkas 1999; Gordon et al. 2004; Mumford 2019); for clinical practice, it is therefore recommended to examine both sides.
- vestibular paroxysmia (▶ Chap. 11).

- short-arm pcBPPV (Buki et al. 2011; Buki et al. 2014; Ping et al. 2020).
- syndrome of the third mobile windows (▶ Chap. 12), most often superior canal dehiscence syndrome.

2. Central disorders, namely
   - central positional vertigo/nystagmus, for instance due to cerebellar lesions (for details, see below and ◘ Table 9.2).

◘ Table 9.2 Clinical features differentiating benign peripheral paroxysmal positioning vertigo (BPPV) from central positional vertigo or nystagmus (CPV)

Features	BPPV	CPV
Latency following precipitating positioning maneuvers	1–15 s (shorter in hcBPPV)	No latency or 1–5 s
Vertigo	Typical	Typical
Duration of attack	5–40 s (longer in hc-BPPV and much longer in rare cupulolithiasis)	5–>60 s
Direction of nystagmus	Torsional-vertical with head positioning in the plane of the posterior (pcBPPV) or the anterior (acBPPV) canal, horizontal with head positioning in the plane of the horizontal (hcBPPV) canal	Purely vertical or torsional, combined torsional/linear, direction of nystagmus does not correspond with the plane of the canal stimulated by the head movement
Course of vertigo and nystagmus in the attack	Crescendo/decrescendo (with typical canalolithiasis)	Crescendo/decrescendo is rare but possible
Nausea and vomiting	Rare with single head-positioning maneuvers (if so, then associated with intense positioning nystagmus); frequent with repeated maneuvers	Frequent with single head-positioning maneuvers (not necessarily associated with intense nystagmus)
Natural course	Spontaneous recovery within days to months in 70–80%	Dependent on etiology, spontaneous recovery within weeks in most cases
Associated neurological signs and symptoms	None (in idiopathic BPPV)	Frequent cerebellar and ocular motor signs, such as ataxia, saccadic pursuit, gaze-evoked nystagmus, downbeat nystagmus, impaired fixation suppression of the VOR
Brain imaging	Normal	Lesions dorsolateral from the fourth ventricle and/or of the dorsal ocular motor vermis, nodulus due to tumor, hemorrhage, infarction, or multiple sclerosis plaque. Less specific lesions (cerebellar degeneration, paraneoplastic syndromes, encephalopathy, intoxication)

Adapted from (Buttner et al. 1999)

- vestibular migraine, which may also be associated with positional vertigo (Dieterich and Brandt 1999; von Brevern et al. 2005; Radtke et al. 2012; Neugebauer et al. 2013; Beh 2018); in addition there is a high comorbidity between migraine, vestibular migraine (▶ Chap. 14) and BPPV.

3. Other disorders, in particular orthostatic dizziness (for diagnostic criteria, see (Kim et al. 2019a)). In these patients, the symptoms typically occur when the patient gets up from lying or sitting down and not when he/she is lying down. This is also helpful when performing the diagnostic positioning maneuvers, because these patients often complain of dizziness when they get up from lying down on the right and left side.

It should also be noted that BPPV occurs more frequently with other vestibular disorders. Examples are acute unilateral vestibulopathy (Büchele and Brandt 1988; Karlberg et al. 2000), where about 15% of patients have so-called post-infectious BPPV, Menière's disease, or vestibular migraine. Therefore, all of these patients should undergo diagnostic positional maneuvers so that comorbidities are not overlooked ("vertigo squared/cubed"). In patients who do not respond to treatment, it is important to rule out bilateral BPPV, which occurs more frequently after head trauma (Gordon et al. 2004) or to consider a transition from pcBPPV to hcBPPV and vice versa.

9.2.2.1 Central Positional Vertigo/Nystagmus

Central positional vertigo and central positional nystagmus (e.g., Buttner et al. 1999; Macdonald et al. 2017; Lemos and Strupp 2022) are caused by infra-tentorial lesions that affect connections between the vestibular nuclei in the medulla oblongata, cerebellar structures close to the midline, namely the nodulus (e.g., Nam et al. 2009; Kim et al. 2012a; Choi et al. 2015; Tateno and Sakakibara 2019) or the dorsal ocular motor vermis (e.g., Shoman and Longridge 2007; Lee et al. 2014a; Kremmyda et al. 2013; see also ▶ Chap. 13). It is important to distinguish between peripheral and central positional nystagmus, as the latter require further laboratory diagnostics, in particular imaging. A systematic clinical examination is as least as relevant as imaging (De Schutter et al. 2019); for details, see below. Four characteristic forms of central positional vertigo/nystagmus can be distinguished, although the symptoms overlap and combinations occur:

- Central downbeat nystagmus, in the head-hanging position (with or without accompanying vertigo), typically in lesions of the nodulus
- Central positional nystagmus (without vertigo)
- Central paroxysmal positional vertigo with nystagmus, typically in nodulus lesions
- "Central positional vomiting"

When patients with pcBPPV have their typical history and patterns, they will almost never be mixed up with a central vestibular lesion. Imaging and additional vestibular testing are not necessary in patients who meet the diagnostic criteria for BPPV in the absence of additional vestibular/neurological signs and/or symptoms inconsistent with BPPV (for references, see Bhattacharyya et al. 2017).

On the other hand, one must distinguish the apogeotropic variant of hcBPPV from a central (usually vestibulocerebellar) lesion. Migraine may also present with horizontal direction-changing positional nystagmus and vertigo (Dieterich and Brandt 1999; von Brevern et al. 2005; Radtke et al. 2012; Neugebauer et al. 2013; Beh 2018). Finally, acBPPV—which can look like a positional downbeat nystagmus—also has to be distinguished from central vestibular disorders (see below, ▶ Sect. 9.4).

These central vestibular disorders occur much more rarely than the typical BPPV which is the second most frequent vestibular disease. However, it can be difficult to distinguish peripheral and central function disorders in the individual patient (◘ Table 9.2). The following six clinical rules are important for diagnosing a *central* positional vertigo/nystagmus (Buttner et al. 1999; Lemos and Strupp 2022):

- Positional nystagmus that does *not* correspond to the plane of the semicircular canal stimulated by the head positioning (e.g., torsional nystagmus after stimulation of the horizontal canal). In clinical practice, this seems to be the most important feature by which a central positional nystagmus can be identified (Buttner et al. 1999).
- Positional vertigo with a purely vertical nystagmus (most often downbeat, rarely upbeat) or purely torsional nystagmus is central. However, a purely horizontal nystagmus is also typical for hcBPPV (see ▶ Sect. 9.3) and the differential diagnosis can be difficult, in particular in apogeotropic nystagmus. According to one systematic study, the intensity of spontaneous nystagmus was similar while sitting and supine in the apogeotropic type of central positional nystagmus, but greater when supine in apogeotropic nystagmus of BPPV (Choi et al. 2018a) (◘ Fig. 9.7).

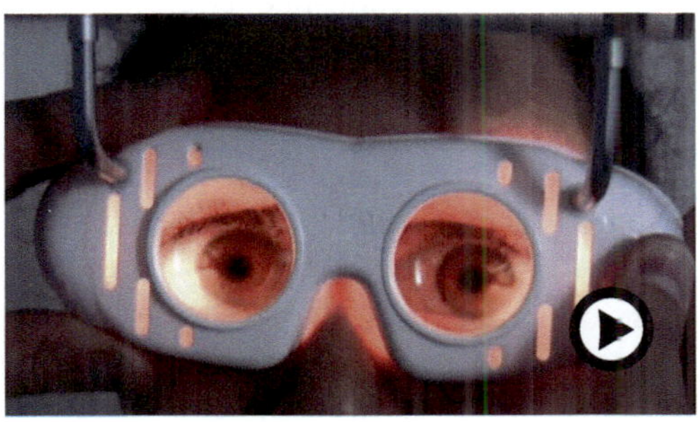

◘ **Fig. 9.7** Central positional downwardly beating nystagmus in all positions
(▶ https://doi.org/10.1007/000-95d)

- Persisting positional nystagmus (slow-phase velocity > 5°/s) without associated vertigo.
- Positioning-induced vomiting after single head movements without any substantial vertigo or nystagmus.
- Associated central cerebellar ocular motor disorders such as saccadic smooth pursuit, gaze-evoked or downbeat nystagmus.
- No or only miminal response to the liberatory maneuvers.

9.2.3 Diagnosis: The Essentials for Clinical Practice

Independent of the patient history, the diagnostic positional maneuvers must be performed in all patients with vertigo and dizziness. In cases with a typical history and correct performance of the diagnostic positional maneuvers, the diagnosis, the affected side and canal (posterior > horizontal >> anterior) and, in horizontal canal BPPV (see below), the mechanism (canalolithiasis >> cupulolithiasis) can be determined. The most important differential diagnosis is central positional vertigo/nystagmus, which can most often be differentiated by the direction of the nystagmus which does not correspond to an affected canal. In unclear cases, in particular if—despite a typical history—vertigo and nystagmus cannot be induced during the diagnostic maneuvers, it is helpful for the patient to use a smartphone to video his/her nystagmus during the diagnostic positional maneuvers (Strupp et al. 2023). Clinical practice shows that BPPV is, on the one hand, still often overlooked, but on the other hand, it is nowadays also diagnosed too frequently. Thus, doctors must assure themselves of the diagnosis in each case. In particular in the elderly, BPPV is often not considered as a differential diagnosis and therefore not diagnosed, because the affected individuals perform head and body movements very slowly so they do not induce attacks of spinning vertigo, but just complain of postural imbalance and dizziness and are therefore not examined for BPPV.

9.2.4 Pathophysiology and Therapeutic Principles

Posterior canal BPPV is, in almost all cases, caused by canalolithiasis (Brandt and Steddin 1993; Brandt et al. 1994). According to this hypothesis, the attacks are induced by otoconia that move freely in the semicircular canal (Brandt and Steddin 1993; Brandt et al. 1994; Hall et al. 1979; Parnes and McClure 1992) (◘ Fig. 9.8). Depending on the direction of sedimentation, the movement of the agglomerate causes an ampullofugal or ampullopetal deflection of the cupula and thus leads to a stimulation or inhibition of the vestibular hair cells. This mechanism was already supported by histopathological studies in 1992 (Parnes and McClure 1992) and more recently by biophysical models of the labyrinth, which allow further detailed evaluation (Obrist et al. 2010; Obrist et al. 2016). Canalolithiasis can predict all features of the BPPV which are as follows (Brandt et al. 1994):

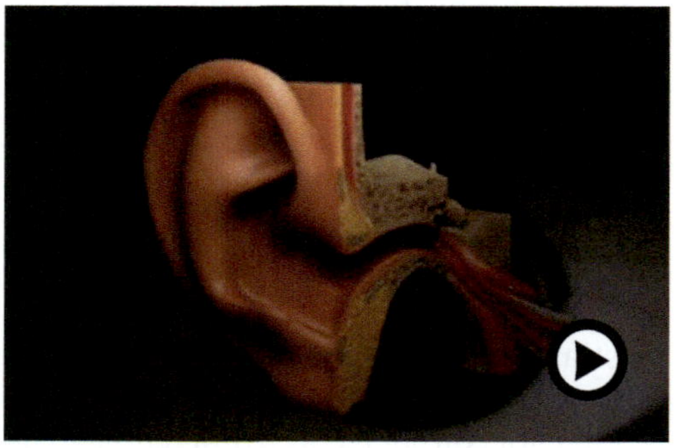

◘ **Fig. 9.8** Animation of the movement of the otoconia in BPPV (► https://doi.org/10.1007/000-95e)

▪▪ Direction of the positional nystagmus

The ampullofugal stimulation of the posterior canal causes eye movements in the plane of the canal via the VOR, according to Ewald's first law. To the examiner, this will appear to be a combination of a vertical (toward the forehead) and a torsional nystagmus (toward the undermost ear) with the fast phase of the nystagmus beating toward the excited canal.

▪▪ Latency

Spinning vertigo and nystagmus appear as soon as the particles in the canal precipitate as a result of gravity. This causes a deflection of the cupula, which exceeds the stimulus threshold of the sensory epithelium after 1–5 s.

▪▪ Duration

After the change in position, the particles move toward the lowest point within the canal and precipitate. Depending on their size and composition, this takes about 10–40 s (Obrist et al. 2010; Obrist et al. 2016).

▪▪ Time course of attacks

After the positioning, the particles fall away from the curved canal wall. They are accelerated from standstill by the forces of gravity, reach a maximal speed during their fall, and return to a standstill at the lowest point in the canal. This explains the temporal crescendo–decrescendo-like course of the attacks; the cupula time constant increases the duration of the nystagmus and vertigo of up to 60 s.

▪▪ Reversal of the direction of the nystag mus

If the direction of the positioning movement is reversed, for instance, when sitting up, the particles move in the opposite direction. Now, the cupula is deflected in the opposite (ampullopetal) direction. This results in a reversal of both the spinning vertigo and the direction of nystagmus due to inhibition of the vestibular hair cells of the posterior canal.

■ ■ Fatigability

The particles can form a agglomerate. During changes in head position or other head movement, they may increasingly fall apart (Dix and Hallpike 1952; Hornrubia et al. 1999). During head movements, small particles cause less movement of the endolymph and thus the cupula, as does a agglomerate, which was confirmed by biophysical experiments (Obrist et al. 2010). If the patient holds his/her head still for several hours (e.g., during sleep), the particles, which had fallen apart before, coalesce into a clump in the lowest place within the canal and again induce spinning vertigo when the head position is changed relative to gravity. This also explains why the symptoms typically begin and are more severe in the early morning and improve during daytime.

■ ■ Effects of the liberatory maneuver

- The mechanism of action and the efficacy of the liberatory/repositioning maneuvers can also be explained by the canalolithiasis hypothesis, i.e., the crystals move freely within the canal, finally moving in the direction of the utricle (see below).

9.2.5 Etiology and Associated Factors

There are two types of BPPV: idiopathic and secondary or symptomatic BPPV. However, a discrimination between the two is not always possible. More than 95% of all cases are classified as idiopathic (women: men = 2:1) (e.g., (Karlberg et al. 2000)); in these cases, degeneration of the otolith organs and otoconia seems to be relevant.

Several epidemiological studies and meta-analyses have evaluated associated factors of BPPV. In a epidemiological study with 1240 individuals, a multivariate analysis showed that age, history of falls, and reduced physical activity are significantly associated with BPPV (Park et al. 2019). Other epidemiological studies showed an increased risk of BPPV in individuals with migraine with an odds ratio of 2.54 (Kim et al. 2019b) and sensorineural hearing loss (after exclusion of patients with Menière's disease) with an odds ratio of 2.9 (Lee et al. 2019). Another epidemiological study found that poor levels of physical activity, unhealthy lifestyles, and prolonged time spent in a recumbent position may be independent risk factors for BPPV (Fu et al. 2020). In a meta-analysis (19 studies published between 2006 and 2019, including 2618 patients with BPPV and 11,668 participants without BPPV), female gender, vitamin D deficiency, osteoporosis, migraine, head trauma, and high total cholesterol level were risk factors for the occurrence of BPPV (Chen et al. 2020).

The role of vitamin D deficiency and osteoporosis has been extensively discussed. First, studies showed decreased bone mineral density and a higher incidence of osteoporosis in patients with BPPV compared with controls (for references, see Yu et al. 2014). Second, there is a seasonal variation of BPPV with a higher prevalence from December to May with a negative correlation to the serum 25-hydroxyvitamin D concentration (for references, see Whitman and Baloh 2015). Third, there are—partially contradictory—results for an association of the vitamin D level with the development of BPPV and the rate of recurrence. In several publications, a low vitamin D level was identified as a risk factor for BPPV, with a particular significance in female, postmenopausal patients (e.g., Song et al. 2020). Reduced vitamin D levels were also found in patients with recurrent BPPV (Rhim 2016; Rhim 2019). However, other publications reported that the coexistence of BPPV with osteoporosis and vitamin D deficiency may be coincidental (Karatas et al. 2017). A meta-analysis of 37 studies failed to establish a relationship between the occurrence of BPPV and a low vitamin D level (AlGarni et al. 2018). Further meta-analysis with subgroup analysis by geographical area highlighted variations in different ethnic groups between Chinese and non-Chinese (Korea, Turkey) patients: Significantly lower blood levels of vitamin D were seen in individuals with BPPV than in controls compared to studies outside China with no significant difference (Yang et al. 2020). Finally, in another study the serum vitamin D concentration was measured in 680 patients (661 Caucasians). 158 patients had BPPV (Goldschagg et al. 2021); 221 had other vestibular diseases and 301 patients had other neurological non-vestibular diseases. There was no significant difference in the serum vitamin concentration between patients with BPPV and those with other vestibular disorders. Patients with other neurological disorders had even lower concentrations than patients with BPPV or other vestibular disorders. This did not support the theory of a specific relationship between serum vitamin D concentration and the occurrence of BPPV or other vestibular disorders.

Secondary or symptomatic cases (women: men = 1: 1):

- Are most often caused by head injury (Karlberg et al. 2000; Balatsouras et al. 2017; Mumford 2019; Di Cesare et al. 2021).
- Can occur after AUVP/vestibular neuritis (Büchele and Brandt 1988) ("post-infectious BPPV" in up to 15% patients with AUVP (Karlberg et al. 2000; Balatsouras et al. 2014)). This can be explained by the preservation of the function of the posterior semicircular canal in AUVP in most patients (Büchele and Brandt 1988) and by the evidence that the labyrinth can also be impaired by the HSV-1 virus inflammation (Arbusow et al. 2000) (see also ▶ Chap. 8.6).

9

9.2.6 Course of the Disease and Its Consequences

We found that the history of the disorder until its diagnosis had lasted more than 4 weeks in 50% of our patients and more than 6 months in 10% (Brandt et al. 2010). It is called "benign" because it generally resolves spontaneously within weeks to months without persisting deficits and can theoretically be well treated (see below). The symptoms recover spontaneously after 1 month in about 20% of cases and after 3 months in about 50% of cases (Lynn et al. 1995; Burton et al. 2012). If not treated, BPPV persists in about 30% of patients (Imai et al., 2005).

The consequences of undiagnosed and untreated BPPV are, however, not at all benign (Lopez-Escamez et al. 2003; Benecke et al. 2013), because they are associated with an increased risk of falls and considerable limitations in daily life in up to 86% of patients with BPPV (Li et al. 2022).

9.2.7 Treatment: Principles, Aims, and Pragmatic Therapy

9.2.7.1 Therapeutic Principles

The mechanism of action of the treatment by liberatory *maneuvers* can be explained by means of the canalolithiasis hypothesis, i.e., freely moving otoconia or an agglomerate of otoconia in the affected canal (Brandt and Steddin 1993; Brandt et al. 1994). Changes of head position relative to gravity can move the otoconia out of the affected canal.

In 1980, Brandt and Daroff first devised an exercise program, which, by means of the simple physical measure of head positioning, loosens the heavy degenerative otolithic material and distributes it into other areas of the labyrinth, where it comes to rest and no longer impairs canal function (Brandt and Daroff 1980).

In 1988, Semont and co-workers (Semont et al. 1988) published liberatory maneuvers that consider the three-dimensional orientation of the posterior canal: The patient's head is turned 45° toward the non-affected side and then the patient's body is moved 90° toward the affected side, followed by a 180° movement of the whole body toward the non-affected side, then the patient returns to an upright sitting position (◘ Fig. 9.9).

In 1992, Epley described the so-called repositioning maneuver (Epley 1992). This requires turns of the patient's head in a supine position with overextension of the head (◘ Fig. 9.10).

In 1994, Brandt and co-workers recommended the Semont maneuvers with movements of the whole body toward the non-affected side by 195° (Brandt et al. 1994).

Finally, based on biophysical experiments (Obrist et al. 2016), the so-called SemontPLUS maneuver was recommended that was more effective than the regular Semont maneuver (Strupp et al. 2021) as well as the Epley maneuver (Strupp et al., Abstract, FP1127, Barany Society meeting, Madrid, 2022) in two prospective randomizied multi-center trials.

For all diagnostic and therapeutic maneuvers it is important that the canal is oriented in parallel to the gravitational vector. Deviations of more than 20° will lead to a failure of the maneuvers (Gebhart et al. 2021). In summary, the Semont, the SemontPLUS and Epley maneuvers are the gold standard treatments for pcBPPV. These treatments are classified with level 1 efficacy based on evidence-based medicine with a high success rate of up to 95%+ (Hilton and Pinder 2014; for references, see also Bhattacharyya et al. 2017), if performed correctly. The efficacy of treatment does not depend on the age of the patients or pre-existing neurological disorders (Chen et al. 2018). Finally, a single maneuver is not sufficient to treat patients (see below).

The efficacy of the Semont maneuver appears to be somewhat less well documented than that of the Epley maneuver (see below), since there are only a few studies with non-treated or sham-treated controls. A randomized study with an untreated control group showed that after one or multiple treatments, 94% of the patients were symptom-free as opposed to only 36% of the untreated controls (Salvinelli et al. 2003). In another double-blind sham-controlled study, 1 h after one Semont maneuver 79% and 24 h later 87% were symptom-free compared to none within the sham group (Mandala et al. 2012). According to retrospective case series, the success rate of the Semont maneuver is around 50–70% after one treatment and over 90–98% after several treatments (Semont et al. 1988; Coppo et al. 1996; Serafini et al. 1996; Levrat et al. 2003; Steenerson and Cronin 1996). Many studies showed that a single Semont maneuver is not able to cure the majority of patients with BPPV with a wide range of reported success rates of a single Semont maneuver in the literature (e.g., 37.5% (Lee et al. 2014b) or 79.3% (Mandala et al. 2012)). Therefore, we recommend that the patient performs self-maneuvers three times in the morning, three times in the afternoon, and three times at night until he/she is no longer able to induce positional vertigo in the morning on three consequtive days.

The efficacy of Epley's maneuver has been proven by several controlled, randomized studies and meta-analyses (Lynn et al. 1995; Froehling et al. 2000; Yimtae et al. 2003; Cohen and Kimball 2004; von Brevern et al. 2006b; Strupp et al. 2007). Another meta-analysis has shown that patients in the first follow-ups were 4.6-times more symptom-free than untreated patients (Woodworth et al. 2004). A randomized study shows that a single maneuver is as effective as multiple maneuvers (Isaradisaikul et al. 2021). This, however, is not our experience. Therefore, we recommend multiple maneuvers (see above). For a comparision of the normal Semont and the Epley versus the SemontPLUS maneuver see below.

Treating BPPV with vestibular suppressant medications (antihistamines and/or benzodiazepines) as well as post-maneuver restrictions of head movements or sleeping positions is not recommended

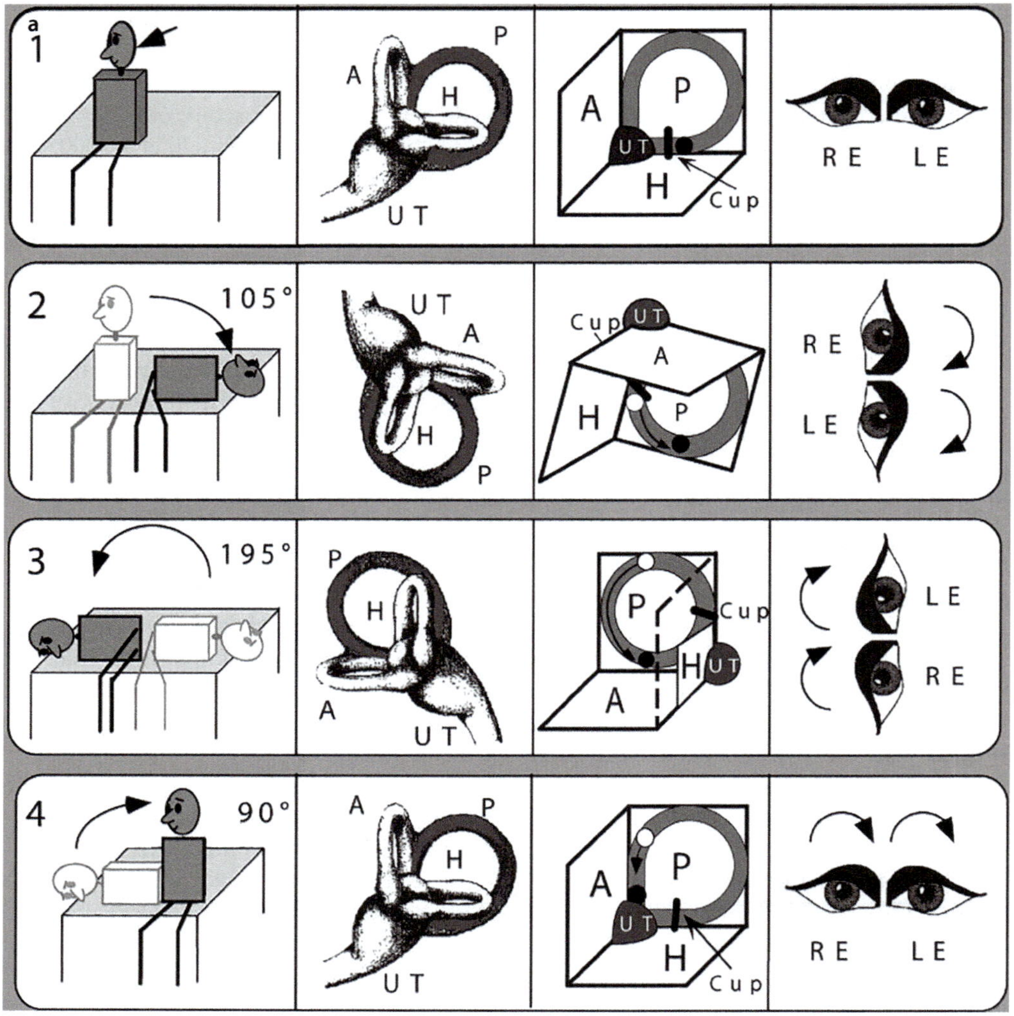

Fig. 9.9 **a** Schematic drawing of the Semont liberatory maneuver of a patient with benign paroxysmal positional vertigo of the left posterior semicircular canal. Panels from left to right: position of body and head, position of labyrinth in space, position and movement of the cristals in the posterior canal (which causes cupula deflection), and the direction of the nystagmus. The agglomerate is depicted as an open circle within the canal; a black circle represents the final resting position of the clot. (1) In the sitting position, the head is turned horizontally 45° to the unaffected ear. The agglomerate, which is heavier than endolymph, settles at the base of the left posterior semicircular canal. (2) The patient is tilted 90° to the left (affected) ear. The change in head position, relative to gravity, causes the clot to gravitate to the lowermost part of the canal and the cupula to deflect downward, inducing BPPV with torsional nystagmus beating toward the undermost ear. The patient maintains this position for 1 min. (3) The patient is turned 180° with the nose down, causing the clot to move toward the exit of the canal. The endolymphatic flow again deflects the cupula so that the nystagmus beats toward the left ear, now uppermost. The patient remains in this position for 1 min. (4) The patient is slowly moved into the sitting position; this causes the clot to enter the utricular cavity (Adapted from (Brandt et al. 1994)). A, P, H anterior, posterior, horizontal semicircular canals, Cup cupula, UT utricular cavity, RE right eye, LE left eye. **b** Semont liberatory maneuver of a patient with typical benign paroxysmal positional vertigo of the left posterior canal

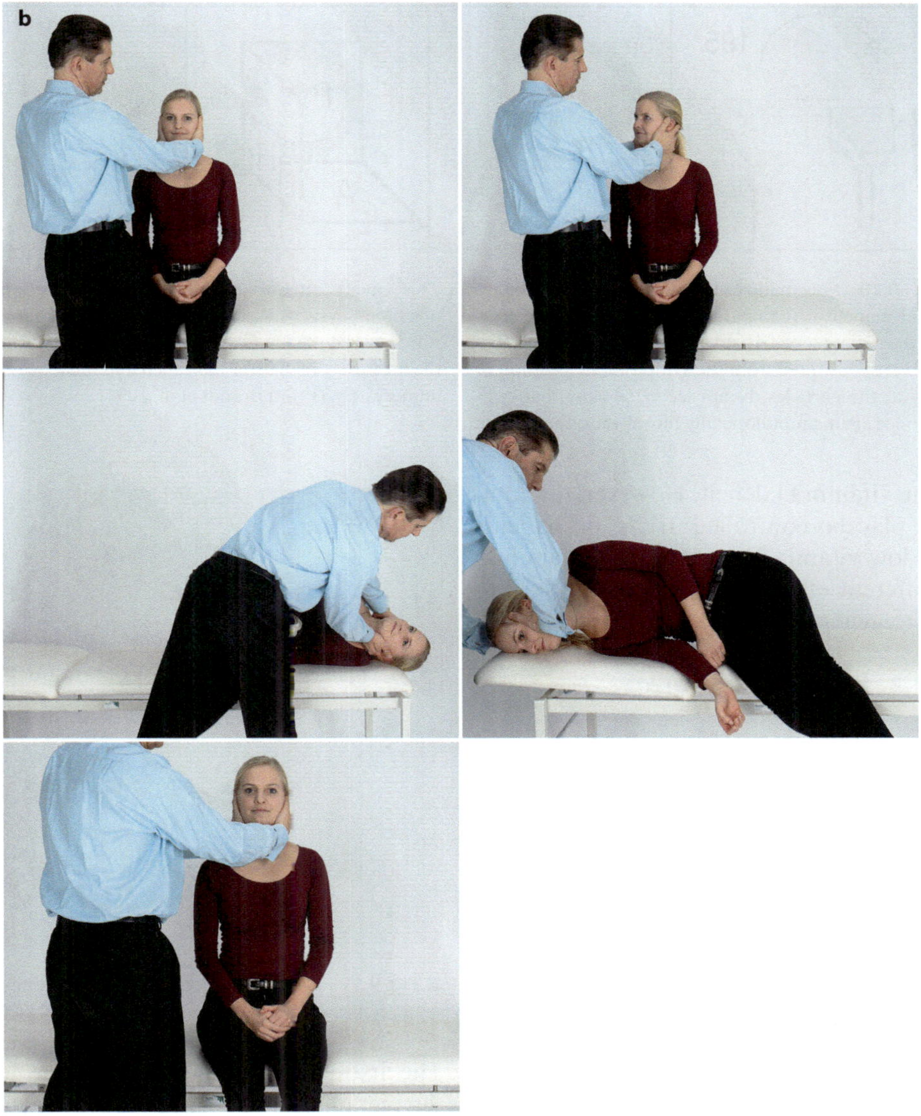

Fig. 9.9 (continued)

(Bhattacharyya et al. 2017). Betahistine may have an impact on the improvement of symptoms after the liberatory maneuvers but not on the efficacy of the repositioning maneuvers (Bhattacharyya et al. 2017; Jalali et al. 2020; Sayin et al. 2020).

Some studies showed that supplementation with vitamin D led to a lower recurrence rate of BPPV (Sheikhzadeh et al. 2016; Jeong et al. 2020) (for references for recurrent BPPV, see Jeong et al. 2022). Another study, however, did not find an effect of vitamin supplementation (Rhim 2020). All in all, there is some evidence that patients with BPPV and low vitamin D should receive a supplementation, mainly because

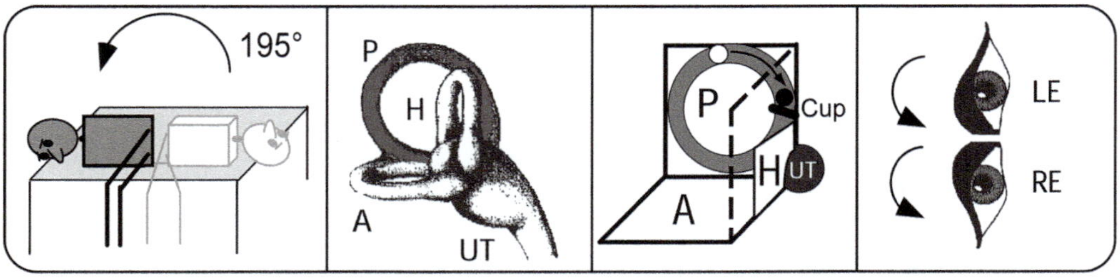

Fig. 9.10 Schematic drawing of an ineffective Semont maneuver (compare with Fig. 9.9, panel 3). After the patient with left-sided benign paroxysmal positional vertigo is tilted from the symptomatic position to the right, the particles do not leave the canal but sediment once again ampullopetally moves onto the cupula. This causes an ampullopetal cupula deflection with positional nystagmus, which in this position beats downward toward the unaffected right ear. This indicates that the liberatory maneuver has failed and must be repeated immediately. (From Brandt et al. 1994)

of the vitamin D deficit. However, randomized placebo-controlled trials in patients with low vitamin D and normal vitamin D in different ethnic groups are necessary to lead to general recommendations.

9.2.7.2 Pragmatic Therapy

Semont Liberatory Maneuver

According to the liberatory maneuver described by Alain Semont, the patient's head is first rotated by 45° to the side of the non-affected labyrinth, in order to bring the posterior canal into the plane of the positional maneuver (Semont et al. 1988) (Figs. 9.9 and 9.11). Then, the patient is turned 90° to the side of the affected labyrinth; he/she holds this position for 1 min (Obrist et al. 2016). Afterward comes the so-called great toss: The patient is turned by 180° to the side of the unaffected labyrinth, where he/she again has to remain lying for 1 min:

- Positional nystagmus to the uppermost ear indicates that the plug has left the canal; i.e., the therapy is successful.
- Conversely, positional nystagmus to the lowermost healthy ear indicates that the liberatory maneuver failed (Fig. 9.10) and the procedure must be repeated immediately.
- Finally, the patient sits up and has to maintain this position for 1 min.

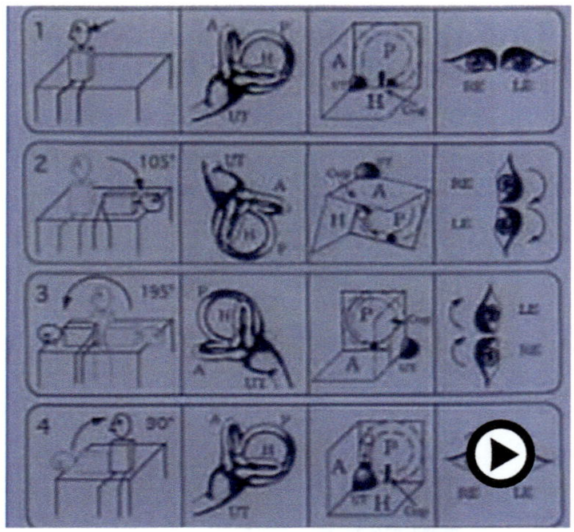

Fig. 9.11 Semont manoeuvre for the left posterior semicircular canal (► https://doi.org/10.1007/000-959)

The first maneuvers should be performed by the therapist and should then be repeated by the patient three times in the morning, three times in the afternoon, and three times in the evening as self-maneuvers until the patient is symptom-free. The use of an app with detailed patient-oriented instructions (e.g., "positional vertigo app") may be helpful. In cases of pronounced fear or nausea, we recommend administering premedication with 50–100 mg dimenhydrinate or other antivertiginous drugs about 30 min before beginning the exercises. The recommendation to remain upright for 48 h after a successful treatment

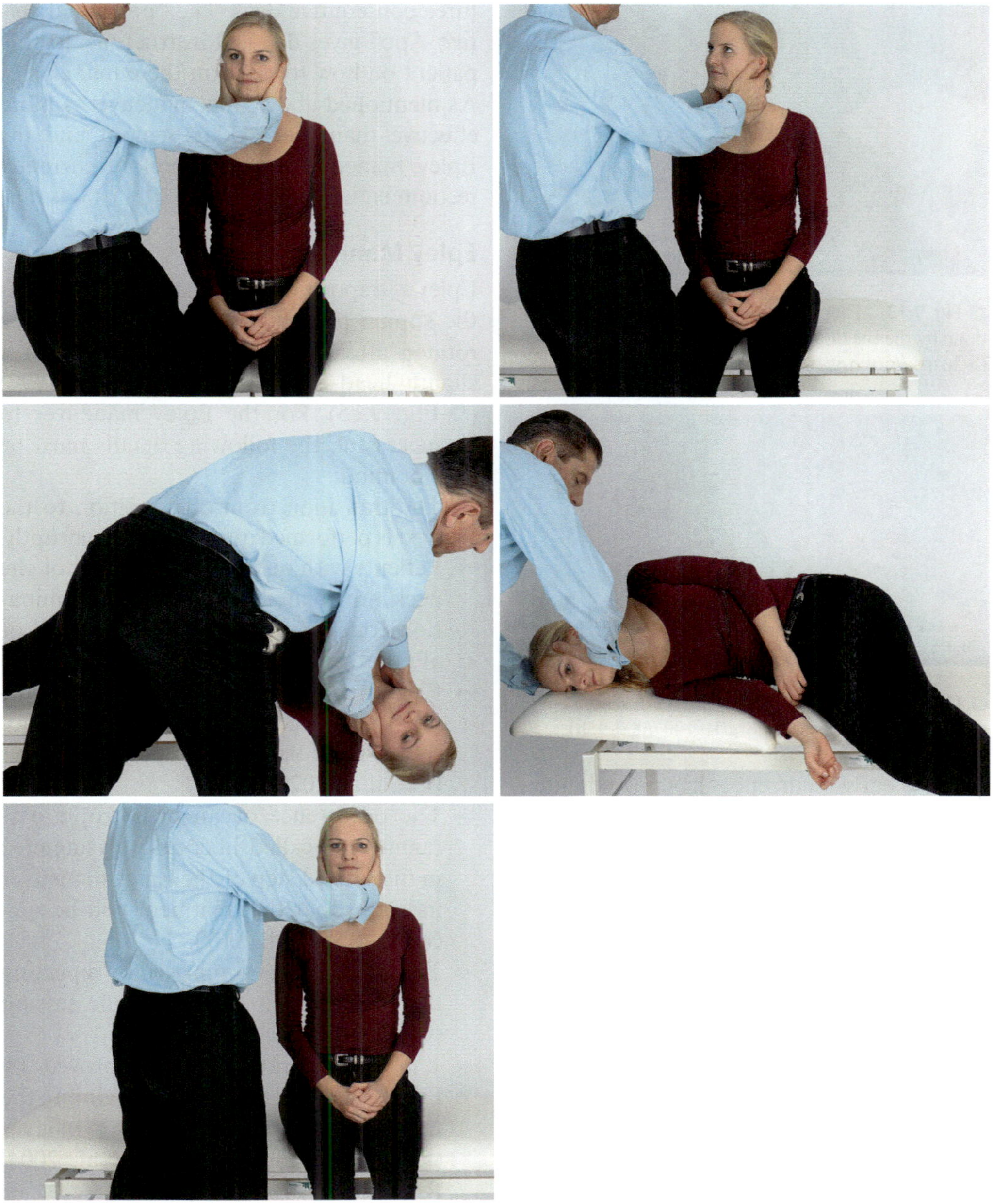

Fig. 9.12 SemontPLUS maneuver. In this modification, the head of the patient is moved at least 60° below earth horizontal (third image). Based on a biophysical model and two randomized trials, this significantly increased the efficacy of the maneuver in comparison with the normal Semont maneuver and the Epley maneuver. Each position should be maintained for 1 min. The maneuvers should be repeated by the patient three times in the morning, three times in the afternoon, and three times at night until the patient is not able to induce spinning vertigo on three consequtive days

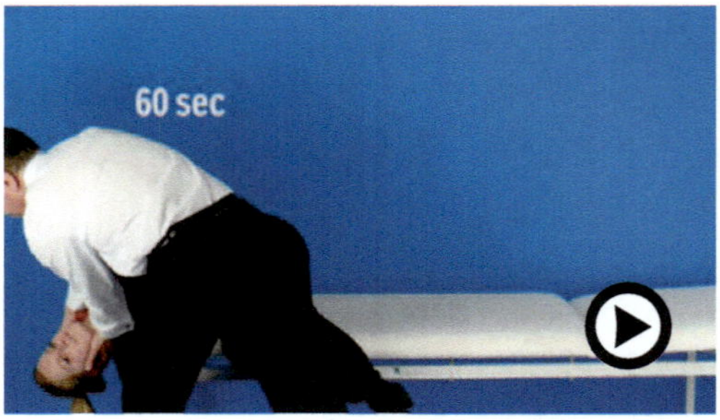

■ **Fig. 9.13** Therapeutic SemontPLUS maneuver done by the the doctor (▶ https://doi.org/10.1007/000-95g)

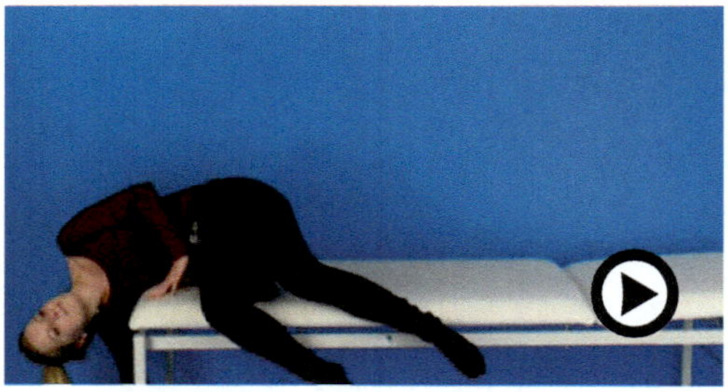

■ **Fig. 9.14** Therapeutic SemontPLUS self-manoeuvre (▶ https://doi.org/10.1007/000-95h)

9

to avoid early recurrences has proved unnecessary (Massoud and Ireland 1996).

SemontPLUS maneuver

A modification of the Semont maneuver is the so-called SemontPLUS maneuver, which is based on the results of a biophysical model of BPPV (Obrist et al. 2016): When the patient's body is moved toward the affected side, the angle should be at least 150°, i.e., at least 60° below earth horizontal (■ Figs. 9.12, 9.13 and 9.14); in this way, the otoconia move much further in the direction of the utricle. After 60 sec the patient is moved at least 240° toward the non-affected side and the clot of otoconia is then already beyond the vertex of the canal, which increases the efficacy of the maneuver. After another 60 sec the patient should sit upright and maintain this position for another 60 sec. These maneuvers should be performed by the patient three times in the morning, at noon and at night until the patient cannot induce spinning vertigo on three consequtive days. The "positional vertigo App" gives detailed instructions for the patient on how to perform these maneuvers. As mentioned above, this maneuver is more effective than the regular Semont and the Epley maneuver and is therefore currently recommended (Strupp et al. 2021).

Epley Maneuver

Epley's repositioning maneuver requires the supine patient's head and trunk to be rotated after being tilted backward into a slightly head-hanging position (Epley 1992) (■ Fig. 9.15). For the Epley maneuver to be successful, the following details must be kept in mind:

- The transition from one position to the next is performed quickly but not abruptly.
- Patients with restricted movement of the neck are treated either on an examination couch with the headrest lowered or alternatively with the Semont maneuver.
- Placing a pillow under the shoulders during this therapeutic maneuver can reduce the discomfort of the Epley maneuver (Lee et al. 2020).
- The occurrence of an orthotropic nystagmus (so-called liberatory nystagmus) in the second step of the Epley maneuver indicates that the treatment will be successful (Oh et al. 2007).
- The success rate is improved by repeating the maneuver 2–3 times in one session (Gordon and Gadoth 2004).
- The success rate is not improved by Epley's original suggestion to vibrate the mastoid bone during the maneuver (Hain et al. 2000; Macias et al. 2004; Ruckenstein and Shepard 2007).
- The recommendation to remain upright for 48 h after a successful treatment to avoid early recurrences has proved unnecessary (Marciano and Marcelli 2002; Roberts et al. 2005).

Self-treatment The Semont, SemontPLUS and Epley maneuvers can be successfully applied by the patient himself/herself (Radtke

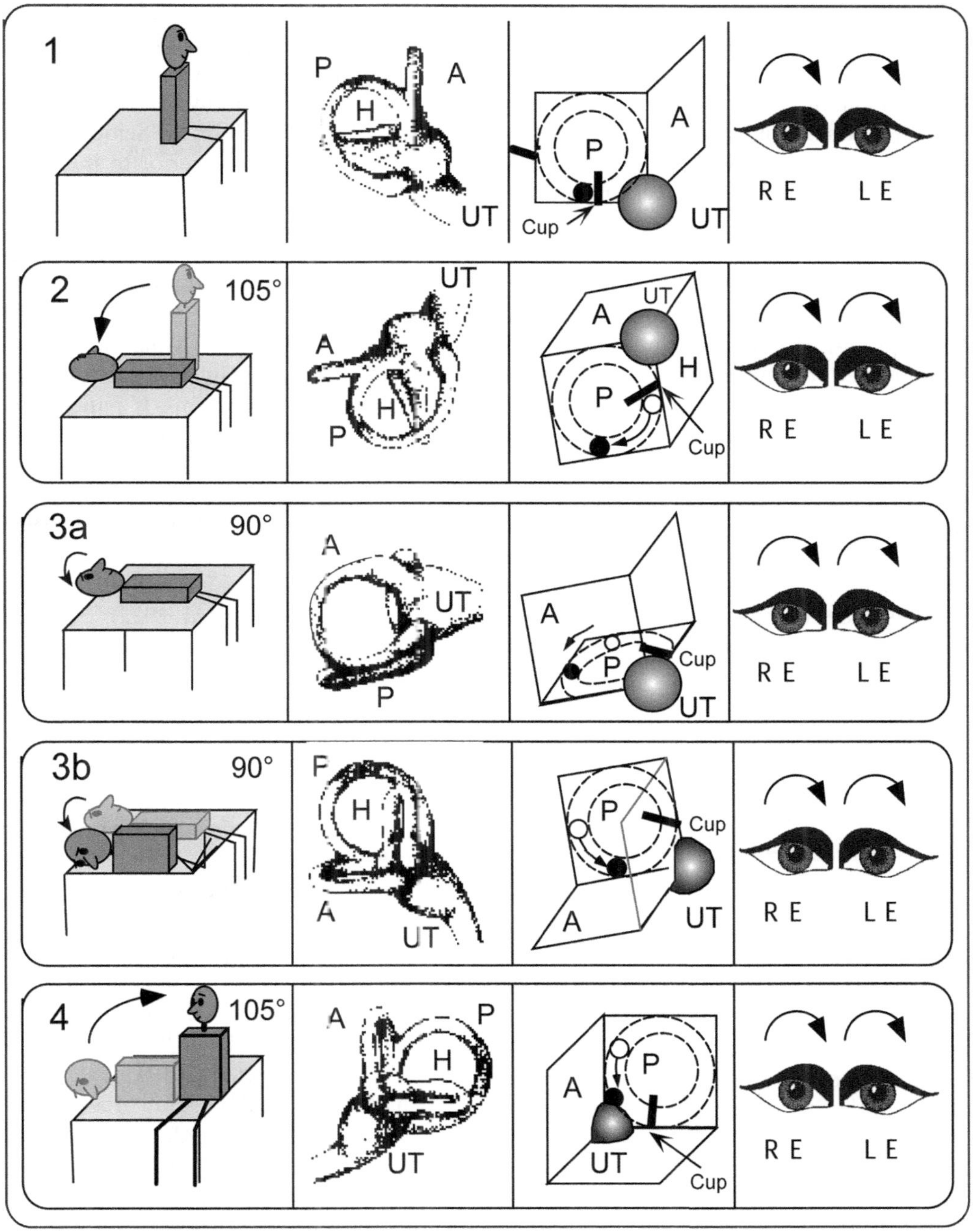

Fig. 9.15 Schematic drawing of modified Epley maneuver. Patient characteristics and abbreviations are as in Fig. 9.9. **1** In the sitting position, the head is turned horizontally 45° to the affected (left) ear. **2** The patient is tilted approximately 105° backward into a slightly head-hanging position, causing the clot to move in the canal, deflecting the cupula downward, and inducing the paroxysmal positioning vertigo. The patient remains in this position for 1 min. **3a** The head is turned 90° to the unaffected ear, now undermost, and **3b** the head and trunk continue turning another 90° to the right, causing the clot to move toward the exit of the canal. The patient remains in this position for 1 min. The positional nystagmus beating toward the affected (uppermost) ear in positions 3a and 3b indicates effective therapy. **4** The patient is moved into the sitting position (adapted from (Brandt et al. 1994))

et al. 2004). The treatment is performed three times in the morning, three times at noon and three times at night until the patients cannot induce spinning vertigo on three consequtive days. Thorough guidance by demonstration and pictures is necessary; the "positional vertigo App" has proved to be very helpful for patients. The success rates (50–90% after 1 week = 21 treatment sessions) are not as high as when a therapist performs the maneuver. As a rule, it takes longer until the patient is symptom-free (Radtke et al. 1999). Self-administered maneuvers in the treatment of recurrent BPPV may not be effective because recurrences may not be from the same canal (same side and same canal in only 24%) (Kim and Kim 2017). In clinical practice, self-treatment follows treatment by a therapist until the patient is free of symptoms. Finally, we recommend a follow-up examination of patients under treatment for BPPV after one to two weeks to check the efficacy of the maneuvers (see below).

9.2.7.3 Comparison of the Semont, SemontPLUS and Epley Maneuvers, Additional Measures, Follow-up Examinations, and Secondary Functional Dizziness

Direct comparisons of the two methods found no differences in their efficacy (Cohen and Jerabek 1999; Herdman and Tusa 1996; Massoud and Ireland 1996; Soto-Varela et al. 2001; Steenerson and Cronin 1996; Hilton and Pinder 2014). In two more recent prospective randomized trials (with more than 190 patients each), the efficacy of the SemontPLUS maneuver with an overextension of the head by at least 60° below earth horizontal when the patient is moved toward the affected side showed the following results: In comparison to the Semont maneuver the days until recovery could be significantly reduced from 3.6 to 1.8 by the SemontPLUS maneuver (Strupp et al. 2021); in comparison to the Epley maneuver the days until recovery could be significantly reduced from 3.3 to 1.9 days (Strupp et al., Abstract, FP1127, Barany Society meeting, Madrid, 2022). Therefore, the SemontPLUS maneuver is evidently superior to the other two. The choice of the maneuver to be used should depend on which maneuver the therapist has the most experience with or if there are any individual contraindications. Very obese patients are easier to treat with the Epley maneuver, while the Semont maneuver is more suitable for patients with shoulder and neck problems. If patients do not respond to treatment (e.g., very obese individuals), special 3D chairs can be used to perform the liberatory maneuvers (Luryi et al. 2018). However, they are not superior to correctly performed maneuvers by doctors as was shown in a randomized trial (Schuricht and Hougaard 2022). Surgical intervention (see above) is not recommended.

Post-traumatic BPPV, which is bilateral in 10% of cases, requires a longer duration of treatment (Gordon et al. 2004), but can also be treated very effectively (Aron et al. 2015); one should begin with treatment of the more affected side.

Although the treatment maneuvers per se are effective for the treatment of positional vertigo and positional nystagmus, a meta-analysis showed that elderly subjects in particular suffer much longer and are much more impaired by BPPV than previously assumed (Sim et al. 2019).

Unilateral surgical plugging of a semicircular canal (e.g., Hotta et al. 2017) can lead to serious adverse events, such as deafness or loss of vestibular function (for references, see Maas et al. 2020). There was not an indication for surgery for any of our patients with BPPV over the last 30 years. Thus, we do not recommend it.

It should be noted that current guidelines recommend a follow-up after 2–4 weeks (Bhattacharyya et al. 2017). Finally, residual dizziness (see below) and anxiety (Lahmann et al. 2015; Vaduva et al. 2018; Wei et al. 2018) are common findings in BPPV patients and their specific treatment improves long-term quality of life. A successful therapy also reduces anxiety after 1–4 weeks (Best et al. 2009a, b; Gunes and Yuzbasioglu 2019).

9.2.7.4 Side Effects of the Therapeutic Maneuvers

Potential side effects of the diagnostic and therapeutic maneuvers are nausea and vomiting, in particular after repeated maneuvers; this requires treatment with antivertiginous drugs, e.g., 50–100 mg dimenhydrinate half an hour before the maneuvers.

About 20–40% of patients develop dizziness and postural imbalance for about 1–3 weeks after successful treatment maneuvers. This is caused by a partial repositioning of the otoconia to the utricle (von Brevern et al. 2006a; Bremova et al. 2013) and is called post-repositional otolith dizziness. Patients should be informed in advance about this positive side effect, because it indicates that the otoconia are falling back onto the utricle, which is a good sign.

There may occasionally be a transition from posterior canal BPPV to horizontal canal BPPV and vice versa, which requires specific treatment maneuvers (Herdman and Tusa 1996).

9.2.7.5 Recurrences after Successful Treatment Maneuvers

According to follow-up observations made over an average of 10 years, the recurrence rate in treated patients is about 50%. Of these patients, 80% have recurrences in the first year independently of the type of treatment maneuver applied (Brandt et al. 2006). Women have a recurrence rate of 58% and thus are more often affected than men who have a recurrence rate of 39%. The recurrence rate is less in the 7th decade than in the 6th decade. A meta-analysis identified the following risk factors for the recurrence of BPPV: female gender, age (≥65 years), hyperlipidemia, diabetes, hypertension, migraine, osteopenia/osteoporosis, head trauma, otitis media, abnormal vestibular-evoked myogenic potential, and long use of computers (Li et al. 2022). Treatment in such cases is again an appropriate treatment maneuver of the affected canal.

9.3 Benign Paroxysmal Positional Vertigo of the Horizontal Canal (hcBPPV)

BPPV of the horizontal canal (McClure 1985) is much rarer than pcBPPV (5–15% of patients with BPPV ((Bhattacharyya et al. 2017). The following features differ from those of pcBPPV:

1. The positional nystagmus is linear and horizontal and corresponds to a stimulation or inhibition of the affected horizontal canal.
2. The nystagmus changes its direction depending on the head position, the underlying mechanisms, the inital position of the otoconia in the horizontal canal and the sequence of the manuevers (Bhandari et al. 2022):

   Geotropic: This is typical of canalolithiasis, i.e., freely moving otoconia within the affected horizontal canal.
   Apogeotropic: This is typical of cupulolithiasis, i.e., otoconia attached to the cupula.
3. During clinical examination, positional vertigo and positional nystagmus should be induced in the patient, who lies supine with the head elevated by 25° to bring the horizontal canal parallel to the gravitational vector, by head turns of 60–90° to the left and the right (◘ Fig. 9.16). For clinical practice, we now recommend beginning with the diagnostic maneuvers for hcBPPV and then for pcBPPV so as not to overlook hcBPPV:

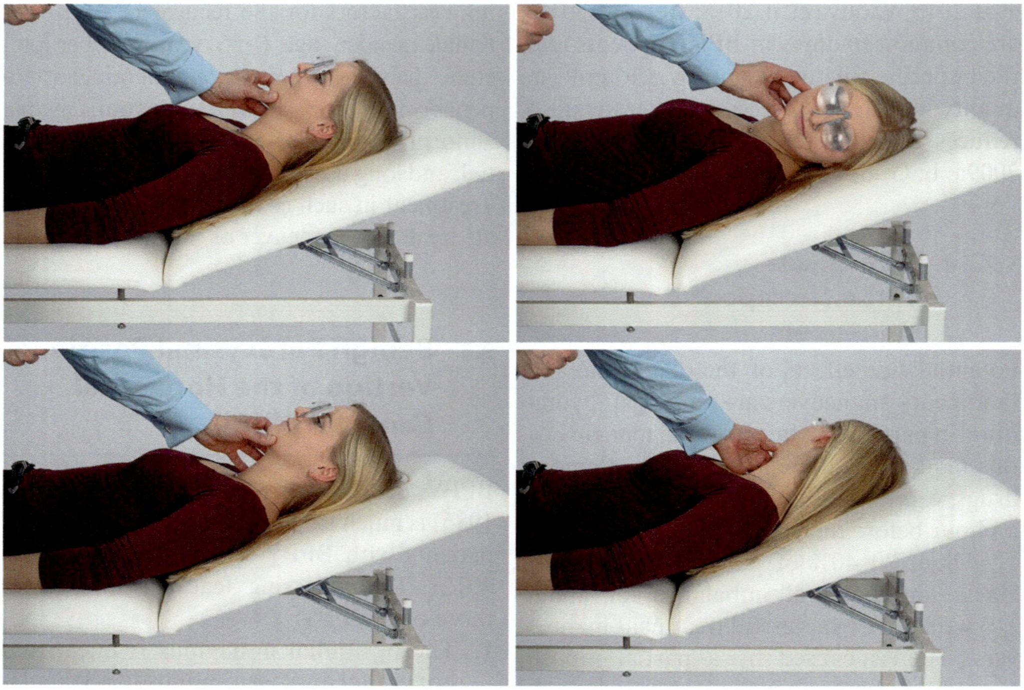

■ **Fig. 9.16** Diagnostic positional maneuvers for suspected horizontal canal BPPV (hcBPPV). The head of the patient is turned to the right and to the left along the longitudinal axis of the body while the subject is supine with the head elevated by 25° to bring the horizontal canal into a vertical position (similar to caloric testing). This leads to a linear horizontal nystagmus. If the nystagmus beats geotropically, this indicates canalolithiasis. In canalolithiasis, the affected side is the side with the higher intensity and the more severe spinning vertigo (due to an ampullopetal movement of the cupula, which leads to an excitation of the horizontal canal). If the nystagmus beats apogeotropically, this indicates cupulolithiasis with a lower intensity of nystagmus and vertigo on the affected side (due to an ampullofugal movement of the cupula, which leads to an inhibition)

4. The duration of the attacks and the nystagmus is longer than in pcBPPV because of the horizontal canal's velocity storage mechanism. Severe positional nystagmus in canalolithiasis can also show a reversal of direction during the attacks; this corresponds to post-rotatory nystagmus (so-called P I and P II). In cupulolithiasis, the duration of the attacks and the nystagmus is much longer because of a permanent deflection of the cupula.
5. The spontaneous recovery rate is higher than in pcBPPV (Imai et al. 2011). In another study with 106 patients (43 with geotropic nystagmus, 63 with apogeotropic nystagmus), it took a mean of 6.7 days for the geotropic nystagmus and 3.7 days for the apogeotropic nystagmus to recover (Shim et al. 2015). This high spontaneous recovery rate evidently also explains the different relative prevalence rates of hcBBPV and pcBPPV, depending on the delay between symptom onset and diagnosis.

9.3.1 Canalolithiasis of Horizontal Canal BPPV

BPPV due to a canalolithiasis of the horizontal semicircular canal is defined as follows (von Brevern et al. 2015):

1. Recurrent attacks of positional vertigo or positional dizziness provoked by lying down or turning over in the supine position.
2. Duration of attacks <1 min.
3. Positional nystagmus elicited after a brief latency or no latency by the supine roll test, beating horizontally toward the *undermost* ear with the head turned to either side (geotropic direction-changing nystagmus) and lasting <1 min.
4. Not attributable to another disorder.

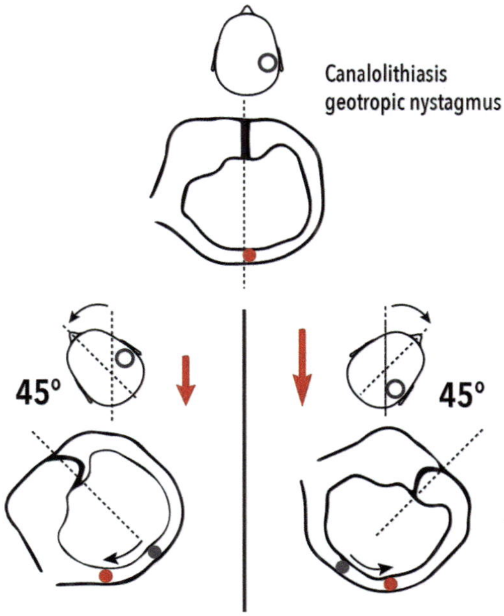

Fig. 9.17 Canalolithiasis of the right horizontal canal leading to a horizontal linear geotropic nystagmus. Schematic drawing of the pathomechanism: The agglomerate of otoconia (red dot) moves within the affected semicircular canal. Turning the head to the left leads to an ampullofugal deviation of the cupula, which causes an inhibition. Turning the head toward the affected right side leads to an ampullopetal deviation of the cupula, which causes an excitation. Since excitation is—according to Ewald's second law—much stronger than inhibition, a head turn toward the affected side leads to a higher intensity of the nystagmus (red arrow on the right) than on the opposite side

9.3.1.1 Clinical Examination

- The diagnostic positional maneuvers are carried out with the patient lying supine with his/her head elevated by 25° by performing head turns by 60–90° to the right and left (Fig. 9.16).
- In the case of canalolithiasis, one is able to induce a linear horizontal direct-changing nystagmus, which beats toward the undermost ear (*geotropically*).
- The affected side is indicated by the higher intensity of the nystagmus and the spinning vertigo. Explanation: If, in canalolithiasis, the head is turned toward the affected side, there is an ampullopetal deviation of the cupula, leading to an excitation of the horizontal canal, which is stronger than an inhibition on the opposite side according to Ewald's second law (Fig. 9.17).
- The clinical findings also depend on the inital position of the otoconia in the the horizontal canal (ampullary versus nonampullary part) and the sequence of the diagnostic maneuvers which can make the interpretation difficult (Bhandari et al. 2022).
- As mentioned above the duration of the attack and the nystagmus is typically longer than in pcBPPV because of the velocity storage mechanism; if there is a very intense nystagmus, one often observes a direction changing of the nystagmus during the attack, corresponding to the post-rotatory nystagmus PI in the initial phase and PII subsequently.
- In contrast to pcBPPV, there is often less fatigability after repeated maneuvers.

In order to carry out a specific therapy, it is necessary to identify the affected side, which, however, it not always possible. The following can be additionally helpful:

1. If there is a transition from pcBPPV to hcBPPV, the same side is most likely affected.
2. The bow and lean test: If the head is bent forward (face down), the nystagmus beats toward the affected side; if the head is overextended (face upward), the nystagmus beats toward the non-affected side (Choung et al. 2006; Choi et al. 2018b).

9.3.1.2 Therapy of Horizontal Canal Canalolithiasis

Before starting treatment, it is important to know and to inform the patient that the spontaneous recovery rate in hcBPPV is higher than in pcBPPV (see above). Over the years, many different types of treatment maneuvers for canalolithiasis of the horizontal canal have been described (for references, see Zuma e Maia et al. 2020):

9

- Roll and modified roll maneuver: The patient lies supine, ideally with the head elevated by 25° and turns the head toward the non-affected side in steps of 90°, maintaining each position for 30 s (Lempert and Tiel-Wilck 1996; White et al. 2005) (Fig. 9.18). This maneuver is more effective than a sham treatment (RCT: 61% versus 35% (Kim et al. 2012b)). It is helpful for the patient to perform these maneuvers while lying on the ground and to turn his/her body toward the non-affected, healthy side as many times as possible. Nevertheless, it often takes a few days until patients recover. The simulation of the various therapeutic maneuvers for the treatment of hcBPPV (Bhandari et al. 2021a) showed that the modified roll maneuver with an initial 90° head turn towards the affected side and then 90° turns towards the non-affected side is theoretically more effective than the normal one. Based on anatomical considerations, the efficacy of the roll maneuvers can be improved by a special pillow which keeps the position of the horizontal canal permanently vertical during these maneuvers.

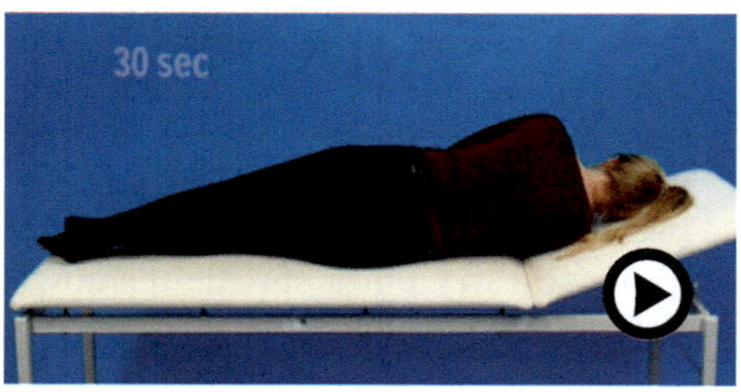

Fig. 9.18 Roll-over maneuver for horizontal canal canalithiasis (▶ https://doi.org/10.1007/000-95j)

- Forced prolonged position: The patient rests on the non-affected side for at least 12 h (Vannucchi et al. 1997). A study showed success rates of about 70% in comparison with 30% for non-treated patients; this was also true for the roll maneuver (Nuti et al. 1998). In a controlled study, the success rate was 77% versus 11% for sham treatment (Mandala et al. 2021).
- Combination of the two previous methods, with a success rate of about 90% (Casani et al. 2002).
- Gufoni maneuver (Gufoni et al. 1998): This can be applied to treat patients with canalolithiasis and those with cupulolithiasis (see below). The advantage of this maneuver is that one does not need to differentiate between the two forms of BPPV. The maneuver is easy because one simply places the patient on the side on which the intensity of the nystagmus is lower. Subsequently, the patient's head is turned 45° downward (Gufoni et al. 1998; Casani et al. 2002; Asprella 2005). The Gufoni maneuver is effective (RCT: 69% versus 35% with sham treatment (Kim et al. 2012b)).
- Modified Zuma maneuver (Zuma e Maia et al. 2020): a 45° head turn to the unaffected side in the sitting position (step I). The patient is then asked to lie down on the affected side (step II). Next, the patient moves into dorsal decubitus and the head is turned 45° toward the unaffected side (step III). The head is then

turned 90° toward the unaffected side (step IV). Finally, the patient's head is tilted slightly forward, followed by a slow return to the sitting position (step V).

9.3.1.3 Pragmatic Therapy

Although several maneuvers have been developed and show efficacy, we recommend the simple combination of repeated modified roll-manuevers (Bhandari et al. 2021a) with the head elevated by 25° (Fig. 9.16) with subsequent forced prolonged rest on the non-affected side for 12 h.

9.3.2 Cupulolithiasis of Horizontal Canal BPPV

The much rarer cupulolithiasis of hcBPPV is defined as follows (von Brevern et al. 2015):

1. Recurrent attacks of positional vertigo or positional dizziness provoked by lying down or turning over in the supine position.
2. Positional nystagmus elicited after a brief latency or no latency by the supine roll test, beating horizontally toward the *uppermost* ear with the head turned to either side (apogeotropic direction-changing nystagmus) and *lasting > 1 min.*
3. Not attributable to another disorder.

9.3.2.1 Clinical Examination

- In cupulolithiasis of hcBPPV, patients often already have linear horizontal nystagmus in an upright position, which can lead to misdiagnosis as AUVP. This linear horizontal nystagmus can be explained by the fact that the horizontal canal is tilted upward by 25° in a head upright position, which leads to a permanent deflection of the cupula with persisting spinning vertigo and linear horizontal nystagmus.
- When performing the diagnostic positional maneuvers in the supine position with the head elevated by 25°, one can induce apogeotropic nystagmus, which is very long-lasting, when the head is turned to the right or the left (Bisdorff and Debatisse 2001) (Figs. 9.19) and 9.20).
- The affected side is the side with the lower intensity of the nystagmus, which is caused by an ampullofugal movement of the cupula (Fig. 9.19).
- Bow and lean test: If the head is tilted downward (face down), the nystagmus beats toward the non-affected side. If the

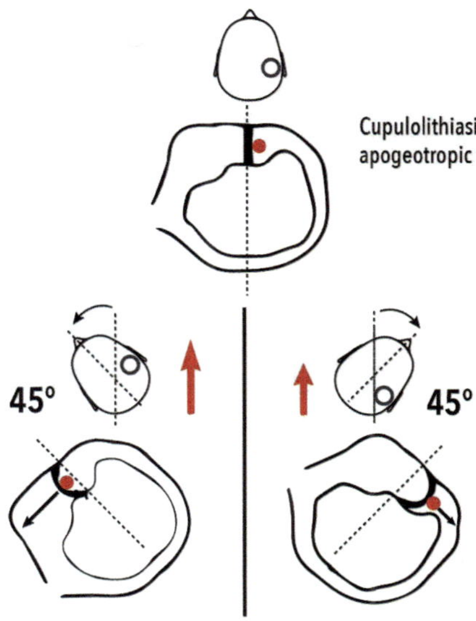

Fig. 9.19 Cupulolithiasis of the right horizontal canal with linear horizontal apogeotropic nystagmus. Schematic drawing of the movement of the agglomerate of otoconia attached to the cupula (red dot). Turning the head to the left in the supine position leads to an ampullopetal deviation of the cupula, which causes excitation with a higher intensity of the nystagmus. Turning the head to the affected right side in the supine position causes an ampullofugal deviation of the cupula, which leads to an inhibition with a lower intensity of the nystagmus. In conclusion, since inhibition is less strong than excitation according to Ewald's second law, turning the head toward the affected side leads to a nystagmus with a lower intensity (red arrow on the right)

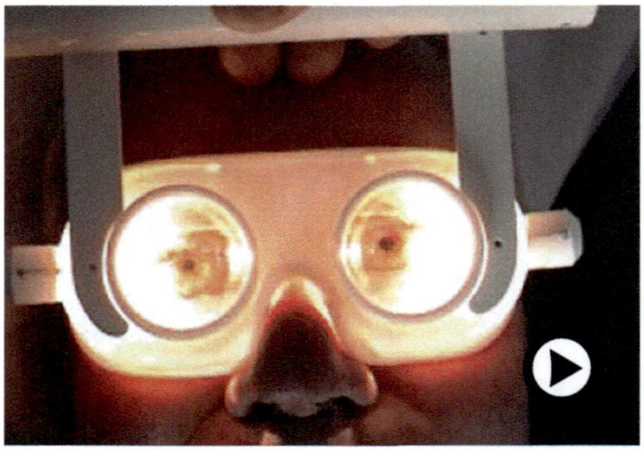

Fig. 9.20 Cupulolithiasis of the left horizontal canal with linear horizontal apogeotropic nystagmus (▶ https://doi.org/10.1007/000-95k)

head is overextended (face up), the nystagmus beats toward the affected side (Choi et al. 2018b); this is the mirror image of the canalolithiasis.

9

All in all, the findings concerning the direction and the intensity of the nystagmus are the reverse of the canalolithiasis. As mentioned above, because of the persisting spinning vertigo and the spontaneous nystagmus in an upright position, cupulolithiasis is often misdiagnosed as AUVP. The positional maneuvers and the response to treatment are helpful to discriminate between the two.

An important differential diagnosis for horizontal apogeotropic nystagmus is central positional nystagmus, most often due to lesions of the vestibulocerebellum. The major difference between the two forms is as follows: the intensity of spontaneous nystagmus is similar while sitting and supine in the apogeotropic type of central positional nystagmus, but greater when supine in apogeotropic nystagmus of hcBPPV (Choi et al. 2015, 2018a). Linear horizontal direction-changing nystagmus was also described in vestibular migraine, which is another differential diagnosis during an attack of spinning vertigo (see above).

9.3.2.2 Treatment of Cupulolithiasis of hcBPPV

Several maneuvers have been described and examined for cupulolithiasis of hcBPPV (for references, see (Zuma e Maia et al. 2020)). We recommend the following two maneuvers:

- Transformation of cupulolithiasis into canalolithiasis by shaking the head with the head bent forward by 120° (Fig. 9.21) with a frequency of about 3 Hz and subsequent treatment similar to that for canalolithiasis (see above) (Kim et al. 2012c).
- Gufoni maneuver: One places the patient on the side on which the intensity of the nystagmus is lower. Subsequently, the patient's head is turned 45° downward (Gufoni et al. 1998; Casani et al. 2002; Asprella 2005).

Both maneuvers are effective, as was shown in a randomized controlled trial: 35% recovery rate with sham treatment, 62% recovery rate with head shaking, 69% recovery rate with the Gufoni maneuver (Kim et al. 2012c). More recently, three maneuvers for the treatment of cupulolithiasis of hcBPPV were compared in a prospective randomized study: head shaking only, Gufoni maneuver, and the roll maneuver. There was no difference in the efficacy of the three maneuvers (Kong et al. 2020).

9.3.2.3 Pragmatic Therapy

We recommend a combination of head shaking for the transition to canalolithiasis and (Fig. 9.22) then the modified roll-maneuver with forced prolonged bed rest.

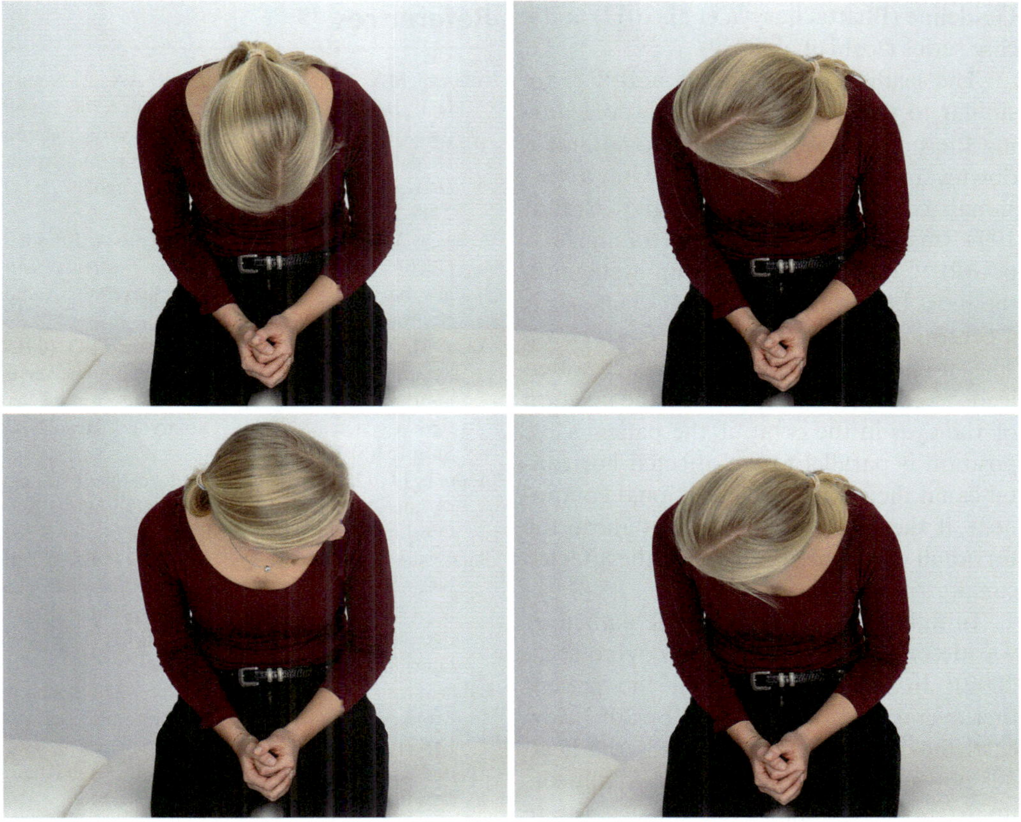

Fig. 9.21 Therapy of cupulolithiasis of hcBPPV to transform cupulolithiasis into canalolithiasis by head shaking. The patient bends his/her head 120° downwards and then shakes his/her head with a frequency of about 3 Hz about 100 times a day. The transition from cupulolithiasis to canalolithiasis can be identified by the transformation of apogeotropic nystagmus into geotropic nystagmus, which is then treated as mentioned above

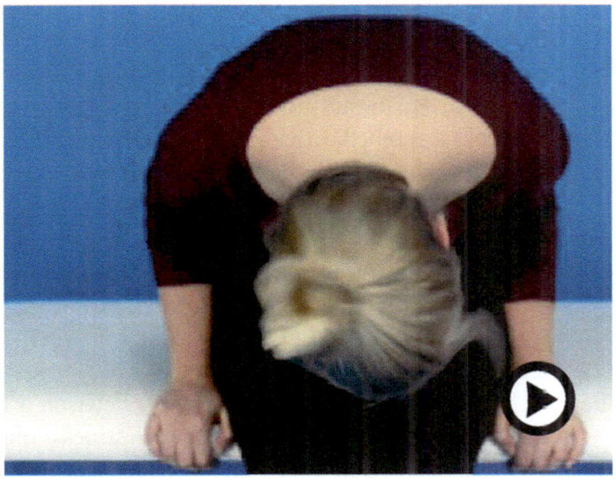

Fig. 9.22 Head shaking manoeuvre to transform a cupulolithiasis in a canalithiasis in horizontal canal BPPV (▶ https://doi.org/10.1007/000-95m)

9.4 BPPV of the Anterior Canal (acBPPV)

The relative frequency of acBPPV (Bertholon et al. 2002; Herdman and Tusa 1996) is very low which can probably be explained by the anatomical position of this canal (also called the superior canal) (Bhandari et al. 2021b), leading to a high spontaneous recovery rate. In a study on 577 patients with BPPV, only 2.2% had acBPPV (Yacovino et al. 2009). Many of our patients who had been diagnosed with acBPPV turned out to have central positional nystagmus. This in line with the Clinical Practice

Guideline (Bhattacharyya et al. 2017) and a case series (Joshi et al. 2020).

The leading symptoms of acBPPV are similar to those of pcBPPV. However, during the positioning maneuvers, one finds a downward-beating nystagmus with a torsional component (Steddin and Brandt 1994; Imai et al. 2006), i.e., a mirror image of pc-BPPV. In downward-beating nystagmus, the most important differential diagnosis is a central positional nystagmus (see above). The torsional component - which often leads to confusion - depends on the position of the eyes in the orbit: if the patient's eye position is parallel to the affected horizontal canal there will be not torsional component, if the patient looks straight ahead the torsional component is towards the affected canal.

Initially a simple therapeutic maneuver was described for acBPPV (Yacovino et al. 2009): In a supine position, the patient first overextends his/her head by 30° below earth horizontal and then bends the head 30° above earth horizontal and finally sits up. After a single maneuver, the success rate was 85%; these findings are supported by a case series (Yang et al. 2019). A simulation of the various maneuvers showed that the Yacovino maneuver theoretically might fail and should be modified to increase its efficacy: The modified Yacovino maneuver. In this even simpler variation, the subject is brought directly from the head-hanging position to the sitting position with the head upright. After an interval of 30 seconds, the subject's neck is flexed forward at an angle of 45°. This modification brings a better repositioning of the otoconial debris into the utricle. The initially recommended chin-to-chest position has to be omitted to avoid the risk of moving the debris from crus commune to posterior canal (Bhandari et al. 2021b).

References

AlGarni MA, Mirza AA, Althobaiti AA, Al-Nemari HH, Bakhsh LS (2018) Association of benign paroxysmal positional vertigo with vitamin D deficiency: a systematic review and meta-analysis. Eur Arch Otorhinolaryngol 275(11): 2705–2711

Arbusow V, Theil D, Strupp M, Mascolo A, Brandt T (2000) HSV-1 not only in human vestibular ganglia but also in the vestibular labyrinth. Audiol Neurootol 6(5):259–262

Aron M, Lea J, Nakku D, Westerberg BD (2015) Symptom resolution rates of posttraumatic versus nontraumatic benign paroxysmal positional vertigo: a systematic review. Otolaryngol Head Neck Surg 153(5):721–730

Asprella LG (2005) Diagnostic and treatment strategy of lateral semicircular canal canalolithiasis. Acta Otorhinolaryngol Ital 25(5):277–283

Balatsouras DG, Koukoutsis G, Ganelis P, Economou NC, Moukos A, Aspris A, Katotomichelakis M (2014) Benign paroxysmal positional vertigo secondary to vestibular neuritis. Eur Arch Otorhinolaryngol 271(5):919–924

Balatsouras DG, Koukoutsis G, Aspris A, Fassolis A, Moukos A, Economou NC, Katotomichelakis M (2017) Benign paroxysmal positional vertigo secondary to mild head trauma. Ann Otol Rhinol Laryngol 126(1):54–60

Beh SC (2018) Horizontal direction-changing positional nystagmus and vertigo: a case of vestibular migraine masquerading as horizontal canal BPPV. Headache 58(7):1113–1117

Benecke H, Agus S, Kuessner D, Goodall G, Strupp M (2013) The burden and impact of vertigo: findings from the REVERT patient registry. Front Neurol 4:136

Bertholon P, Bronstein AM, Davies RA, Rudge P, Thilo KV (2002) Positional down beating nystagmus in 50 patients: cerebellar disorders and possible anterior semicircular canalithiasis. J Neurol Neurosurg Psychiatry 72(3):366–372

Best C, Eckhardt-Henn A, Tschan R, Dieterich M (2009a) Psychiatric morbidity and comorbidity in different vestibular vertigo syndromes. Results of a prospective longitudinal study over one year. J Neurol 256(1):58–65

Best C, Tschan R, Eckhardt-Henn A, Dieterich M (2009b) Who is at risk for ongoing dizziness and psychological strain after a vestibular disorder? Neuroscience 164(4):1579–1587

Bhandari A, Bhandari R, Kingma H, Zuma e Maia, Strupp M (2021a) Three-dimensional simulations of six treatment maneuvers for horizontal canal benign paroxysmal positional vertigo canalithiasis. Eur J Neurol 28:4178–4183

Bhandari A, Bhandari R, Kingma H, Strupp M (2021b) Diagnostic and therapeutic maneuvers for anterior canal BPPV canalithiasis: three-dimensional simulations. Front Neurol 12:740599

Bhandari A, Bhandari R, Kingma H, Strupp M (2022) Modified interpretations of the supine roll test in horizontal canal BPPV based on simulations: How the initial position of the debris in the canal and the sequence of testing affects the direction of the nystagmus and the diagnosis. Front Neurol 13:881156

Bhattacharyya N, Gubbels SP, Schwartz SR, Edlow JA, El-Kashlan H, Fife T, Holmberg JM, Mahoney K, Hollingsworth DB, Roberts R, Seidman MD, Steiner RW, Do BT, Voelker CC, Waguespack RW, Corrigan MD (2017) Clinical practice guideline: benign paroxysmal positional vertigo (update). Otolaryngol Head Neck Surg 156(3_suppl):S1–S47

Bisdorff AR, Debatisse D (2001) Localizing signs in positional vertigo due to lateral canal cupulolithiasis. Neurology 57(6):1085–1088

Brandt T, Daroff RB (1980) Physical therapy for benign paroxysmal positional vertigo. Arch Otolaryngol 106:484–485

Brandt T, Steddin S (1993) Current view of the mechanism of benign paroxysmal positioning vertigo: cupulolithiasis or canalolithiasis? J Vestib Res 3(4):373–382

Brandt T, Steddin S, Daroff RB (1994) Therapy for benign paroxysmal positioning vertigo, revisited. Neurology 44:796–800

Brandt T, Huppert D, Hecht J, Karch C, Strupp M (2006) Benign paroxysmal positioning vertigo: a long-term follow-up (6-17 years) of 125 patients. Acta Otolaryngol 126(2):160–163

Brandt T, Huppert T, Hufner K, Zingler VC, Dieterich M, Strupp M (2010) Long-term course and relapses of vestibular and balance disorders. Restor Neurol Neurosci 28(1):69–82

Bremova T, Bayer O, Agrawal Y, Kremmyda O, Brandt T, Teufel J, Strupp M (2013) Ocular VEMPs indicate repositioning of otoconia to the utricle after successful liberatory maneuvers in benign paroxysmal positioning vertigo. Acta Otolaryngol 133(12):1297–1303

Büchele W, Brandt T (1988) Vestibular neuritis--a horizontal semicircular canal paresis? Adv Otorhinolaryngol 42:157–161

Buki B, Simon L, Garab S, Lundberg YW, Junger H, Straumann D (2011) Sitting-up vertigo and trunk retropulsion in patients with benign positional vertigo but without positional nystagmus. J Neurol Neurosurg Psychiatry 82(1):98–104

Buki B, Mandala M, Nuti D (2014) Typical and atypical benign paroxysmal positional vertigo: literature review and new theoretical considerations. J Vestib Res 24(5):415–423

Burton MJ, Eby TL, Rosenfeld RM (2012) Extracts from the Cochrane Library: modifications of the Epley (canalith repositioning) maneuver for posterior canal benign paroxysmal positional vertigo. Otolaryngol Head Neck Surg 147(3): 407–411

Buttner U, Helmchen C, Brandt T (1999) Diagnostic criteria for central versus peripheral positioning nystagmus and vertigo: a review. Acta Otolaryngol 119(1):1–5

Casani AP, Vannucci G, Fattori B, Berrettini S (2002) The treatment of horizontal canal positional vertigo: our experience in 66 cases. Laryngoscope 112(1):172–178

Chen CC, Cho HS, Lee HH, Hu CJ (2018) Efficacy of repositioning therapy in patients with benign paroxysmal positional vertigo and preexisting central neurologic disorders. Front Neurol 9:486

Chen J, Zhao W, Yue X, Zhang P (2020) Risk factors for the occurrence of benign paroxysmal positional vertigo: a systematic review and meta-analysis. Front Neurol 11:506

Choi JY, Kim JS (2019) Central positional nystagmus: characteristics and model-based explanations. Prog Brain Res 249:211–225

Choi JY, Kim JH, Kim HJ, Glasauer S, Kim JS (2015) Central paroxysmal positional nystagmus: characteristics and possible mechanisms. Neurology 84(22):2238–2246

Choi JY, Glasauer S, Kim JH, Zee DS, Kim JS (2018a) Characteristics and mechanism of apogeotropic central positional nystagmus. Brain 141(3):762–775

Choi S, Choi HR, Nahm H, Han K, Shin JE, Kim CH (2018b) Utility of the bow and lean test in predicting subtype of benign paroxysmal positional vertigo. Laryngoscope 128(11):2600–2604

Choi HG, Kim G, Kim BJ, Hong SK, Kim HJ, Lee HJ (2020) How rare is benign paroxysmal positional vertigo in children? A review of 20 cases and their epidemiology. Int J Pediatr Otorhinolaryngol 132:110008

Choung YH, Shin YR, Kahng H, Park K, Choi SJ (2006) 'Bow and lean test' to determine the affected ear of horizontal canal benign paroxysmal positional vertigo. Laryngoscope 116(10):1776–1781

Cohen HS, Jerabek J (1999) Efficacy of treatments for posterior canal benign paroxysmal positional vertigo. Laryngoscope 109(4):584–590
Cohen HS, Kimball KT (2004) Treatment variations on the Epley maneuver for benign paroxysmal positional vertigo. Am J Otolaryngol 25(1):33–37
Coppo GF, Singarelli S, Fracchia P (1996) Benign paroxysmal positional vertigo: follow-up of 165 cases treated by Semont's liberating maneuver. Acta Otorhinolaryngol Ital 16(6):508–512
De Schutter E, Adham ZO, Kattah JC (2019) Central positional vertigo: a clinical-imaging study. Prog Brain Res 249:345–360
Di Cesare T, Tricarico L, Passali GC, Sergi B, Paludetti G, Galli J, Picciotti PM (2021) Traumatic benign paroxysmal positional vertigo: personal experience and comparison with idiopathic BPPV. Int J Audiol 60:393–397
Dieterich M, Brandt T (1999) Episodic vertigo related to migraine (90 cases): vestibular migraine? J Neurol 246(10):883–892
Dix MR, Hallpike CS (1952) The pathology, symptomatology, and diagnosis of certain common disorders of the vestibular system. Ann Otol 61:987–991
Ekvall HE, Mansson NO, Hakansson A (2005) Benign paroxysmal positional vertigo among elderly patients in primary health care. Gerontology 51(6):386–389
Epley JM (1992) The canalith repositioning procedure: for treatment of benign paroxysmal positional vertigo. Otolaryngol Head Neck Surg 107(3):399–404
Feil K, Feuerecker R, Goldschagg N, Strobl R, Brandt T, Von MA, Grill E, Strupp M (2018) Predictive capability of an iPad-based medical device (medx) for the diagnosis of vertigo and dizziness. Front Neurol 9:29
Froehling DA, Bowen JM, Mohr DN, Brey RH, Beatty CW, Wollan PC, Silverstein MD (2000) The canalith repositioning procedure for the treatment of benign paroxysmal positional vertigo: a randomized controlled trial. Mayo Clin Proc 75(7):695–700
Fu CY, Zhang ZZ, Chen J, Jaiswal SK, Yan FL (2020) Unhealthy lifestyle is an important risk factor of idiopathic BPPV. Front Neurol 11:950
Gebhart I, Götting C, Hool SL, Morrison M, Korda A, Caversaccio M, Obrist D, Mantokoudis G (2021) Semont maneuver for benign paroxysmal positional vertigo treatment: moving in the correct plane matters. Otol Neurotol 42:e341–e347
Goldschagg N, Teupser D, Feil K, Strupp M (2021) No evidence for a specific vitamin D deficit in benign paroxysmal positional vertigo. Eur J Neurol 28:3182–3186
Gordon CR, Gadoth N (2004) Repeated vs single physical maneuver in benign paroxysmal positional vertigo. Acta Neurol Scand 110(3):166–169
Gordon CR, Levite R, Joffe V, Gadoth N (2004) Is posttraumatic benign paroxysmal positional vertigo different from the idiopathic form? Arch Neurol 61(10):1590–1593
Gufoni M, Mastrosimone L, Di NF (1998) Repositioning maneuver in benign paroxysmal vertigo of horizontal semicircular canal. Acta Otorhinolaryngol Ital 18(6):363–367
Gunes A, Yuzbasioglu Y (2019) Effects of treatment on anxiety levels among patients with benign paroxysmal positional vertigo. Eur Arch Otorhinolaryngol 276(3):711–718
Hain TC, Helminski JO, Reis IL, Uddin MK (2000) Vibration does not improve results of the canalith repositioning procedure. Arch Otolaryngol Head Neck Surg 126(5):617–622
Hall SF, Ruby RR, McClure JA (1979) The mechanics of benign paroxysmal vertigo. J Otolaryngol 8(2):151–158
Herdman SJ, Tusa RJ (1996) Complications of the canalith repositioning procedure. Arch Otolaryngol Head Neck Surg 122(3):281–286
Hilton MP, Pinder DK (2014) The Epley (canalith repositioning) manoeuvre for benign paroxysmal positional vertigo. Cochrane Database Syst Rev 12:CD003162
Honrubia V, Baloh RW, Harris MR, Jacobson KM (1999) Paroxysmal positional vertigo syndrome. Am J Otol 20(4):465–470
Hotta S, Imai T, Higashi-Shingai K, Okazaki S, Okumura T, Uno A, Ohta Y, Morihana T, Sato T, Inohara H (2017) Unilateral posterior canal-plugging surgery for intractable bilateral posterior canal-type benign paroxysmal positional vertigo. Auris Nasus Larynx 44(5):540–547
Hulse R, Biesdorf A, Hormann K, Stuck B, Erhart M, Hulse M, Wenzel A (2019) Peripheral vestibular disorders: an epidemiologic survey in 70 million individuals. Otol Neurotol 40:88–95
Imai T, Ito M, Takeda N, Uno A, Matsunaga T, Sekine K, Kubo T (2005) Natural course of the remission of vertigo in patients with benign paroxysmal positional vertigo. Neurology 64:920–921
Imai T, Takeda N, Ito M, Nakamae K, Sakae H, Fujioka H, Kubo T (2006) Three-dimensional analysis of benign paroxysmal positional nystagmus in a patient with anterior semicircular canal variant. Otol Neurotol 27(3):362–366
Imai T, Takeda N, Ito M, Inohara H (2011) Natural course of positional vertigo in patients with apogeotropic variant of horizontal canal benign paroxysmal positional vertigo. Auris Nasus Larynx 38(1):2–5
Isaradisaikul SK, Chowsilpa S, Hanprasertpong C, Rithirangsriroj T (2021) Single cycle versus multiple cycles of Canalith repositioning procedure for treatment of posterior canal benign paroxysmal positional vertigo: a randomized controlled trial. Otol Neurotol 42(1):121–128

Jalali MM, Gerami H, Saberi A, Razaghi S (2020) The impact of betahistine versus dimenhydrinate in the resolution of residual dizziness in patients with benign paroxysmal positional vertigo: a randomized clinical trial. Ann Otol Rhinol Laryngol 129(5):434–440

Jeong SH, Kim JS, Kim HJ, Choi JY, Koo JW, Choi KD, Park JY, Lee SH, Choi SY, Oh SY, Yang TH, Park JH, Jung I, Ahn S, Kim S (2020) Prevention of benign paroxysmal positional vertigo with vitamin D supplementation: a randomized trial. Neurology 95(9):e1117–e1125

Jeong SH, Lee SU, Kim JS (2022) Prevention of recurrent benign paroxysmal positional vertigo with vitamin D supplementation: a meta-analysis. J Neurol 269:619–626

Joshi P, Mossman S, Luis L, Luxon LM (2020) Central mimics of benign paroxysmal positional vertigo: an illustrative case series. Neurol Sci 41(2):263–269

Karatas A, Acar YG, Yuce T, Haci C, Cebi IT, Salviz M (2017) Association of benign paroxysmal positional vertigo with osteoporosis and vitamin D deficiency: a case controlled study. J Int Adv Otol 13(2):259–265

Karlberg M, Hall K, Quickert N, Hinson J, Halmagyi GM (2000) What inner ear diseases cause benign paroxysmal positional vertigo? Acta Otolaryngol 120(3):380–385

Katsarkas A (1999) Benign paroxysmal positional vertigo (BPPV): idiopathic versus post-traumatic. Acta Otolaryngol 119(7):745–749

Kim HJ, Kim JS (2017) The patterns of recurrences in idiopathic benign paroxysmal positional vertigo and self-treatment evaluation. Front Neurol 8:690

Kim HA, Yi HA, Lee H (2012a) Apogeotropic central positional nystagmus as a sole sign of nodular infarction. Neurol Sci 33(5):1189–1191

Kim JS, Oh SY, Lee SH, Kang JH, Kim DU, Jeong SH, Choi KD, Moon IS, Kim BK, Kim HJ (2012b) Randomized clinical trial for geotropic horizontal canal benign paroxysmal positional vertigo. Neurology 79(7):700–707

Kim JS, Oh SY, Lee SH, Kang JH, Kim DU, Jeong SH, Choi KD, Moon IS, Kim BK Oh HJ, Kim HJ (2012c) Randomized clinical trial for apogeotropic horizontal canal benign paroxysmal positional vertigo. Neurology 78(3):159–166

Kim HA, Bisdorff A, Bronstein AM, Lempert T, Rossi-Izquierdo M, Staab JP, Strupp M Kim JS (2019a) Hemodynamic orthostatic dizziness/vertigo: diagnostic criteria. J Vestib Res 29(2–3):45–56

Kim SK, Hong SM, Park IS, Choi HG (2019b) Association between migraine and benign paroxysmal positional vertigo among adults in South Korea. JAMA Otolaryngol Head Neck Surg 145(4):307–312

Kim HJ, Song JM, Zhong L, Yang X, Kim JS (2020) Questionnaire-based diagnosis of benign paroxysmal positional vertigo. Neurology 94(9):e942–e949

Kollen L, Frandin K, Moller M, Fagevik OM, Moller C (2012) Benign paroxysmal positional vertigo is a common cause of dizziness and unsteadiness in a large population of 75-year-olds. Aging Clin Exp Res 24(4):317–323

Kong TH, Song MH, Kang JW, Shim DB (2020) Double-blind randomized controlled trial on efficacy of cupulolith repositioning maneuver for treatment of apogeotropic horizontal canal benign paroxysmal positional vertigo. Acta Otolaryngol 140:473–478

Kremmyda O, Zwergal A, la FC, Brandt T, Jahn K, Strupp M (2013) 4-Aminopyridine suppresses positional nystagmus caused by cerebellar vermis lesion. J Neurol 260(1):321–323

Lahmann C, Henningsen P, Brandt T, Strupp M, Jahn K, Dieterich M, Eckhardt-Henn A, Feuerecker R, Dinkel A, Schmid G (2015) Psychiatric comorbidity and psychosocial impairment among patients with vertigo and dizziness. J Neurol Neurosurg Psychiatry 86(3):302–308

Lee HJ, Kim ES, Kim M, Chu H, Ma HI, Lee JS, Koo JW, Kim HJ, Hong SK (2014a) Isolated horizontal positional nystagmus from a posterior fossa lesion. Ann Neurol 76(6):905–910

Lee JD, Shim DB, Park HJ, Song CI, Kim MB, Kim CH, Byun JY, Hong SK, Kim TS, Park KH, Seo JH, Shim BS, Lee JH, Lim HW, Jeon EJ (2014b) A multicenter randomized double-blind study: comparison of the Epley, Semont, and sham maneuvers for the treatment of posterior canal benign paroxysmal positional vertigo. Audiol Neurootol 19(5):336–341

Lee SY, Kong IG, Oh DJ, Choi HG (2019) Increased risk of benign paroxysmal positional vertigo in patients with a history of sudden sensory neural hearing loss: a longitudinal follow-up study using a national sample cohort. Otol Neurotol 40(2):e135–e141

Lee HJ, Jeon EJ, Lee DH, Seo JH (2020) Therapeutic efficacy of the modified Epley maneuver with a pillow under the shoulders. Clin Exp Otorhinolaryngol 13(4):376–380

Lemos J, Strupp M (2022) Central positional nystagmus: an update. J Neurol 269:1851–1860

Lempert T, Tiel-Wilck K (1996) A positional maneuver for treatment of horizontal-canal benign positional vertigo. Laryngoscope 106(4):476–478

Levrat E, Van Melle G, Monnier P, Maire R (2003) Efficacy of the Semont maneuver in benign paroxysmal positional vertigo. Arch Otolaryngol Head Neck Surg 129(6):629–633

Li S, Wang Z, Liu Y, Cao J, Zheng H, Jing Y, Han L, Ma X, Xia R, Yu L (2022) Risk factors for the recurrence of benign paroxysmal positional vertigo: a systematic review and meta-analysis. Ear Nose Throat J 1101:NP112–NP134

Lindell E, Finizia C, Johansson M, Karlsson T, Nilson J, Magnusson M (2018) Asking about dizziness when turning in bed predicts examination findings for benign paroxysmal positional vertigo. J Vestib Res 28(3–4):339–347

Lopez-Escamez JA, Gamiz MJ, Finana MG, Perez AF, Canet IS (2002) Position in bed is associated with left or right location in benign paroxysmal positional vertigo of the posterior semicircular canal. Am J Otolaryngol 23(5):263–266

Lopez-Escamez JA, Gamiz MJ, Fernandez-Perez A, Gomez-Finana M, Sanchez-Canet I (2003) Impact of treatment on health-related quality of life in patients with posterior canal benign paroxysmal positional vertigo. Otol Neurotol 24(4):637–641

Luryi AL, Lawrence J, LaRouere M, Babu S, Bojrab DI, Zappia J, Sargent EW, Schutt CA (2018) Treatment of patients with benign paroxysmal positional vertigo and severe immobility using the particle repositioning chair: a retrospective cohort study. Ann Otol Rhinol Laryngol 127(6):390–394

Lynn S, Pool A, Rose D, Brey R, Suman V (1995) Randomized trial of the canalith repositioning procedure. Otolaryngol Head Neck Surg 113(6):712–720

Maas BDPJ, van der Zaag-Loonen HJ, van Benthem PPG, Bruintjes TD (2020) Effectiveness of canal occlusion for intractable posterior canal benign paroxysmal positional vertigo: a systematic review. Otolaryngol Head Neck Surg 162(1):40–49

Macdonald NK, Kaski D, Saman Y, Al-Shaikh SA, Anwer A, Bamiou DE (2017) Central positional nystagmus: a systematic literature review. Front Neurol 8:141

Macias JD, Ellensohn A, Massingale S, Gerkin R (2004) Vibration with the canalith repositioning maneuver: a prospective randomized study to determine efficacy. Laryngoscope 114(6):1011–1014

Mandala M, Santoro GP, Asprella LG, Casani AP, Faralli M, Giannoni B, Gufoni M, Marcelli V, Marchetti P, Pepponi E, Vannucchi P, Nuti D (2012) Double-blind randomized trial on short-term efficacy of the Semont maneuver for the treatment of posterior canal benign paroxysmal positional vertigo. J Neurol 259(5):882–885

Mandala M, Califano L, Casani AP, Faralli M, Marcelli V, Neri G, Pecci R, Scasso F, di SL S, Vannucchi P, Giannoni B, Dasgupta S, Bindi I, Salerni L, Nuti D (2021) Double-blind randomized trial on the efficacy of the forced prolonged position for treatment of lateral canal benign paroxysmal positional vertigo. Laryngoscope 131:E1296–E1300

Marciano E, Marcelli V (2002) Postural restrictions in labyrintholithiasis. Eur Arch Otorhinolaryngol 259(5):262–265

Massoud EA, Ireland DJ (1996) Post-treatment instructions in the nonsurgical management of benign paroxysmal positional vertigo. J Otolaryngol 25(2):121–125

McClure JA (1985) Horizontal canal BPV. J Otolaryngol 14:30–35

Mumford CJ (2019) Post-traumatic benign paroxysmal positional vertigo. Pract Neurol 19(4):354–355

Nam J, Kim S, Huh Y, Kim JS (2009) Ageotropic central positional nystagmus in nodular infarction. Neurology 73(14):1163

Neugebauer H, Adrion C, Glaser M, Strupp M (2013) Long-term changes of central ocular motor signs in patients with vestibular migraine. Eur Neurol 69(2):102–107

Neuhauser HK (2016) The epidemiology of dizziness and vertigo. Handb Clin Neurol 137:67–82

Nuti D, Agus G, Barbieri MT, Passali D (1998) The management of horizontal-canal paroxysmal positional vertigo. Acta Otolaryngol 118(4):455–460

Obrist D, Hegemann S, Kronenberg D, Hauselmann O, Rosgen T (2010) In vitro model of a semicircular canal: design and validation of the model and its use for the study of canalithiasis. J Biomech 43(6):1208–1214

Obrist D, Nienhaus A, Zamaro E, Kalla R, Mantokoudis G, Strupp M (2016) Determinants for a successful semont maneuver: an in vitro study with a semicircular Canal model. Front Neurol 7:150

Oghalai JS, Manolidis S, Barth JL, Stewart MG, Jenkins HA (2000) Unrecognized benign paroxysmal positional vertigo in elderly patients. Otolaryngol Head Neck Surg 122(5):630–634

Oh HJ, Kim JS, Han BI, Lim JG (2007) Predicting a successful treatment in posterior canal benign paroxysmal positional vertigo. Neurology 68(15):1219–1222

Park MK, Lee DY, Kim YH (2019) Risk factors for positional vertigo and the impact of vertigo on daily life: the Korean National Health and nutrition examination survey. J Audiol Otol 23(1): 8–14

Parnes LS, McClure JA (1992) Free-floating endolymph particles: a new operative finding during posterior semicircular canal occlusion. Laryngoscope 102(9):988–992

Ping L, Yi-Fei Z, Shu-Zhi W, Yan-Yan Z, Xiao-Kai Y (2020) Diagnosis and treatment of the short-arm type posterior semicircular canal BPPV. Braz J Otorhinolaryngol. https://doi.org/10.1016/j.bjorl.2020.10.012

Radtke A, Neuhauser H, von Brevern M, Lempert T (1999) A modified Epley's procedure for self-

9

treatment of benign paroxysmal positional vertigo. Neurology 53(6):1358–1360
Radtke A, von BM, Tiel-Wilck K, Mainz-Perchalla A, Neuhauser H, Lempert T (2004) Self-treatment of benign paroxysmal positional vertigo: Semont maneuver vs Epley procedure. Neurology 63(1): 150–152
Radtke A, von BM, Neuhauser H, Hottenrott T, Lempert T (2012) Vestibular migraine: long-term follow-up of clinical symptoms and vestibulo-cochlear findings. Neurology 79(15):1607–1614
Rhim GI (2016) Serum vitamin D and recurrent benign paroxysmal positional vertigo. Laryngoscope Investig Otolaryngol 1(6):150–153
Rhim GI (2019) Serum vitamin D and long-term outcomes of benign paroxysmal positional vertigo. Clin Exp Otorhinolaryngol 12(3) 273–278
Rhim GI (2020) Effect of vitamin D injection in recurrent benign paroxysmal positional vertigo with vitamin D deficiency. Int Arch Otorhinolaryngol 24(4):e423–e428
Roberts RA, Gans RE, DeBoodt JL, Lister JJ (2005) Treatment of benign paroxysmal positional vertigo necessity of postmaneuver patient restrictions. J Am Acad Audiol 16(6):357–366
Ruckenstein MJ, Shepard NT (2007) The canalith repositioning procedure with and without mastoid oscillation for the treatment of benign paroxysmal positional vertigo. ORL J Otorhinolaryngol Relat Spec 69(5):295–298
Salvinelli F, Casale M, Trivelli M, D'Ascanio L, Firrisi L, Lamanna F, Greco F, Costantino S (2003) Benign paroxysmal positional vertigo: a comparative prospective study on the efficacy of Semont's maneuver and no treatment strategy. Clin Ter 154(1):7–11
Sayin I, Koç RH, Temirbekov D, Gunes S, Cirak M, Yazici ZM (2020) Betahistine add-on therapy for treatment of subjects with posterior benign paroxysmal positional vertigo: a randomized controlled trial. Braz J Otorhinolaryngol S1808-8694(20)30141–30145
Schuricht A, Hougaard DD (2022) Is a mechanical rotational chair superior to manual treatment maneuvers on an examination bed in the treatment of benign paroxysmal positional vertigo? Otol Neurotol 43:e235–e242
Semont A, Freyss G, Vitte E (1988) Curing the BPPV with a liberatory maneuver. Adv Otorhinolaryngol 42:290–293
Serafini G, Palmieri AM, Simoncelli C (1996) Benign paroxysmal positional vertigo of posterior semicircular canal: results in 160 cases treated with Semont's maneuver. Ann Otol Rhinol Laryngol 105(10):770–775
Shah MU, Lotterman S, Roberts D, Eisen M (2019) Smartphone telemedical emergency department consults for screening of nonacute dizziness. Laryngoscope 129(2):466–469
Sheikhzadeh M, Lotfi Y, Mousavi A, Heidari B, Bakhshi E (2016) The effect of serum vitamin D normalization in preventing recurrences of benign paroxysmal positional vertigo: a case-control study. Caspian J Intern Med 7(3):173–177
Shim DB, Ko KM, Lee JH, Park HJ, Song MH (2015) Natural history of horizontal canal benign paroxysmal positional vertigo is truly short. J Neurol 262(1):74–80
Shoman N, Longridge N (2007) Cerebellar vermis lesions and tumours of the fourth ventricle in patients with positional and positioning vertigo and nystagmus. J Laryngol Otol 121(2):166–169
Sim E, Tan D, Hill K (2019) Poor treatment outcomes following repositioning maneuvers in younger and older adults with benign paroxysmal positional vertigo: a systematic review and meta-analysis. J Am Med Dir Assoc 20(2):224
Song P, Zhao X, Xu Y, Zhao Z, Wang L, Liu Y, Gao Q (2020) Correlation between benign paroxysmal positional vertigo and 25-hydroxyvitamin D. Front Neurol 11:576
Soto-Varela A, Bartual-Magro J, Santos-Perez S, Velez-Regueiro M, Lechuga-Garcia R, Perez-Carro-Rios A, Caballero L (2001) Benign paroxysmal vertigo: a comparative prospective study of the efficacy of Brandt and Daroff exercises, Semont and Epley maneuver. Rev Laryngol Otol Rhinol (Bord) 122(3):179–183
Steddin S, Brandt T (1994) Benign paroxysmal positional vertigo. Differential diagnosis of posterior, horizontal and anterior canalolithiasis. Nervenarzt 65(8):505–510
Steenerson RL, Cronin GW (1996) Comparison of the canalith repositioning procedure and vestibular habituation training in forty patients with benign paroxysmal positional vertigo. Otolaryngol Head Neck Surg 114(1):61–64
Strupp M, Cnyrim C, Brandt T (2007) Vertigo and dizziness: treatment of benign paroxysmal positioning vertigo, vestibular neuritis and Menère's disease. In: Candelise L (ed) Evidence-based neurology – management of neurological disorders. Blackwell Publishing, Oxford, pp 59–69
Strupp M, Goldschagg N, Vinck AS, Bayer O, Vandenbroeck S, Salerni L, Hennig A, Obrist D, Mandala M (2021) BPPV: Comparison of the SemontPLUS with the semont maneuver: a prospective randomized trial. Front Neurol 12:652573
Strupp M, Mavrodiev V, Goldschagg N (2023) Triple benign paroxysmal positional vertigo and the stremgth of video-based remote management. JAMA Neurol https://doi.org/10.1001/jamaneurol.2022.4861

Tateno F, Sakakibara R (2019) Positional vertigo after isolated cerebellar nodulus stroke: a report of 3 cases. J Stroke Cerebrovasc Dis 28(2):487–489
Vaduva C, Esteban-Sanchez J, Sanz-Fernandez R, Martin-Sanz E (2018) Prevalence and management of post-BPPV residual symptoms. Eur Arch Otorhinolaryngol 275(6):1429–1437
van der Zaag-Loonen H, van Leeuwen RB, Bruintjes TD, van Munster BC (2015) Prevalence of unrecognized benign paroxysmal positional vertigo in older patients. Eur Arch Otorhinolaryngol 272(6):1521–1524
Vannucchi P, Giannoni B, Pagnini P (1997) Treatment of horizontal semicircular canal benign paroxysmal positional vertigo. J Vestib Res 7(1):1–6
von Brevern M, Zeise D, Neuhauser H, Clarke AH, Lempert T (2005) Acute migrainous vertigo: clinical and oculographic findings. Brain 128(Pt 2): 365–374
von Brevern M, Schmidt T, Schonfeld U, Lempert T, Clarke AH (2006a) Utricular dysfunction in patients with benign paroxysmal positional vertigo. Otol Neurotol 27(1):92–96
von Brevern M, Seelig T, Radtke A, Tiel-Wilck K, Neuhauser H, Lempert T (2006b) Short-term efficacy of Epley's manoeuvre: a double-blind randomised trial. J Neurol Neurosurg Psychiatry 77(8):980–982
von Brevern M, Radtke A, Lezius F, Feldmann M, Ziese T, Lempert T, Neuhauser H (2007) Epidemiology of benign paroxysmal positional vertigo: a population based study. J Neurol Neurosurg Psychiatry 78(7):710–715
von Brevern M, Bertholon P, Brandt T, Fife T, Imai T, Nuti D, Newman-Toker D (2015) Benign paroxysmal positional vertigo: Diagnostic criteria. J Vestib Res 25(3–4):105–117
Wei W, Sayyid ZN, Ma X, Wang T, Dong Y (2018) Presence of anxiety and depression symptoms affects the first time treatment efficacy and recurrence of benign paroxysmal positional vertigo. Front Neurol 9:178
White J, Savvides P, Cherian N, Oas J (2005) Canalith repositioning for benign paroxysmal positional vertigo. Otol Neurotol 26(4):704–710
Whitman GT, Baloh RW (2015) Seasonality of benign paroxysmal positional vertigo. JAMA Otolaryngol Head Neck Surg 141(2):188–189
Woodworth BA, Gillespie MB, Lambert PR (2004) The canalith repositioning procedure for benign positional vertigo: a meta-analysis. Laryngoscope 114(7):1143–1146
Yacovino DA, Hain TC, Gualtieri F (2009) New therapeutic maneuver for anterior canal benign paroxysmal positional vertigo. J Neurol 256(11):1851–1855
Yang X, Ling X, Shen B, Hong Y, Li K, Si L, Kim JS (2019) Diagnosis strategy and Yacovino maneuver for anterior canal-benign paroxysmal positional vertigo. J Neurol 266(7):1674–1684
Yang B, Lu Y, Xing D, Zhong W, Tang Q, Liu J, Yang X (2020) Association between serum vitamin D levels and benign paroxysmal positional vertigo: a systematic review and meta-analysis of observational studies. Eur Arch Otorhinolaryngol 277(1):169–177
Yimtae K, Srirompotong S, Srirompotong S, Sae-Seaw P (2003) A randomized trial of the canalith repositioning procedure. Laryngoscope 113(5):828–832
Yu S, Liu F, Cheng Z, Wang Q (2014) Association between osteoporosis and benign paroxysmal positional vertigo: a systematic review. BMC Neurol 14:110
Zuma e Maia, Ramos BF, Cal R, Brock CM, Mangabeira Albernaz PL, Strupp M (2020) Management of lateral semicircular canal benign paroxysmal positional vertigo. Front Neurol 11:1040

Menière's Disease

Contents

Supplementary Information The online version contains supplementary material available at [https://doi.org/10.1007/978-3-030-78260-3_10]. The videos can be accessed by scanning the related images with the SN More Media App.

M. Strupp et al., *Vertigo and Dizziness*, https://doi.org/10.1007/978-3-030-78260-3_10

Menière's disease (MD) is an episodic vertigo syndrome typically combining vestibular and cochlear symptoms and signs. It is the second most frequent cause of peripheral vestibular vertigo and known as an inner ear disease since 1861 (for references, see Lustig and Lalwani 1997). The pathognomonic histopathological finding is endolymphatic hydrops. However, the etiology and pathophysiology of MD are, despite many studies, so far not fully understood (for references, see Nakashima et al. 2016). The current diagnostic criteria for MD are as follows (adapted from Lopez-Escamez et al. 2015) (▶ Box 10.1):

Box 10.1 Diagnostic Criteria of MD

MD

1. Two or more spontaneous episodes of vertigo, each lasting 20 min to 12 h
2. Audiometrically documented low- to medium-frequency sensorineural hearing loss (SNHL) in one ear
3. Defining the affected ear on at least one occasion before, during, or after one of the episodes of vertigo (± 24 h)
4. Fluctuating aural symptoms (hearing, tinnitus, or fullness) in the affected ear
5. Not better accounted for by another vestibular diagnosis

Probable MD

1. Two or more episodes of vertigo or dizziness, each lasting 20 min to 24 h
2. Fluctuating aural symptoms (hearing, tinnitus, or fullness) in the affected ear
3. Not better accounted for by another vestibular diagnosis

For its diagnosis, it is important to document low- to medium-frequency sensorineural hearing loss in the affected ear; the hearing loss should ideally be related to an episode of vertigo (± 24 h). Without this, only the diagnosis of *probable* MD can be made. This underlines the importance of the use of portable tablet- or smartphone-based audio apps for the measurement of hearing by the patient before, during, and after an episode of vertigo (Tse et al. 2019).

10.1 Epidemiology

The reported prevalence of MD ranges—depending on the ethnic group—from 35/100,000 in Japan (Shojaku et al. 2005) to 513/100.000 in Finland (Havia et al. 2005; for references, see Harris and Alexander 2010), which supports the relevance of genetic and environmental factors (see below). The typical age of onset ranges from the third to the seventh decades of life. MD can also begin in early childhood (Choung et al. 2006; Brantberg et al. 2012; Chen et al. 2020). An epidemiological study showed a rapid yearly increase of the incidence rate of MD from 2013 to 2017 in Korea which the authors explain by an aging society, an increase in medical accessibility, and lifestyle changes (Kim and Cheon 2020). The often-published preponderance of females could not be confirmed and might be due to the misdiagnosis of vestibular migraine as MD (Becker-Bense et al. 2019). The odds of MD are higher for older subjects (adjusted OR per 10-year increase: 1.5), white ethnicity (OR 1.7), and severe obesity (OR 1.7) (Alexander and Harris 2010; Tyrrell et al. 2014). An association with several other diseases was reported, e.g., migraine (OR 2.0), arthritis (OR 1.8), or psoriasis (OR 1.8) (Tyrrell et al. 2014); the latter two may indicate the relevance of immune processes (see below).

10.2 Diagnosis

10.2.1 Patient History

The leading symptoms of MD are recurrent episodes of vertigo, lasting at least 20 min to many hours, accompanied by impairment of hearing, tinnitus, or aural fullness in the affected ear (◘ Fig. 10.1). The attacks most often occur without any provoking factors. In at least one third of cases, tinnitus and ear pressure increase and hearing impairment becomes more severe before the attacks.

The duration of the episodes is defined as the time that the patient has to be at rest and cannot move. It may last less than 20 min or more than 12 h, but neither is a common finding, and other disorders should be considered when such durations are noted (Perez-Garrigues et al. 2008). The duration of an episode may be difficult to define as patients may have residual symptoms after an episode, because the attacks with spinning or non-spinning vertigo can be followed by postural imbalance and impairment of gait, which may last longer until the peripheral vestibular deficit recovers or is centrally compensated.

A temporal association between hearing loss and the vertigo episode often occurs as a change in hearing within ±24 h of the vertigo episode, which is an important diagnostic criterion. In the first years of the disease, hearing often fluctuates considerably. After recurrent episodes of vertigo, there is often a progression of hearing loss which persists; then, the episodes of vertigo are often no longer associated with other ear symptoms.

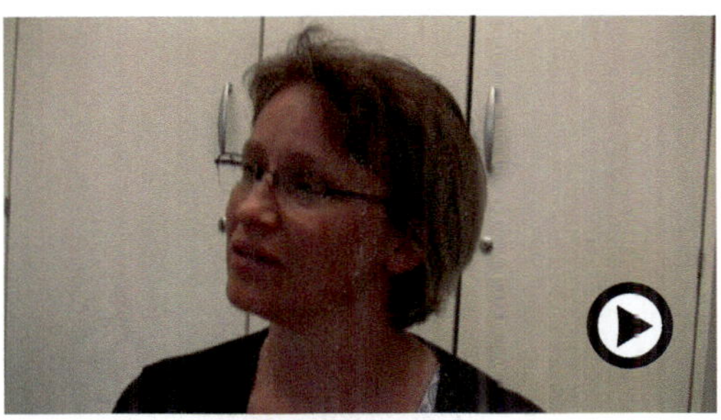

◘ **Fig. 10.1** Menière's disease: patient history (▶ https://doi.org/10.1007/000-95r)

Monosymptomatic pure vestibular or pure cochlear episodes may occur at the beginning of the disease. Overall, there is a high level of variability of the vestibular and audiological symptoms, which may make the diagnosis in the initial phase challenging, in particular the differential diagnosis between MD and vestibular migraine and autoimmune and inherited inner ear diseases. The latter two differential diagnoses are of particular relevance in patients with bilateral MD. Episodic vertigo may precede the onset of hearing loss by several weeks or months, but tinnitus or aural fullness is usually associated with the first episode of vertigo. Conversely, sensorineural hearing loss may precede the onset of vertigo episodes by several months or years (Belinchon et al. 2012). This clinical variant is called delayed MD. The affected ear is mainly determined by the hearing loss (see below for details).

Since the phenotype of MD is characterized by a variable combination of vestibular and audiological symptoms, a clinical sub-classification of MD seems to be relevant for the diagnosis and for future therapeutic studies, because different pathomechanisms may underlie these various subtypes (Phillips et al. 2018). The "MD Consortium" (a European ENT initiative for large-scale clinical and genomic research in MD) has recommended five major clinical groups of patients with unilateral and bilateral MD (▶ Box 10.2). This was mainly based on cluster analyses using clinical variables, such as the onset of hearing, migraine, familial history, or a comorbid autoimmune disorder, to identify subgroups of patients with MD (Frejo et al. 2016, 2017).

Box 10.2 Clinical Subgroups of Patients with MD (Frejo et al. 2017)

Unilateral MD

- Type 1 Sporadic MD (if concurrent migraine, autoimmune disease, or familial MD is observed, patients do not belong to this subgroup)
- Type 2 Delayed MD (hearing loss precedes vertigo attacks by months or years)
- Type 3 Familial MD (at least two patients in the first or second degree)
- Type 4 Sporadic MD with migraine (temporal relationship not required)
- Type 5 Sporadic MD with an autoimmune disease

Bilateral MD

- Type 1 Unilateral hearing loss becomes bilateral
- Type 2 Sporadic, simultaneous hearing loss (usually symmetric)
- Type 3 Familial MD (most families have bilateral hearing loss, but unilateral patients may coexist in the same family)
- Type 4 Sporadic MD with migraine
- Type 5 Sporadic MD with an autoimmune disease

Tumarkin's otolithic catastrophe (Tumarkin 1936), also called vestibular drop attacks: This is another manifestation of MD (◘ Fig. 10.2). It is characterized by sudden attacks with falls out of the blue, which are due to a sudden loss of vestibulospinal tone. Patients may also fall to one side. The attacks last just a few seconds, rarely longer, most often without loss of consciousness (Black et al. 1982); if the latter occurs, it is also called vestibular syncope (Pyykko et al. 2018b). These attacks are associated with a considerable reduction of quality of life (Pyykko et al. 2018a).

Patients with MD may also develop symptoms of the syndrome of the third mobile windows: Changes in pressure or low-frequency sounds (Tullio phenomenon) can induce short attacks lasting seconds to minutes. These symptoms often occur during the course of the disease, probably due to pronounced endolymphatic hydrops, which brings the endolymphatic labyrinth close to the stapes footplate.

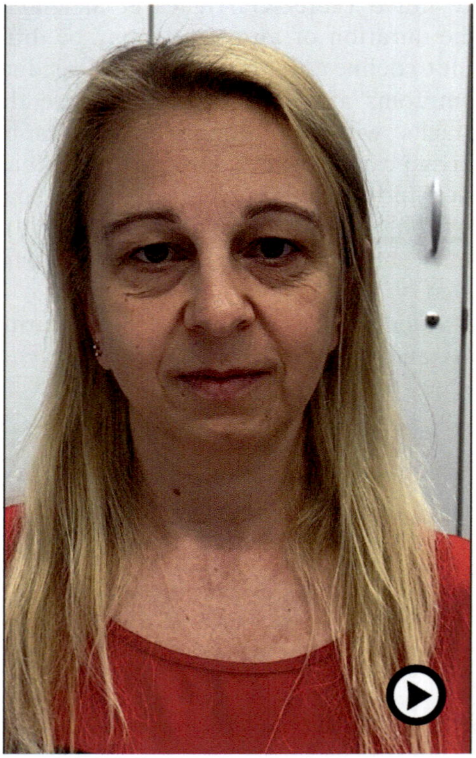

◘ **Fig. 10.2** Tumarkin's otolithic catastrophes (▶ https://doi.org/10.1007/000-95p)

10.2.2 Clinical Examination

In the attack-free interval:

- Testing of hearing, including the finger rub test, Rinne and Weber. Additional audiometry is indicated (see below). Otoscopy: There should be no evidence for herpes zoster, otitis media, or other pathology.
- Bedside examination of the vestibular and the ocular motor systems to look for other peripheral or central disorders as differential diagnoses. It should be noted that the head impulse test is often normal in MD despite reduced caloric irrigation (see below).

During an attack:

Pathophysiologically, there is a unilateral, transient vestibular excitation—lasting minutes—and subsequently a longer-lasting vestibulocochlear inhibition/deficit with the following clinical findings:

- During the initial period with excitation associated with spinning or non-spinning vertigo: nystagmus with the fast phase beating toward the affected labyrinth.
- Subsequently, there is a reversal of the direction with the fast phase now beating toward the non-affected labyrinth. This reversal (first excitation, then conduction block) is typically found in MD during the first many minutes (Fig. 10.3 and 10.4).

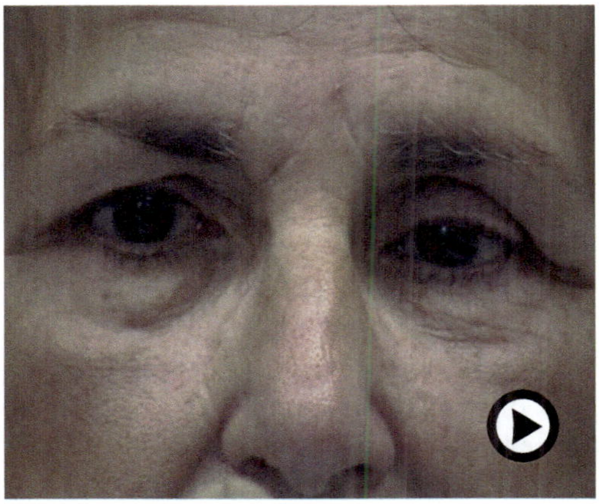

Fig. 10.3 Initial phase of an acute attack in MD: nystagmus beats towards the affected side (► https://doi.org/10.1007/000-95q)

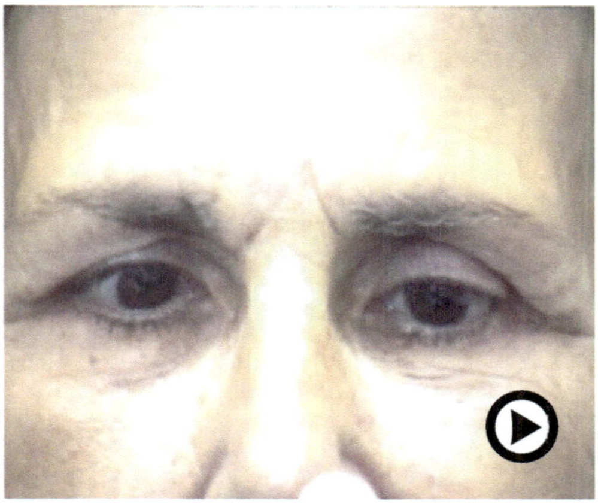

Fig. 10.4 Late phase of an attack in MD: nystagmus beats towards the non-affected side (► https://doi.org/10.1007/000-95n)

Diagnostically, it has been shown to be very helpful for patients to video their eye movements during an attack of vertigo and use an audio app to document hearing (Tse et al. 2019).

10.2.3 Laboratory Examinations

Audiometry According to the current diagnostic criteria of MD, audiometry is the most important laboratory examination. Sensorineural hearing loss in the low- and medium-frequency range is required for the diagnosis and to identify the affected ear (Lopez-Escamez et al. 2015).

Low-frequency SNHL is defined as increases in pure tone thresholds for bone-conducted sound that are higher (i.e., worse) in the affected ear than the contralateral ear by at least 30 dB HL at each of two contiguous frequencies below 2000 Hz (Figs. 10.5 and 10.6). In cases of bilateral low-frequency sensorineural hearing loss, the absolute thresholds for bone-conducted sound must be 35 dB HL or higher at each of two contiguous frequencies below 2000 Hz. If multiple audiograms are available, demonstration of recovery of low-frequency sensorineural

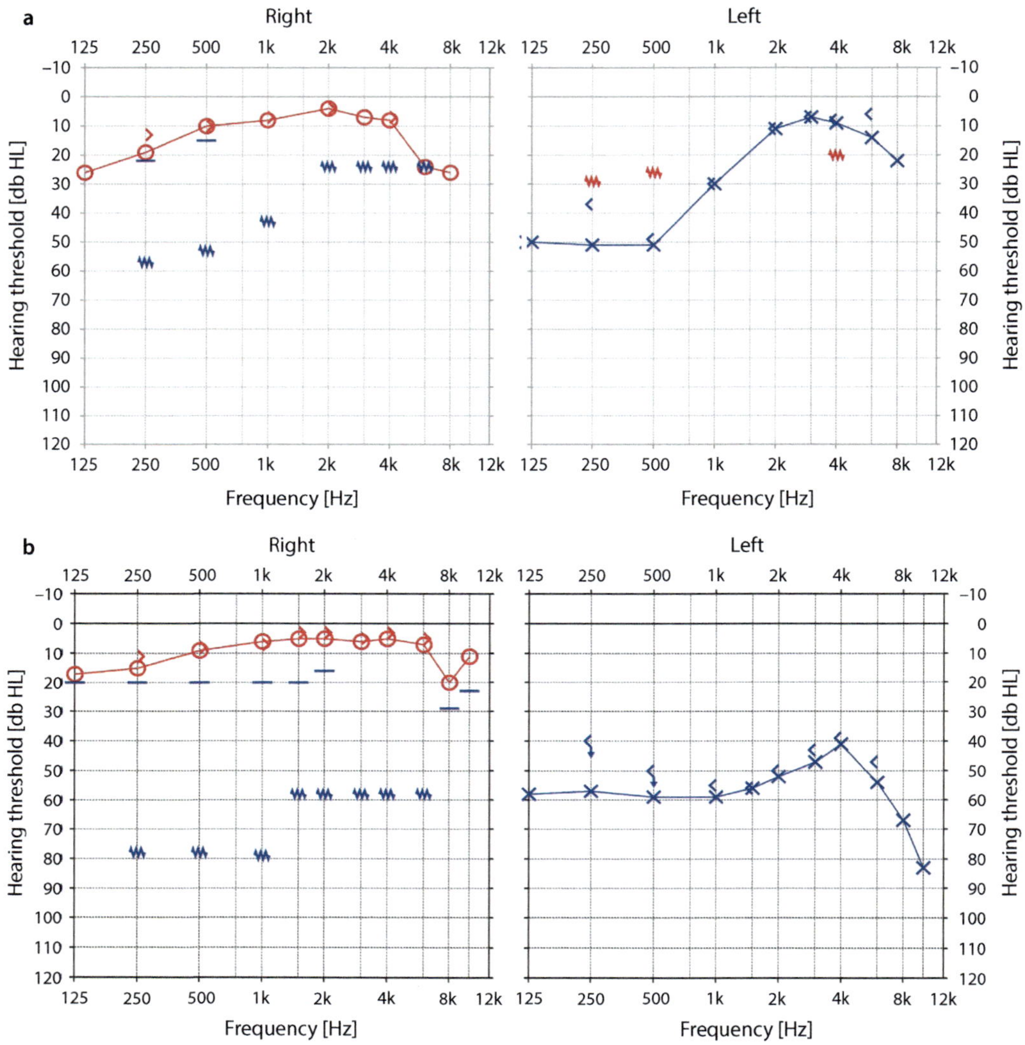

10

Fig. 10.5 **a**, **b** Pure tone audiogram in two patients with left-sided MD (red o: air conduction on the right; blue x: air conduction on the left, red >: bone conduction on the right; blue <: bone conduction on the left). **a** Left-sided sensorineural hearing loss in the low-frequency range. There must be a reduction of hearing of at least 30 dB in two neighboring frequencies below 2000 Hz (Lopez-Escamez et al. 2015). **b** Left-sided sensorineural pantonal hearing loss

hearing loss at some point in time further supports the diagnosis of MD. In many cases, audiological testing allows a differentiation between MD and vestibular migraine, although there is a clear overlap (Battista 2004; Cha et al. 2007; De Valck et al. 2007).

Bilateral synchronous (symmetric or asymmetric) sensorineural hearing loss can occur in some patients (Nabi and Parnes 2009; Belinchon et al. 2011) although such a pattern should raise concern for the possibility of autoimmune inner ear disease (see differential diagnoses) as an alternative explanation for the vertigo episodes or a comorbid condition. Sensorineural hearing loss in MD can also involve medium and high frequencies after several episodes of vertigo, leading to pantonal hearing loss.

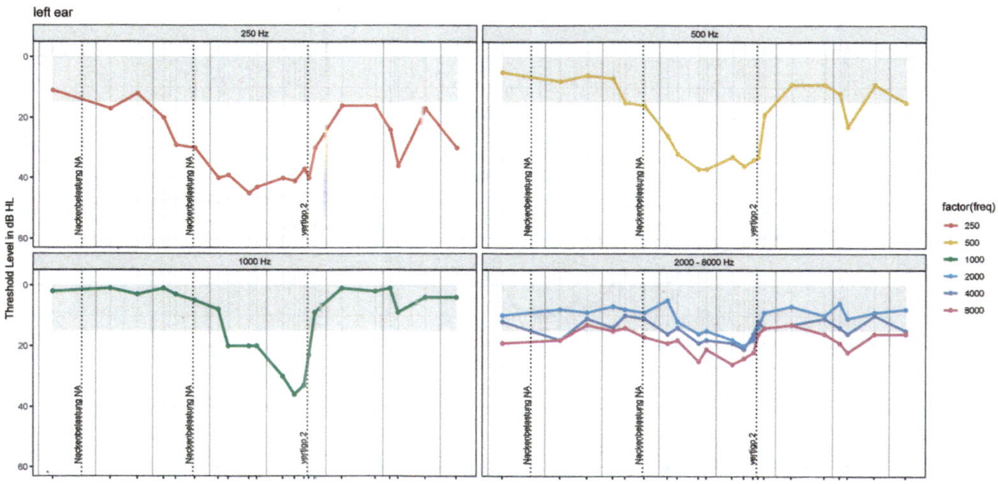

Fig. 10.6 Audiogram for four different frequency spectra recorded by a patient using an audio app before, during, and after an attack. There was a decrease of hearing in the low-frequency range before and during the attack with an improvement after the attack

10.2.4 Complementary Laboratory Testing

Vestibular testing In patients with MD, there is typically a pathological caloric response with a pseudo-normal video-HIT (Fig. 10.7) (McGarvie et al. 2015; Jerin et al. 2019; Hannigan et al. 2019). This dissociation is helpful for the diagnosis and differential diagnosis (Kaci et al. 2020; Shugyo et al. 2020). The cause of this typical dissociation is not yet completely understood (Shaw and Raghavan 2018; Rey-Martinez et al. 2020); it is probably caused by the increase of the diameter of the endolymphatic space with a change in the hydrodynamics, leading to a pseudo-normal HIT.

The vestibular deficit and the course of the disease can be documented by means of caloric testing. The video-HIT or VEMP are less often impaired. The combination of these examinations is useful to better identify the affected side, in particular to identify whether there is bilateral MD.

10.3 Imaging

10.3.1 Contrast MRI of the Inner Ear and Endolymphatic Hydrops

In most patients with MD, contrast MRI—after intratympanic gadolinium injection (first description 2007: (Nakashima et al. 2007; Gurkov et al. 2011)) or after intravenous application of gadolinium (Naganawa et al. 2010; Kirsch et al. 2019)—demonstrates an enlargement of the endolymphatic space, into which gadolinium does not diffuse: endolymphatic hydrops (ELH) (Fig. 10.8) (for references, see Bernaerts and De 2019; Loureiro et al. 2020; Connor and Pai 2021). ELH was, for instance, examined in a study with 148 patients with MD and healthy controls (Bernaerts et al. 2019): The sensitivity for the diagnosis was 84.6% and the specificity was 92.3%. These findings were supported by other studies focusing on volumetry of ELH (Ito et al. 2019); however, in

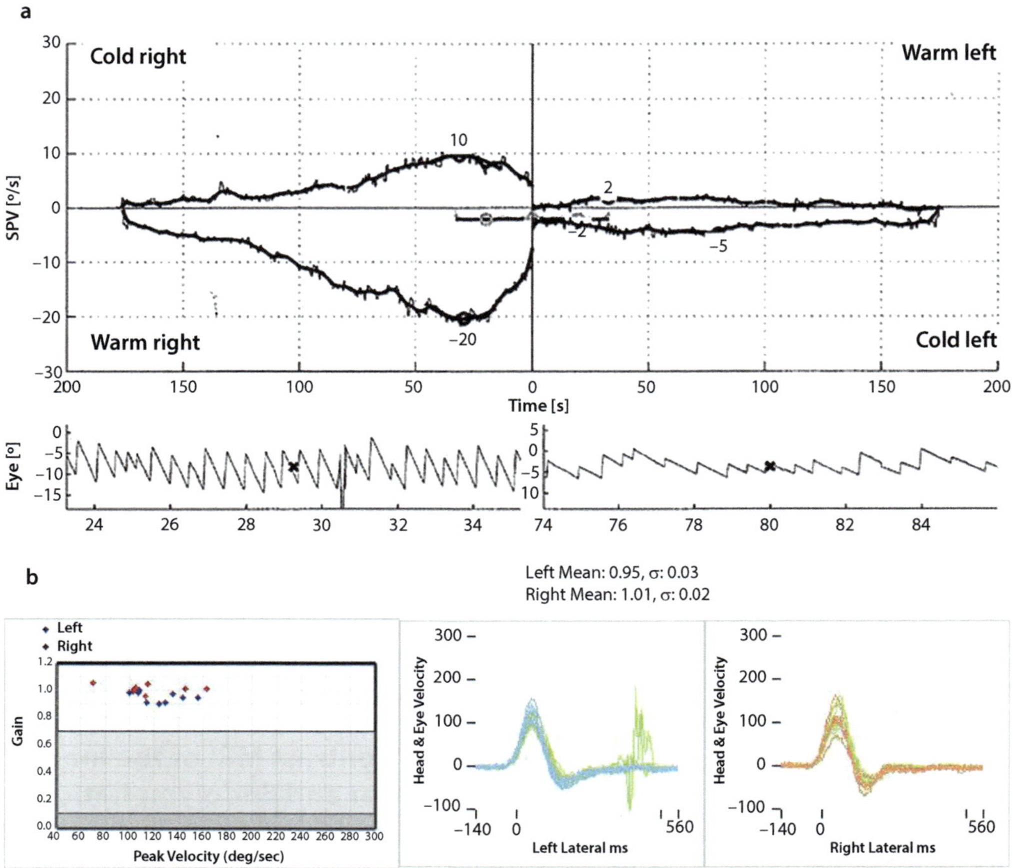

Fig. 10.7 a, b Vestibular testing in a patient with left-sided MD. **a** Caloric testing: partial deficit on the left side in the low-frequency range. **b** Video-HIT: normal (or pseudo-normal) VOR gain in the high-frequency range. This dissociation is typical of MD, probably due to the increase in the diameter of the endolymphatic duct, which leads to the pseudo-normal video-HIT

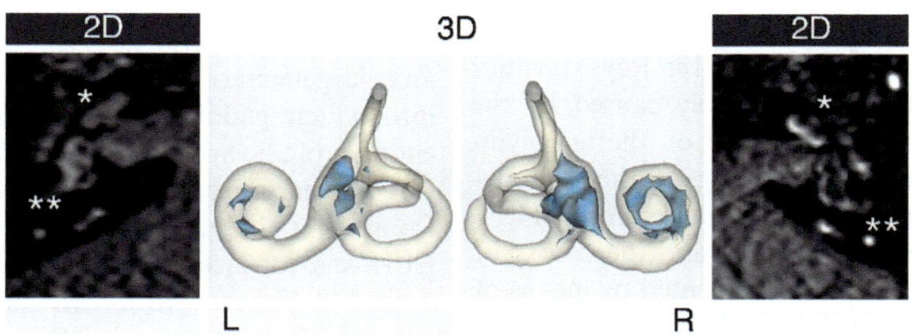

Fig. 10.8 High-resolution MRI of the inner ear, after intravenous injection of gadolinium, showing both labyrinths in a patient with bilateral MD with more pronounced symptoms from the right ear and asymmetrical ELH on the right side (R) with normal findings on the left (L). Gadolinium diffuses into the perilymphatic space only (white, *cochlea, **labyrinth), which explains why ELH is only indirectly visualized by contrast sparing. In 2D imaging, ELH can only be visualized on certain slices depending on the size and orientation of the ELH. 3D reconstruction (middle) can demonstrate the whole extent of the ELH (blue) (Kindly provided by V. Kirsch)

these studies, ELH was also found in healthy subjects (see below). A significant correlation was also found between ELH and the impairment of hearing, but not the vestibular deficit (Zhang et al. 2020).

The role of ELH in the diagnosis of MD has been under discussion since the 1980s (Rauch et al. 1989) and is still a matter of debate (see also below: pathological anatomy, pathophysiology, and etiology) (Lopez-Escamez and Attye 2019; Kay-Rivest et al. 2020). ELH is also found in inner ear imaging in healthy subjects (Ito et al. 2019), e.g., in 10% in the sacculus as well as in 40% of patients with a sensorineural hearing loss >45 dB without vestibular symptoms (Attye et al. 2018). On the one hand, almost all patients with MD have ELH on imaging. On the other hand, ELH also occurs in other vestibular syndromes with involvement of the inner ear, such as vestibular migraine with hearing problems (in about 20%) (Gurkov et al. 2014; Kirsch et al. 2018). In a narrative review, it was reported that radiologically ELH was found in 99.4% of patients with MD, but also in 31% of healthy subjects, 28.1% of patients with vestibular migraine, and 25.9% of patients with vestibular schwannoma (van der Lubbe et al. 2020). In another imaging study on vestibular migraine and concurrent MD, ELH was seen in 80% in MD, in 25% of patients presenting with both MD and vestibular migraine, and in 8% of vestibular migraine patients (Oh et al. 2021). One can conclude from these studies that the radiological demonstration of ELH is a necessary, but not sufficient condition for the diagnosis of MD. Therefore, there is no general recommendation for a radiological demonstration of ELH to diagnose MD (Kay-Rivest et al. 2020). The combination of the radiological demonstration of ELH and contrast enhancement of the perilymphatic space (Nahmani et al. 2020) probably makes a greater contribution to the diagnosis of MD (van Steekelenburg et al. 2020).

A contrast MRI of the brain should, of course, be performed to exclude other pathologies, particularly vestibular schwannoma which can also be associated with episodes of vertigo, impairment of hearing and tinnitus.

10.4 Differential Diagnoses and Clinical Problems

The typical patient history in combination with a typical audiogram is the key to the diagnosis. The relevant differential diagnoses are summarized in ► Box 10.3.

Box 10.3 Important Differential Diagnoses for MD (in Alphabetical Order)

- Autosomal dominant sensorineural hearing loss
- Autoimmune inner ear disease
- Benign recurrent vestibulopathy
- Cerebrovascular disease (stroke/TIA in the vertebrobasilar system, namely AICA territoty) (see ► Chap. 13)
- Cogan's syndrome
- Endolymphatic sac tumor
- Meningiomas and other masses of the cerebellopontine angle
- Otosyphilis
- Susac syndrome (low-frequency hearing loss, tinnitus, visual loss, and/or central neurological/psychiatric symptoms due to an autoimmune microangiopathy)
- Syndrome of the third mobile windows (see ► Chap. 12)
- Vestibular migraine (see ► Chap. 14)
- Vestibular paroxysmia (see ► Chap. 11)
- Vestibular schwannoma

The two most important differential diagnoses are as follows:

- In patients with recurrent episodes: vestibular migraine (see ► Chap. 14): It should be noted that there are patients

who fulfill the criteria for *both* diseases (Murofushi et al. 2018) (see also ▶ Box 10.2.), which can also be explained pathophysiologically.
- In patients with a first attack of MD without evident acute hearing problems: AUVP (see ▶ Chap. 8) or stroke (see ▶ Chap. 13)

In patients with recurrent episodes of vertigo, *vestibular migraine* is the most important differential diagnosis, because the variable duration of attacks from 5 min to 72 h overlaps with the duration of attacks in MD (Lempert et al. 2012). As mentioned above, patients can fulfill the criteria for both diseases. An association between MD and headache was already described by Prosper Menière and later reinforced (Moshtaghi et al. 2016; Atkinson 1962).

There is also a pathophysiological association between MD and vestibular migraine (Liu and Xu 2016), because vestibular migraine can also lead to dysfunction in the inner ear and thus to ELH (Gurkov et al. 2014; Kirsch et al. 2018); this is similar to, for instance, retinal migraine.

10

The diagnosis of *vestibular migraine* as a differential diagnosis is supported by:
- No evidence of significant hearing impairment (in particular <2000 Hz) despite several episodes. Mild unilateral hearing disturbances were observed in 3–12% (Kayan and Hood 1984; Cass et al. 1997; Battista 2004) and bilaterally in 18% in a longitudinal study over 9 years (Radtke et al. 2012) in patients with vestibular migraine. Impairment of hearing and vestibular function was even described in patients with migraine (Benjamin et al. 2022).
- Typical migrainous symptoms during >50% of the attacks.
- Migraine in the patient history or concurrent migraine.
- Mild-to-moderate central ocular motor dysfunction in the attack-free interval, which is found in up to 60% of patients (Dieterich and Brandt 1999).
- A convincing response to treatment of the attacks and to prophylactic treatment with anti-migrainous drugs.

In terms of the differential diagnosis of *AUVP* one should ask the patient about and examine for audiological symptoms and signs as well as the duration of the symptoms, which typically last >24 h in AUVP.

Another rare but serious differential diagnosis is *Cogan's syndrome*, which manifests with a double triad: vertigo, hearing and eye problems, as well as impaired vestibular function, sensorineural hearing loss, and interstitial keratitis, typically affecting both sides, which if untreated often leads to bilateral vestibulopathy and deafness (for references, see Durtette et al. 2017). In such cases, examination for eye symptoms and signs and laboratory tests that show evidence of a generalized inflammation (erythrocytes sedimentation rate, CRP, and leukocytes) are of particular interest. Even if Cogan's syndrome is only suspected, an immediate and aggressive immunosuppressive therapy is fully indicated: initially, for instance, methylprednisolone i.v. 1 g/d for 5 days to preserve audiovestibular function (Durtette et al. 2017).

Another differential diagnosis is *benign recurrent vestibulopathy*, which also overlaps with vestibular migraine (van Esch et al. 2017; Ducroz et al. 2022). In patients with recurrent short attacks of vertigo, *vestibular paroxysmia* is another differential diagnosis (see ▶ Chap. 11); it may also be associated with audiological symptoms and signs. Typically, the duration of the attacks is much shorter and the audiological and vestibular deficits are only minor. Here, the response to treatment with a sodium channel blocker also supports the diagnosis of vestibular paroxysmia.

In patients with Tumarkin's otolithic catastrophe, paroxysmal brainstem attacks, TIA in the vertebrobasilar territory or cardiovascular diseases should be considered as differential diagnoses.

Another relevant differential diagnosis, in particular in patients with a first attack, is an *AICA infarction*. This also manifests with acute spinning or non-spinning vertigo and other ear symptoms; however, there is often a pronouced or even complete audiovestibular deficit, which one rarely finds during a first attack in MD, and there are also central symptoms and signs (see ▶ Chap. 13).

10.4.1 Diagnosis: The Essentials for Clinical Practice

The current diagnostic criteria (▶ Box 10.1), which require a pure tone audiometry with sensorineural hearing loss in the low- and medium-frequency range associated with an attack of vertigo, allow a reliable diagnosis in most cases. Testing of hearing has several clinical implications: in an acute vestibular syndrome it can discriminate between MD and AUVP and in case of an audiological deficit it may support the diagnosis of a acute central vestibular syndrome to due an AICA-infarction. Devices including audio apps can also contribute to the diagnosis because they allow testing of hearing by the patient during an episode of vertigo. There are different clinical subtypes of unilateral and bilateral MD. It should be noted that there is a considerable overlap between MD and vestibular migraine which is also the most important differential diagnosis. A contrast MRI of the inner ear is indicated, particularly to exclude vestibular schwannoma; the radiological demonstration of ELH requires further evaluation as a diagnostic tool.

10.5 Pathological Anatomy, Pathophysiology, and Etiology

The etiology and pathophysiology of MD are, despite many studies, so far not fully understood (for references, see Nakashima et al. 2016). The pathognomonic histological finding is ELH, which was already suspected by the German physiologist Hensen in 1880 ("glaucoma of the inner ear") and was histopathologically described in 1938 (Hallpike and Cairns 1938; Yamakawa 1938). In temporal bone studies, ELH was found to be a highly prevalent feature in MD (99.4%) (for references, see van der Lubbe et al. 2020).

Pathophysiologically, ELH evidently occurs due to a relatively too high production or a relatively too low reabsorption of endolymph. The increased endolymphatic pressure can lead to a rupture of the endolymph membrane (Schuknecht and Gulya 1983) and/or an opening of tension-sensitive unselective ion channels (Yeh et al. 1998). This leads to an increase in the potassium concentration in the perilymphatic space with potassium-induced depolarization, which initially causes a transient excitation and subsequently a conduction block, leading to the episodes of vertigo and hearing problems in association with direction-changing nystagmus (see above).

As mentioned above, ELH may also be found in patients who do not suffer from MD. This was already shown in 1989 in a blinded histopathological study (Rauch et al. 1989). Since then, there has been a lively discussion about the role of ELH, which was revived after radiological demonstration of ELH in 2007 (Nakashima et al. 2007; Naganawa et al. 2010; Gurkov et al. 2011; Kirsch et al. 2019; van der Lubbe et al. 2020) (◘ Fig. 10.6) (see above).

The assumed etiologies that can ultimately lead to ELH are very wide-ranging (for references, see Nakashima et al. 2016). A complex impairment of ion homeostasis caused by a multifactorial pathogenesis, involving the possible combination of different factors ranging from genetic to autoimmune diseases with the final endpoint of ELH is assumed. Of particular relevance are autoimmunological factors (Caulley et al. 2018; Tyrrell et al. 2014; Frejo and Lopez-Escamez 2022) and genetic factors (Escalera-Balsera et al. 2020; Gallego-Martinez and Lopez-Escamez 2020) with familial cases in 6–9% of cases (Lee et al. 2015; Requena et al. 2014), which also lead to the above-mentioned sub-classification (▶ Box 10.2).

10.6 Course of the Disease

MD is characterized by an intra- and inter-individually very variable course and the development of audiological and vestibular deficits. As mentioned above, the age of onset ranges from the third to the seventh decades of life, rarely in childhood (Choung et al. 2006; Brantberg et al. 2012; Chen et al. 2020). At first, the patients are without symptoms in the interval between attacks; then, they develop increasing tinnitus and loss of deep tones and vestibular deficits if attacks are not prevented.

The other ear can also become affected over time. The longer one follows these patients, the more often one sees a bilateral involvement (Nabi and Parnes 2009). In the early stage of the disease (up to 2 years), 15% of the cases are bilateral. After 10 years about 35% develop a bilateral form, and after 20 years, up to 47% (Takumida et al. 2006; Huppert et al. 2010. This also explains why the disease is the second most frequent cause of a bilateral vestibulopathy (Zingler et al. 2007) (see ▶ Chap. 7). A lower incidence of bilateral MD was reported in an Asian population (Suh et al. 2019). Bilateral MD with early bilateral progression exhibited poorer prognosis compared with late bilateral progression (Lee et al. 2019).

The long-term course of the disease in many patients is more benign than previously assumed (Huppert et al. 2010): the frequency of attacks declines in the first 5–10 years.

Turmarkin's otolithic catastrophe (see above) occurs in about 3–7% of patients with MD; it may occur in the early and the late course of the disease. There is often a spontaneous remission, although the other symptoms and signs may progress (Huppert et al. 2010).

10.7 Treatment

The treatment of MD consists of prophylactic measures, symptomatic treatment of the attacks, and, if patients complain of postural imbalance, vestibular exercises (for the latter two, see also ▶ Chap. 5).

10.7.1 Prophylactic Therapy: Aims and Principles

The aim of a prophylactic treatment in MD is to prevent the episodes of vertigo, hearing loss, tinnitus, and ear pressure as well as a progression of the vestibular and audiological deficits. Ideally, this can be achieved by a reduction of ELH.

However, methodologically the efficacy of individual treatments in MD is hard to assess because of the clinical heterogeneity of the disease, its fluctuating course, its high rate of response to placebo (up to 70% (Adrion et al. 2016; Otonomy, press release 30.8.2017)) and the potential overlap with VM. Further, there are very few state-of-the-art placebo-controlled studies (see for references van Esch et al., 2022a, 2022b) and a comparison of just two treatments without a placebo-group is not justified as long as there is not at least one clearly approved and safe treatment. These are some of the reasons why there is no general consensus yet on the preventive treatment of MD, which leads to various recommendations (Sharon et al. 2015; Magnan et al. 2018; Quaranta et al. 2019; Espinosa-Sanchez and Lopez-Escamez 2020).

Many treatment options have been proposed. There is, however, *no* evidence to date for the efficacy of a low-salt diet, abstinence from coffee or alcohol (Hussain et al. 2018), diuretics (Thirlwall and Kundu 2006), endolymphatic sac surgery (Pullens et al. 2013), the “Meniett device” (Russo et al. 2017), and betahistine in dosages of up to 144 mg/d, which is not superior to placebo (Adrion et al. 2016; Devantier et al. 2020; see for Ref. van Esch et al., 2021, 2022). This is also true for intratympanic dexamethasone (Otonomy, press release 30.8.2017).

10.7.1.1 Oral Treatment

Betahistine This is a weak H1 agonist and an H3 antagonist. Direct or indirect activation of the H1-receptor, which was found in a high density in the human endolymphatic membrane (Moller et al. 2016), increases membrane permeability and can thereby theoretically reduce ELH. As an inverse agonist of the H3 receptor, it also increases dose-dependent cochlear blood flow, which may contribute to its effects in MD (Ihler et al. 2012; Bertlich et al. 2017; Bertlich et al. 2015). The combination of betahistine with the monoamine oxidase inhibitor selegiline (see below) increases cochlear blood even with low dosages of betahistine (Kloos et al. 2022).

While some reviews or meta-analyses concluded that there is a positive effect of betahistine in MD (Nauta 2014; Ramos et al. 2015; Ahmadzai et al. 2020) and its use was recommended (Casani et al. 2018), others found no evidence for its efficacy in the dosages of up to 144 mg/d examined (Devantier et al. 2020; see for references van Esch et al., 2022a, 2022b). According to a randomized, controlled trial on 221 patients—in which a strong placebo effect of about 70% was found—betahistine in a dose of 48 or 144 mg/d was not superior to placebo (Adrion et al. 2016); however, the methodology of this study was criticized by others (Ernst et al. 2017). (◘ Fig. 10.9).

Un-controlled observational studies have shown that higher doses are associated with higher efficacy (Lezius et al. 2011). A basic pharmacokinetic problem is that 99% of orally ingested betahistine is metabolized in the gastrointestinal tract by MAO-B/A (Sternson et al. 1974), which can be inhibited, for instance, by the MAO-B inhibitor selegiline (Myllyla et al. 1992) or rasagiline. This approach has received support from experimental studies in animal models (Tighilet et al. 2018; Kloos et al. 2022). Off-label treatment of individual patients suggests that combining orally administered betahistine with the MAO-B inhibitor selegiline may enhance its efficacy (◘ Fig. 10.10). A phase I pharmacokinetic study in 15 healthy individuals (Pk-Best study) showed that the bioavailability of betahistine can be increased by 5 mg selegiline by a factor of 100 (Strupp et al., Abstract, FP1126, Barany Society meeting, Madrid, 2022). These findings can be the basis for a placebo-controlled prospective randomized clinical trial.

In the future, there is an urgent need for state-of-the-art randomized, placebo-controlled trials, which also consider the different subtypes (see ► Box 10.2), with clinical relevant endpoints to study its efficacy and e.g., the effects of a combined therapy with MAO-B inhibitors.

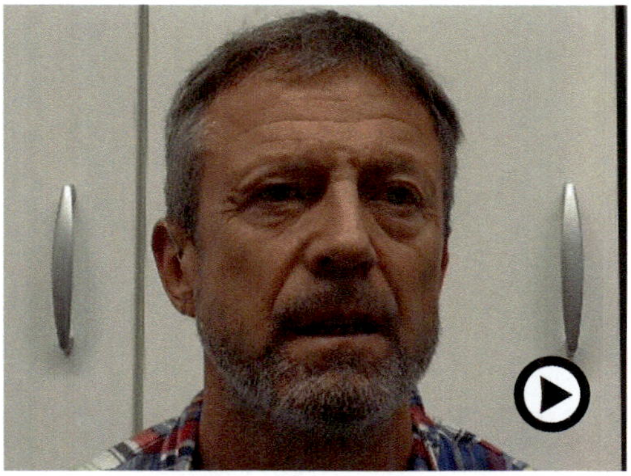

◘ **Fig. 10.9** Treatment with oral betahistine (► https://doi.org/10.1007/000-95s)

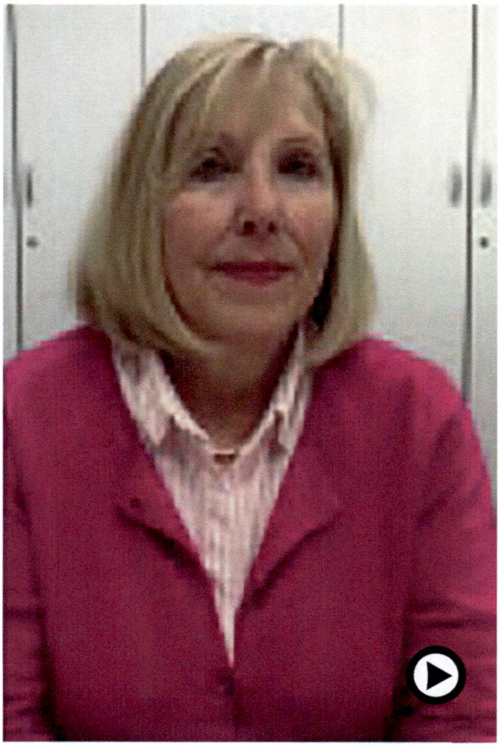

Fig. 10.10 Treatment with the combination of betahistine and oral selegiline (▶ https://doi.org/10.1007/000-95t)

10.7.1.2 Intratympanic Administration of Steroids and Gentamicin

The studies published so far on intratympanic application of corticosteroids and gentamicin are heterogeneous and, to some extent, contradictory (for references, see Schoo et al. 2017; for meta-analyses see van Esch et al. 2022a).

Intratympanic corticosteroids Steroids are neither vestibulotoxic nor cochleotoxic; their mechanism of action in MD is, however, not known. A double-blind, placebo-controlled study showed a positive effect of intratympanic dexamethasone (82% versus 57% in the placebo group) (Garduno-Anaya et al. 2005). A state-of-the-art study with a high dosage and long-term (3 months) application of dexamethasone, however, did not find a difference in the primary endpoint in comparison to placebo (Otonomy, press release 30.8.2017); the placebo-effect after three months was about 60%. A basic methodological problem is that the pharmacokinetics of the steroids are highly variable and that there is a lack of precision in nomenclature in the inner ear drug delivery field which makes it very difficult to compare studies (Salt and Plontke 2020; Salt et al. 2019).

Intratympanic gentamicin The intratympanic administration of gentamicin reduces the frequency of the vertigo attacks (several RCT and meta-analyses (for references, see (Schoo et al. 2017) and a Cochrane review (Pullens and van Benthem 2011)). An extensive meta-analysis, however, came to a different conclusion: "Overall, our results seem to provide the limited evidence about efficacy and toxicity effects of (intratympanic gentamicin)" (Zhang et al. 2019) A metaanalysis also concluded that there is only low evidence for the efficacy of gentamicin in MD (van Esch et al. 2022a). Therefore, here also further state-of-the-art placebo-controlled trials with clinically meaningful endpoints are necessary.

The basis of effective gentamicin therapy is its ototoxicity, which leads to a reduction of vestibular function (Nicolas et al. 2019). Gentamicin accumulates and damages mainly type I hair cells (Lyford-Pike et al. 2007). The ototoxic effect of aminoglycosides develops with a delay of weeks (Magnusson et al. 1991); therefore, the therapeutic regimen was changed many years ago: either individual injection with an interval of at least 4 weeks or one single injection and follow-up checks with an individualized dosing depending on the response (Lange et al. 2004). It should also be noted that about 20% of patients—depending on the dosage and the frequency of the application—develop an impairment of hearing (Colletti et al. 2007; Flanagan et al. 2006). This is a limitation of the use of gentamicin. Therefore, it should only be given to patients who already have a significant impairment of hearing. One should also note that the utility of gentamicin is further limited because 47% of patients with MD develop the condition bilaterally (Takumida et al. 2006; Huppert et al. 2010).

Comparison of intratympanic corticosteroids and gentamicin Such studies are currently not recommended because of the above-mentioned strong placebo effect of about 70% and the fact that there is so far no established, well-tolerated gold standard for the treatment of MD as a comparator, which also explains the contradictory results of such studies.

An RCT came to the conclusion that gentamicin is superior to dexamethasone (response rate of 93% for gentamicin and 61% for dexamethasone) (Casani et al. 2012). However, another RCT found no difference between the efficacy of methylprednisolone and gentamicin (Patel et al. 2016), also not during the long-term course of the disease (Harcourt et al. 2019); one must, however, always take into account placebo-effects when comparing two measures in non-controlled trials. According to a meta-analysis (Jiang et al. 2020), intratympanic gentamicin was superior to intratympanic steroids in reducing the number of vertigo attacks (odds ratio 3.08, $p < 0.01$), however, the quality of the studies included was low. For hearing, there was no difference between the two treatments. In a systematic review, it was stated that, for subjective outcomes, intratympanic gentamicin was slightly favored compared to intratympanic corticosteroids, but for objective outcomes and complications, no significant differences were seen (Yaz et al. 2020). This means the findings are non-conclusive, which is most likely due to the methodological limitations of the underlying studies.

Combined intratympanic therapies In a placebo-controlled study, intratympanic dexamethasone was compared with 48 mg t.i.d. betahistine or placebo. The combined therapy was significantly better than the monotherapy (Albu et al. 2016). In another study, it was found that an intratympanic injection of a mixture of gentamicin and dexamethasone is superior to intratympanic dexamethasone only (Otzturk and Ata 2019).

10.7.1.3 Surgical Treatment

Although endolymphatic sac surgery has been recommended by many surgeons (Lim et al. 2015; Sood et al. 2014), a Cochrane review showed that its efficacy is not proven (Pullens et al. 2013); this is supported by a detailed metaanalysis (van Esch et al. 2022a). In advanced MD with a prominent loss of vestibular and audiological function, labyrinthectomy and simultaneous cochlear implantation leads to the cessation of the vertigo attacks (if the patient is suffering from unilateral MD with certainty) and to an improvement of hearing.

10.7.2 Pragmatic Therapy

10.7.2.1 Symptomatic Treatment of the Attacks

The attacks are typically self-limiting, although they often last many hours. Vertigo, nausea, and vomiting can be treated by antivertiginous drugs, as in the treatment of an acute vestibular syndrome. We recommend dimenhydrinate 50–100 mg orally, as a suppository or intravenously (1–3 × 100 mg/d); if patients do not respond, ondansetron (4–8 mg) or benzodiazepines (e.g., lorazepam 0.5–1.0 mg sublingually) can be given.

10.7.2.2 Prophylactic Therapy

If patients have two or more relevant attacks per month, a prophylactic treatment is indicated. At present, an incremental approach is recommended, beginning with conservative treatment (e.g., betahistine, see below), then semi-invasive non-destructive techniques (e.g., intratympanic cortisone application), semi-invasive destructive measures (intratympanic gentamicin), and, finally, in very rare cases with hearing loss, invasive destructive techniques (e.g., labyrinthectomy in combination with a cochlea implant) as a last resort.

As pointed out above, there is so far insufficient evidence for the efficacy of most prophylactic therapies. Therefore, the recommendations below are also based on personal experience, which is the lowest level of evidence.

10.7.2.3 Betahistine Dihydrochloride

Betahistine dihydrochloride, at least 3 × 4 tablets per day, each tablet containing 24 mg, i.e., at least 96 mg/t.i.d. for at least 12 months. If the patient is free of attacks or almost free of attacks for 6 months, the dosage can be reduced: by one tablet every 3 months. Since MD is a chronic relapsing disease, it is most often a long-term prophylactic treatment. These recommendations are based on observational studies. If the frequency of attacks does not decrease after 3 months of treatment, the dosage can be increased to up to 480 mg/d (i.e., 20 24 mg-tablets per day) or even higher. A potential alternative, which is based on "individual cases of off-label use" is the combined treatment with betahistine dihydrochloride (e.g., 4 × 48 mg/d) and 5 mg selegiline per day or 1 mg rasagiline per day, with strict consideration of contraindications and interactions of these MAO-B inhibitors.

10.7.2.4 Intratympanic Treatment

We very rarely see an indication for intratympanic treatment. If it is indicated, one can start with glucocorticoids, which are not ototoxic: 50 mg methyl-prednisolone or 2 mg dexamethasone, two injections with a latency of 2 weeks. If this not sufficient even after 3 months and there is a considerable impairment of vestibular and audiological function and the affected ear can be identified with certainty, gentamicin can be given: 12–40 mg intratympanically as a single dosage, then observation of the effects over a period of at least 4–8 weeks (Stokroos and Kingma 2004; Postema et al. 2008; Pullens and van Benthem 2011). If this is not effective, one or more additional injections can be performed. In parallel, audiological and vestibular function must be monitored.

10.7.2.5 Surgical Treatment

If none of the above therapeutic options is effective, which is, in our experience, extremely rare, surgical treatment may be considered. In cases of advanced MD with considerable vestibular and cochlear deficits, labyrinthine destruction with simultaneous cochlear implantation can lead to suspension of the attacks of vertigo and an improvement of hearing (Westhofen 2013). With all destructive measures one has to consider the high frequency of bilateral MD.

10.7.2.6 Treatment of Tumarkin's Otolithic Catastrophe

Recurrent vestibular drop attacks (Tumarkin's otolithic catastrophe) are very dangerous for patients and lead to a significant reduction of functioning and quality of life (see above). If even a very high dosage of betahistine and the combination with a MAO-B inhibitor does not lead to an improvement of the symptoms, intratympanic steroids or gentamicin can be used. As is true for all intratympanic treatments, the affected ear has to be identified with certainty using various measures, e.g., the combination of audiogram, caloric irrigation, HIT, and VEMP. There are so far no controlled studies on this.

10.7.2.7 Physiotherapy

Daily balance and life-long training (for references, see (Hall et al. 2022 and ► Chap. 5) is indicated in patients who suffer from postural imbalance and dizziness due to a functionally relevant peripheral vestibular deficit, in particular in patients with bilateral MD. It is also indicated to improve central compensation in patients who have had a severe attack of MD with a transient peripheral vestibular deficit.

References

Adrion C, Fischer CS, Wagner J, Gurkov R, Mansmann U, Strupp M (2016) Efficacy and safety of betahistine treatment in patients with Meniere's disease: primary results of a long term, multicentre, double blind, randomised, placebo controlled, dose defining trial (BEMED trial). BMJ 352:h6816

Ahmadzai N, Cheng W, Kilty S, Esmaeilisaraji L, Wolfe D, Bonaparte J, Schramm D, Fitzpatrick E, Lin V, Skidmore B, Hutton B (2020) Pharmacologic and surgical therapies for patients with Meniere's disease: a systematic review and network meta-analysis. PLoS One 15(9):e0237523

Albu S, Nagy A, Doros C, Marceanu L, Cozma S, Musat G, Trabalzini F (2016) Treatment of Meniere's disease with intratympanic dexamethasone plus high dosage of betahistine. Am J Otolaryngol 37(3):225–230

Alexander TH, Harris JP (2010) Current epidemiology of Meniere's syndrome. Otolaryngol Clin N Am 43(5):965–970

Atkinson M (1962) Migraine and Meniere's disease. Arch Otolaryngol 75:220–225

Attye A, Eliezer M, Medici M, Tropres I, Dumas G, Krainik A, Schmerber S (2018) In vivo imaging of saccular hydrops in humans reflects sensorineural hearing loss rather than Meniere's disease symptoms. Eur Radiol 28(7):2916–2922

Battista RA (2004) Audiometric findings of patients with migraine-associated dizziness. Otol Neurotol 25(6):987–992

Becker-Bense S, Wittmann C, Dieterich M (2019) Balanced sex distribution in patients with Meniere's disease. J Neurol 266(Suppl 1):42–46

Belinchon A, Perez-Garrigues H, Tenias JM, Lopez A (2011) Hearing assessment in Meniere's disease. Laryngoscope 121(3):622–626

Belinchon A, Perez-Garrigues H, Tenias JM (2012) Evolution of symptoms in Meniere's disease. Audiol Neurootol 17(2):126–132

Benjamin T, Gillard D, Abouzari M, Djalilian HR, Sharon JD (2022) Vestibular and auditory manifestations of migraine. Curr Opin Neurol 35:84–89

Bernaerts A, De FB (2019) Imaging of Meniere disease. Neuroimaging Clin N Am 29(1):19–28

Bernaerts A, Vanspauwen R, Blaivie C, van DJ, Zarowski A, Wuyts FL, Vanden Bossche S, Offeciers E, Casselman JW, De FB (2019) The value of four stage vestibular hydrops grading and asymmetric perilymphatic enhancement in the diagnosis of Meniere's disease on MRI. Neuroradiol 61(4):421–429

Bertlich M, Ihler F, Freytag S, Weiss BG, Strupp M, Canis M (2015) Histaminergic H-heteroreceptors as a potential mediator of betahistine-induced increase in Cochlear blood flow. Audiol Neurootol 20(5):283–293

Bertlich M, Ihler F, Weiss BG, Freytag S, Strupp M, Canis M (2017) Cochlear pericytes are capable of reversibly decreasing capillary diameter in vivo after tumor necrosis factor exposure. Otol Neurotol 38(10):e545–e550

Black FO, Effron MZ, Burns DS (1982) Diagnosis and management of drop attacks of vestibular origin: Tumarkin's otolithic crisis. Otolaryngol Head Neck Surg 90(2):256–262

Brantberg K, Duan M, Falahat B (2012) Ménière's disease in children aged 4-7 years. Acta Otolaryngol 132(5):505–509

Casani AP, Piaggi P, Cerchiai N, Seccia V, Franceschini SS, Dallan I (2012) Intratympanic treatment of intractable unilateral Meniere disease: gentamicin or dexamethasone? A randomized controlled trial. Otolaryngol Head Neck Surg 146(3):430–437

Casani AP, Guidetti G, Schoenhuber R (2018) Report from a consensus conference on the treatment of Ménière's disease with betahistine: rationale, methodology and results. Acta Otorhinolaryngol Ital 38(5):460–467

Cass SP, Furman JM, Ankerstjerne K, Balaban C, Yetiser S, Aydogan B (1997) Migraine-related vestibulopathy. Ann Otol Rhinol Laryngol 106(3):182–189

Caulley L, Quimby A, Karsh J, Ahrari A, Tse D, Kontorinis G (2018) Autoimmune arthritis in Meniere's disease: a systematic review of the literature. Semin Arthritis Rheum 48(1):141–147

Cha YH, Brodsky J, Ishiyama G, Sabatti C, Baloh RW (2007) The relevance of migraine in patients with Meniere's disease. Acta Otolaryngol 127:1241–1245

Chen W, Chen Y, Geng Y, Lin N, Luo S, Wang Z, Yu S, Sha Y (2020) The value of 3D-real IR MRI with intravenous gadolinium injection in the diagnosis of suspected Meniere's disease in children. Acta Otolaryngol 141:117–121

Choung YH, Park K, Kim CH, Kim HJ, Kim K (2006) Rare cases of Meniere's disease in children. J Laryngol Otol 120(4):343–352

Colletti V, Carner M, Colletti L (2007) Auditory results after vestibular nerve section and intratympanic gentamicin for Meniere's disease. Otol Neurotol 28(2):145–151

Connor SEJ, Pai I (2021) Endolymphatic hydrops magnetic resonance imaging in Ménière's disease. Clin Radiol 76(1):76.e1–76.e19

De Valck CF, Claes GM, Wuyts FL, Van de Heyning PH (2007) Lack of diagnostic value of high-pass noise masking of auditory brainstem responses in Meniere's disease. Otol Neurotol 28(5):700–707
Devantier L, Hougaard D, Handel MN, Liviu-Adelin GF, Schmidt JH, Djurhuus B, Callesen HE (2020) Using betahistine in the treatment of patients with Ménière's disease: a meta-analysis with the current randomized-controlled evidence. Acta Otolaryngol 140(10):845–853
Dieterich M, Brandt T (1999) Episodic vertigo related to migraine (90 cases): vestibular migraine? J Neurol 246(10):883–892
Ducroz C, Dumas G, Quatre R, Attyai A, Fabre C, Schmerber S (2022) Benign recurrent vestibulopathy: MRI and vestibular tests results in a series of 128 cases. Eur Arch Otorhinolaryngol 279:169–173
Durtette C, Hachulla E, Resche-Rigon M, Papo T, Zenone T, Lioger B, Deligny C, Lambert M, Landron C, Pouchot J, Kahn JE, Lavigne C, De WB, Dhote R, Gondran G, Pertuiset E, Quemeneur T, Hamidou M, Seve P, Le GT, Grasland A, Hatron PY, Fain O, Mekinian A (2017) Cogan syndrome: characteristics, outcome and treatment in a French nationwide retrospective study and literature review. Autoimmun Rev 16(12):1219–1223
Ernst A, Schlattmann P, Waldfahrer F, Westhofen M (2017) Die Behandlung des M. Menière mit Betahistin: Kritische Anmerkungen zur BEMED-Studie. Laryngorhinootol 96(8):519–521
Escalera-Balsera A, Roman-Naranjo P, Lopez-Escamez JA (2020) Systematic review of sequencing studies and gene expression profiling in familial meniere disease. Genes (Basel) 11:(12)
Espinosa-Sanchez JM, Lopez-Escamez JA (2020) The pharmacological management of vertigo in Meniere disease. Expert Opin Pharmacother 21(14):1753–1763
Flanagan S, Mukherjee P, Tonkin J (2006) Outcomes in the use of intra-tympanic gentamicin in the treatment of Meniere's disease. J Laryngol Otol 120(2):98–102
Frejo L, Lopez-Escamez JA (2022) Cytokines and inflammation in meniere disease. Clin Exp Otorhinolaryngol 15:(1)49–59
Frejo L, Soto-Varela A, Santos-Perez S, Aran I, Batuecas-Caletrio A, Perez-Guillen V, Perez-Garrigues H, Fraile J, Martin-Sanz E, Tapia MC, Trinidad G, Garcia-Arumi AM, Gonzalez-Aguado R, Espinosa-Sanchez JM, Marques P, Perez P, Benitez J, Lopez-Escamez JA (2016) Clinical subgroups in bilateral Meniere disease. Front Neurol 7:182
Frejo L, Martin-Sanz E, Teggi R, Trinidad G, Soto-Varela A, Santos-Perez S, Manrique R, Perez N, Aran I, Almeida-Branco MS, Batuecas-Caletrio A, Fraile J, Espinosa-Sanchez JM, Perez-Guillen V, Perez-Garrigues H, Oliva-Dominguez M, Aleman O, Benitez J, Perez P, Lopez-Escamez JA (2017) Extended phenotype and clinical subgroups in unilateral Meniere disease: a cross-sectional study with cluster analysis. Clin Otolaryngol 42(6):1172–1180
Gallego-Martinez A, Lopez-Escamez JA (2020) Genetic architecture of Meniere's disease. Hear Res 397:107872
Garduno-Anaya MA, Couthino De TH, Hinojosa-Gonzalez R, Pane-Pianese C, Rios-Castaneda LC (2005) Dexamethasone inner ear perfusion by intratympanic injection in unilateral Meniere's disease: a two-year prospective, placebo-controlled, double-blind, randomized trial. Otolaryngol Head Neck Surg 133(2):285–294
Gurkov R, Flatz W, Louza J, Strupp M, Krause E (2011) In vivo visualization of endolyphatic hydrops in patients with Meniere's disease: correlation with audiovestibular function. Eur Arch Otorhinolaryngol 268(12):1743–1748
Gurkov R, Kantner C, Strupp M, Flatz W, Krause E, Ertl-Wagner B (2014) Endolymphatic hydrops in patients with vestibular migraine and auditory symptoms. Eur Arch Otorhinolaryngol 271(10):2661–2667
Hall CD, Herdman SJ, Whitney SL, Anson ER, Carender WJ, Hoppes CW, Cass SP, Christy JB, Cohen HS, Fife TD, Furman JM, Shepard NT, Clendaniel RA, Dishman JD, Goebel JA, Meldrum D, Ryan C, Wallace RL, Woodward NJ (2022) Vestibular rehabilitation for peripheral vestibular hypofunction: an updated clinical practice guideline from the academy of neurologic physical therapy of the american physical therapy association. J Neurol Phys Ther 46:(2)118–177
Hallpike CS, Cairns H (1938) Observations on the pathology of Meniere's syndrome: (section of otology). Proc R Soc Med 31(11):1317–1336
Hannigan IP, Welgampola MS, Watson SRD (2019) Dissociation of caloric and head impulse tests: a marker of Meniere's disease. J Neurol 268:431–439
Harcourt JP, Lambert A, Wong PY, Patel M, Agarwal K, Golding JF, Bronstein AM (2019) Long-term follow-up of Intratympanic methylprednisolone versus gentamicin in patients with unilateral Meniere's disease. Otol Neurotol 40(4):491–496
Harris JP, Alexander TH (2010) Current-day prevalence of Meniere's syndrome. Audiol Neurootol 15(5):318–322
Havia M, Kentala E, Pyykko I (2005) Prevalence of Meniere's disease in general population of Southern Finland. Otolaryngol Head Neck Surg 133(5):762–768
Huppert D, Strupp M, Brandt T (2010) Long-term course of Meniere's disease revisited. Acta Otolaryngol 130(6):644–651
Hussain K, Murdin L, Schilder AG (2018) Restriction of salt, caffeine and alcohol intake for the treat-

ment of Meniere's disease or syndrome. Cochrane Database Syst Rev (12):CD012173
Ihler F, Bertlich M, Sharaf K, Strieth S, Strupp M, Canis M (2012) Betahistine exerts a dose-dependent effect on cochlear stria vascularis blood flow in Guinea pigs in vivo. PLoS One 7(6) e39086
Ito T, Inui H, Miyasaka T, Shiozaki T, Hasukawa A, Yamanaka T, Kichikawa K, Kitahara T (2019) Endolymphatic volume in patients with meniere's disease and healthy controls: three-dimensional analysis with magnetic resonance imaging. Laryngoscope Investig Otolaryngol 4(5):653–658
Jerin C, Maxwell R, Gurkov R (2019) High-frequency horizontal semicircular canal function in certain Meniere's disease. Ear Hear 40(1):128–134
Jiang M, Zhang Z, Zhao C (2020) What is the efficacy of gentamicin on the incidence of vertigo attacks and hearing in patients with Meniere's disease compared with steroids? A meta-analysis. J Neurol 268:3717–3727
Kaci B, Nooristani M, Mijovic T, Maheu M (2020) Usefulness of video head impulse test results in the identification of Meniere's disease. Front Neurol 11:581527
Kayan A, Hood JD (1984) Neuro-otological manifestations of migraine. Brain 107(Pt 4):1123–1142
Kay-Rivest E, Friedmann DR, Roland JT (2020) Imaging for Menière disease. AJNR Am J Neuroradiol 41(11):1964–1965
Kim MH, Cheon C (2020) Epidemiology and seasonal variation of Ménière's disease: data from a population-based study. Audiol Neurootol 25(4):224–230
Kirsch V, Becker-Bense S, Berman A, Kierig E, Ertl-Wagner B, Dieterich M (2018) Transient endolymphatic hydrops after an attack of vestibular migraine: a longitudinal single case study. J Neurol 265(Suppl 1):51–53
Kirsch V, Nejatbakhshesfahani F, Ahmadi SA, Dieterich M, Ertl-Wagner B (2019) A probabilistic atlas of the human inner ear's bony labyrinth enables reliable atlas-based segmentation of the total fluid space. J Neurol 266(Suppl 1):52–61
Kloos B, Bertlich M, Spiegel JL, Freytag S, Lauer SK, Canis M, Weiss BG, Ihler F (2022) Low dose betahistine in combination with selegiline increases cochlear blood flow in guinea pigs. Ann Otol Rhinol Laryngol 34894221098803
Lange G, Maurer J, Mann W (2004) Long-term results after interval therapy with intratympanic gentamicin for Meniere's disease. Laryngoscope 114(1):102–105
Lee JM, Kim MJ, Jung J, Kim HJ, Seo YJ, Kim SH (2015) Genetic aspects and clinical characteristics of familial Meniere's disease in a South Korean population. Laryngoscope 125(9):2175–2180
Lee HJ, Lee JM, Shim DB, Jung J, Kwak SH, Kim SH (2019) Is early progression to bilateral involvement in Ménière's disease a poor prognostic indicator? Otol Neurotol 40(10):1333–1338
Lempert T, Olesen J, Furman J, Waterston J, Seemungal B, Carey J, Bisdorff A, Versino M, Evers S, Newman-Toker D (2012) Vestibular migraine: diagnostic criteria. J Vestib Res 22(4):167–172
Lezius F, Adrion C, Mansmann U, Jahn K, Strupp M (2011) High-dosage betahistine dihydrochloride between 288 and 480 mg/day in patients with severe Meniere's disease: a case series. Eur Arch Otorhinolaryngol 268(8):1237–1240
Lim MY, Zhang M, Yuen HW, Leong JL (2015) Current evidence for endolymphatic sac surgery in the treatment of Meniere's disease: a systematic review. Singap Med J 56(11):593–598
Liu YF, Xu H (2016) The intimate relationship between vestibular migraine and Meniere disease: a review of pathogenesis and presentation. Behav Neurol 2016:3182735
Lopez-Escamez JA, Attye A (2019) Systematic review of magnetic resonance imaging for diagnosis of Meniere disease. J Vestib Res 29(2–3):121–129
Lopez-Escamez JA, Carey J, Chung WH, Goebel JA, Magnusson M, Mandala M, Newman-Toker DE, Strupp M, Suzuki M, Trabalzini F, Bisdorff A (2015) Diagnostic criteria for Meniere's disease. J Vestib Res 25(1):1–7
Loureiro RM, Sumi DV, Tames HLVC, Soares CR, Salmito MC, Gomes RLE, Daniel MM (2020) Endolymphatic hydrops evaluation on MRI: practical considerations. Am J Otolaryngol 41(2):102361
Lustig LR, Lalwani A (1997) The history of Meniere's disease. Otolaryngol Clin N Am 30(6):917–945
Lyford-Pike S, Vogelheim C, Chu E, Della Santina CC, Carey JP (2007) Gentamicin is primarily localized in vestibular type I hair cells after intratympanic administration. J Assoc Res Otolaryngol 8(4):497–508
Magnan J, Ozgirgin ON, Trabalzini F, Lacour M, Escamez AL, Magnusson M, Guneri EA, Guyot JP, Nuti D, Mandala M (2018) European position statement on diagnosis, and treatment of Meniere's disease. J Int Adv Otol 14(2):317–321
Magnusson M, Padoan S, Karlberg M, Johansson R (1991) Delayed onset of ototoxic effects of gentamicin in patients with Meniere's disease. Acta Otolaryngol Suppl Stockh 485:120–122
McGarvie LA, Curthoys IS, MacDougall HG, Halmagyi GM (2015) What does the dissociation between the results of video head impulse versus caloric testing reveal about the vestibular dysfunction in Ménière's disease? Acta Otolaryngol 135(9): 859–865
Moller MN, Kirkeby S, Vikesa J, Nielsen FC, Caye-Thomasen P (2016) Expression of histamine receptors in the human endolymphatic sac: the molecular rationale for betahistine use in Menieres disease. Eur Arch Otorhinolaryngol 273(7):1705–1710

Moshtaghi O, Sahyouni R, Lin HW, Ghavami Y, Djalilian HR (2016) A historical recount: discovering Ménière's disease and its association with migraine headaches. Otol Neurotol 37(8):1199–1203

Murofushi T, Tsubota M, Kitao K, Yoshimura E (2018) Simultaneous presentation of definite vestibular migraine and definite Meniere's disease: overlapping syndrome of two diseases. Front Neurol 9:749

Myllyla VV, Sotaniemi KA, Vuorinen JA, Heinonen EH (1992) Selegiline as initial treatment in de novo parkinsonian patients. Neurology 42(2):339–343

Nabi S, Parnes LS (2009) Bilateral Meniere's disease. Curr Opin Otolaryngol Head Neck Surg 17(5):356–362

Naganawa S, Yamazaki M, Kawai H, Bokura K, Sone M, Nakashima T (2010) Visualization of endolymphatic hydrops in Meniere's disease with single-dose intravenous gadolinium-based contrast media using heavily T(2)-weighted 3D-FLAIR. Magn Reson Med Sci 9(4):237–242

Nahmani S, Vaussy A, Hautefort C, Guichard JP, Guillonet A, Houdart E, Attye A, Eliezer M (2020) Comparison of enhancement of the vestibular perilymph between variable and constant flip angle-delayed 3D-FLAIR sequences in Meniere disease. AJNR Am J Neuroradiol 41:706–711

10

Nakashima T, Naganawa S, Sugiura M, Teranishi M, Sone M, Hayashi H, Nakata S, Katayama N, Ishida IM (2007) Visualization of endolymphatic hydrops in patients with Meniere's disease. Laryngoscope 117(3):415–420

Nakashima T, Pyykko I, Arroll MA, Casselbrant ML, Foster CA, Manzoor NF, Megerian CA, Naganawa S, Young YH (2016) Meniere's disease. Nat Rev Dis Primers 2:16028

Nauta JJ (2014) Meta-analysis of clinical studies with betahistine in Meniere's disease and vestibular vertigo. Eur Arch Otorhinolaryngol 271(5):887–897

Nicolas S, Kmeid M, Mansour C, Fraysse B, Deguine O, Marx M, Fraysse ME (2019) Long-term vertigo control and vestibular function after low-dose on-demand transtympanic gentamicin for refractory Meniere's disease. Otol Neurotol 40(2):218–225

Oh S-Y, Dieterich M, Lee B, Boegle R, Kang J-J, Lee N-R, Gerb J, Hwang S-B, Kirsch V (2021) Endolymphatic hydrops in patients with vestibular migraine and concurrent Meniere's disease. Front Neurol 12:594481

Otzturk K, Ata N (2019) Intratympanic mixture gentamicin and dexamethasone versus dexamethasone for unilateral Meniere's disease. Am J Otolaryngol 40(5):711–714

Patel M, Agarwal K, Arshad Q, Hariri M, Rea P, Seemungal BM, Golding JF, Harcourt JP, Bronstein AM (2016) Intratympanic methylprednisolone versus gentamicin in patients with unilateral Meniere's disease: a randomised, double-blind, comparative effectiveness trial. Lancet 388(10061):2753–2762

Perez-Garrigues H, Lopez-Escamez JA, Perez P, Sanz R, Orts M, Marco J, Barona R, Tapia MC, Aran I, Cenjor C, Perez N, Morera C, Ramirez R (2008) Time course of episodes of definitive vertigo in Meniere's disease. Arch Otolaryngol Head Neck Surg 134(11):1149–1154

Phillips JS, Murdin L, Rea P, Sutton L (2018) Clinical subtyping of Meniere's disease. Otolaryngol Head Neck Surg 159(3):407–409

Postema RJ, Kingma CM, Wit HP, Albers FW, Van Der Laan BF (2008) Intratympanic gentamicin therapy for control of vertigo in unilateral Meniere's disease: a prospective, double-blind, randomized, placebo-controlled trial. Acta Otolaryngol 128(8):876–880

Pullens B, van Benthem PP (2011) Intratympanic gentamicin for Meniere's disease or syndrome. Cochrane Database Syst Rev (3):CD008234

Pullens B, Verschuur HP, van Benthem PP (2013) Surgery for Meniere's disease. Cochrane Database Syst Rev (2):CD005395

Pyykko I, Manchaiah V, Zou J, Levo H, Kentala E (2018a) Impact of Tumarkin attacks on complaints and work ability in Meniere's disease. J Vestib Res 28(3–4):319–330

Pyykko I, Manchaiah V, Zou J, Levo H, Kentala E (2018b) Vestibular syncope: a disorder associated with drop attack in Ménière's disease. Auris Nasus Larynx 45(2):234–241

Quaranta N, Picciotti P, Porro G, Sterlicchio B, Danesi G, Petrone P, Asprella LG (2019) Therapeutic strategies in the treatment of Meniere's disease: the Italian experience. Eur Arch Otorhinolaryngol 276:1943–1950

Radtke A, von BM, Neuhauser H, Hottenrott T, Lempert T (2012) Vestibular migraine: long-term follow-up of clinical symptoms and vestibulo-cochlear findings. Neurology 79(15):1607–1614

Ramos AR, Ledezma Rodriguez JG, Navas RA, Cardenas Nunez JL, Rodriguez MV, Deschamps JJ, Liviac Ticse JA (2015) Use of betahistine in the treatment of peripheral vertigo. Acta Otolaryngol 135(12):1205–1211

Rauch SD, Merchant SN, Thedinger BA (1989) Meniere's syndrome and endolymphatic hydrops. Double-blind temporal bone study. Ann Otol Rhinol Laryngol 98(11):873–883

Requena T, Espinosa-Sanchez JM, Cabrera S, Trinidad G, Soto-Varela A, Santos-Perez S, Teggi R, Perez P, Batuecas-Caletrio A, Fraile J, Aran I, Martin E, Benitez J, Perez-Fernandez N, Lopez-Escamez JA (2014) Familial clustering and genetic heterogeneity in Meniere's disease. Clin Genet 85(3):245–252

Rey-Martinez J, Altuna X, Cheng K, Burgess AM, Curthoys IS (2020) Computing endolymph hydrodynamics during head impulse test on normal and hydropic vestibular labyrinth models. Front Neurol 11:289

Russo FY, Nguyen Y, De SD, Bouccara D, Sterkers O, Ferrary E, Bernardeschi D (2017) Meniett device in meniere disease: randomized, double-blind, placebo-controlled multicenter trial. Laryngoscope 127(2):470–475

Salt AN, Plontke SK (2020) Steroid nomenclature in inner ear therapy. Otol Neurotol 41(6):722–726

Salt AN, Hartsock JJ, Hou J, Piu F (2019) Comparison of the pharmacokinetic properties of triamcinolone and dexamethasone for local therapy of the inner ear. Front Cell Neurosci 13:347

Schoo DP, Tan GX, Ehrenburg MR Pross SE Ward BK, Carey JP (2017) Intratympanic (IT) therapies for Meniere's disease: some consensus among the confusion. Curr Otorhinolaryngol Rep 5(2): 132–141

Schuknecht HF, Gulya AJ (1983) Endolymphatic hydrops: an overview and classification. Ann Otol 92(Suppl 106):1–20

Sharon JD, Trevino C, Schubert MC Carey JP (2015) Treatment of Meniere's disease. Curr Treat Options Neurol 17(4):341

Shaw B, Raghavan RS (2018) Dissociation between caloric and head impulse testing in patients with congenital abnormalities of the semicircular canals. J Laryngol Otol 132(10):932–935

Shojaku H, Watanabe Y, Fujisaka M, Tsubota M, Kobayashi K, Yasumura S, Mizukoshi K (2005) Epidemiologic characteristics of definite Meniere's disease in Japan. A long-term survey of Toyama and Niigata prefectures. ORL J Otorhinolaryngol Relat Spec 67(5):305–309

Shugyo M, Ito T, Shiozaki T, Nishikawa D, Ohyama H, Fujita H, Yamanaka T, Kitahara T (2020) Comparison of the video head impulse test results with caloric test in patients with Meniere's disease and other vestibular disorders. Acta Otolaryngol 140(9):728–735

Sood AJ, Lambert PR, Nguyen SA, Meyer TA (2014) Endolymphatic sac surgery for Meniere's disease: a systematic review and meta-analysis. Otol Neurotol 35(6):1033–1045

Sternson LA, Tobia AJ, Walsh GM, Sternson AW (1974) The metabolism of betahistine in the rat. Drug Metab Dispos 2(2):123–128

Stokroos R, Kingma H (2004) Selective vestibular ablation by intratympanic gentamicin in patients with unilateral active Meniere's disease: a prospective, double-blind, placebo-controlled, randomized clinical trial. Acta Otolaryngol 124(2):172–175

Suh MJ, Jeong J, Kim HJ, Jung J, Kim SH (2019) Clinical characteristics of bilateral Meniere's disease in a single Asian ethnic group. Laryngoscope 129(5):1191–1196

Takumida M, Kakigi A, Takeda T, Anniko M (2006) Meniere's disease: a long-term follow-up study of bilateral hearing levels. Acta Otolaryngol 126(9):921–925

Thirlwall AS, Kundu S (2006) Diuretics for Meniere's disease or syndrome. Cochrane Database Syst Rev (3):CD003599

Tighilet B, Leonard J, Watabe I, Bernard-Demanze L, Lacour M (2018) Betahistine treatment in a cat model of vestibular pathology: pharmacokinetic and pharmacodynamic approaches. Front Neurol 9:431

Tse D, Ramsay T, Lelli DA (2019) Novel use of portable audiometry to track hearing fluctuations in Meniere's disease: a pilot study. Otol Neurotol 40(2):e130–e134

Tumarkin A (1936) The otolithic catastrophe: a new syndrome. Br Med J 2(3942):175–177

Tyrrell JS, Whinney DJ, Ukoumunne OC, Fleming LE, Osborne NJ (2014) Prevalence, associated factors, and comorbid conditions for Meniere's disease. Ear Hear 35(4):e162–e169

van der Lubbe MFJA, Vaidyanathan A, Van RV, Postma AA, Bruintjes TD, Kimenai DM, Lambin P, van HM, van de Berg R (2020) The "hype" of hydrops in classifying vestibular disorders: a narrative review. J Neurol 267(Suppl 1):197–211

van Esch BF, van WE, van der Zaag-Loonen HJ, PPGV B, van Leeuwen RB (2017) Clinical characteristics of benign recurrent Vestibulopathy: clearly distinctive from vestibular migraine and Ménière's disease? Otol Neurotol 38(9):e357–e363

van Esch BF, Zaag-Loonen H, Bruintjes T, Kuijpers T, van Benthem PPG (2022a) Interventions for Meniere's disease: an umbrella systematic review. BMJ Evid Based Med 27:(4)235–245

van Esch BF, Zaag-Loonen H, Bruintjes T, van Benthem PP (2022b) Betahistine in Meiniere's Disease or Syndrome: A Systematic Review. Audiol Neurootol 27:(1)1–3

van Steekelenburg JM, van WA, LMH d P, Vijlbrief OD, Bommelje CC, Koopman JP, Verbist BM, Blom HM, Hammer S (2020) Value of endolymphatic hydrops and perilymph signal intensity in suspected Meniere disease. AJNR Am J Neuroradiol 41(3):529–534

Westhofen M (2013) Indications for operative therapy of vestibular vertigo and the associated success rates. HNO 61(9):752–761

Yamakawa K (1938) Über die pathologische Veränderung bei einem Meniere-Kranken. J Otorhinolaryngol Soc (Jpn) 44:2310–2312

Yaz F, Ziylan F, Smeeing DPJ, Thomeer HGXM (2020) Intratympanic treatment in Ménière's disease, efficacy of aminoglycosides versus corticosteroids in comparison studies: a systematic review. Otol Neurotol 41(1):1–10

Yeh TH, Herman P, Tsai MC, Tran-Ba-Huy P, Van-den-Abbeele T (1998) A cationic nonselective stretch-activated channel in the Reissner's membrane of the Guinea pig cochlea. Am J Phys 274(3 Pt 1):C566–C576

Zhang Y, Fu J, Lin H, Shen C, Wang X, Wu J (2019) The clinical outcomes after intratympanic gentamicin injection to treat Meniere's disease: a meta-analysis. Otol Neurotol 40(4):419–429

Zhang W, Hui L, Zhang B, Ren L, Zhu J, Wang F, Li S (2020) The correlation between endolymphatic hydrops and clinical features of Meniere disease. Laryngoscope 131:E144–E150

Zingler VC, Cnyrim C, Jahn K, Weintz E, Fernbacher J, Frenzel C, Brandt T, Strupp M (2007) Causative factors and epidemiology of bilateral vestibulopathy in 255 patients. Ann Neurol 61(6):524–532

10

Vestibular Paroxysmia

Contents

Supplementary Information The online version contains supplementary material available at [https://doi.org/10.1007/978-3-030-78260-3_11]. The videos can be accessed by scanning the related images with the SN More Media App.

M. Strupp et al., *Vertigo and Dizziness*, https://doi.org/10.1007/978-3-030-78260-3_11

The leading symptom of vestibular paroxysmia (VP) (Brandt and Dieterich 1994), a rare vestibular disorder, is recurrent short-lasting spontaneous attacks of spinning or non-spinning vertigo. This disease was re-classified with two subtypes: VP and probable VP with the major difference being the response to a sodium channel blocker (Strupp et al. 2016b) (▶ Box 11.1).

Box 11.1 Modified Diagnostic Criteria for Vestibular Paroxysmia According to the Classification Committee of the Bárány Society (Strupp et al. 2016b)

Vestibular paroxysmia (each point needs to be fulfilled):

1. At least ten attacks of spontaneous spinning or non-spinning vertigo
2. Duration less than 1 min
3. Stereotyped phenomenology in a particular patient
4. Response to treatment with a sodium channel blocker
5. Not better accounted for by another diagnosis

Probable vestibular paroxysmia (each point needs to be fulfilled):

1. At least five attacks of spinning or non-spinning vertigo
2. Duration less than 5 min
3. Spontaneous occurrence or provoked by certain head movements
4. Stereotyped phenomenology in a particular patient
5. Not better accounted for by another diagnosis

11.1 Epidemiology

Although there are no data on the life-prevalence of VP, it can be considered a rare disease. A few case series and single cases have been published (e.g., Best et al. 2013; Brandt and Dieterich 1994; Chang et al. 2013; He et al. 2009; Hüfner et al. 2008a; Lehnen et al. 2015; Strupp et al. 2013; Steinmetz et al. 2022; Hanskamp et al. 2022). The relative frequency of VP in a group of 39,918 patients with vertigo and dizziness in a tertiary care center was around 3.1%.

The mean age of the patients, for instance, in the three case series with more than ten patients, was 51 years (range 25–67 years) (Brandt and Dieterich 1994), 48.0 ± 15.3 years (± SD) (Hüfner et al. 2008a), and 47.2 ± 14.7 years (Best et al. 2013). Vestibular paroxysmia was also described in children, with features similar to those in adults (Lehnen et al. 2015). From the three studies in adults mentioned above, a total number of 63 patients, 32 were female.

11.2 Diagnosis

11.2.1 Patient History

The leading symptom of VP is recurrent short attacks of spinning or non-spinning vertigo, which typically last for seconds to a minute, but occasionally longer (◘ Figs. 11.1 and 11.2). In extreme cases, up to 70 attacks per day can occur. In the vast majority of cases, the attacks occur spontaneously. In some patients, attacks can be induced, for instance, by head turns to the right and to the left. In these cases, one should make sure that the head turns occurred in an upright body and head position, which is important for differentiating VP from BPPV. Attacks can also be induced by hyperventilation (Hüfner et al. 2008a; Lee et al. 2020), which is another relevant clinical symptom. In a study (Steinmetz et al. 2022) with 146 patients (73 with VP and 73 with probable VP), the frequency of the attacks ranged between 5 and 30 attacks per day. Spinning vertigo was the most frequent

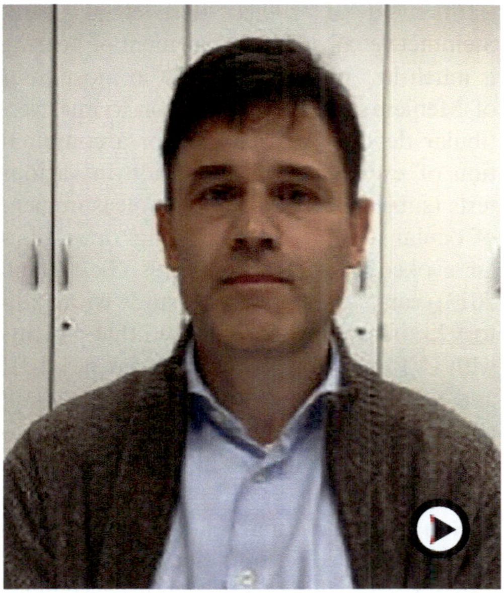

Fig. 11.1 Probable vestibular paroxymia: patient history (▶ https://doi.org/10.1007/000-95x)

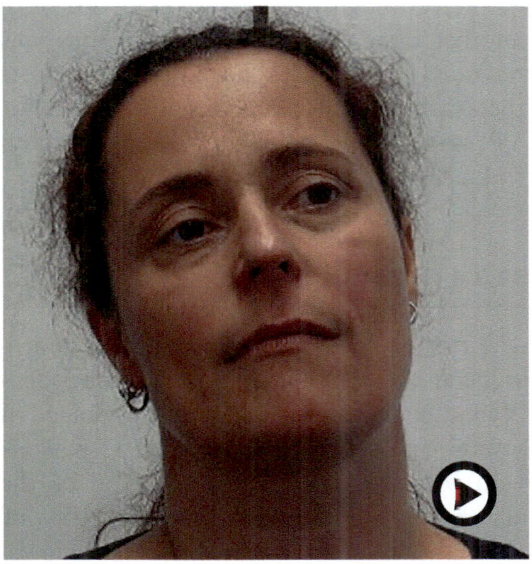

Fig. 11.2 Probable vestibular paroxymia: patient history (▶ https://doi.org/10.1007/000-95w)

type; this was more frequent in patients with VP than in those with probable VP. In two-thirds of patients, attacks occurred spontaneously; in one-quarter, they were triggered by head movements. The majority (approximately 70%) did not report accompanying symptoms; in those with symptoms, mild unilateral cochlear symptoms prevailed. One-third of patients initially showed hyperventilation-induced nystagmus.

In some patients, the attacks are associated with hyperacusis or hypacusis and/or tinnitus in the affected ear (e.g. Kim and Choi 2021). If the attacks are regularly associated with such hearing symptoms or other unilateral symptoms (see below), the affected side can be identified, which is particularly important in rare patients who need surgery.

As mentioned above, a convincing response to treatment with sodium channel blockers, such oxcarbazepine, carbamazepine, or lacosamide (see below), in adequate dosages is important for the diagnosis, i.e., the diagnosis can only be made *ex juvantibus*. As long as the effect of the treatment is not known, only the diagnosis of probable VP can be made. If the patient does not respond to an adequate pharmacotherapy, the diagnosis is doubtful (see differential diagnosis below (▶ Box 11.2)).

There are also patients who have – in addition to the recurrent attacks of vertigo – other neurological symptoms and signs, e.g., facial hemispasm (Straube et al. 1994; Silva-Hernandez et al. 2019), which is due to a combined irritation of cranial nerves VIII and VII in the meatus acusticus internus where both nerves lie close to each other. The combination of trigeminal neuralgia and facial hemispasm – two types of neurovascular compression of a cranial nerve – was also described (Han et al. 2018) as well

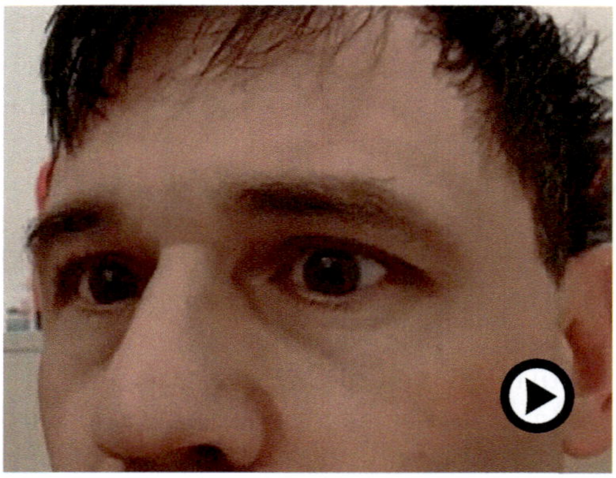

Fig. 11.3 Spontaneous nystagmus during an attack in vestibular paroxysmia (▶ https://doi.org/10.1007/000-95v)

as other combinations (Goldschagg et al. 2022). There is an analogous disease due to a compression of the cochlear nerve characterized by recurrent short attacks of tinnitus (so-called typewriter tinnitus) (Russell and Baloh 2009; Sunwoo et al. 2017); here again the diagnosis can only be made *ex juvantibus*.

11

11.2.2 Bedside Examination

Between the attacks In about 20% of patients, there is evidence of a mild unilateral peripheral vestibular hypofunction (pathological head-impulse test, head-shaking nystagmus) or a slight impairment of hearing. In some patients, hyperventilation can induce vertigo and nystagmus, which can change its direction (Hüfner et al. 2008a; Lee et al. 2020; Steinmetz et al. 2022).

During an attack There is typically spontaneous nystagmus, which can be recorded by the patient using a video camera, which significantly helps the diagnosis (Fig. 11.3) (see also ▶ Sect. 11.2.3).

11.2.3 Laboratory Examinations

Between the attacks About 45–50% of patients have evidence of mild to moderate peripheral vestibulo-cochlear deficits (Hüfner et al. 2008a; Best et al. 2013; Steinmetz et al. 2022); impairment of hearing is much less pronounced than in most cases of Menière's disease. In addition to mild vestibular deficits, an excitation or a combination of excitation and inhibition in various tests (subjective visual vertical, measurement of ocular torsion, caloric testing, or vestibular evoked myogenic potentials (Best et al. 2013)) can also be present. A study with auditory brainstem response showed that patients with VP had longer interpeak latency I-III and wave III latency compared to non-VP patients which also supports the pathophysiology (see below) (Sun et al. 2022).

During an attack In a well-documented case with right-sided neurovascular cross-compression, initially a left-beating nystagmus was recorded by videooculography, which, after 47 s, beat to the right for 10 s; this is compatible with an inhibition and excitation of the vestibular nerve (Choi et al. 2018). In another case, an excitatory nystagmus was recorded (Young et al. 2019), which supports the assumed pathophysiology (see below) of VP and the response to treatment with sodium channel blockers.

11.2.4 Imaging

The role of MRI in demonstrating a neurovascular compression (Fig. 11.4) and identifying the affected side has been evaluated in several case series. In a study of 32 patients with VP, neurovascular compression of the eighth cranial nerve was detected in 95% of the patients; bilateral neurovascular compression was found in 42% of the patients (Hüfner et al. 2008a). In another study of 20 patients with VP, neurovascular compression of the eighth cranial nerve was found in all patients, but also in 7 out of 20 control subjects (sensitivity: 100%, specificity: 65% for the diagnosis of VP by MRI) (Best et al. 2013). The distance between the brainstem and compressing vessels varied between 0.0 and 10.2 mm. This part

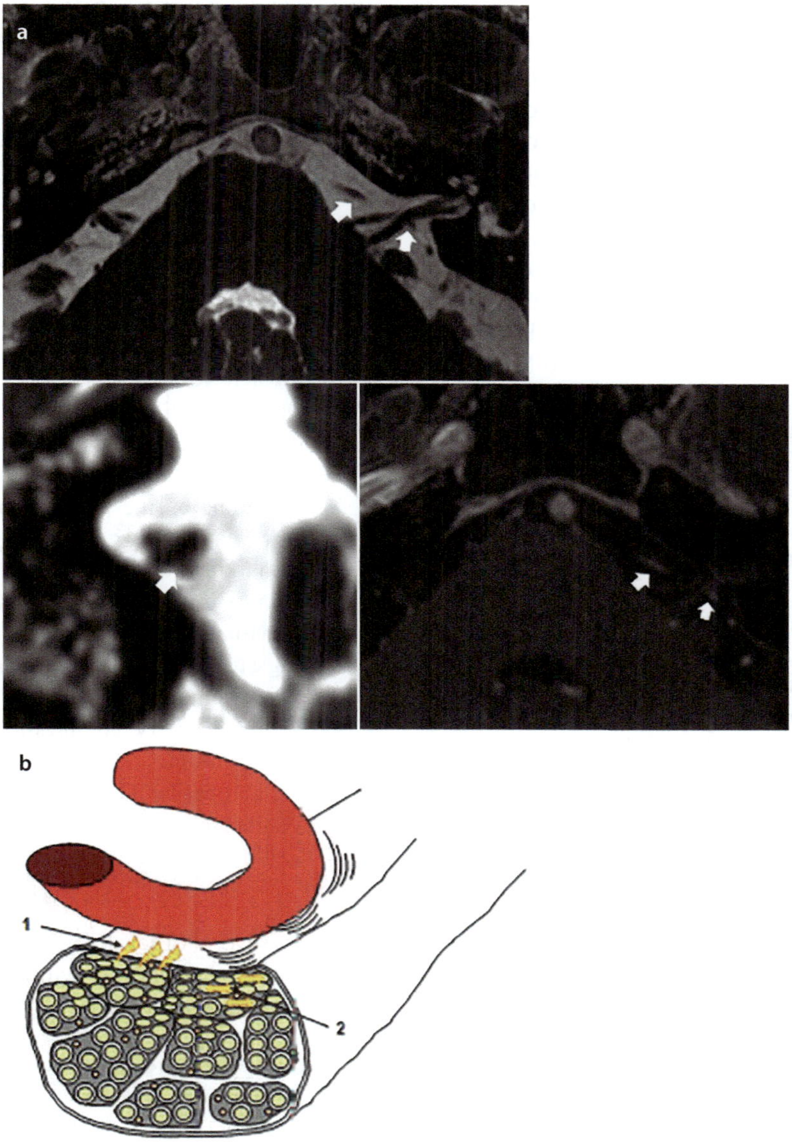

Fig. 11.4 Neurovascular compression in vestibular paroxysmia (VP). (**a**) MRI of the cerebellopontine angle. Neurovascular cross-compression of the AICA (white arrows) with the left eighth cranial nerve. (**b**) Pathophysiology of VP in analogy to other neurovascular compression syndromes. (1) Schematic drawing of the affected axonal transmission in partially demyelinated axons due to pulsatile compression, (2) Schematic drawing of the site of intraaxonal ephaptic transmission, i.e., a pathological paroxysmal transmission between neighboring partially demyelinated axons. (Adapted from Hüfner et al. (2009))

of the nerve is proximal to the transition zone (up to 15 mm (Lang 1982)) and covered by oligodendrocytes. The compressing vessel was the anterior inferior cerebellar artery in 15 cases (75%), the posterior inferior cerebellar artery in one (5%), a vein in two (10%), and the vertebral artery (10%) in another two cases (Best et al. 2013). Thus, a high-resolution MRI with 3D-CISS/FIESTA sequences of the brainstem may support the diagnosis (for reference, see

Karamitros et al 2022). In a third case series, a neurovascular compression of the eighth cranial nerve was also found in 45% of healthy subjects (Sivarasan et al. 2019); however, this study included only 20 healthy controls and nine patients with VP. Nerve angulation at the point of contact occurred in 5 of the cases (44%), but in none of the controls. This study supports the concept of neurovascular compression in VP and suggests that nerve angulation may be a specific feature. In a fourth imaging study with a total of 470 MRI scans, the authors also concluded that the vascular loop is a normal variant which may or may not give rise to audiovestibular symptoms or VP and that clinical assessment is still the most important tool in deriving a diagnosis of VP and MRI may be useful to rule out other central causes (Teh et al. 2022). Finally in a study with 18 patients with VP and 18 age-matched healthy controls even the combination of various imaging techniques did not suffice to diagnose VP on a single-subject level due to individual variability and lack of diagnostic specificity (Kierig et al. 2022). All in all, it is important to note that neurovascular contact is a common phenomenon in asymptomatic patients, has a low specificity and therefore the correlation with symptoms and signs remains essential (Sivarasan et al. 2019).

Since recurrent attacks of vertigo can also have other causes, a cranial MRI should be performed to exclude the presence of a tumor in the area of the cerebellopontine angle, arachnoid cysts (Arbusow et al. 1998), megalodolichobasilaris, brainstem plaques in multiple sclerosis, brainstem infarctions (both can lead to paroxysmal brainstem attacks), or other brainstem lesions such as brainstem melanocytoma (Lee et al. 2018).

11.2.5 Differential Diagnosis

As stated above, it is important for making the diagnosis that the recurrent spontaneous short attacks of vertigo respond to treatment with a sodium channel blocker and that other pathologies are excluded by MRI (see above). The important differential diagnoses of VP are summarized in ► Box 11.2.

Box 11.2 The Most Relevant Differential Diagnoses for Vestibular Paroxysmia (in Alphabetical Order)

- BPPV
- Central positional vertigo
- Episodic ataxias
- Functional dizziness
- Menière's disease
- Orthostatic dizziness
- Panic attacks
- Paroxysmal brainstem attacks
- Syndrome of the third mobile windows
- Tumarkin's otolithic catastrophe
- Tumors in the brainstem (e.g., melanocytoma) or the cerebellopontine angle (e.g., vestibular schwannoma or meningioma)
- Vertebral artery compression/occlusion syndrome
- Vertebrobasilar TIAs
- Vestibular epilepsy
- Vestibular migraine

There are several other disorders, which may present with the leading symptom of recurent spontaneous short attacks of vertigo:

Paroxysmal brainstem or cerebellar attacks Such attacks with vertigo, dysarthria, or ataxia (after stroke or in MS) may be difficult to distinguish, as they can also lead to ephaptic discharges of neighboring fibers of the brainstem paths and can respond to low doses of sodium channel blockers (for reference, see (Li et al. 2011). In such cases, the use of MRI with thin brainstem slices is useful for establishing the diagnosis.

Tumors in the cerebellopontine angle Recurrent short attacks of vertigo, which may also be induced by hyperventilation and may be associated with nystagmus, can also occur in patients with a vestibular schwannoma (e.g., Minor et al. 2000). A rare cause of short and head position-dependent attacks of vertigo is an arachnoidal cyst, which leads to an extension of the nerve (Arbusow et al. 1998). In such a case, the symptoms could be explained by a conduction block of the nerve, lasting hours to days in combination with additional head position-dependent excitation of the nerve, which leads to direction-changing nystagmus.

Positional vertigo A differentiation between BPPV (see ► Chap. 9) can be made based on the patient history with recurrent attacks of vertigo that are induced by changes of head or body position relative to gravity, the typical nystagmus during the diagnostic positional maneuvers corresponding to the affected canal and the effect of the liberatory maneuvers. In patients with VP, attacks can also be induced by head movements, typically when turning the head to the right and to the left in an upright head and body position, which is not typical of BPPV. Another differential diagnosis is central positional vertigo and nystagmus (see ► Chap. 13), which is often associated with a central positional downbeat nystagmus.

Menière's Disease and Tumarkin's Otolithic Catastrophe (see ► Chap. 10) In patients with longer-lasting attacks of vertigo, one differential diagnosis is Menière's disease. However, the duration of attacks typically ranges from 20 min to 12 h and one finds a low- to medium-frequency sensorineural hearing loss (>30 dB, <2000 Hz) (Lopez-Escamez et al. 2015). Tumarkin's otolithic catastrophe ("vestibular drop attacks") occurs most often in patients with known Menière's disease, typically while standing, whereas in VP the attacks occur in any body positions.

Vestibular Migraine (see ► Sect. 14.1) Another differential diagnosis is vestibular migraine (VM) (Dieterich and Brandt 1999; Lempert et al. 2012). Even very short attacks of vertigo can occur in VM. It should be noted for the differential diagnosis that, in most patients with VM, there is a history of migraine and/or typical additional migrainous features during the attacks of vertigo.

Vertebrobasilar transient ischemic attacks (TIAs) These can also manifest with short oligosymptomatic attacks of vertigo (Paul et al. 2013), but the frequency is much lower than in most patients with VP. In patients with severe vertebrobasilar stenosis, attacks of vertigo can also manifest, but they are often dependent on blood pressure or body position; in these cases, CT-, MR-, or conventional angiography help to make the diagnosis.

Panic attacks According to DSM-5, the diagnostic criteria for a panic attack include a discrete period of intense fear or discomfort, in which four (or more) of the following symptoms develop abruptly and reach a peak within minutes: feeling dizzy, unsteady, lightheaded, or faint; nausea or abdominal distress; palpitations, and/or accelerated heart rate; sweating; trembling or shaking; sensations of shortness of breath or being smothered; feeling of choking; chest pain or discomfort; derealization or depersonalization; fear of losing control or going insane; sense of impending death; paresthesias; chills or hot flashes. Panic attacks are often longer than typical attacks of VP. It may be helpful to ask the patient which of the symptoms come first to differentiate between the two. Finally, videoing of eye movements during an episode (◘ Fig. 11.4) considerably helps the differentiation.

Syndrome of the third mobile windows (see ► Chap. 12) Here the leading symptom is recurrent attacks of vertigo, which are induced by changes of pressure (such as sneezing, coughing, pressing, or lifting heavy weights) or certain sounds (Minor et al. 1998); in addition, many of these patients also have autophony. Rarely, patients also have attacks during changes of head position.

Episodic ataxias (EA; see ► Sects. 13.4 and 16.3) In the most frequent subtype, EA2, the duration of the attacks varies from several minutes to hours and more than 90% of the patients have cerebellar signs, in particular cerebellar gaze-evoked nystagmus and downbeat nystagmus (Jen and Wan 2018). The onset of manifestations after the age of 20 is unusual. The much rarer EA1 is another differential diagnosis. It is characterized by recurrent attacks of ataxia, dizziness, and visual blurring, provoked by abrupt postural changes, emotion, vestibular stimulation, and lasting minutes. These patients also have neuromyotonia, i.e., continuous spontaneous muscle fiber activity (Jen and Wan 2018).

Epilepsy with vestibular aura Vestibular auras can manifest with short attacks of vertigo often lasting a few seconds (Tarnutzer et al. 2015) and nystagmus (Pfefferkorn et al. 2004). Vestibular aura with additional symptoms, so-called non-isolated vestibular aura, is much more prevalent than isolated vestibular aura, which is rare. Vestibular aura is primarily associated with temporal lobe seizures.

Vertebral artery compression/occlusion syndrome The short attacks of vertigo are typically provoked by head turns that lead to vertebral artery compression and transiently reduced blood flow to the brainstem and labyrinth (Kim et al. 2022). They may also be associated with a nystagmus indicating an excitation (Strupp et al. 2000; Choi et al. 2005).

Hemodynamic orthostatic dizziness/vertigo The leading symptom is recurrent attacks of dizziness, rarely vertigo, which are induced by changes of body position from lying or sitting down to an upright position. Orthostatic hypotension must be demonstrated for the diagnosis to be made (Kim et al. 2019).

11.2.6 Diagnosis: The Essentials

As mentioned above, the leading symptom of VP is recurrent, most often spontaneous, short attacks of vertigo, which are intraindividually uniform and respond to treatment with a sodium channel blocker. This means that the diagnosis is made *ex juvantibus* and after exclusion of other etiologies only, because there is no proving test. It can be helpful for the patient to video his or her eye movements during an attack, so that one can look for a nystagmus. In some patients, neurootological examination reveals subtle peripheral vestibular and/or audiological deficits. Demonstration of a neurovascular compression of the eighth nerve by MRI has a high sensitivity, but only a very low specificity because up to 45% of healthy subjects also have a neurovascular contact. Therefore, imaging is mainly required to exclude other pathologies.

11.3 Course of the Disease

There are two studies on the long-term course of the disease with contrary conclusions. In one study with 61 patients with a mean follow-up was 3.4 years, 44 (72%) still experienced vertigo attacks at follow-up and 71% reported having limitations of their quality of life (Hanskamp et al. 2022). The authors concluded that there is a rather unfavorable prognosis in patients with VP in terms of vertigo attacks and quality of life and recommended that after the initial diagnosis follow-up is warranted to monitor clinical outcomes. In the second study (Steinmetz et al. 2022) with 146 patients, three-quarters of the patients with VP remained attack-free during a mean follow-up of 4.8 years, more than half of them even without any medication. The authors concluded that the long-term prognosis of VP

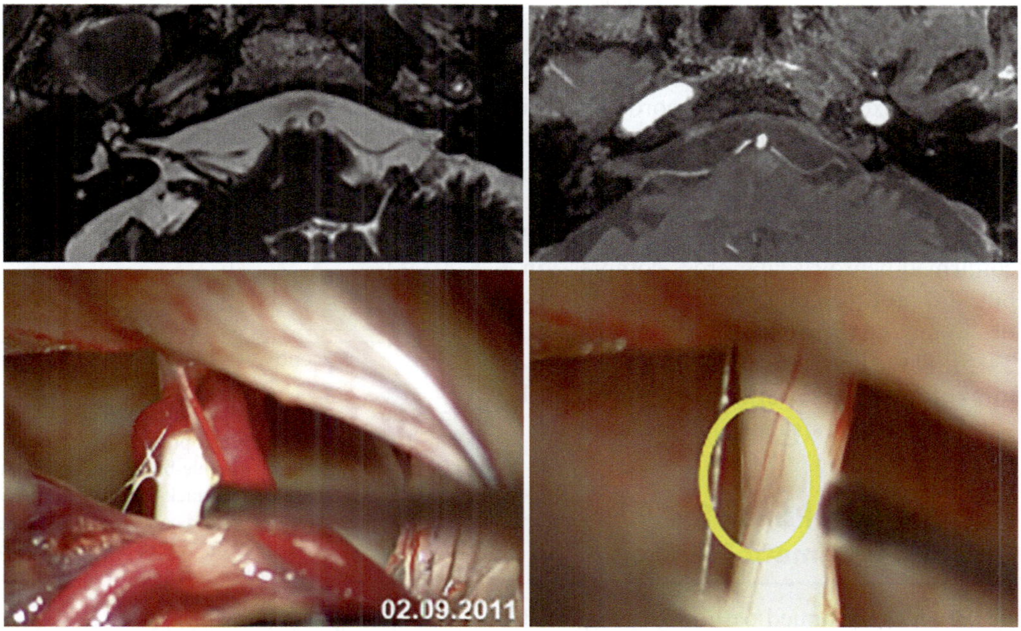

Fig. 11.5 Patient with right-sided vestibular paroysmia with attacks of vertigo and buzzing in the right ear. Cranial MRI (left upper corner: constructive interference in steady-state sequence, right upper corner: time-of-flight) shows contact between the right eighth cranial nerve and the anterior inferior cerebellar artery. Intraoperative micrographs demonstrate vascular contact (left lower corner) and considerable compression of the eighth nerve after removal of the arteries (right lower corner, circle). The patient has been free of symptoms since surgery in 2011. (Adapted from Strupp et al. (2013))

appears favorable, not necessarily requiring ongoing treatment. We recommend regular follow-up examinations to evaluate the course of the disease as well as the effects and side-effects of the treatment (see below) to adjust the dosage.

11.4 Pathophysiology and Etiology

Already in 1975 Jannetta and colleagues described the pathophysiology of VP: "neurovascular cross-compression in patients with hyperactive dysfunction symptoms of the eighth cranial nerve" (Jannetta 1975). In analogy to the brief recurrent symptoms in trigeminal neuralgia, hemifacial spasm, glossopharyngeal neuralgia, or myokymia of the superior oblique muscle (Yousry et al. 2002; Hüfner et al. 2008b), it is assumed that the short attacks of vertigo are caused by compression of the vestibular nerve (Fig. 11.5). Pathophysiologically, the compression can cause partial demyelination of axons, which can lead to ephaptic discharges, i.e., pathological paroxysmal inter-axonal transmissions between neighboring axons which can be further triggered by the pulsations of the artery and by sensory input during head movements similar to senory input in trigeminal neuralgia. The hypothesis of excitation of the vestibular nerve is supported by cases in which a nystagmus caused by hyperexcitability was found during an attack (Young et al. 2019), a transition of nystagmus caused by hypo- and hyperexcitability was recorded (Choi et al. 2018) and by evidence for hyperexcitability and vestibular deficits found even between the attacks (Best et al. 2013).

A seven Tesla MRI in six patients with VP confirmed neurovascular cross-compression but did not detect structural abnormalities in any of these patients (Rommer et al. 2015). These findings suggest that the symptoms of VP in these patients were not caused at least by major structural nerve lesions.

11.5 Therapy: Principles and Pragmatic Therapy

Based on the assumed pathophysiology and in analogy to other neurovascular cross syndromes, primarily a prophylactic therapy of the attacks of vertigo with sodium channel blockers has been recommended (Brandt and Dieterich 1994) because they reduce the excitability of the peripheral nerves (for references, see Strupp et al. 2016a).

11

If the diagnosis is proven with a convincing response to treatment and fulfillment of the current diagnostic criteria (▶ Box 11.1) and the affected side is definitely identified and the patient does not tolerate pharmacotherapy, surgical treatment (Jannetta 1975) can be considered in rare individual cases.

Pharmacotherapy The therapeutic effect of carbamazepine has been described in non-controlled case series. In one of these case series, 11 out of 11 patients responded (Brandt and Dieterich 1994). In another, 7 out 8 patients showed an improvement (Kanashiro et al. 2005). In an observational study in 32 patients with a mean observational period of 3 years, a significant and persistent reduction of the frequency of attacks to 10% of the initial frequency and a reduction of the intensity and duration of the attacks were found during treatment with carbamazepine or oxcarbazepine (Hüfner et al. 2008a).

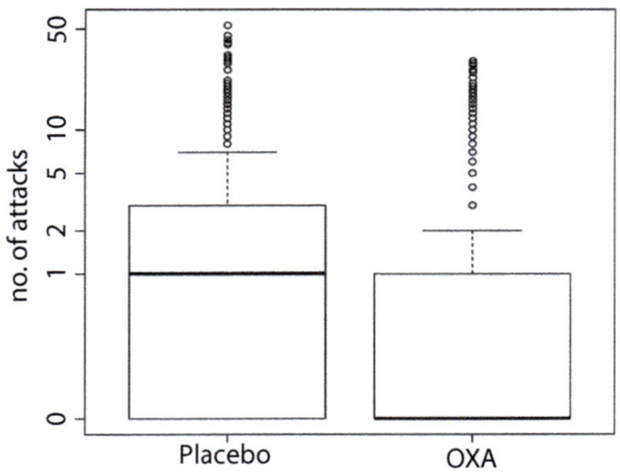

■ **Fig. 11.6** Therapy with oxcarbazepine (OXA: 300 mg 1-1-1 vs. placebo). In a prospective, randomized, placebo-controlled, double-blind study, OXA reduced the mean number of attacks per day from 5.9 to 3.2. The probability of one day with at least one attack of vertigo was 0.62 on placebo and 0.41 on OXA; thus, the relative risk was reduced to 0.67 (95% CI 0.47–0.95, $p = 0.025$). The drop-out rate, however, was 60%: 43 patients were randomized, 18 patients did not complete the study because of adverse events (Bayer et al. 2018)

In a randomized, placebo-controlled trial, a significant therapeutic effect of oxcarbazepine (900 mg/d), which has fewer side effects and interactions than carbamazepine, was found (reduction to 0.53, $p < 0.001$) (■ Fig. 11.6). However, the drop-out rate due to adverse events was 60% (Bayer et al. 2018). Since there are several contraindications and several side effects and interactions for carbamazepine and oxcarbazepine, the compliance, persistence and adherence of patients can be quite low. A well-tolerated (Li et al. 2020) and evidently effective alternative is lacosamide (100–400 mg/d), as was shown in an observational study in 7 patients (Strupp et al. 2019): the mean number of attacks per month was reduced from 13 to 3 and all patients tolerated the medication well.

Surgical Treatment In 1986, Jannetta and colleagues (Møller et al. 1986) reported a case series of 21 patients treated by microvascular decompression, 16 of whom benefited from this procedure. These results were confirmed by larger case series on 41 patients (Møller and Møller 1990) and 207 patients (Møller et al. 1993) with a success rate between 73% and 80%. Later it was criticized that the selection criteria for surgery were variable and that no standardized outcome measures were used (Yap et al. 2008).

11.5.1 Pragmatic Therapy

11.5.1.1 Pharmacotherapy

A therapeutic trial of low dose of oxcarbazepine (300–900 mg/d) or carbamazepine (200–800 mg/d) is often effective (for references, see Brandt et al. 2016; Strupp et al. 2016a). To evaluate the efficacy of the drugs, a treatment period of at least 4 weeks is recommended and the effects should be documented by a patient's diary in which the number of attacks per day is noted. Moreover, a positive response supports the diagnosis.

In case of intolerance to these drugs, lacosamide (100–400 mg/d) can be given (Strupp et al. 2019), which is well tolerated (Li et al. 2020). Other sodium channel blockers, which are theoretically effective, are phenytoin (300–900 mg/d) or lamotrigine (25 mg/d with slow increase up to a daily dosage of 100–200 mg/d); for the latter two, there are neither case series nor clinical studies yet.

11.5.1.2 Surgical Treatment

Despite the reports of partial successes (see above Møller et al. 1986, 1993; Møller and Møller 1990) and clinically well-documented single cases (e.g., Strupp et al. 2013) operative microvascular decompression should be reserved for cases with VP with the following prerequisites: (1) the diagnosis is certain with a convincing response to pharmacotherapy; (2) various medications are not tolerated; and (3) the affected side is clearly identified. These restrictions also have to be considered because of the risk of a brainstem and/or cerebellar infarction due to intra- or post-operative vasospasm (1–3%). Since the labyrinthine artery originates from the anterior inferior cerebellar artery (AICA) and the AICA is in 75% the compressing vessel that has to be moved, an infarction can also cause hearing and/or vestibular loss.

References

Arbusow V, Strupp M, Dieterich M, Jäger L, Hischa A, Schulz P, Brandt T (1998) Alternating episodes of vestibular nerve excitation and failure. Neurology 51(5):1480–1483

Bayer O, Bremova T, Strupp M, Hüfner K (2018) A randomized double-blind, placebo-controlled, cross-over trial (Vestparoxy) of the treatment of vestibular paroxysmia with oxcarbazepine. J Neurol 265(2):291–298

Best C, Gawehn J, Kramer HH, Thömke F, Ibis T, Müller-Forell W, Dieterich M (2013) MRI and neurophysiology in vestibular paroxysmia: contradiction and correlation. J Neurol Neurosurg Psychiatry 84(12):1349–1356

Brandt T, Dieterich M (1994) Vestibular paroxysmia: vascular compression of the eighth nerve? Lancet 343(8900):798–799

Brandt T, Huppert T, Hüfner K, Zingler VC, Dieterich M, Strupp M (2010) Long-term course and relapses of vestibular and balance disorders. Restor Neurol Neurosci 28(1):69–82

Brandt T, Strupp M, Dieterich M (2016) Vestibular paroxysmia: a treatable neurovascular cross-compression syndrome. J Neurol 263 Suppl 1:90–96

Chang TP, Wu YC, Hsu YC (2013) Vestibular paroxysmia associated with paroxysmal pulsatile tinnitus: a case report and review of the literature. Acta Neurol Taiwanica 22(2):72–75

Choi KD, Shin HY, Kim JS, Kim SH, Kwon OK, Koo JW, Park SH, Yoon BW, Roh JK (2005) Rotational vertebral artery syndrome: oculographic analysis of nystagmus. Neurology 65(8):1287–1290

Choi SY, Choi JH, Choi KD (2018) The nystagmus of vestibular paroxysmia. J Neurol 265(7):1711–1713

Dieterich M, Brandt T (1999) Episodic vertigo related to migraine (90 cases): vestibular migraine? J Neurol 246(10):883–892

Goldschagg N, Brem C, Strupp M (2022) Case report: bitter vertigo. Front Neurol 13:1028597

Han J, Wang T, Xie Y, Cao D, Kang Z, Song X (2018) Successive occurrence of vertebrobasilar dolichectasia induced trigeminal neuralgia, vestibular

paroxysmia and hemifacial spasm: a case report. Medicine (Baltimore) 97(25):e11192
Hanskamp LAJ, Schermer TR, van Leeuwen RB (2022) Long-term prognosis of vertigo attacks and health-related quality of life limitations in patients with vestibular paroxysmia. Otol Neurotol 43:e475–e481
He LY, Dong WW, Huang W, Luo Y, Lu FJ (2009) [Clinical manifestations and imaging features of peripheral vestibular paroxysmia: a report of 7 cases]. Zhonghua Yi Xue Za Zhi 89(13):909–911
Hüfner K, Barresi D, Glaser M, Linn J, Adrion C, Mansmann U, Brandt T, Strupp M (2008a) Vestibular paroxysmia: diagnostic features and medical treatment. Neurology 71(13):1006–1014
Hüfner K, Linn J, Strupp M (2008b) Recurrent attacks of vertigo with monocular oscillopsia. Neurology 71(11):863
Hüfner K, Jahn K, Linn J, Strupp M, Brandt T (2009) Vestibularisparoxysmie Nervenheilkunde 28:26–30
Jannetta PJ (1975) Neurovascular cross-compression in patients with hyperactive dysfunction symptoms of the eighth cranial nerve. Surg Forum 26:467–468
Jen JC, Wan J (2018) Episodic ataxias. Handb Clin Neurol 155:205–215
Kanashiro AM, Alexandre PL, Pereira CB, Melo AC, Scaff M (2005) [Vestibular paroxysmia: clinical study and treatment of eight patients]. Arq Neuropsiquiatr 63(3A):643–647

11

Karamitros A, Kalamatianos T, Stranjalis G, Anagnostou E (2022) Vestibular paroxysmia: Clinical features and imaging findings; a literature review. J Neuroradiol 49:225–233
Kierig E, Gerb J, Boegle R, Ertl-Wagner B, Dieterich M, Kirsch V (2022) Vestibular paroxysmia entails vestibular nerve function, microstructure and endolymphatic space changes linked to root-entry zone neurovascular compression. J Neurol. https://doi.org/10.1007/s00415-022-11399-y
Kim HA, Bisdorff A, Bronstein AM, Lempert T, Rossi-Izquierdo M, Staab JP, Strupp M, Kim JS (2019) Hemodynamic orthostatic dizziness/vertigo: diagnostic criteria. J Vestib Res 29(2–3):45–56
Kim CH, Choi KD (2021) Periodic Tinnitus and Direction-Changing Nystagmus in Vestibular Paroxysmia. J Clin Neurol 17:493–495
Kim JS, Newman-Toker DE, Kerber KA, Jahn K, Bertholon P, Waterston J, Lee H, Bisdorff A, Strupp M (2022) Vascular vertigo and dizziness: Diagnostic criteria. J Vestib Res 32:(3)205–222
Lang J (1982) [Anatomy, length and blood vessel relations of "central" and "peripheral" paths of intracisternal cranial nerves]. Zentralbl Neurochir 43:217–258
Lee SU, Kim HJ, Choi JY, Kim JS (2018) Lower brainstem melanocytoma masquerading as vestibular paroxysmia. J Neurol 265(5):1222–1225
Lee SM, Oh EH, Choi SY, Jo JW, Choi JH, Choi KD (2020) Hyperventilation-triggered vertigo and nystagmus in vestibular paroxysmia. J Clin Neurol 16(3):507–509
Lehnen N, Langhagen T, Heinen F, Huppert D, Brandt T, Jahn K (2015) Vestibular paroxysmia in children: a treatable cause of short vertigo attacks. Dev Med Child Neurol 57(4):393–396
Lempert T, Olesen J, Furman J, Waterston J, Seemungal B, Carey J, Bisdorff A, Versino M, Evers S, Newman-Toker D (2012) Vestibular migraine: diagnostic criteria. J Vestib Res 22(4):167–172
Li Y, Zeng C, Luo T (2011) Paroxysmal dysarthria and ataxia in multiple sclerosis and corresponding magnetic resonance imaging findings. J Neurol 258(2):273–276
Li J, Sun M, Wang X (2020) The adverse-effect profile of lacosamide. Expert Opin Drug Saf 19:131–138
Lopez-Escamez JA, Carey J, Chung WH, Goebel JA, Magnusson M, Mandala M, Newman-Toker DE, Strupp M, Suzuki M, Trabalzini F, Bisdorff A (2015) Diagnostic criteria for Meniere's disease. J Vestib Res 25(1):1–7
Minor LB, Solomon D, Zinreich JS, Zee DS (1998) Sound- and/or pressure-induced vertigo due to bone dehiscence of the superior semicircular canal. Arch Otolaryngol Head Neck Surg 124(3):249–258
Minor LB, Haslwanter T, Straumann D, Zee DS (2000) Hyperventilation-induced nystagmus in patients with vestibular schwannoma. Neurology 53(9):2158–2168
Møller MB, Møller AR (1990) Vascular compression syndrome of the eighth nerve. Clinical correlations and surgical findings. Neurol Clin 8(2):421–439
Møller MB, Møller AR, Jannetta PJ, Sekhar L (1986) Diagnosis and surgical treatment of disabling positional vertigo. J Neurosurg 64:21–28
Møller MB, Møller AR, Jannetta PJ, Jho HD, Sekhar LN (1993) Microvascular decompression of the eighth nerve in patients with disabling positional vertigo: selection criteria and operative results in 207 patients. Acta Neurochir 125(1–4):75–82
Paul NL, Simoni M, Rothwell PM (2013) Transient isolated brainstem symptoms preceding posterior circulation stroke: a population-based study. Lancet Neurol 12(1):65–71
Pfefferkorn T, Holtmannspotter M, Querner V, Dudel C, Noachtar S, Strupp M, Brandt T (2004) Epileptic nystagmus. Neurology 63(7):E14
Rommer PS, Wiest G, Kronnerwetter C, Zach H, Loader B, Elwischger K, Trattnig S (2015) 7-Tesla MRI demonstrates absence of structural lesions in patients with vestibular paroxysmia. Front Neuroanat 9:81
Russell D, Baloh RW (2009) Gabapentin responsive audiovestibular paroxysmia. J Neurol Sci 281(1–2):99–100

Silva-Hernandez L, Silva-Hernandez M, Gutierrez-Viedma A, Yus M, Cuadrado ML (2019) Hemifacial spasm and vestibular paroxysmia: co-presence of two neurovascular compression syndromes in a patient. Neurologia 34(2):131–133

Sivarasan N, Touska P, Murdin L, Connor S (2019) MRI findings in vestibular paroxysmia - an observational study. J Vestib Res 29(2–3):137–145

Steinmetz K, Becker-Bense S, Strobl R, Grill E, Seelos K, Huppert D (2022) Vestibular paroxysmia: clinical characteristics and long-term course. J Neurol https://doi.org/10.1007/s00415-022-11151-6

Straube A, Büttner U, Brandt T (1994) Recurrent attacks with skew deviation, torsional nystagmus, and contraction of the left frontalis muscle. Neurology 44:177–178

Strupp M, Planck JH, Arbusow V, Steiger HJ, Brückmann H, Brandt T (2000) Rotational vertebral artery occlusion syndrome with vertigo due to "labyrinthine excitation". Neurology 54(6):1376–1379

Strupp M, von Stuckrad-Barre S, Brandt T, Tonn JC (2013) Teaching NeuroImages: compression of the eighth cranial nerve causes vestibular paroxysmia. Neurology 80(7):e77

Strupp M, Dieterich M, Brandt T, Feil K (2016a) Therapy of vestibular paroxysmia, superior oblique myokymia, and ocular neuromyotonia. Curr Treat Options Neurol 18(7):34

Strupp M, Lopez-Escamez JA, Kim JS, Straumann D, Jen JC, Carey J, Bisdorff A, Brandt T (2016b) Vestibular paroxysmia: diagnostic criteria. J Vestib Res 26:409–415

Strupp M, Elger C, Goldschagg N (2019) Treatment of vestibular paroxysmia with lacosamide. Neurol Clin Pract 9(6):539–541

Sun H, Tian X, Zhao Y, Jiang H, Gao Z, Wu H (2022) Application of ABR in pathogenic neurovascular compression of the 8th cranial nerve in vestibular paroxysmia. Acta Neurochir (Wien) https://doi.org/10.1007/s00701-022-05157-2

Sunwoo W, Jeon YJ, Bae YJ, Jang JH, Koo JW, Song JJ (2017) Typewriter tinnitus revisited: the typical symptoms and the initial response to carbamazepine are the most reliable diagnostic clues. Sci Rep 7(1):10615

Tarnutzer AA, Lee SH, Robinson KA, Kaplan PW, Newman-Toker DE (2015) Clinical and electrographic findings in epileptic vertigo and dizziness: a systematic review. Neurology 84(15):1595–1604

Teh CS, Noordiana SH, Shamini S, Prepageran N (2022) Vascular loops: the innocent bystander for vestibular paroxysmia. Ann Otol Rhinol Laryngol 131:604-608

Yap L, Pothula VB, Lesser T (2008) Microvascular decompression of cochleovestibular nerve. Eur Arch Otorhinolaryngol 265(8):861–869

Young AS, Jonker B, Welgampola MS (2019) Vestibular paroxysmia presenting with irritative nystagmus. Neurology 92(15):723–724

Yousry I, Dieterich M, Naidich TP, Schmid UD, Yousry TA (2002) Superior oblique myokymia: magnetic resonance imaging support for the neurovascular compression hypothesis. Ann Neurol 51(3):361–368

Syndrome of the Third Mobile Windows

Contents

Supplementary Information The online version contains supplementary material available at [https://doi.org/10.1007/978-3-030-78260-3_12]. The videos can be accessed by scanning the related images with the SN More Media App.

M. Strupp et al., *Vertigo and Dizziness*, https://doi.org/10.1007/978-3-030-78260-3_12

The leading symptom of these rare diseases is recurrent attacks of vertigo which may be associated with oscillopsia and which are induced by changes in pressure or sounds. In addition, many patients can hear the sounds of their own body louder in the affected ear (autophony) or external sounds louder. These symptoms are caused by a pathological transduction of pressure to the inner ear due to a bony defect, which leads to a "third mobile window." The most frequent subtypes are canal dehiscence syndromes such as the superior semicircular canal dehiscence syndrome (SCDS) which was first described by Minor and co-workers (Minor et al. 1998 see for Ref. Eberhard et al. 2021). The posterior (Chien et al. 2011; Philip et al. 2019; Lee et al. 2020) and the horizontal canal (Zhang et al. 2011) can also be affected; very few patients have bilateral SCDS. Similar symptoms can also occur due to an enlarged vestibular duct (Stahl and Otteson 2022). A very rare entity is "perilymphatic fistula" (this term is not strictly correct, because it is not a fistula; one might call it Transient Perilymphatic Leakage (TPL); see ▶ Sect. 12.2).

12.1 Superior Semicircular Canal Dehiscence Syndrome (SCDS)

The current criteria for SCDS are as follows:

Box 12.1 Diagnostic Criteria for Superior Canal Dehiscence Syndrome (SCDS)

The diagnosis of superior semicircular canal dehiscence syndrome requires all of the following criteria:

1. At least one of the following symptoms consistent with a third window lesion of the inner ear:
    1. Bone conduction hyperacusis
    2. Sound-induced vertigo and/or oscillopsia time-locked to the stimulus
    3. Pressure-induced vertigo and/or oscillopsia time-locked to the stimulus
    4. Pulsatile tinnitus
2. At least 1 of the following signs or diagnostic tests indicating a "third mobile window" of the inner ear:
    1. Nystagmus characteristic of excitation or inhibition of the affected superior canal evoked by sound, or by changes in middle ear pressure or intracranial pressure
    2. Low-frequency negative bone conduction thresholds on pure tone audiometry
    3. Enhanced VEMP responses (low cervical VEMP thresholds or high ocular VEMP amplitudes)
3. High-resolution temporal bone CT imaging with multiplanar reconstruction demonstrating dehiscence of the superior canal
4. Not better accounted for by another vestibular disease or disorder

Adapted from (Ward et al. 2021)

12

12.1.1 Diagnosis

12.1.1.1 Patient History

In patients with a syndrome of the third mobile windows, there is a wide spectrum of possible vestibular and auditory symptoms (for reference, see Ward et al. 2017; Steenerson et al. 2020; Naert et al. 2021; Ward et al. 2021), which often makes the diagnosis difficult. There are also patients who have only attacks of vertigo or only hearing problems (Watson et al. 2000). The leading symptoms are:

- Attacks, lasting seconds to minutes, of spinning or non-spinning vertigo induced by changes in pressure, e.g., sneezing, coughing, pressing, lifting heavy weights, and/or sounds (Tullio phenomenon) most often of a low frequency or fremitus (Morrison et al. 2022). These attacks can be associated with oscillopsia or postural imbalance. Other potential inducing factors are: significant changes in altitude (e.g., using a ski lift, mountain hikes, flights), changes in pressure when entering or leaving a tunnel, changes in body position (e.g., bending over), or pressing a finger on the external auditory canal of the affected ear. Sometimes patients also report pulsatile tinnitus or pulsatile oscillopsia. Other patients complain of movement-induced postural imbalance and gait disorder (most likely due to movement-induced changes of intracranial pressure). A patient with recurrent positional vertigo was also reported (Young et al. 2019).

- Autophony, i.e., the patient hears the sounds of his/her own body, e.g., pulse, swallowing, speaking, eye movements, blinking, and even bowel movements can be heard in the affected ear.
- In addition, some patients can hear external sounds also louder, namely in the low frequency range which can lead to a severe impairment.

The disease most often occurs spontaneously. When taking the patient history, it is important to ask about traumas that could cause or trigger such attacks, for example, barotrauma, head trauma (McCrary et al. 2021), ear trauma (also operations of the ear), or excessive Valsalva maneuvers due to lifting of heavy weights. A syndrome of the third mobile windows can also occur in children, often with only auditory symptoms (Lee et al. 2011).

12.1.1.2 Physical Examination

Clinical Examination of the Vestibular System

Typically, changes in intracranial pressure or in the pressure in the middle ear cause the symptoms and signs: short attacks of spinning or non-spinning vertigo, oscillopsia, and/or nystagmus in the plane of the affected canal. Clinical examination can also reveal a pulse-synchronous vertical torsional nystagmus (Karam et al. 2021; Milenkovic et al. 2021). The provoking factors are as follows:

Changes in pressure via the external auditory canal by the Politzer balloon or pressure on the tragus (Hennebert's sign); the increase in pressure should persist for at least 30 seconds. In parallel, one observes the patient's eye movement using Frenzel's glasses or M-glasses or video-oculography (see below). Nystagmus can occur during the increase and/or the subsequent decrease in pressure. In SCDS, one typically finds a vertical torsional nystagmus in the plane of the superior canal (for horizontal and posterior canals, see below): Hennebert's sign (◘ Fig. 12.1). Positive pressure from the outside leads – via the oval window – to an excitation of the affected superior canal due to an ampullofugal movement of the cupula. These tests allow the affected side and the affected semicircular canal to be identified because the change in pressure is only from one side.

Valsalva maneuver Increase of intracranial pressure by abdominal pressing against the closed vocal cord. Here also one can observe a vertical torsional nystagmus (◘ Fig. 12.2). This maneuver leads to increased pressure in the direction of the oval window with an inhibition of the superior semicircular canal (ampullopetal deviation of the cupula). Pressing against

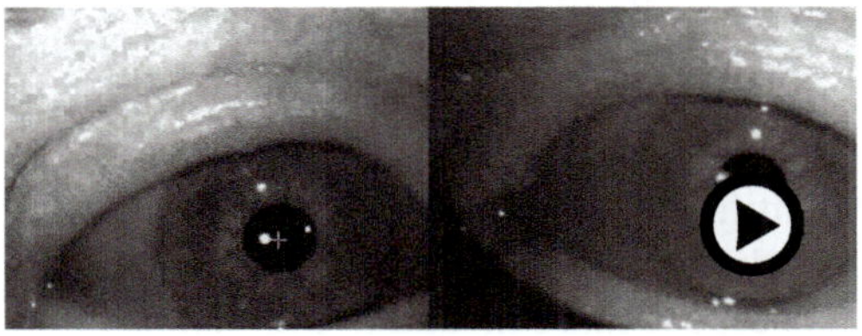

◘ Fig. 12.1 Pressure induced nystagmus (Hennebert's sign) in left sided SCDS (▶ https://doi.org/10.1007/000-961)

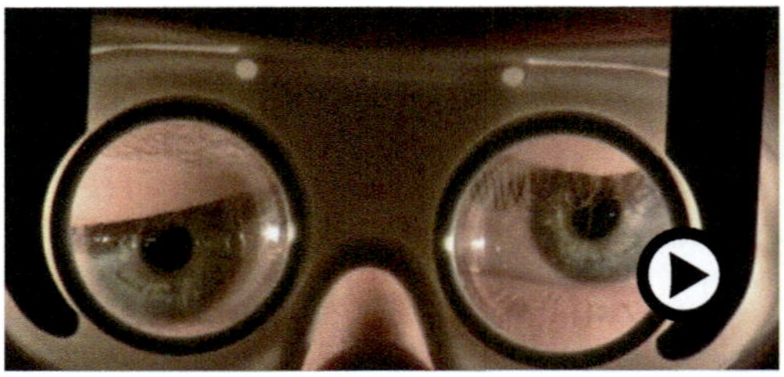

■ **Fig. 12.2** Vertical torsional nystagmus in a patient with left-sided superior canal dehiscence syndrome during the Valsalva maneuver (► https://doi.org/10.1007/000-960)

the closed nostril leads to a combined increase of intracranial and middle ear pressure, which can also induce nystagmus. The two latter maneuvers, however, do not allow clear identification of the affected side because they cause bilateral changes in pressure.

Clinical Testing of Hearing and ENT Examination

During the Weber test (512 Hz), the sound is typically louder on the affected side, which correlates with autophony. The Rinne test can provide evidence of impaired bone conduction on the affected side in the low-frequency range.

When vibratory sensation is tested with a tuning fork on the extremities or the sternum, patients can hear the vibration in the affected ear, which allows easy identification of the affected side (Strupp and Zwergal 2019) (■ Fig. 12.3). Tympanoscopy can provide evidence of a hypermobile stapes.

12.1.1.3 Laboratory Examinations

Patients with suspected SCDS require combined vestibular and audiological testing and a high-resolution bone CT before the diagnosis can be made and the affected side identified. The application of vibration to the skull can also contribute to the diagnosis because this can lead to nystagmus in the plane of the affected canal (Dumas et al. 2019).

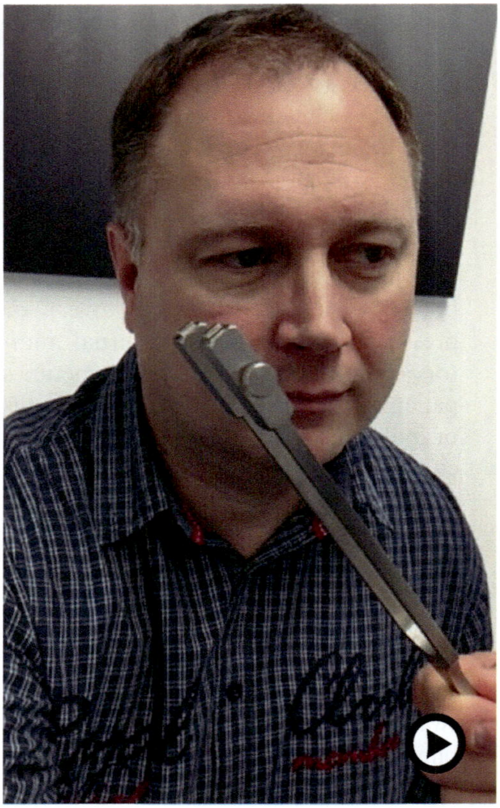

■ **Fig. 12.3** Use of the tuning fork to diagnose and localize the affected side in SCDS from (Strupp and Zwergal 2019) (► https://doi.org/10.1007/000-95z)

Vestibular Laboratory Testing

Videooculography This allows the recording of eye movements induced by changes in pressure or by certain sounds in order to determine the direction of the nystagmus induced. The nystagmus occurs in the plane of the affected semicircular canal, due to either excitation or inhibition depending on the stimulation method (see above). In patients with SCDS, it is helpful for the patient to look in the direction of the plane of the superior canal (e.g., 45° to the left if one expects left-sided SCDS) during such a recording, because a pure vertical nystagmus will be induced, which supports the diagnosis (■ Fig. 12.4).

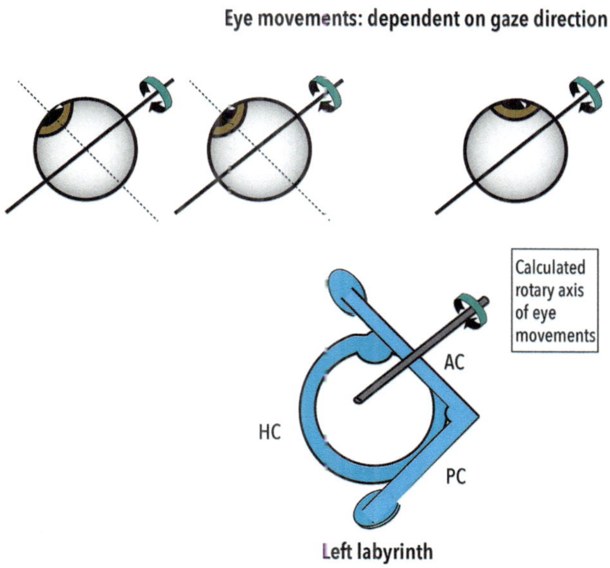

Fig. 12.4 Dependence of the direction of the nystagmus on the gaze direction in a patient with left-sided SCDS. If the patient looks 45° to the left, there will be a pure vertical nystagmus (top left). If the patient looks straight ahead (top right), there will be a vertical torsional nystagmus

Vestibular-evoked potentials (VEMP) Many studies (for references, see Fife et al. 2017; Papathanasiou and Straumann 2019) have demonstrated that VEMP can considerably contribute to the diagnosis of SCDS because the amplitudes are typically increased on the affected side. For ocular VEMP (oVEMP), it was shown that the optimal stimulation frequency is 4 kHz (Tran et al. 2020). Another study showed that if the amplitude of the oVEMP is higher than 16.7 μV, the sensitivity is 100% and the specificity is 39% (Verrecchia et al. 2019). An example is given in Fig. 12.5. However, oVEMP can also be elevated in patients without SCDS, namely in Menière's disease (Hassannia et al. 2021) which underlines that for the diagnosis several consistent criteria have to be fullfilled. For the cervical VEMP (cVEMP) with threshold recording, the best stimulation frequency is 2 kHz; under these conditions a specificity of almost 100% and a sensitivity of 92% was reported (Noij et al. 2019). Since oVEMP are easier to perform and do not depend on threshold measurements, they are recommended for clinical routine. In addition, a review of published papers showed that they are evidently more sensitive and more specific than cVEMP (Fife et al. 2017).

***Testing for Tullio phenomenon* using an audiometer** Sounds of certain frequencies can induce vertigo and nystagmus in the plane of the affected canal, which should ideally be recorded by videooculography.

The other vestibular laboratory examinations are mainly used for the exclusion of other diseases.

12.1.1.4 Audiological Examination

Patients often have negative bone conduction in the low-frequency range (≤500 Hz) (Fig. 12.6), which corresponds to autophony and supports the diagnosis.

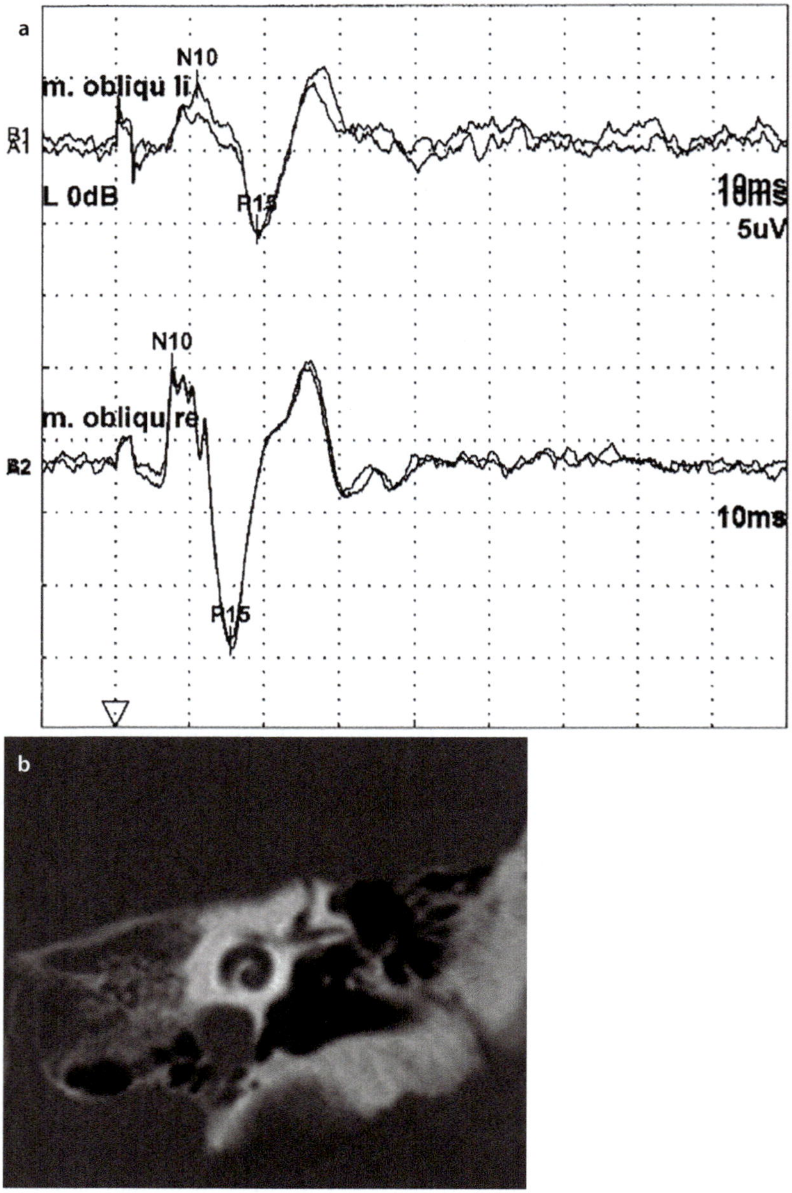

Fig. 12.5 **a** Ocular vestibular-evoked myogenic potentials (oVEMP) in a patient with left-sided SCDS. When recording from the right inferior oblique muscle (lower trace) during the stimulation of the left labyrinth, the amplitude of the N10-P15 is 19.8 μV compared to 10.1 μV on the non-affected side (upper trace). **b** High-resolution CT of the temporal bone shows the bony defect on top of the superior canal

12.1.2 Imaging

The bony defect on the superior canal (Fig. 12.7) can be visualized by a high-resolution temporal bone CT. The resolution must be ≤0.6 mm with 3D reconstruction perpendicular ("Stenvers") and parallel ("Poschel") to the affected semicircular canal (Fig. 12.7) (Mau et al. 2018; Ho 2019; Duman and Dogan

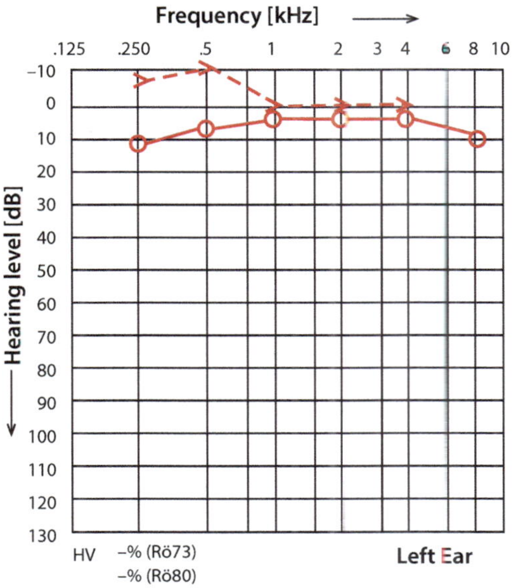

■ **Fig. 12.6** Pure tone audiometry with negative bone conduction in the low-frequency range of the affected right ear

2020), ideally with a flat panel CT (Tunkel et al. 2019). It is important not to generate false pathological findings. It should be noted that healthy subjects can also have a bony defect on a temporal bone CT of the superior canal. In a study on 500 healthy subjects, this was found on one side in 2% and on both sides in 0.6%; in 110 patients who had audiological and/or vestibular symptoms, 14% had a unilateral and 1.8% a bilateral bony defect without symptoms of SCDS (Berning et al. 2019). This clearly shows that a "pathological CT" alone is not sufficient for the diagnosis of SCDS. On the other hand, even small punctiform bony defects, which can hardly be visualized by CT, can lead to SCDS (Niesten et al. 2015). MRI should be used to exclude other pathologies (Spear et al. 2016).

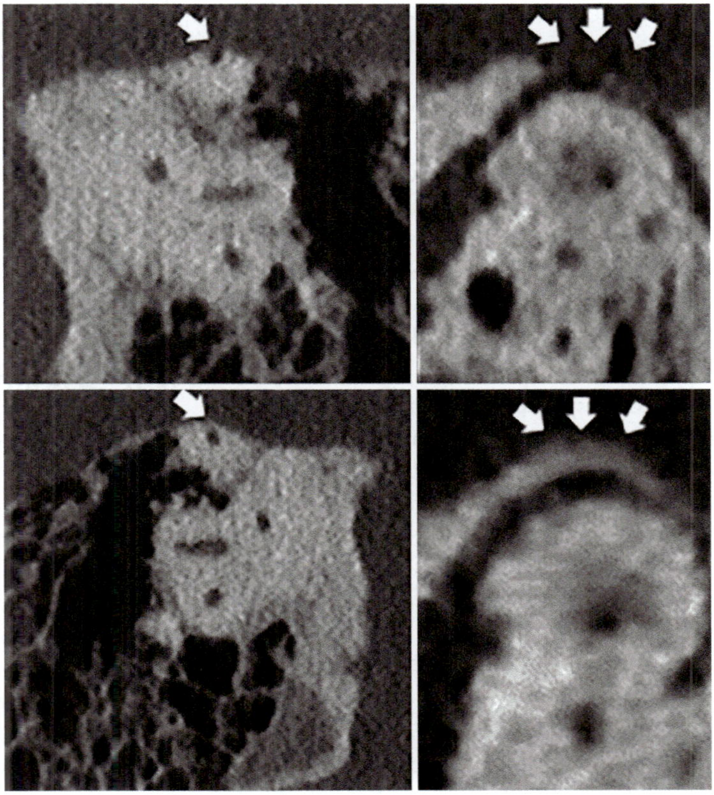

■ **Fig. 12.7** High-resolution CT of the temporal bone in two planes. **Top:** Bony defect of the left superior canal. This, however, is not sufficient for the diagnosis, because about 2% of all healthy subjects may show similar CT findings without any symptoms. **Bottom:** Normal temporal bone CT of the superior canal on the right side

12.1.3 Syndrome of Different Third Mobile Windows, Differential Diagnoses and Clinical Problems

The following types are also relevant:

Horizontal canal dehiscence syndrome (Zhang et al. 2011) *or posterior semicircular canal dehiscence syndrome* (Chien et al. 2011; Philip et al. 2019). The symptoms are similar to SCDS. However, analysis of the direction of the induced nystagmus and imaging allow a differentiation between the three subtypes. It is important to note that an elarged vestibular duct can lead to similar symptoms (Stahl and Otteson, 2022), namely autophony and a negative bone conduction. Therefore, this entity must always be considered as a subtype of the syndrome of the third mobile windows which can be seen on CT.

Bilateral SCDS Up to 50% of patients with SCDS anatomically have a very thin roof of the superior canal bilaterally (Carey et al. 2000), without necessarily having bilateral symptoms. Therefore, to make a correct diagnosis of symptomatic bilateral SCDS, not only the imaging, but also the other above-mentioned criteria should be fulfilled for both sides. Bilateral SCDS can lead to vertical oscillopsia and a vertical nystagmus (Deutschlander et al. 2004).

12

Secondary syndrome of the third mobile windows The above-mentioned symptoms and signs can also occur in other inner ear diseases that impair the integrity of the temporal bone, in particular cholesteatomas, meningiomas, or meningoceles and after head trauma (McCrary et al. 2021). Patients with Menière's disease can also develop a secondary syndrome of third mobile window.

Near dehiscence syndrome (N-SCDS) (i.e., roof of the superior semicircular canal thin, but not missing). In a study, the clinical and neurophysiological findings and predictors of successful surgical treatment in 17 N-SCDS patients were analyzed and compared to 16 patients with SCDS (Baxter et al. 2019). It was found that patients with N-SCDS had less frequent pressure- or sound-induced nystagmus, the cVEMP thresholds were higher and the oVEMP amplitudes were lower. In both cohorts, the results of the surgery were similar. One can thus conclude that SCDS and N-SCDS are part of a broad clinical spectrum, which may explain the diversity of this disease.

Perilymphatic fistula (see below, ▶ Sect. 12.2)

Box 12.2 Alphabetical List of the Important Differential Diagnoses of Syndrome of the Third Mobile Windows

- Bilateral syndrome of the third mobile windows
- Bilateral vestibulopathy
- BPPV
- Central positional vertigo
- Functional dizziness
- Menière's disease
- Panic attacks
- Vertebral artery compression/occlusion syndrome
- Vestibular paroxysmia
- Vestibular migraine

12.1.4 Diagnosis: The Essentials

As summarized in ▶ Box 12.1, the diagnosis of syndrome of the third mobile windows (in most cases, SCDS) relies on consistent findings, i.e., the combination of typical symptoms, clinical findings, and laboratory examinations, in particular o/cVEMP and a high-resolution CT of the temporal bone with 3D reconstruction. A systematic approach leads to a high consistency and reliability of the diagnosis (Naert et al. 2021). In this way, unnecessary operations can be avoided. A systematic approach, however, is often not yet the case in clinical practice (Cozart et al. 2021).

In addition, over the last 20 years, there has been a change of thinking: the above-mentioned symptoms were often wrongly attributed to a "perilymphatic fistula" (see ► Sect. 12.2); now there is a consensus that the vast majority of patients with syndrome of the third mobile windows do *not* have a fistula. Finally, many patients with a syndrome of the third mobile windows are misdiagnosed as having a functional disorder.

12.1.5 Pathophysiology and Etiology

Pathophysiology The above-mentioned symptoms and signs are caused by a pathological transduction of pressure via a third window (in addition to the round and oval windows) (◘ Fig. 12.7). This explains both the vestibular and audiological symptoms and signs and the findings of the laboratory examinations (for references, see Iversen and Rabbitt 2020). In healthy subjects, there is a transduction of pressure from the oval window to the inner ear and a conduction via the round window. The third window changes the biomechanics of the inner ear considerably (Rosowski et al. 2004): Pressure changes and sounds are partially transducted in the direction of the third window, which leads to pressure-induced symptoms and, for instance, the Tullio phenomenon, i.e., sound-induced nystagmus in the plane of the affected semicircular canal. SCD facilitates the flow of sound volume velocity through the cochlear partition at low frequencies, resulting in bone hyperacusis (Guan et al. 2020) which can also explain autophonia (Mikulec et al. 2004) as well as the increased amplitudes of the oVEMP and reduced cVEMP thresholds (Overview in Ward et al. 2017).

Etiology The precise etiology is still unclear. It is assumed that there is a primary congenital delay in bone growth above the superior canal (Carey et al. 2000). In addition, there is some evidence for destructing osteoclastic processes (Kamakura and Nadol Jr. 2017). There are also cases in which the symptoms begin after head trauma, barotrauma, or changes of pressure after lifting heavy weights, coughing, or pressing, which may lead to a rupture of the bone due to increased intracranial pressure.

12.1.6 Therapy: Principles and Pragmatic Treatment

In patients with only mild symptoms and signs, it is often sufficient to explain the mechanism of the disease and to recommend that they avoid changes in pressure. In cases with a more severe impairment, surgical treatment may be discussed and recommended.

12.1.6.1 Pragmatic Therapy

1. Explanation of the mechanism and the cause of the disease.
2. In mild cases with tolerable symptoms, a conservative approach is justified, i.e., recommendation to avoid changes in pressure as much as possible.
3. In cases with severe signs and symptoms and impairment of quality of life, surgery is possible (◘ Fig. 12.8):
   1. Canal plugging
   2. Resurfacing, i.e., restoring the surface of the superior semicircular canal
   3. Capping, i.e., simply covering the bony defect.

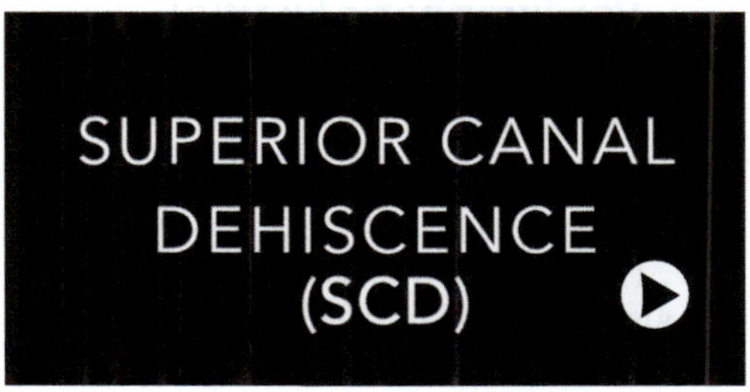

◘ **Fig. 12.8** Case of SCDS with different treatment options (courtesy of Louis Hofmeyr, Cape Town, SA) (► https://doi.org/10.1007/000-962)

Possible surgical approaches are via the middle fossa or through the mastoid; large case series have been published (e.g., Romiyo et al. 2019). In a retrospective study in ten patients, it was demonstrated that transmastoid resurfacing of the SCDS with cartilage is associated with many complications (33%), in particular CSF leaks, and the long-term results were not promising: 33% of the patients required a second operation (Al et al. 2019). In a study in 118 patients, it was shown that canal plugging can lead to significantly more vestibular symptoms due to the defect in the superior canal function, but with a lower incidence of tinnitus (Wung et al. 2019). In conclusion, there is so far no consensus about the best surgical methods and approach (Ward et al. 2017; Ossen et al. 2017). It should be noted that an estimation of the quality of life should be part of the evaluation of the therapeutic interventions (Allsopp et al. 2020), which is indeed improved by surgery (de Wolf et al. 2021).

Alternatively, a fixation of the stapes or a stabilization of the oval window can also be performed (Gona and Phillips 2020) which reduces the resonance oscillations. This, however, causes an improvement in only a small number of patients (Ahmed et al. 2019); but it also explains why in the past some patients with canal dehiscence syndromes, who were misdiagnosed with "perilymphatic fistula", responded to this treatment (see below).

12.2 Perilymphatic Fistula/Transient Perilymphatic Leakage

The leading symptom of "perilymphatic fistula" (PLF), which is very rare and which can also be called transient perilymph leakage (TPL, see below), is recurrent attacks of vertigo induced by changes in pressure or certain sounds, which are thus also caused by a third mobile window (for an overview, see Deveze et al. 2018; Weinreich and Carey 2019; Sarna et al. 2020). Most patients who were previously misdiagnosed with a PLF and had surgery most likely had SCDS, in particular since the fixation of the stapes (see above) can also result in an improvement of symptoms of SCDS. All in all, PLF is a very rare subtype of syndrome of the third mobile windows.

Although PLF was first described more than 100 years ago, there is still an ongoing discussion about the diagnostic criteria and the therapy. The current classification is summarized in ▶ Box 12.3. In addition to the above-mentioned tests for SCDS and the imaging studies of the temporal bone, measurement of Cochlin-tomoprotein has proved to be helpful to support the diagnosis of PLF (Ikezono et al. 2018).

Box 12.3 Suggested Japanese Classification of the Subtypes and Possible Etiologies of Perilymphatic Fistula (2017)

- Category 1 In the history, trauma, diseases of the middle or inner ear, operations:
  - (1a) Direct labyrinthine trauma (luxation of the stapes, fracture of the capsula otocius, etc.)
  - (1b) Other trauma (brain trauma, polytrauma, etc.)
  - (2a) Diseases of the middle or inner ear (cholesteatoma, other tumors, malformations, dehiscence, etc.)
  - (2b) Iatrogenic (surgery or other medical treatment, etc.)
- Category 2 External barotrauma: history of massive pressure changes (e.g., scuba diving or flying)
- Category 3 Internal barotrauma: history of internal pressure changes (e.g., physical exertion, sneezing, coughing, pressing)
- Category 4 No evident cause in the history

12.2.1 Terminology, Pathophysiology, and Therapeutic Principles

12.2.1.1 Terminology

A fistula (Latin *fistula*, i.e., a tube or pipe) is, by definition, a pathological tube-like connection between two hollow organs or between a hollow organ and the surface of the body. If one transfers this terminology to the perilymphatic space, one can assume that there is a leak of the perilymph, which leads to a impairment of function or a persisting loss of function of the inner ear. Therefore, one can also call this "transient perilymph leakage" (TPL).

12.2.1.2 Pathophysiology

The perilymphatic and the endolymphatic space lie within the bony labyrinth. The border of tissue between the bony labyrinth and the middle ear forms the annular ligament of the base of the stapes and the membrane of the round window. The TPL can be localized at the round or the oval window or may be due to bony defects, such as fractures, erosion of the bone, or microfissures of the labyrinth. A TPL is thus caused by a pathological connection between the perilymphatic space of the inner ear and the middle ear, the mastoid, or even in an intracranial direction.

12.2.1.3 Etiology

Possible causes are head trauma, barotrauma, chronic inflammation with erosion of the bone, tumors, in particular cholesteatomas, or surgical procedures such as stapedectomy or a cochlear implantation. However, simple traumas due to sneezing, coughing, or pressing or lifting heavy weights can lead to a TPL if the membranes or the bone covering are thin (see ► Box 12.3). Specific causes can be:

1. A bony defect in the direction of the epidural space, as in SCDS (see ► Sect. 12.1).
2. A pathological hypermobility of the stapes or the membrane of the oval or round window or the ossicular chain with a hypermotility of the stapes footplate (Dieterich et al. 1989).
3. A congenitally pathological bulging/prominence of the oval window causing a trans-stapedial CSF fistula, which leads to a perilymphatic hydrops and sensorineural hearing loss in children.
4. Fractures or microfissures, which extend, for instance, from the ampulla of the posterior canal to the round window.
5. Bony defects in the region of the lateral wall of the labyrinth (toward the middle ear) together with a partial collapse of the perilymphatic space ("floating labyrinth" (Nomura et al. 1992)) or
6. Chronic otitis media, which can also lead to a dehiscence of the horizontal canal (Chien et al. 2011).

All of these can lead to a pathological pressure transduction from the middle ear to the labyrinth, which leads to symptoms during the Valsalva maneuver. The therapeutic principles derive from the pathophysiology: conservative (spontaneous) or operative closure of the leakage.

12.2.2 Pragmatic Therapy

The therapy of the first choice for TPL is conservative, as most fistulas close spontaneously.

12.2.3 Conservative Therapy

Conservative therapy consists of 1–3 weeks of bed rest with moderate elevation of the head, if necessary a mild sedative, the administration of laxatives (to avoid pressing during bowel movements), and several weeks of limited physical activity that avoids all heavy lifting, abdominal pressing, strong coughing, or sneezing, even after improvement. This often leads to recovery. If conservative therapy fails and disturbing vestibular symptoms persist, exploratory tympanoscopy has been recommended to examine the oval and round windows. A retrospective analysis and review of the literature, however, questions the benefit of the frequently used tympanoscopy in patients with sudden hearing loss and suspected TPL: only 11–14% were identified with a leakage. It was concluded that there was no significant improvement after exploratory tympanostomy and sealing of the membranes for patients with a TPL (Heilen et al. 2020).

12.2.4 Surgical Therapy

Surgical closure of the leakage successfully relieves vertigo in only up to 70% of patients (overview in Deveze et al. 2018); the pre-existing hearing loss generally does not improve at all. The operative procedure involves the removal of the mucous membrane in the region of the fistula and its substitution with autologous material (perichondral tissue of the tragus or fascia by means of gel foam). Leakage of the oval window adjacent to the stapes footplate require a stapedectomy and prosthesis. Even if the operation is successful, the postoperative sensitivity of the patients to extreme physical strain (abdominal pressing, barotrauma) is greater than that of healthy subjects. Consequently, relapses occur not infrequently.

References

Ahmed W, Rajagopal R, Lloyd G (2019) Systematic review of round window operations for the treatment of superior semicircular canal dehiscence. J Int Adv Otol 15(2):209–214

Al AA, Farmer R, Bance M (2019) Outcomes of transmastoid resurfacing for superior canal dehiscence using a cartilage overlay technique. Laryngoscope 129(9):2164–2169

Allsopp T, Kim AH, Robbins AM, Page JC, Dornhoffer JL (2020) Quality of life outcomes after transmastoid plugging of superior semicircular canal dehiscence. Am J Otolaryngol 41(2):102287

Baxter M, McCorkle C, Trevino GC, Zuniga MG, Carter AM, Della Santina CC, Minor LB, Carey JP, Ward BK (2019) Clinical and physiologic predictors and postoperative outcomes of near dehiscence syndrome. Otol Neurotol 40(2):204–212

Berning AW, Arani K, Branstetter BF (2019) Prevalence of superior semicircular canal dehiscence on high-resolution CT imaging in patients without vestibular or auditory abnormalities. AJNR Am J Neuroradiol 40(4):709–712

Carey JP, Minor LB, Nager GT (2000) Dehiscence or thinning of bone overlying the superior semicircular canal in a temporal bone survey. Arch Otolaryngol Head Neck Surg 126(2):137–147

Chien WW, Carey JP, Minor LB (2011) Canal dehiscence. Curr Opin Neurol 24(1):25–31

Cozart AC, Kennedy JT, III, Seidman MD (2021) A basis for standardizing superior semicircular canal dehiscence management. Ear Nose Throat J 100:NP444–NP453

Deveze A, Matsuda H, Elziere M, Ikezono T (2018) Diagnosis and treatment of perilymphatic fistula. Adv Otorhinolaryngol 81:133–145

de Wolf MJF, Dawe N, Jervis S, Kumar R, Dalton CL, Lindley K, Irving R (2021) Transmastoid occlusion surgery for superior semicircular canal dehiscence syndrome improves patient-reported quality-of-life measures and corrects cVEMP thresholds and amplitudes. Otol Neurotol 42:1534–1543

Deutschlander A, Strupp M, Jahn K, Jager L, Quiring F, Brandt T (2004) Vertical oscillopsia in bilateral superior canal dehiscence syndrome. Neurology 62:784–787

Dieterich M, Brandt T, Fries W (1989) Otolith function in man: results from a case of otolith Tullio phenomenon. Brain 112:1377–1392

Duman IS, Dogan SN (2020) Contribution of reformatted multislice temporal computed tomography images in the planes of Stenvers and Poschl to the diagnosis of superior semicircular canal dehiscence. J Comput Assist Tomogr 44(1):53–58

Dumas G, Tan H, Dumas L, Perrin P, Lion A, Schmerber S (2019) Skull vibration induced nystagmus in patients with superior semicircular canal dehiscence. Eur Ann Otorhinolaryngol Head Neck Dis 136(4):263–272

Eberhard KE, Chari DA, Nakajima HH, Klokker M, Cayo-Thomasen P, Lee DJ (2021) Current trends, controversies, and future directions in the evaluation and management of superior canal dehiscence syndrome. Front Neurol 12:638574

Fife TD, Colebatch JG, Kerber KA, Brantberg K, Strupp M, Lee H, Walker MF, Ashman E, Fletcher

J, Callaghan B, Gloss DS (2017) Practice guideline: cervical and ocular vestibular evoked myogenic potential testing: report of the guideline development, dissemination, and implementation Subcommittee of the American Academy of Neurology. Neurology 89(22):2288–2296

Gona A, Phillips JS (2020) 'Soft reinforcement' of the round window for superior semi-circular canal dehiscence syndrome. J Laryngol Otol 134:366–368

Guan X, Cheng YS, Galaiya DJ, Rosowski JJ, Lee DJ, Nakajima HH (2020) Bone-conduction hyperacusis induced by superior canal dehiscence in human: the underlying mechanism. Sci Rep 10(1):16564

Hassannia F, Misale P, Harvey K, Yu E, Rutka JA (2021) Elevated ocular VEMP responses in the absence of a superior semicircular canal dehiscence. Am J Otolaryngol 42:102789

Heilen S, Lang CP, Warnecke A, Lenarz T, Durisin M (2020) Exploratory tympanotomy in sudden sensorineural hearing loss for the identification of a perilymphatic fistula - retrospective analysis and review of the literature. J Laryngol Otol 134(6):501–508

Ho ML (2019) Third window lesions. Neuroimaging Clin N Am 29(1):57–92

Ikezono T, Matsumura T, Matsuda H, Shikaze S, Saitoh S, Shindo S, Hasegawa S, Oh SH, Hagiwara Y, Ogawa Y, Ogawa H, Sato H, Tono T, Araki R, Maeda Y, Usami SI, Kase Y (2018) The diagnostic performance of a novel ELISA for human CTP (Cochlin-tomoprotein) to detect perilymph leakage. PLoS One 13(1):e0191498

Iversen MM, Rabbitt RD (2020) Biomechanics of third window syndrome. Front Neurol 11:891

Kamakura T, Nadol JB Jr (2017) Evidence of osteoclastic activity in the human temporal bone. Audiol Neurootol 22(4–5):218–225

Karam EZ, Moreno AF, Benavides MA (2021) Slit lamp demonstration of heartbeat nystagmus due to superior canal dehiscence. Neurology 97:642–643

Lee GS, Zhou G, Poe D, Kenna M, Amin M, Ohlms L, Gopen Q (2011) Clinical experience in diagnosis and management of superior semicircular canal dehiscence in children. Laryngoscope 121(10):2256–2261

Lee JA, Liu YF, Nguyen SA, McRackan TR, Meyer TA, Rizk HG (2020) Posterior Semicircular Canal Dehiscence: Case Series and Systematic Review. Otol Neurotol 41:511–521

Mau C, Kamal N, Badeti S, Reddy R Ying YM, Jyung RW, Liu JK (2018) Superior semicircular canal dehiscence: diagnosis and management. J Clin Neurosci 48:58–65

McCrary HC, Babajanian E, Patel N, Yang S, Kircher M, Carlson ML, Gurgel RK (2021) Superior semicircular canal dehiscence syndrome following head trauma: a multi-institutional review. Laryngoscope 131:E2810–E2818

Mikulec AA, McKenna MJ, Ramsey MJ, Rosowski JJ, Herrmann BS, Rauch SD, Curtin HD, Merchant SN (2004) Superior semicircular canal dehiscence presenting as conductive hearing loss without vertigo. Otol Neurotol 25(2):121–129

Milenkovic I, Sycha T, Berger-Sieczkowski E, Rommer P, Czerny C, Wiest G (2021) Pulse-synchronous torsional nystagmus. Pract Neurol 21:445–447

Minor LB, Solomon D, Zinreich JS, Zee DS (1998) Sound- and/or pressure-induced vertigo due to bone dehiscence of the superior semicircular canal. Arch Otolaryngol Head Neck Surg 124(3): 249–258

Morrison M, Korda A, Wagner F, Caversaccio MD, Mantokoudis G (2022) Case report: fremitus nystagmus in superior canal dehiscence syndrome. Front Neurol 13:844687

Naert L, Ocak I, Griet M, van de Berg R, Stultiens JJA, Van de Heyning P, Bisdorff A, Sharon JD, Ward BK, Van Rompaey V (2021) Prospective analysis of an evidence-based symptom set in superior canal dehiscence syndrome. Otol Neurotol 42(2): e186–e192

Niesten ME, Stieger C, Lee DJ, Merchant JP, Grolman W, Rosowski JJ, Nakajima HH (2015) Assessment of the effects of superior canal dehiscence location and size on intracochlear sound pressures. Audiol Neurootol 20(1):62–71

Noij KS, Herrmann BS, Guinan JJ Jr, Rauch SD (2019) Toward optimizing cVEMP: 2,000-Hz tone bursts improve the detection of superior canal dehiscence. Audiol Neurootol 23(6):335–344

Nomura Y, Okuno T, Hara M, Young YH (1992) "Floating" labyrinth. Pathophysiology and treatment of perilymph fistula. Acta Otolaryngol 112(2):186–191

Ossen ME, Stokroos R, Kingma H, van Tongeren J, Van Rompaey V, Temel Y, van de Berg R (2017) Heterogeneity in reported outcome measures after surgery in superior canal dehiscence syndrome-a systematic literature review. Front Neurol 8:347

Papathanasiou ES, Straumann D (2019) Why and when to refer patients for vestibular evoked myogenic potentials: a critical review. Clin Neurophysiol 130(9):1539–1556

Philip A, Mammen MD, Lepcha A, Alex A (2019) Posterior semicircular canal dehiscence: a diagnostic and surgical conundrum. BMJ Case Rep 12(7):e229573

Romiyo P, Duong C, Ng E, Wung V, Udawatta M, Nguyen T, Sheppard JP, Preet K, Alemnew M, Seo D, Gopen Q, Yang I (2019) Superior semicircular canal dehiscence postoperative outcomes: a case series of 156 repairs. J Clin Neurosci 68:69–72

Rosowski JJ, Songer JE, Nakajima HH, Brinsko KM, Merchant SN (2004) Clinical, experimental, and theoretical investigations of the effect of superior

semicircular canal dehiscence on hearing mechanisms. Otol Neurotol 25(3):323–332
Sarna B, Abouzari M, Merna C, Jamshidi S, Saber T, Djalilian HR (2020) Perilymphatic fistula: a review of classification, etiology, diagnosis, and treatment. Front Neurol 11:1046
Spear SA, Jackson NM, Mehta R, Morel CE, Miller LS, Anderson D, Arriaga MA (2016) Is MRI equal to CT in the evaluation of thin and dehiscent superior semicircular canals? Otol Neurotol 37(2):167–170
Stahl MC, Otteson T (2022) Systematic review on vestibular symptoms in patients with enlarged vestibular aqueducts. Laryngoscope 132:873–880
Steenerson KK, Crane BT, Minor LB (2020) Superior semicircular canal dehiscence syndrome. Semin Neurol 40(1):151–159
Strupp M, Zwergal A (2019) Teaching video NeuroImages: use your tuning fork to diagnose vertigo. Neurology 93(15):e1497
Tran ED, Swanson A, Sharon JD, Vaisbuch Y, Blevins NH, Fitzgerald MB, Steenerson KK (2020) Ocular vestibular-evoked myogenic potential amplitudes elicited at 4 kHz optimize detection of superior semicircular canal dehiscence. Front Neurol 11:879
Tunkel AE, Carey JP, Pearl M (2019) Flat panel computed tomography in the diagnosis of superior semicircular canal dehiscence syndrome. Otol Neurotol 40(2):213–217
Verrecchia L, Brantberg K, Tawfique Z, Maoli D (2019) Diagnostic accuracy of ocular vestibular evoked myogenic potentials for superior canal dehiscence syndrome in a large cohort of dizzy patients. Ear Hear 40(2):287–294
Ward BK, Carey JP, Minor LB (2017) Superior canal dehiscence syndrome: lessons from the first 20 years. Front Neurol 8:177
Ward BK., van de Berg R, van Rompaey V, Bisdorff A, Hullar TE, Welgampola MS, Carey JP (2021) Semicircular canal dehiscence syndrome (SCDS): diagnostic criteria of the Bàràny Society 31(3):131–141
Watson SRD, Halmagyi GM, Colebatch JG (2000) Vestibular hypersensitivity to sound (Tullio phenomenon): structural and functional assessment. Neurology 54(3):722–728
Weinreich HM, Carey JP (2019) Perilymphatic fistulas and superior semi-circular canal dehiscence syndrome. Adv Otorhinolaryngol 82:93–100
Wung V, Romiyo P, Ng E, Duong C, Nguyen T, Seo D, Yang I, Gopen Q (2019) Sealing of superior semicircular canal dehiscence is associated with improved balance outcomes postoperatively versus plugging of the canal in middle fossa craniotomy repairs: a case series. J Neurosurg 28:1–5
Young AS, McMonagle B, Pohl DV, Magnussen J, Welgampola MS (2019) Superior semicircular canal dehiscence presenting with recurrent positional vertigo. Neurology 93(24):1070–1072
Zhang LC, Sha Y, Dai CF (2011) Another etiology for vertigo due to idiopathic lateral semicircular canal bony defect. Auris Nasus Larynx 38(3):402–405

Central Vestibular Disorders

Contents

Supplementary Information The online version contains supplementary material available at [https://doi.org/10.1007/978-3-030-78260-3_13]. The videos can be accessed by scanning the related images with the SN More Media App.

M. Strupp et al., *Vertigo and Dizziness*, https://doi.org/10.1007/978-3-030-78260-3_13

13.1 General Survey of Central Vestibular Syndromes

13.1.1 Clinical Synopsis

Central vestibular forms of vertigo are caused by lesions along the vestibular pathways in the brainstem, which extend from the vestibular nuclei in the medulla oblongata to the ocular motor nuclei and integration centers in the rostral midbrain, and to the vestibulocerebellum, the thalamus, and multisensory vestibular cortex areas in the temporoparietal cortex (Brandt and Dieterich 1994; Dieterich and Brandt 1993a; Baier et al. 2008; Baier and Dieterich 2009) (■ Fig. 13.1). In tertiary interdisciplinary outpatient dizziness units, central vestibular disorders including vestibular migraine comprise about 25% of the established diagnoses (Newman-Toker et al. 2008; Kerber et al. 2017; Vanni et al. 2015; Brandt and Dieterich 2017; Zwergal and Dieterich 2020).

On the one hand, central vestibular disorders are clearly defined clinical syndromes of various etiologies, for example, downbeat or upbeat nystagmus. The occurrence of these typical ocular motor findings in only

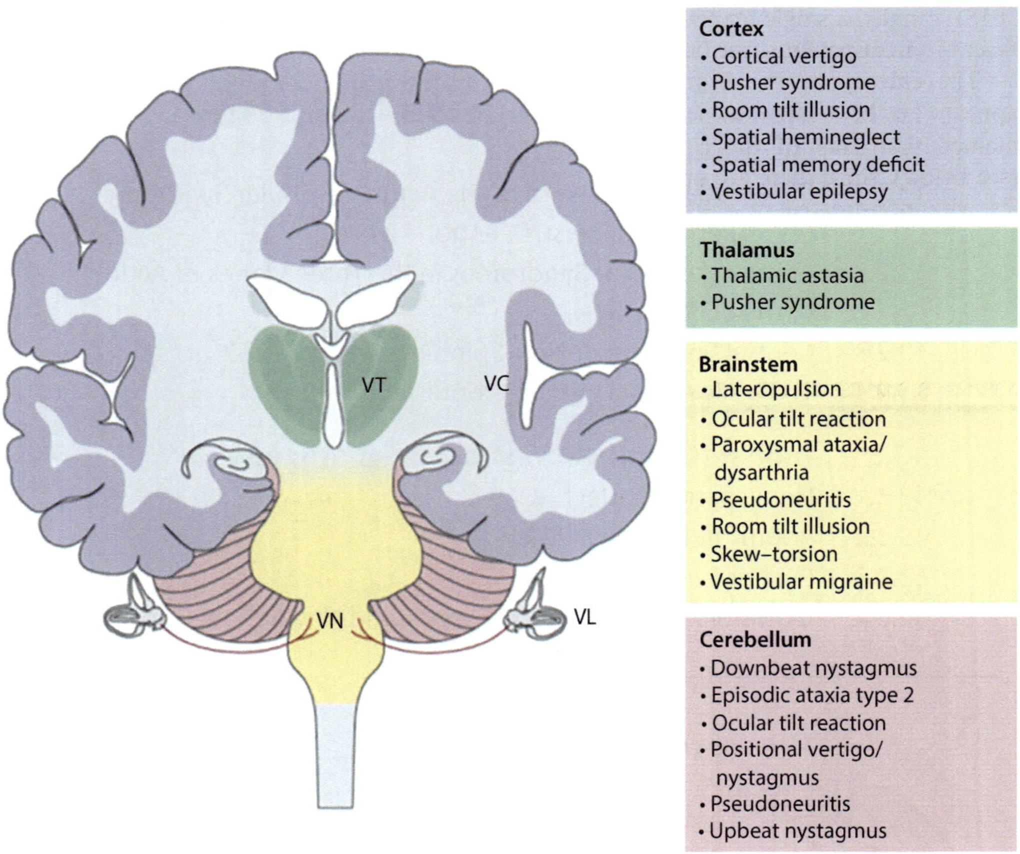

■ **Fig. 13.1** Central vestibular syndromes and disorders of higher vestibular function. The schematic drawing presents an incomplete list of syndromes that have been attributed to cortical, thalamic, brainstem, or cerebellar lesions. Some disorders are linked to central lesions at multiple levels. For example, the ocular tilt reaction can be caused by brainstem or cerebellar lesions. In some conditions, the topographic assignment is uncertain. VC vestibular cortex, VL vestibular labyrinth, VN vestibular nucleus, VT vestibular thalamus. (Brandt and Dieterich 2017) (pseudoneuritis is an acute central vestibular syndrome, ACVS)

cerebellar or brainstem lesions allows their definite localization. On the other hand, central vestibular symptoms can also be a part of a more complex infratentorial clinical syndrome with other symptoms or supranuclear/nuclear/fascicular ocular motor disorders and/or other neurological brainstem deficits (e.g., in Wallenberg's syndrome or midbrain infarction).

The beginning and duration of the symptoms help in the differential diagnosis of central vestibular forms of vertigo:

- **Short attacks of spinning vertigo or postural imbalance lasting seconds to minutes** or for a few hours are caused by transient ischemic attacks within the vertebrobasilar territory, vestibular migraine, episodic ataxia type 2, paroxysmal brainstem attacks with ataxia/dysarthria in MS, and rarely by vestibular epilepsy.
- **Episodes of spinning vertigo or postural imbalance lasting hours to several days**, generally with additional brainstem deficits, can be caused by an infarction, hemorrhage, or MS plaque in the brainstem, rarely by a long-lasting attack of vestibular migraine.
- **Several days to weeks (or even longer periods) of persisting postural imbalance** (seldom persisting spinning vertigo), combined with a tendency to fall in a certain direction, is usually caused by permanent damage to the brainstem or the cerebellum bilaterally, e.g., downbeat nystagmus syndrome (Fig. 13.2) most often due to degenerative cerebellar disease or the temporary upbeat nystagmus syndrome (Fig. 13.3) due to paramedian pontomedullary or pontomesencephalic damage (infarction, hemorrhage, tumor, intoxication).

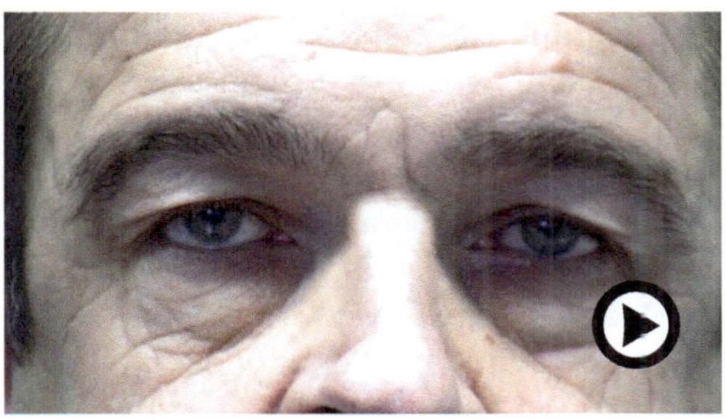

Fig. 13.2 Downbeat nystagmus
(▶ https://doi.org/10.1007/000-966)

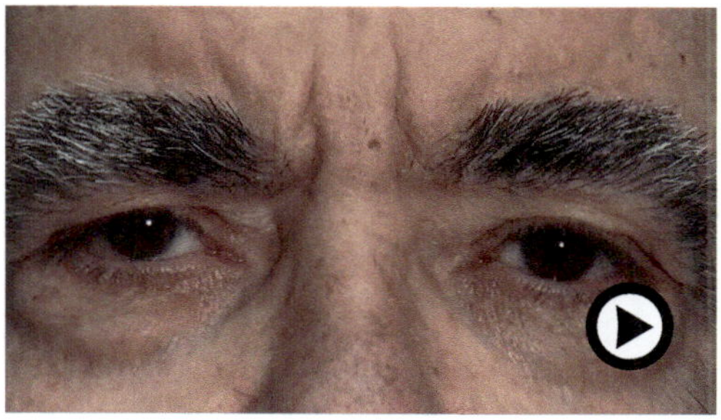

Fig. 13.3 Upbeat nystagmus
(▶ https://doi.org/10.1007/000-964)

In peripheral vestibular disorders, specific dysfunctions like spontaneous or positional nystagmus can be precisely ascribed to the affected labyrinthine structure. For example, canalolithiasis of the vertical or the horizontal canals in benign paroxysmal positional vertigo can be unambiguously identified by the direction of the positional nystagmus elicited by head movements in the plane of the affected canal. In contrast, syndromes that are identical in central vestibular disorders can originate from separate and distinct lesions within the vestibular circuitry, especially in the brainstem and cerebellum (Dieterich and Brandt 1993a; Brandt and Dieterich 1994; Baier et al. 2008, 2012b). This is best illustrated by a central vestibular tone imbalance due to unilateral lesions of the graviceptive pathways. The graviceptive pathways originate from the labyrinthine otoliths and vertical semicircular canals. They mediate our perception of verticality and stabilize gaze, head and body in the upright position. Lesions of the pathways can cause, for example, similar syndromes of a vestibular tone imbalance in the roll plane (Dieterich and Brandt 1993a, b) (Fig. 13.4).

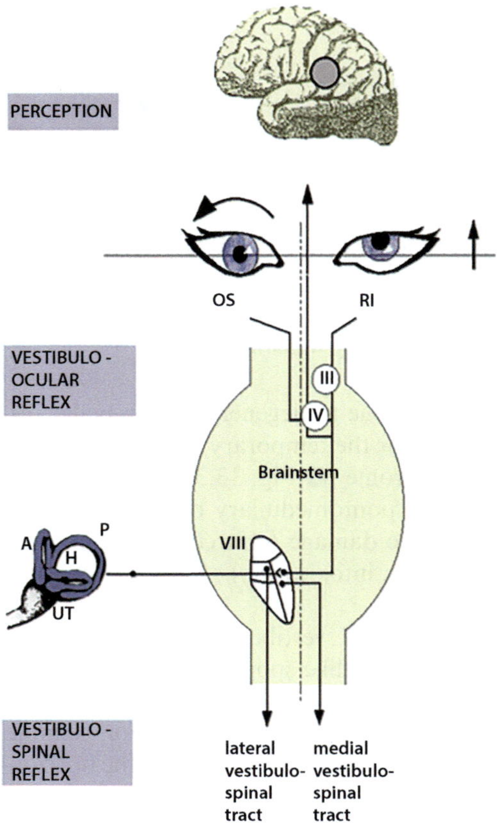

Fig. 13.4 Schematic drawing representing the vestibulo-ocular reflex (VOR) with its three-neuron arc and its mediation of ocular motor, perceptual and postural functions, as well as an ocular tilt reaction with ocular torsion and vertical deviation of the eyes due to a tone imbalance of the graviceptive pathways (see arrows for rotation and upward deviation of the eyes). A, H, P anterior, horizontal, and posterior semicircular canals, RI inferior rectus muscle, OS superior oblique muscle, III, IV, VIII nuclei of cranial nerves, UT utricle

13

Unilateral cortical lesions of the multisensory vestibular network may cause higher cognitive vestibular disorders modulated by a thalamo-cortical vestibular lateralization (dominance of the right hemisphere in right-handers; dominance of the left hemisphere in left-handers). This is reflected by a more frequent manifestation and more severe course of the hemineglect and the pusher syndrome after acute right-sided infarctions of the middle cerebral artery (Brandt et al. 2014).

The examples of central vestibular syndromes mentioned above may be difficult for physicians managing dizzy patients to understand, since signs and symptoms can mimic those of peripheral vestibular disorders. The bilateral structure of the vestibular system helps us to understand its sensorimotor, perceptual and cognitive functions, as well as its disorders.

13.1.2 The Bilateral Central Vestibular Network

The most important structures in central vestibular forms of vertigo are the neuronal pathways mediating the vestibulo-ocular reflex (VOR) (Fig. 13.4). They travel from the peripheral labyrinth over the vestibular nuclei in the medullary brainstem to the ocular motor nuclei (III, IV, VI) and the supranuclear integration centers in the pons and midbrain (interstitial nucleus of Cajal, INC, and rostral interstitial nucleus of the medial longitudinal fascicle, riMLF) (Brandt and Dieterich 1994, 2017) (Figs. 13.4 and 13.5). Compensatory eye movements are generated over this three-neuron reflex arc during rapid head and body movements. Also of importance are the interstitial nucleus of Cajal, the INC, and the rostral interstitial nucleus of the MLF, the riMLF, as integration centers in the midbrain for vertical and torsional eye movements, as well as the nucleus prepositus hypoglossi together with the vestibular nuclei and the cerebellum as integration centers for horizontal eye movements.

Ascending pathways travel both contralaterally and ipsilaterally (Zwergal et al.

2008) over the posterolateral thalamus up to a network of vestibular areas in the parietotemporal cortex and the posterior insula, e.g., the parietoinsular vestibular cortex (PIVC), and areas in the superior temporal gyrus and inferior parietal lobes, which are primarily responsible for perception, self-motion, and orientation in space. Descending pathways lead from the vestibular nuclei along the medial and lateral vestibulospinal tract into the spinal cord to mediate postural control. In addition, there are numerous pathways to the vestibulocerebellum.

Thus, disorders of the VOR are characterized not only by ocular motor deficits, but also by disorders of perception (due to impaired vestibulocortical projections of the VOR) and by disorders of postural control (due to impaired vestibulospinal projections of the VOR) (◘ Fig. 13.4).

The *bilateral* anatomical organization of the vestibular system provides four functional advantages: optimal differentiation of active and passive head motion, spatial orientation, sensory substitution of a unilateral peripheral failure, and central compensation of a peripheral or central vestibular tone imbalance (Dieterich and Brandt 2015a).

The structure is based on bilaterally ascending and descending pathways and at least five crossings, three in the brainstem (first between the vestibular nuclei; second in the pons above the vestibular nuclei; and third in the rostral midbrain tegmentum). There are at least two crossings between the hemispheres: one between the insular-opercular cortices (i.e., the core region of the vestibular cortex) via the splenium of the corpus callosum and the other probably between the multisensory cortical visual motion areas MST (Kirsch et al. 2016; Dieterich and Brandt 2018a, b; Conrad et al. 2022b) (◘ Fig. 13.5).

The resulting sensorimotor and cognitive functions within this network can be

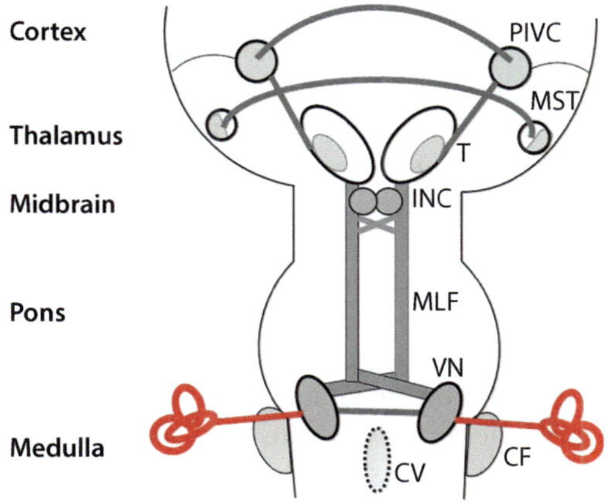

◘ **Fig. 13.5** Schematic drawing of the bilaterally organized anatomical vestibular structures from the labyrinth via the vestibular nerve and the vestibular nucleus (VN) to the multisensory vestibular cortex (parieto-insular vestibular cortex, PIVC) and the medial superior temporal area (MST) of the visual cortex. The vestibular input of the peripheral end organ (in red) is mediated ipsilaterally and contralaterally, in particular, via the medial longitudinal fascicle (MLF) to the midbrain tegmentum with the interstitial nucleus of Cajal (INC). Three important crossings of the ascending vestibular pathways were found in the brainstem: one between the vestibular nuclei, a second in the pons above the vestibular nuclei, and a third in the midbrain at the level of the oculomotor nuclei and the INC. Two crossings are known at the cortical level, the most important one between the core area PIVC of both hemispheres traveling through the corpus callosum in the posterior part of the splenium. Another connects the multisensory areas responsible for motion detection MST in the secondary visual cortex of both hemispheres

subdivided from caudal brainstem to cortex into three major groups (Dieterich and Brandt 2015a):

1. Reflexive control of gaze, head, and body in three spatial planes (yaw, pitch, roll) at brainstem-cerebellar level
2. Perception of self-motion and control of voluntary movement and balance at the cortical/subcortical level
3. Higher vestibular cognitive functions, e.g., spatial memory and navigation.

With respect to descending vestibulospinal pathways, a fourth function can be differentiated: a monosymptomatic axial lateropulsion without additional vestibular signs and symptoms in lateral medullary brainstem lesions (Thömke et al. 2005; Kim et al. 2007, 2015a).

This concept of specific reflexive and voluntary sensorimotor functions and cognition as dependent on the level of the lesion site from the medullary brainstem to the cortex helps the clinician to localize circumscribed disorders.

13.1.3 Anatomical Separation of Peripheral and Central Vestibular Structures

The traditional classification of vestibular disorders is based on the anatomical lesion site and distinguishes between the peripheral vestibular system and the central vestibular system. The former includes the labyrinth and the vestibular nerve, that is, the first-order neurons are classified as peripheral. By contrast, the vestibular nuclei in the pontomedullary brainstem and the vestibular pathways that project from these nuclei to the vestibulocerebellum (via the cerebellar peduncles), brainstem, thalamus, and cortex areas are grouped as central structures (◘ Fig. 13.4). When applied clinically, this simple anatomical distinction suffers from certain weaknesses. The first weakness is the inaccuracy in diagnosing disorders originating at the transition from the peripheral to the central system, i.e., the root entry zone of the eighth nerve. This area is subserved by the peripheral vestibular neuron traversing from the vestibular ganglion to the vestibular nucleus and is "peripheral" by definition. Thus, lesions of the root entry zone of the eighth nerve—although anatomically peripheral—require a neurological approach to disclose lacunar infarctions or MS plaques (acute central vestibular syndrome; formerly named "pseudoneuritis") (Kim and Lee 2010; Brandt et al. 2014). Another weakness of a purely anatomical distinction between peripheral and central vestibular disorders involves the sensitivity and specificity of the attribution of a distinct dysfunction to a lesioned structure, which is easier to do for peripheral than for central disorders (Brandt and Dieterich 2017).

13.1.4 Dominance of the Central Thalamocortical Vestibular System

The bilateral organization of human brain functions is characterized by a hemispheric specialization that is determined by phylogenetic, genetic, and developmental factors (Tzourio-Mazoyer 2016; Tzourio-Mazoyer et al. 2017; Dieterich and Brandt 2018a, b; Brandt and Dieterich 2019). This has been primarily investigated for handedness and the lateralization of language (Ocklenburg et al. 2013a, b). Apparently, language does not strictly depend on handedness, since almost all right-handers and nearly 70% of left-handers have left-hemispheric control for language (Scharoun and Bryden 2014). Hemispheric lateralization of handedness and speech is slowly established in the developing brain, appearing to be relatively determined by age 3 (Hodgson et al. 2016). The input of sensory modalities is mediated in both hemispheres, but lateralization may also depend on context. An fMRI and MEG study showed that the right acoustic cortex was predominantly activated during passive listening to different sound localizations (Brunetti et al. 2005), when applying complex periodic sounds in MEG (Coffey et al. 2016) and in a combination of EEG and fMRI (Coffey et al. 2017).

The vestibular network with two labyrinths is special because it requires a continuous interaction between right and left network structures at different levels—

especially the hemispheres—for a global perception of self-motion, of gravity vector, and spatial orientation. This is necessary for adequate motor responses to body accelerations in order to maintain postural balance (Dieterich and Brandt 2018a, b). Nevertheless, the syndromes and courses of multisensory cortical vestibular syndromes (e.g., spatial hemineglect, pusher syndrome) can only be understood on the basis of specialization and lateralization of hemispheric brain functions.

A PET study found that the vestibular cortical network has a right-hemispheric dominance in right-handers and a left-hemispheric dominance in left-handers (Dieterich et al. 2003) (◘ Fig. 13.6). This study was based on caloric vestibular stimulation and could be confirmed by fMRI during galvanic vestibular stimulation and auditory-evoked vestibular (otolith) stimulation (Fink et al. 2003; Schlindwein et al. 2008; Janzen et al. 2008) (◘ Fig. 13.7). A meta-analytical analysis using activation likelihood estimation for the integration of the so far published neuroimaging results of the vestibular system in humans confirmed the dominance of the right hemisphere in right-handers and found the core region of the vestibular cortical circuitry to be a parietal opercular area, OP2 (Eulenburg zu et al. 2012). Another meta-analysis, which also investigated the precise localization of the vestibular cortical network by using functional MRI studies, identified the posterior insula (short insular gyrus III, long insular gyrus IV), the retroinsular cortex (Ri), and the parietal operculum (OP2) as core regions depending on the vestibular activation by caloric, galvanic, or auditory vestibular stimulation (Lopez et al. 2012a). The latter regions seem to be the human homolog of the core region of the "parieto-insular vestibular cortex" (PIVC), which was first discovered in electrophysiological studies of the monkey (Grüsser et al. 1990a, b; Guldin and Grüsser 1998). The regions of the posterior insular, retroinsular, and opercular cortex within the right hemisphere also showed a volume increase 6 months after damage of the vestibular pathways due to a unilateral pontomedullary brainstem stroke affecting the vestibular nucleus (Conrad et al. 2020, 2021, 2022a, b) (◘ Fig. 13.8). Functional MRI connectivity-based parcellation of the vestibular network in both hemispheres in right-handers and left-handers showed that the vestibular dominance was located in the area of the posterior insula and parietal operculum, whereas the surrounding multisensory vestibular cortical regions (superior temporal gyrus, inferior parietal lobule, inferior frontal gyrus) were organized symmetrically, connecting the other sensory systems (auditory, visual) (Kirsch et al. 2018).

Structural and functional lateralization of the central vestibular system is not restricted to the vestibular cortex but seems to include the thalamus and upper brainstem. MRI diffusion tensor imaging tractography in right-handers was performed on the bilateral vestibular brainstem pathways from the vestibular nuclei via the paramedian and posterolateral thalamic subnuclei to the multisensory vestibular cortex (Dieterich et al. 2017) (◘ Fig. 13.9). Quantitative analysis revealed a rope-ladder-like system of vestibular pathways in the brainstem with crossings at pontine and mesencephalic levels. Three structural types of right-left fiber distributions could be delineated: (i) evenly distributed pathways at the lower pontine level from the vestibular nuclei to the pontine crossing; (ii) a moderate, pontomesencephalic right-sided lateralization between the pontine and mesencephalic crossings; and (iii) a further increase of the right-sided lateralization above the mesencephalic crossing leading to the thalamic vestibular subnuclei. The increasing lateralization along the brainstem was the result of an asymmetric number of pontine and mesencephalic crossing fibers which was higher

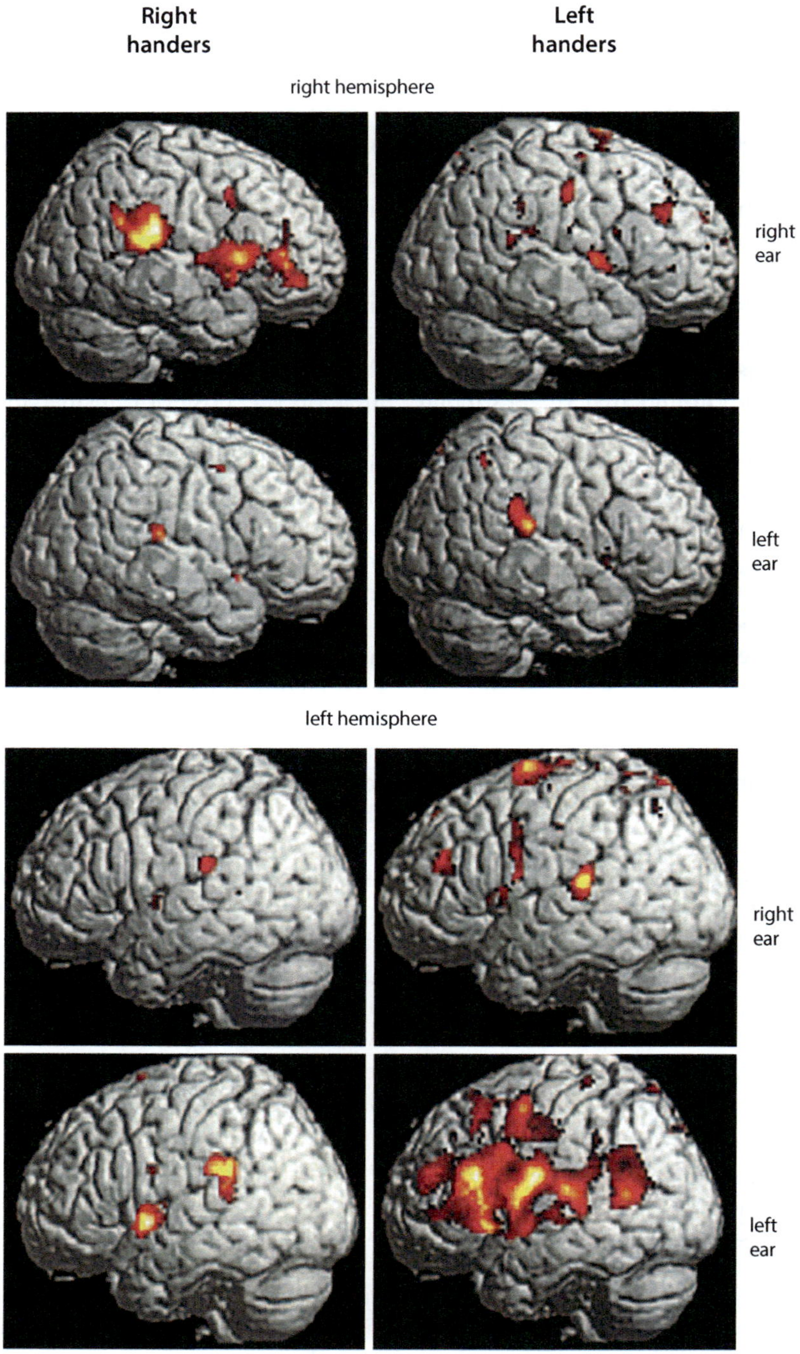

13

Fig. 13.6 PET activation pattern of 12 healthy right-handed and 12 healthy left-handed volunteers during caloric vestibular stimulation of the right or left ear ($H_2{}^{15}O$-PET). Activations were found in the temporo-parieto-insular region of both hemispheres with a dominance within the right hemisphere in right-handers and within the left hemisphere in left-handers. The network of activated areas includes the posterior insular-opercular region, superior temporal gyrus, inferior frontal gyrus, anterior insula, inferior parietal lobule, hippocampus, and cingulum. (Modified from Dieterich et al. 2003)

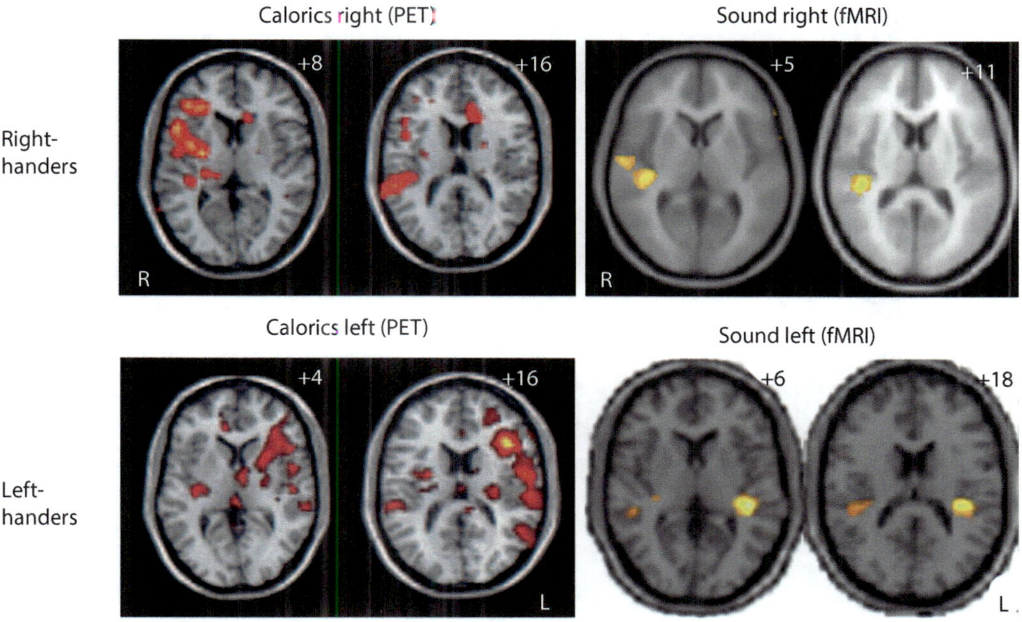

Fig. 13.7 Activation patterns for different PET and fMRI studies during vestibular stimulation in healthy right-handers and left-handers. In PET, a caloric vestibular stimulation of the horizontal semicircular canals was performed. In fMRI, a stimulation of the sacculus by click-induced cervical vestibular evoked myogenic potentials (cVEMP) was performed. Separate presentation for right-handers and left-handers. Activated areas lie in the insular and retroinsular cortex, superior temporal gyrus, and inferior parietal lobe and are more enhanced in the right hemisphere in right-handers and in the left hemisphere in left-handers. (Dieterich and Brandt 2018b)

for left-to-right crossings. The dominance of the right vestibular meso-diencephalic circuitry in right-handers corresponds to the right hemispheric dominance of the vestibular cortical network.

The establishment of vestibular lateralization is based on two separate thalamocortical networks (Brandt and Dieterich 2018, 2019) (Fig. 13.10) which are the structural basis for non-reflexive higher multisensorimotor and cognitive vestibular functions organized in cooperative provincial and connector hubs (Hwang et al. 2017). The absence of direct interconnections between the two thalamic nuclei "separates" the right and left thalamocortical networks. This allows the two hemispheres to operate simultaneously while using different spatial reference systems: egocentric manipulation of objects (handedness) and allocentric spatial orientation of the self. This separation of the two thalamocortical networks may be a precondition for different neuronal networks to develop during maturation in infancy and thus allow the lateralization of certain brain functions such as vestibular dominance (Brandt and Dieterich 2015).

This is compatible with the concept of lateralization of spatial attention: a left hemispheric egocentric focus for categorical recognition of objects and a right-hemispheric global allocentric focus for mediating large-scale spatial coordinates (Van der Ham et al. 2014).

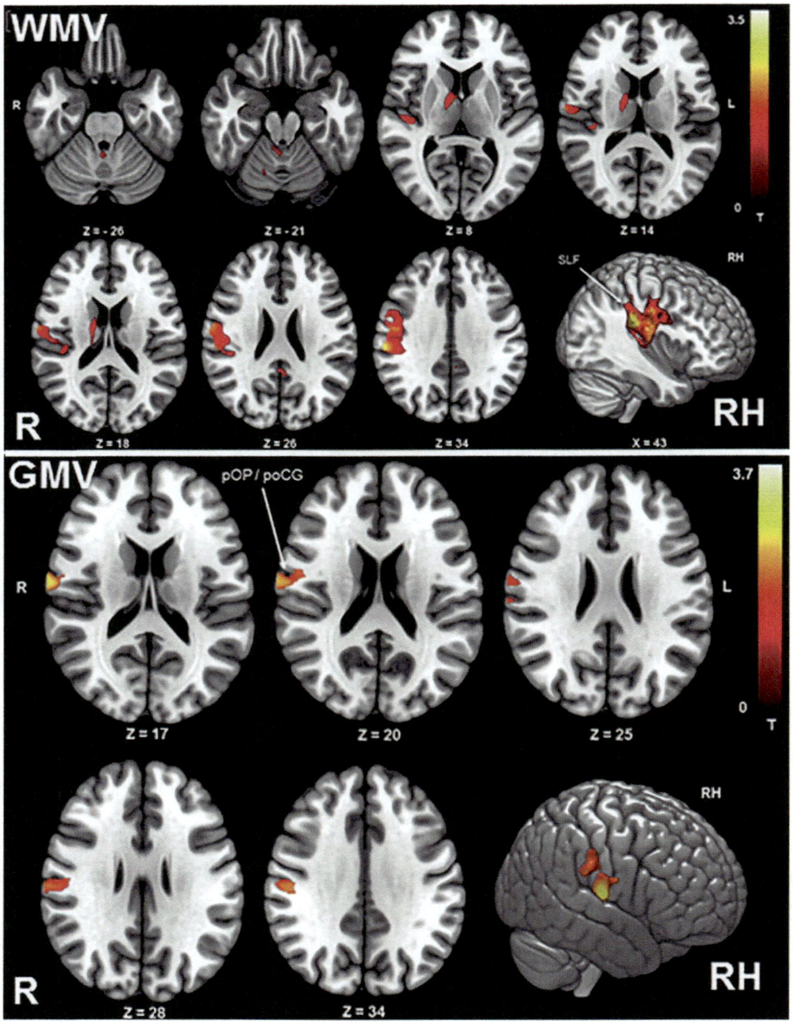

Fig. 13.8 Voxel-based morphometry in 15 patients with acute unilateral pontomedullary infarctions 6 months after stroke onset compared to age-matched healthy volunteers. Grey matter volume increases (GMV) and white matter volume increases (WMV) are shown. GMV and WMV increases are located in the retroinsular cortex, parietal operculum, postcentral gyrus, and superior temporal gyrus predominantly of the right hemisphere (RH). WMV increases and GMV increases in those patients ($n = 9$) who presented with spontaneous nystagmus in the acute phase were found in the parietal opercular cortex and postcentral gyrus of the right hemisphere only as well as the right anterior thalamus (for WMV increases). These data confirm the concept of a vestibular dominance of the right hemisphere in right-handers (Conrad et al. 2020). (OP parietal operculum, poCG postcentral gyrus, SLF superior longitudinal fascicle)

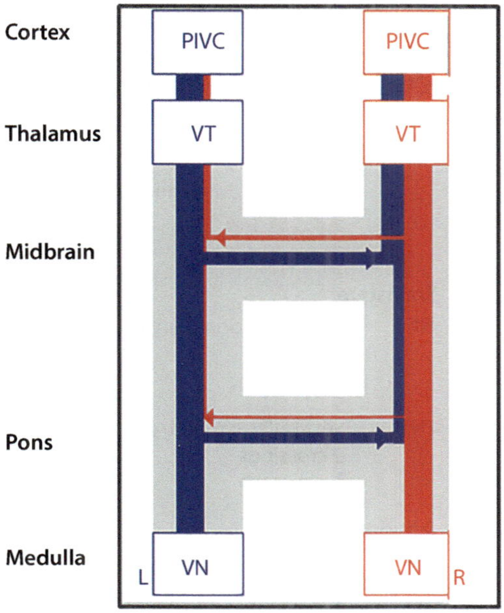

Fig. 13.9 MRI diffusion-weighted tractography of the vestibular pathways from the vestibular nuclei (VN) in the medullary brainstem via the paramedian and posterolateral thalamus (VT) to the parieto-insular vestibular cortex (PIVC) in the posterior insula. The quantitative schematic representation of the ipsilateral (vertical) and contralateral (horizontally crossing) pathways, which were analyzed from the two regions of interest (ROI) of the paramedian and posterolateral thalamus, visualizes the number of fibers by the width of the line. Due to the different number of crossing fibers (more from left, L, to right, R) at pontine and midbrain level, an asymmetry of fibers results with a preponderance of the right side in the upper midbrain, thalamus, and cortex. The arrow direction gives the fiber direction from origin to target, but does not allow differentiation between afferent/ascending and efferent/descending pathways. Pathways from the right vestibular nucleus are depicted in red, those from the left in blue. (Dieterich et al. 2017)

13.1.5 Reciprocal Inhibitory Interaction Between the Vestibular, the Visual, and the Somatosensory Systems

When the neurons within the temporo-parietal vestibular network are activated in both hemispheres, a downregulation (deactivation) occurs within the visual and somatosensory cortex bilaterally (Wenzel et al. 1996; Bense et al. 2001). Since opposite activation-deactivation patterns were found during visually induced self-motion perception, for example, activations of occipital and parietal visual areas co-occurring with deactivations of the multisensory vestibular cortex, e.g., the PIVC (Brandt et al. 1998, 2000; Dieterich et al. 2003), it was assumed that a reciprocal inhibitory cortical interaction takes place between the two sensory systems, the visual and the vestibular systems (Brandt et al. 1998). This interaction provides a powerful means for shifting the sensorial weight from the less to the more reliable modality in order to resolve potential perceptual conflicts in situations with mismatched sensory inputs. A reciprocal inhibitory interaction between sensory systems is a fundamental perceptual mechanism of the cortex (Brandt and Dieterich 1999). Such interactions were also seen between other sensory modalities, e.g., the somatosensory and nociceptive, the nociceptive and the vestibular, the tactile sensory and visual, and the visual and auditory systems (Bense et al. 2001; Laurienti et al. 2002; Maihöfner et al. 2006; Merabet et al. 2007).

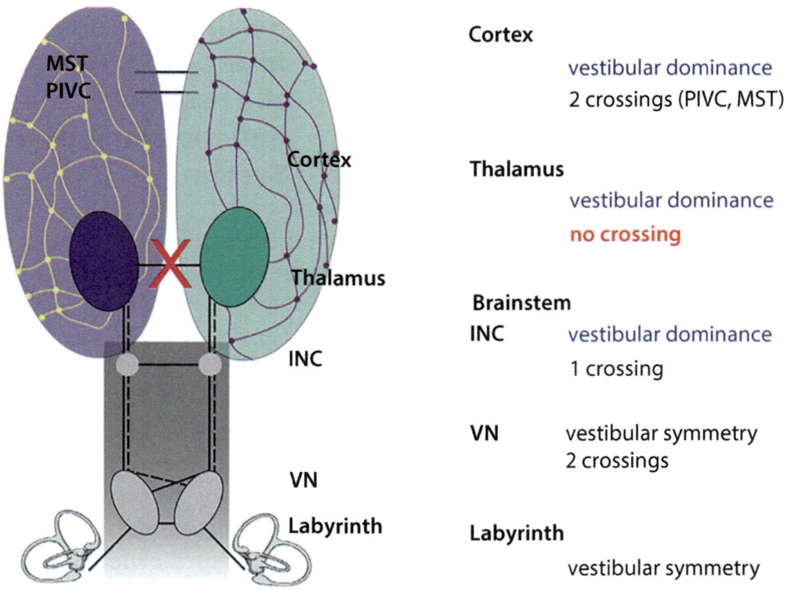

Fig. 13.10 Schematic drawing of the bilateral central vestibular pathways from the labyrinth to the thalamus with their right-left symmetries or asymmetries. Three brainstem crossings of vestibular pathways were found: (i) between the vestibular nuclei (VN), (ii) above the vestibular nuclei in the pons; and (iii) in the midbrain at the level of the interstitial nucleus of Cajal (INC). In the cortex, two transcallosal interhemispheric crossings were described (between the parieto-insular vestibular cortex, PIVC, in the insula, and between the medial superior temporal areas, MST, in the visual cortex). A most important finding is that there is no direct connection between the thalamus of both sides (red cross). The separation of the two widely distributed networks in both hemispheres allows for a simultaneous working of different complex sensorimotor and cognitive functions. Such a separation of thalamo-cortical networks in the two hemispheres is a precondition for brain development in childhood with the growing of different networks for different brain functions such as the lateralization of handedness on one side and that of multisensory orientation in space on the other. (Brandt and Dieterich 2018, 2019)

The clinical relevance of a reciprocal visual-vestibular interaction is best demonstrated by PET studies in patients with unilateral vestibular neuritis causing severe spinning vertigo and spontaneous nystagmus in the acute phase (Bense et al. 2004; Becker-Bense et al. 2014). On the one hand, the beneficial effect of downregulation of the visual cortex can be explained by psychophysical experiments, which demonstrated that the amplitude of oscillopsia in patients with acquired nystagmus is always significantly smaller than the net retinal slip due to the involuntary eye movement (Brandt and Dieterich 1988; Dieterich et al. 1998). In addition, perception of object motion is reduced in these patients with acquired nystagmus (Dieterich et al. 1998) as well as in patients with a deficient VOR due to bilateral vestibular failure (Mesland et al. 1996; Shallo-Hoffmann and Bronstein 2003). Interestingly, the latter patients showed an enhanced activity in the visual cortex bilaterally, including the motion-sensitive area MT/V5 (Dieterich et al. 2007), whereas patients with unilateral vestibular failure showed diminished activations of the visual motion processing areas (Deutschländer et al. 2008).

On the other hand, the deactivation of the visual cortex can depend not only on eye movements (retinal slip due to vestibular nystagmus or defective VOR) but also solely on the vestibular input. The deactivation of the visual cortex appears to be more dependent on the vestibular input, since galvanic stimulation of the vestibular nerve during functional MRI also induced significant bilateral signal decreases of the visual cortex (Bense et al. 2001), although no vestibular nystagmus was elicited. The only eye movement was a mild tonic ocular torsion without oscillopsia.

The rare paroxysmal syndrome of room tilt illusion (see page 270) may serve as a clinical example of a reciprocal inhibitory interaction between the visual and vestibular systems. Transient upside-down inversion of vision has been repeatedly described in patients with unilateral peripheral and central vestibular lesions (Sierra-Hidalgo et al. 2012). Transient upside-down vision or 90° tilts are obviously vestibular signs that indicate a misperception of verticality. Thus, the transient course of room-tilt illusion may reflect the perceptual consequence of a shift of the sensorial weight from the misleading vestibular to the more reliable visual sense. While having to resolve intersensory mismatches between the visual and vestibular systems, the brain also has to resolve potential intrasensory mismatches between the two hemispheres.

13.1.6 Frequent Causes of Central Vestibular Disorders

Central vestibular syndromes are generally the result of lesions or pathological excitations of pathways, nuclei or of core areas. Lesions are most often caused by:

- Infarction
- Hemorrhage
- Multiple sclerosis
- Tumor
- Degenerative brain diseases

Pathological excitations occur rarely in paroxysmal brainstem attacks (with ataxia and dysarthria) in MS or after lacunar infarctions or in vestibular epilepsy. Vestibular epilepsy is even more rarely due to excitation of the temporo-parieto-occipital junction (Brandt 1999; Hewett et al. 2011; Hewett and Bartolomei 2013).

Table 13.1 provides an overview of ischemic lesions caused by lacunar or

Table 13.1 Clinical syndrome and corresponding arterial territory affected by unilateral vascular lesions

Brain site/clinical syndrome		Artery
Medulla oblongata	Wallenberg's syndrome (DVD) with OTR and its features (head tilt, vertical deviation of the eyes, ocular torsion, deviation of the SVV) ipsiversive: lesion of the medial vestibular nuclei	Branches of the vertebral artery or the posterior inferior cerebellar artery (PICA) Rare: posterior spinal artery
	Acute vestibular syndrome (DVD) = "Vestibular pseudo-neuritis": lesion of the vestibular fascicle, medial and/or superior vestibular nuclei or superior cerebellar peduncle	Branches of the vertebral artery or PICA
	OTR ipsiversive: lesion of the superior vestibular nuclei	Anterior inferior cerebellar artery (AICA)
Pons and midbrain	OTR or its components toward the opposite contraversive side: lesion of the MLF	Paramedian arteries from the basilar artery
	UBN in combination with INO: lesion of the superior vestibular nuclei and the CVTT	Paramedian arteries from the basilar artery

(continued)

Table 13.1 (continued)

Brain site/clinical syndrome		Artery
	SVV tilt ipsiversive: lesion of the medial lemniscus (IVTT)	Paramedian arteries from the basilar artery
Rostral midbrain	OTR or its components contraversive: lesion of the INC and riMLF	Paramedian midbrain arteries from the basilar artery
Paramedian thalamus	OTR contraversive to the lesion, only if rostral midbrain is affected (INC lesion)	50% of the paramedian midbrain arteries originate together with the paramedian thalamus arteries from the basilar artery
	Thalamic astasia with contralateral lateropulsion and SVV deviation: lesion of the centromedian thalamus (rare)	Paramedian thalamus arteries from the basilar artery
Posterolateral/ventrolateral thalamus	Tendency to fall to the side, SVV deviation ipsiversive or contraversive	Thalamogeniculate arteries or perhaps branches of the posterior cerebral artery
	Thalamic astasia with backward/ contralateral falls	Thalamogeniculate arteries or perhaps branches of the posterior cerebral artery (more often of the right side)
	Pusher syndrome (rare)	Thalamogeniculate arteries or perhaps branches of the posterior cerebral artery
Temporo-parietal and insular cortex	Tendency to fall to the side, SVV deviation contraversive or ipsiversive	Branches of the middle cerebral artery
	Pusher syndrome (rare)	Branches of the middle cerebral artery
Vestibulo-cerebellum	OTR with its components contraversive (ca. 60%) or ipsiversive (ca. 25%): lesions of the uvula, nodulus, tonsil, dentate nucleus, or parts of the cerebellar hemispheres	Branches of the AICA and PICA
	Acute vestibular syndrome (DVD) = "Vestibular pseudo-neuritis": lesion of the cerebellar peduncle, uvula, nodulus, tonsil; often combined with central positional nystagmus	Branches of the vertebral artery, PICA, AICA

OTR ocular tilt reaction, *MLF* medial longitudinal fasciculus, *riMLF* rostral interstitial nucleus of the MLF, *INC* interstitial nucleus of Cajal, *CVTT* central ventral tegmental tract, *IVTT* ipsilateral vestibulothalamic tract, *SVV* subjective visual vertical, *AICA* anterior inferior cerebellar artery, *PICA* posterior inferior cerebellar artery

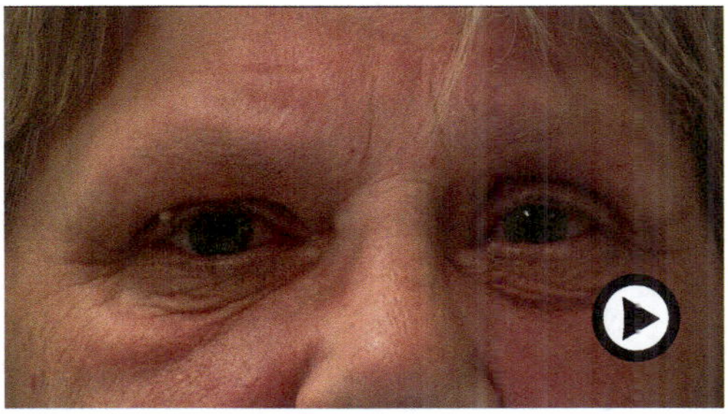

◘ **Fig. 13.11** Wallenberg's syndrome on the right side (▶ https://doi.org/10.1007/000-955)

territorial infarctions in the region of the central vestibular system, giving the typical clinical syndromes and vascular territories (◘ Fig. 13.11).

13.2 Clinical Aspects of Central Vertigo and Dizziness Disorders

13.2.1 Differential Diagnostics of the Acute Vestibular Syndrome (AVS): Peripheral Versus Central

In the acute phase following the sudden occurrence of spinning or postural vertigo/dizziness, the first question concerns the differential diagnosis: Is it an acute peripheral or a central vestibular syndrome (AVS) caused, for example, by an acute stroke (Brandt and Dieterich 2017)? If it is, specific diagnostics and therapy must be begun without delay. Thus, if the main symptom is acute vertigo, the following 6-step procedure is recommended for the first examination:

1. Perform the head impulse test (HIT, ◘ Fig. 3.5) (Cnyrim et al. 2008; Kattah et al. 2009; Newman-Toker et al. 2008) preferably with videooculography for quantification and documentation (video-HIT) (Mantokoudis et al. 2015; Mossman et al. 2015) to test the high-frequency VOR (◘ Fig. 4.1).
2. Look for a skew deviation (vertical deviation) using the cover test (◘ Fig. 3.2).
3. Look for spontaneous peripheral vestibular nystagmus (with Frenzel's goggles or M-glasses) as opposed to central fixation nystagmus (◘ Fig. 3.4).
4. Look for a gaze-evoked nystagmus (◘ Fig. 3.12) in the opposite direction to a possible spontaneous nystagmus or vertically upward/downward.
5. Look for deficits of smooth pursuit (◘ Fig. 3.13) and saccades (◘ Fig. 3.15), in horizontal and vertical directions.
6. Romberg test (◘ Fig. 3.8): a severe body lateropulsion most likely indicates a central rather than a peripheral lesion.

This 6-step procedure is more sensitive than the 3-step HINTS test (HINTS = *H*ead-impulse, *N*ystagmus, *T*est of *S*kew deviation) for detecting central disorders, because additional ocular motor deficits of smooth pursuit and saccades are examined. The HIT, combined with tests for gaze-evoked nystagmus and skew deviation, can quickly distinguish a central from a peripheral AVS. In an AVS, the presence of a skew deviation, a normal head impulse test (Newman-Toker et al. 2008), and a gaze-evoked nystagmus in the opposite direction to that of spontaneous nystagmus indicate a lesion of the brainstem or the cerebellum (◘ Figs. 13.12 and 13.13). The overlap areas of ischemic infarcts concentrate on the medial and superior part of the vestibular nuclei, the inferior cerebellar peduncle (Brandt and Dieterich 2017) and cerebellar midline structures.

If the root entry zone of the vestibular nerve is affected, for example, by lacunar infarctions or MS plaques, the head impulse test may be pathological and therefore suggest a labyrinthine or peripheral nerve disorder. Even a three-step bedside test detects a central ischemia with a sensitivity of 100% and a specifity of 96% and thus is superior to an early MRI with diffusion-weighted sequences (88%) (Kattah et al. 2009). This procedure

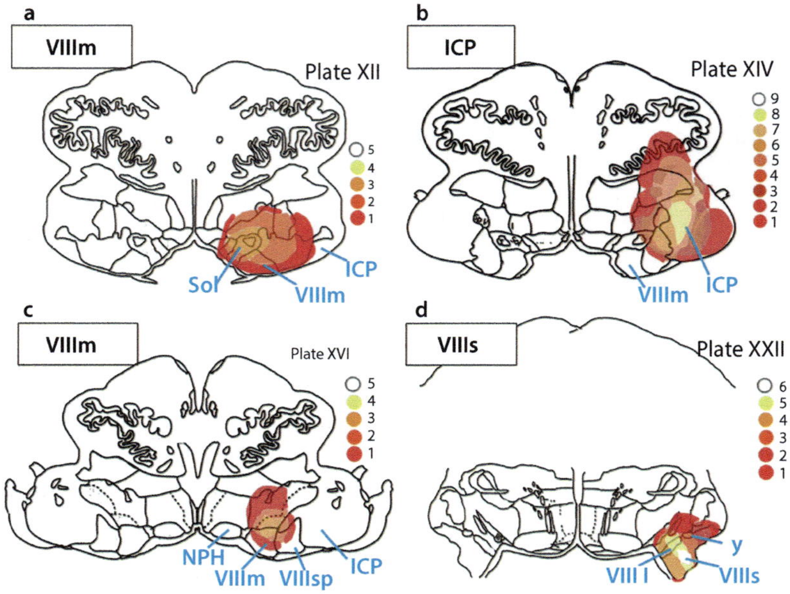

Fig. 13.12 Localization of brainstem lesions that cause an acute *central* vestibular syndrome, formerly named pseudoneuritis. Overlap areas of 23 infarctions from 5 publications show lesion sites superimposed on four slices **a**–**d** of the brainstem atlas from Olszewski and Baxter (1982): **a** medial vestibular nucleus; **b** inferior cerebellar peduncle; **c** medial vestibular nucleus; **d** superior and lateral vestibular nucleus. (ICP: inferior cerebellar peduncle, Sol: nucleus of the solitary tract, NPH: nucleus prepositus hypoglossi, VIII m: medial vestibular nucleus, VIII s: superior vestibular nucleus, VIII sp: spinal (or inferior) vestibular nucleus, VIII l: lateral vestibular nucleus, y: small group of cells in the dorsolateral pontine tegmentum called y group). (Modified after Brandt and Dieterich 2017)

13

allows the general neurologist to detect a central cause of the condition (Halmagyi and Curthoys 1988; Kattah et al. 2009; Mantokoudis et al. 2015; Chen et al. 2011) which requires an instant work-up for further diagnosis, e.g., in cases of monosymptomatic brainstem or cerebellar strokes. If available, a quantitative video-HIT should be performed in the emergency room to help to differentiate the unilateral and highly asymmetrical semicircular canal dysfunction in peripheral AVS from abnormalities seen in central AVS (Chen et al. 2011; Mantokoudis et al. 2015). HIT gain and compensatory saccades may differ between pontine-cerebellar strokes and acute peripheral lesions. Peripheral lesions cause an ipsilateral gain reduction, central lesions caused by PICA strokes are characterized by a contralateral gain bias, whereas anterior inferior cerebellar artery (AICA) strokes are characterized by a more symmetrical bilateral gain reduction (Chen et al. 2011; Mantokoudis et al. 2015). Some AICA strokes with unilateral labyrinthine ischemia are at risk of being misclassified if judged only by VOR gain (Mantokoudis et al. 2015).

Cerebellar infarcts with AVS primarily affect midline cerebellar structures, such as

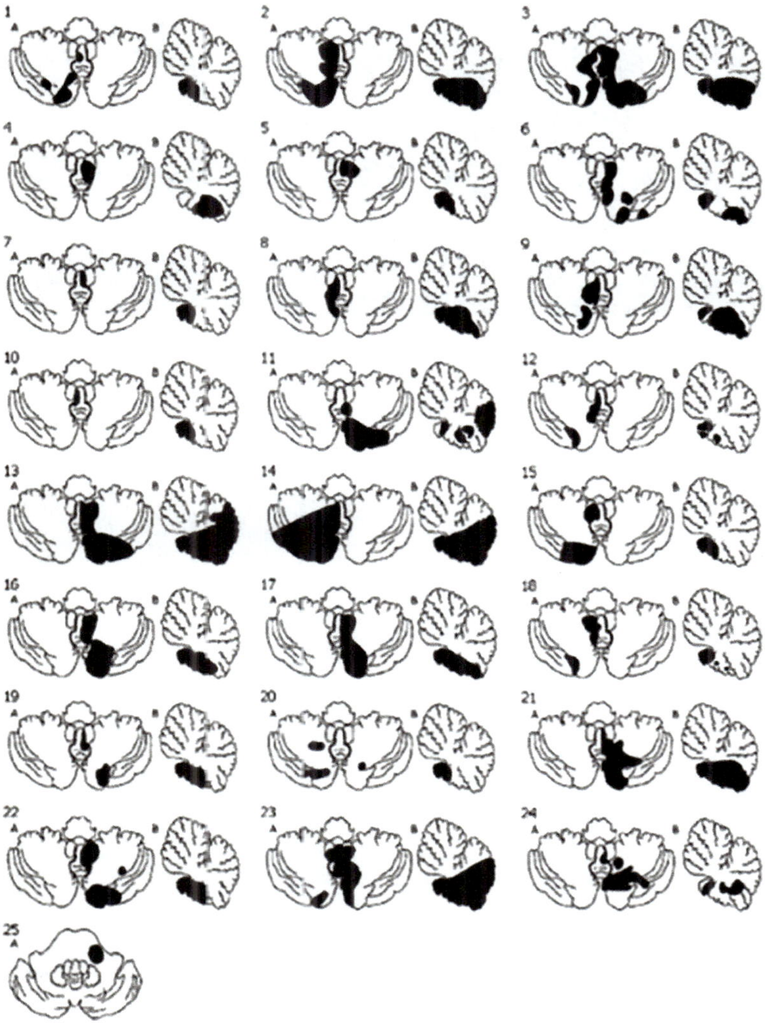

Fig. 13.13 Localization of cerebellar infarctions in 25 patients with an acute central vestibular syndrome. The lesion sites are primarily around the midline in the area of the nodulus, uvula, and tonsil. (Lee et al. 2006)

the uvula, nodulus, and tonsil (Lee et al. 2006; Choi and Kim 2019) (Fig. 13.14), often combined with spontaneous and central positional nystagmus.

It must be stressed that after an acute, isolated episode of vertigo, the risk of having a stroke in the next 4 years is approximately 6%. This is three times higher than the risk in an age-matched control group; if there are additional vascular risk factors, then the risk is even 5.5 times higher (Lee et al. 2011).

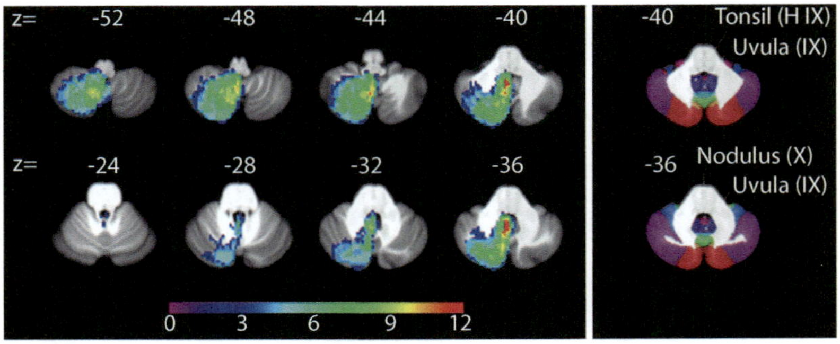

Fig. 13.14 Overlap areas of cerebellar infarctions in patients with an acute central vestibular syndrome who presented with a spontaneous nystagmus and a central positional nystagmus in the acute phase. Lesions are chiefly located in the nodulus, uvula, and tonsil. The number of overlaps is depicted in different colors from violet ($n = 1$) to red ($n = 12$). (Choi and Kim 2019)

Furthermore, careful taking of the patient history is helpful: course (first episode), trigger (spontaneous occurrence), duration (>60 min), together with the ABCD^2-score (age, blood pressure, central accompanying symptoms, duration, diabetes) (Tehrani et al. 2018).

In conclusion, skew deviation is the only specific but not sensitive sign for a central AVS. The horizontal HIT is not specific because it is pathological in 9% of AVS patients with a pontocerebellar infarction near the root entry zone of the eighth nerve (Newman-Toker et al. 2008). However, a normal HIT in AVS patients with spontaneous nystagmus indicates a central lesion in almost all cases (Newman-Toker et al. 2008).

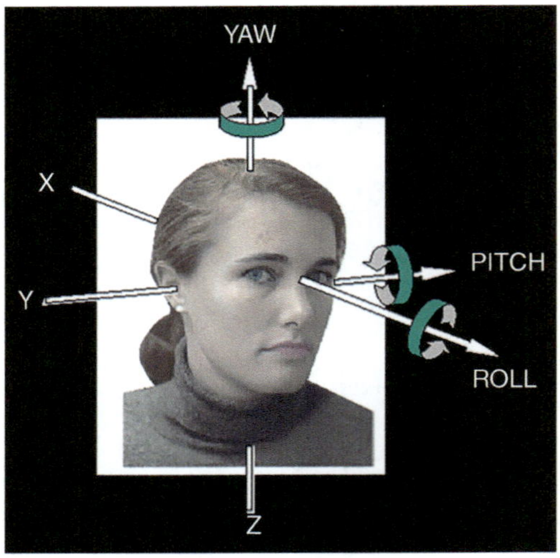

Fig. 13.15 Spatial orientation of the three major planes of action of the vestibulo-ocular reflex (VOR): yaw, pitch, and roll

13.2.2 Central Vestibular Syndromes in the Three Planes of Action of the VOR

For a simple clinical overview, the central vestibular brainstem syndromes can be classified according to the three major planes of action of the VOR (Brandt and Dieterich 1994; Dieterich and Brandt 1995) (Figs. 13.15 and 13.16).

13.2.2.1 Overview 3.2.1 Syndromes of the VOR and Its Clinical Symptoms

Horizontal Plane (Yaw)

- Acute central vestibular syndrome (ACVS), formerly known as "vestibular pseudoneuritis" (Fig. 13.17)
- Spontaneous horizontal nystagmus (most often not suppressed by fixation)

13

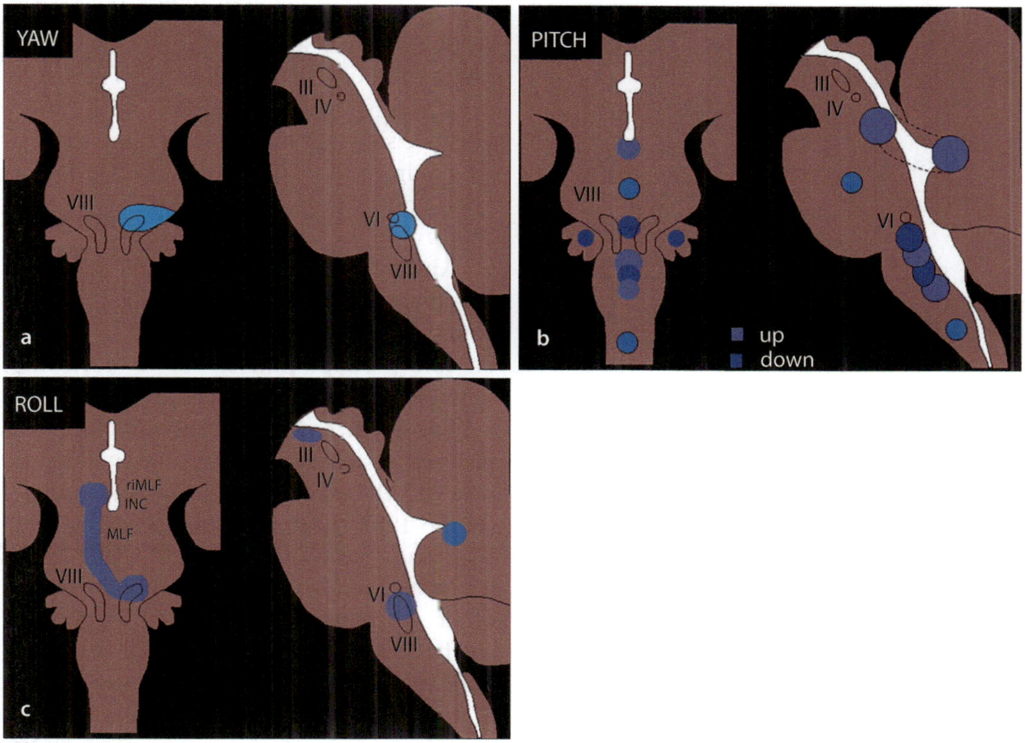

Fig. 13.16 Schematic drawing of the brainstem and cerebellum with the typical sites of lesions that induce vestibular syndromes in the three planes of the VOR: in yaw (**a**), pitch (**b**), and roll (**c**) plane. (III, IV, VI, VIII: cranial nerve nuclei, MLF medial longitudinal fascicle, riMLF rostral interstitial nucleus of the medial longitudinal fascicle, INC interstitial nucleus of Cajal)

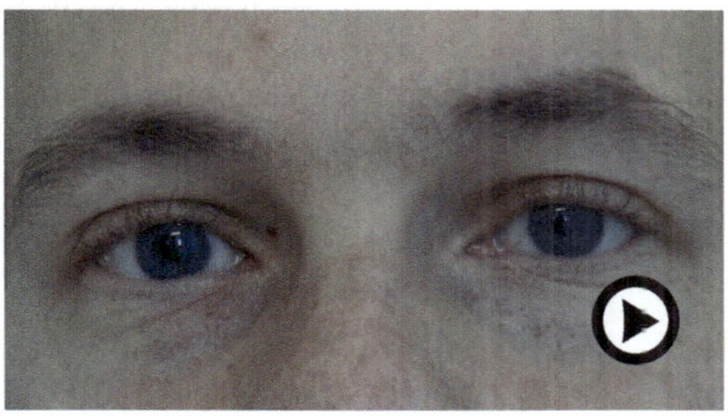

Fig. 13.17 Acute central vestibular syndrome (ACVS) (▶ https://doi.org/10.1007/000-963)

- Horizontal past-pointing to the right/left (subjective straight-ahead)
- Postural instability
- Lateropulsion

Sagittal Plane (Pitch)

- Downbeat/upbeat nystagmus (Fig. 13.2 and 13.3)
- Deviation of the subjective horizontal upwards or downwards
- Past-pointing to up/down ("subjective straight-ahead")
- Postural instability
- Tendency to fall forward or backward

Frontal Plane (Roll)

- Ocular tilt reaction (Fig. 13.18) with
  - Skew deviation
  - Ocular torsion
  - Head tilt and/or
  - Deviation of the SVV
- Postural instability
- Lateropulsion

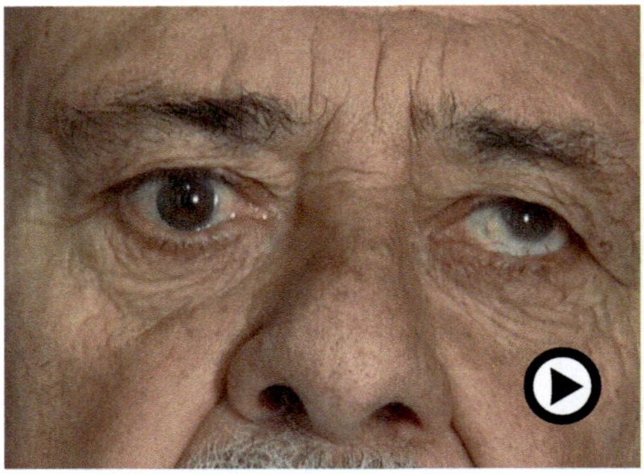

Fig. 13.18 Ocular tilt reaction (▶ https://doi.org/10.1007/000-967)

13.2.2.2 Central Vestibular Syndromes in the Horizontal (Yaw) Plane

As far as we know, central syndromes in the yaw plane (Figs. 13.16 and 13.19) are caused only by lesions in the area of:

- The entry zone of the vestibular nerve in the medulla oblongata
- The medial vestibular nucle
- The neighboring integration centers for horizontal eye movements (nucleus praepositus hypoglossi, NPH, and paramedian pontine reticular formation, PPRF)

13

Other clinical signs are:

- Ipsilateral caloric hyporesponsiveness
- Horizontal gaze deviation
- A tendency to fall to the affected side (lateropulsion)
- Past-pointing, corresponding to a deviation of the "subjective straight-ahead"

The clinical symptoms are similar to those of an acute peripheral vestibular lesion, as occurs in vestibular neuritis, and thus the syndrome was also called "vestibular pseudoneuritis." A purely central yaw plane syndrome is rare, because the area of a lesion that can theoretically cause a pure tone imbalance in the yaw plane adjoins and in part overlaps with structures in the vestibular nuclei, which are also responsible for vestibular function in the roll plane. Thus, skew deviation is the only specific, but not very sensitive sign that indicates an acute vestibular syndrome (vestibular pseudo neuritis) as opposed to vestibular neuritis (Cnyrim et al. 2008).

Among peripheral vestibular disorders, a yaw plane syndrome may manifest as horizontal BPPV (▶ Chap. 9) caused by canalo- or rarely cupulolithiasis of a horizontal semicircular canal (Baloh et al. 1993).

The most common causes include MS plaques or ischemic infarctions within the area of the vestibular nuclei or fascicles (Hopf 1987; Dieterich and Büchele 1989; Kim and Lee 2010) (Fig. 13.19). If the lesion extends beyond the vestibular nuclei, other accompanying brainstem symptoms can be detected. Since a unilateral medullary ischemic or inflammatory brainstem lesion is, as a rule, present, the prognosis is favorable because central compensation takes place over the opposite side. The symptoms can be expected to resolve slowly—as in acute unilateral vestibulopathy—within days to weeks (Dieterich and Brandt 1992; Cnyrim et al. 2007). In such cases, central compensation can be promoted by early balance training together with the simultaneous treatment of the underlying illness.

13.2.2.3 Central Vestibular Syndromes in the Sagittal (Pitch) Plane

Vestibular syndromes in the sagittal (pitch) plane have so far been attributed to lesions in the following sites:

- Paramedially bilaterally in the medullary and pontomedullary brainstem
- Pontomesencephalic brainstem (with the adjacent cerebellar peduncle)
- Paramedian pons
- Flocculus/paraflocculus of the cerebellum, bilaterally

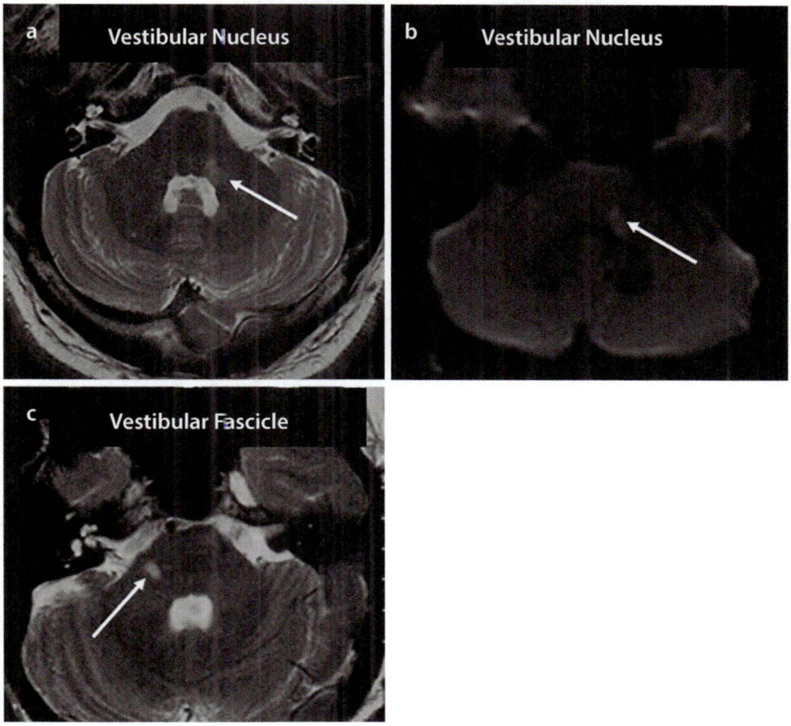

Fig. 13.19 MRI scans of two representative patients with an acute central vestibular syndrome, formerly named pseudoneuritis, presenting with a dysfunction of the VOR particularly in the yaw plane, i.e., rotational vertigo, spontaneous horizontal-torsional nystagmus, postural imbalance with lateral falls. In patient one, **a** T2-weighted and **b** diffusion-weighted sequences show a pontomedullary brainstem stroke that affects the medial vestibular nucleus and the cerebellar peduncle. In the second patient, **c** the infarction causes damage of the eighth nerve fascicle

Despite the numerous clinical studies on upbeat (UBN) and downbeat (DBN) nystagmus as well as the many hypotheses proposed to explain their pathomechanism, so far the pathophysiology of these disorders has not been clarified (Halmagyi and Leigh 2004; Glasauer et al. 2003, 2005; Marti et al. 2005; Pierrot-Deseilligny and Milea 2005). There seem to be various forms of DBN responsible for different aspects of the disorder. Several pathomechanisms that cause an instability in the brainstem-cerebellar networks, which normally stabilize vertical gaze, are currently being discussed: for example, an asymmetry:

- In the vertical neuronal integrator with a disorder of the saccade generator, which is conspicuous in eccentric gaze positions
- In the central connections of the VOR for vertical eye movements, including the otolithic pathways, which explains the frequent dependence on gravity
- In the vertical gaze-pursuit system with spontaneous upward drift

Here the flocculus/paraflocculus seems to play a special role, since its damage leads to a disinhibition of the vestibular pathways of the superior vestibular nucleus to the oculomotor nucleus. This fits with findings from functional imaging studies, which have proven that patients with idiopathic downbeat nystagmus have a hypometabolism or a reduced activity in the flocculus/paraflocculus as well as in the pontomedullary brainstem (Bense et al. 2006; Kalla et al. 2006; Hüfner et al. 2007b) (◘ Figs. 13.20 and 13.21). In contrast, structural MRI found atrophies of the grey matter not in the flocculus/paraflocculus but in the lateral portions of the cerebellar hemispheres (lobule VI) and in the oculomotor vermis (Hüfner et al. 2007b).

The dependence of the intensity of DBN on the head position suggests a disorder of the otolithic pathways in some cases (intensity is less in the upright position than in the prone or supine positions). Similarly, the efficacy of drug treatment with the potassium channel blocker 4-aminopyridine can depend on position (Spiegel et al. 2010; Sander et al. 2011).

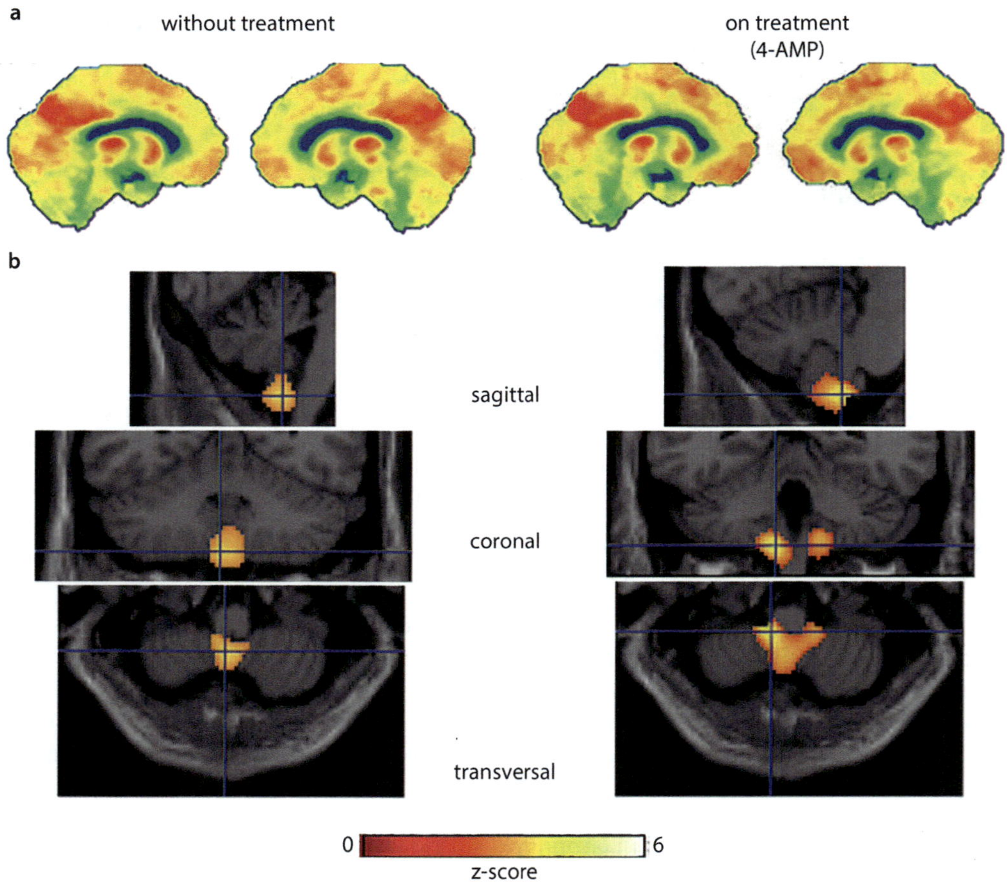

◘ **Fig. 13.20** Imaging downbeat nystagmus in PET and fMRI. **a, b** A patient with idiopathic downbeat nystagmus showed a significantly reduced glucose metabolism (FDG-PET) in the flocculus/paraflocculus (left) which increased together with the improvement of the clinical syndrome after administration of 4-aminopyridine (right) (Bense et al. 2006). **c** A reduction of the activations (fMRI) in the flocculus could also be observed in four patients with downbeat nystagmus during vertical gaze pursuit movements. (Kalla et al. 2006)

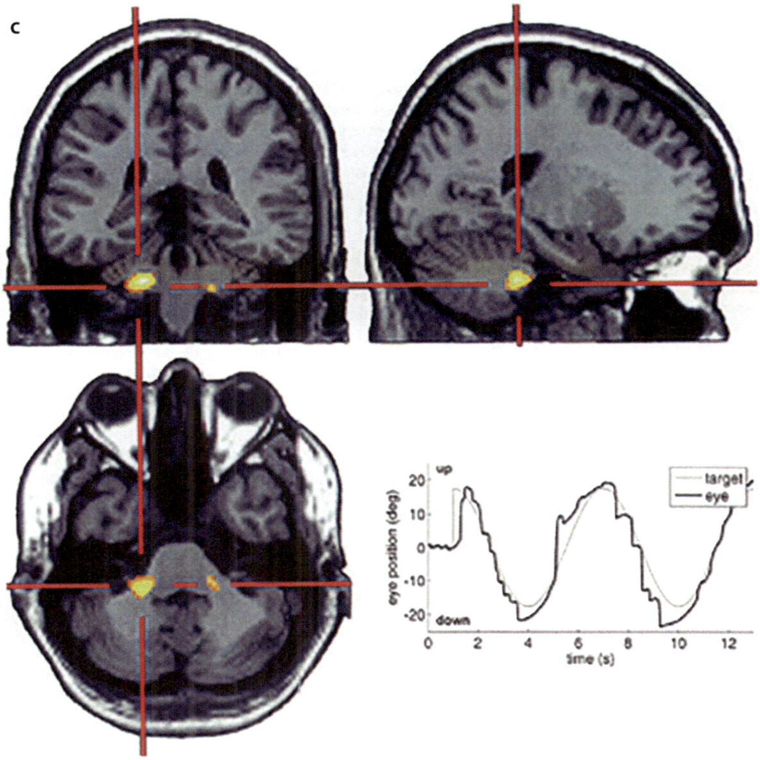

Fig. 13.20 (continued)

13.2.2.4 Downbeat Nystagmus Syndrome (DBN)

Downbeat nystagmus syndrome (DBN) (Fig. 13.2) is the most frequently acquired fixational nystagmus. It beats downward in primary gaze position, is exacerbated on lateral gaze and in the head-hanging position, and can have a spinning component. It is accompanied by a combination of visual and vestibulocerebellar ataxia with:

- A tendency to fall backward (Brandt et al. 1986)
- Past-pointing upward
- A disturbance of vertical gaze pursuit (Leigh and Zee 2016)

DBN is often associated with other ocular motor, cerebellar, and vestibular disorders, e.g., disorders of gaze pursuit, OKN, or the visual suppression of the VOR. The intensity of idiopathic DBN can be dependent on head position and on the time of day: it is stronger in the morning than at noon or in the afternoon (Spiegel et al. 2009). This is in line with reports by patients that the strongest DBN symptoms occur in the morning with an alleviation over the course of the day (Feuerecker et al. 2015). The syndrome is frequently persistent. DBN and UBN directionally specifically impair the perception of object motion (Dieterich et al. 1998).

DBN is often the result of a bilateral lesion of the flocculus or the paraflocculus (Zee et al. 1981; Kalla et al. 2006; Hüfner et al. 2007b) (Figs. 13.20 and 13.21), mostly caused by degenerative cerebellar atrophy, more rarely by intoxication with

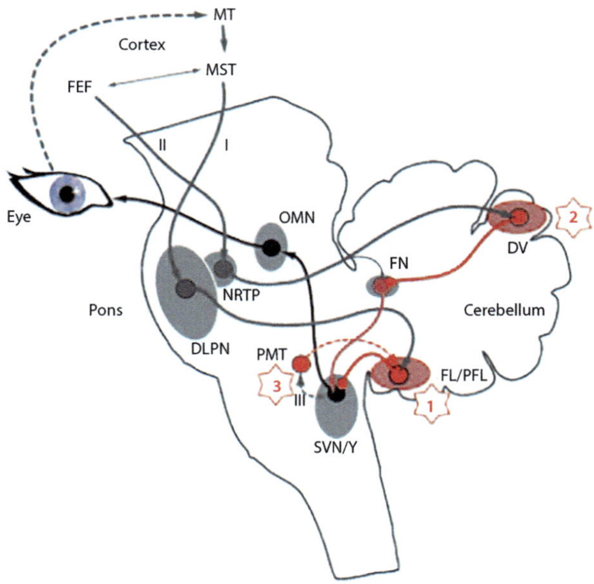

Fig. 13.21 Schematic drawing of a model of the pathomechanism of downbeat nystagmus. The model assumes a common final stretch for the pathways that cause the disinhibition of neurons of the superior vestibular nucleus and of the Y group. Ocular motor connections of the gaze pursuit system (I, II) and of vertical gaze stabilization (III) are affected. Various lesion sites (stars 1–3) can evoke downbeat nystagmus. (FEF frontal eye fields, DLPN dorsolateral pontine nuclei, DV ocular motor dorsal vermis, FN fastigial nucleus, MT middle temporal area, MST middle superior temporal area, NRTP nucleus reticularis tegmenti pontis, OMN ocular motor nuclei, PMT nucleus of the paramedian tract, SVN superior vestibular nucleus, Y neurons of the y-group, FL/PFL flocculus/paraflocculus). (Hüfner et al. 2007b)

13

antiepileptic drugs. It is more rarely induced by a lesion on the floor of the fourth ventricle (Leigh and Zee 2016). Most of the cases are idiopathic (38%), degenerative disorders of the cerebellum (20%), vascular lesions (9%), and malformations (7%). The more rare causes are, in decreasing frequency, toxic drug damage, lesions in MS and paraneoplastic syndromes, vestibular migraine, vitamin B12 deficiency, or traumatic and hypoxic injuries (Wagner et al. 2008). In exceptional cases, however, it may be caused by a paramedian lesion of the medulla oblongata, for example, in MS, hemorrhage, infarction, or tumor.

There are two subgroups of the idiopathic form of DBN:

- One appearing with clear cerebellar signs but *without* cerebellar pathology in MRI.
- The other in combination with bilateral vestibulopathy (Migliaccio et al. 2004; Wagner et al. 2008; Zingler et al. 2007). In these cases, neurodegenerative, in part genetically transmitted, disorders involve the peripheral and central vestibular system including the cerebellum. One variant is a gangliopathy of cranial and peripheral nerves with cerebellar degeneration, cerebellar ataxia with neuropathy, and bilateral vestibular areflexia syndrome (CANVAS syndrome) (Kirchner et al. 2011; Szmulewicz et al. 2011; Pothier et al. 2011; Yacovino et al. 2019). In 89% of patients with CANVAS syndrome, a circumscribed atrophy of the anterior and dorsal vermis and crus I of the cerebellum was seen in MRI (Kirchner et al. 2011; Szmulewicz et al. 2011;

Wagner et al. 2008). In some cases, this is caused by mutations of autosomal recessive RFC1-repeat expansions with a late-onset ataxia (Cortese et al. 2019; Rafehi et al. 2019). Interestingly, chronic coughing is a frequent associated symptom.

13.2.2.5 Upbeat Nystagmus (UBN)

Upbeat nystagmus (◘ Fig. 13.3) is rarer than DBN. It is a fixation-induced nystagmus that abruptly beats upward in primary gaze position (Nakada and Remler 1981) and is partially dependent on head position. UBN is combined with a disorder of the vertical smooth-pursuit eye movements, a visual and vestibulospinal ataxia with a tendency to fall backward, and past-pointing downward. Ocular convergence can transiently reverse its vertical direction (Cox et al. 1981). As distinct to DBN it is not a permanent syndrome but resolves spontaneously within days to months.

Pathoanatomical findings indicate that:

- Most acute lesions are located paramedially in the medulla oblongata, in neurons of the paramedian tract, close to the caudal part of the perihypoglossal nucleus (◘ Figs. 13.22 and 13.23), which is responsible for vertical gaze-holding (Janssen et al. 1998; Pierrot-Deseilligny et al. 2007).
- Lesions have been reported to occur paramedially in the tegmentum of the pontomesencephalic junction, the brachium conjunctivum, and probably in the anterior vermis (Ranalli and Sharpe 1988; Pierrot-Deseilligny et al. 2005; Pierrot-Deseilligny and Milea 2005; Leigh and Zee 2016).
- A lateral lesion in the caudal pons, which includes the superior vestibular nucleus and its connection to the central ventral tegmental tract, CVTT, can also lead to a UBN (Tilikete et al. 2008).

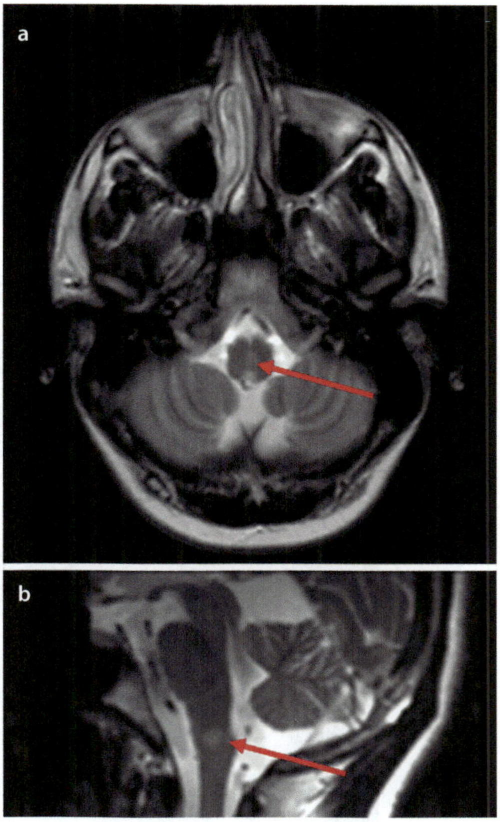

◘ **Fig. 13.22** MRI with contrast medium of a patient with upbeat nystagmus syndrome induced by a contrast-absorbing tumor located paramedially in the medulla oblongata, **a** transversal slice and **b** medial slice

Because the eye movements generally have larger amplitudes, oscillopsia in UBN is very distressing and impairs vision. UBN due to damage of the pontomesencephalic brainstem is frequently combined—especially in MS patients—with a unilateral or bilateral internuclear ophthalmoplegia (INO), indicating that the MLF is affected. In these cases, the main etiologies are bilateral lesions in MS, brainstem ischemia or tumor (◘ Fig. 13.22), Wernicke's encephalopathy, cerebellar degeneration, and dysfunction of the cerebellum due to intoxication.

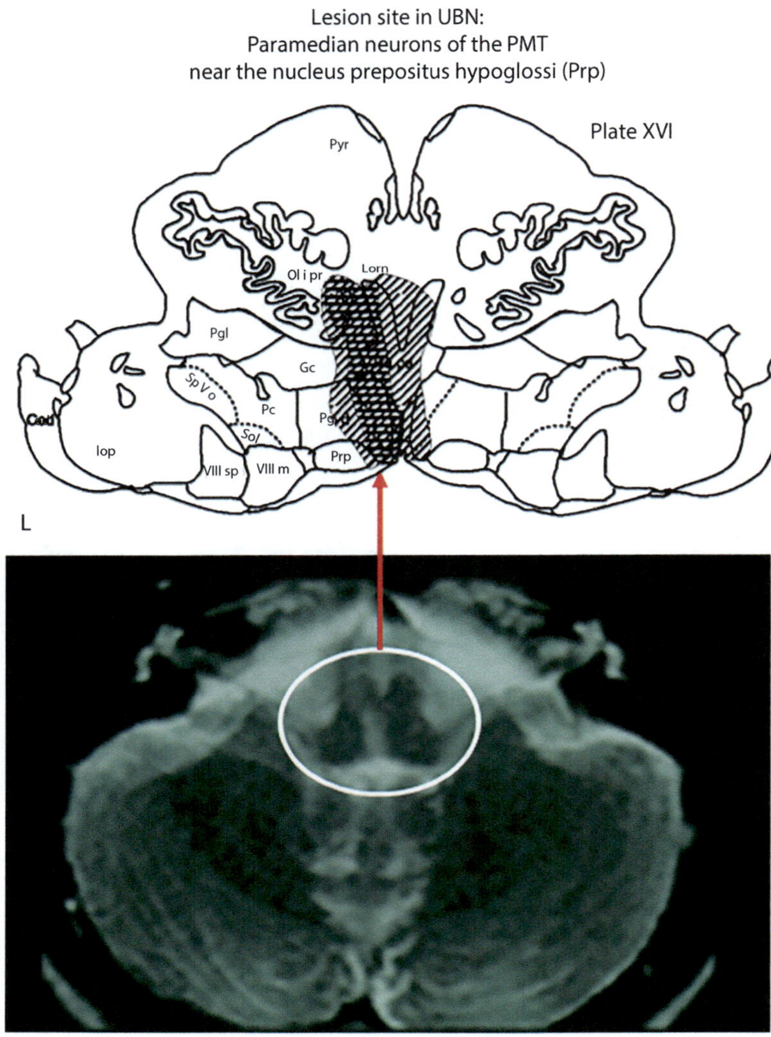

Fig. 13.23 T2-weighted MRI (bottom) of a patient with an acute swaying dizziness, unsteadiness of stance and gait, and blurred vision due to oscillopsia. The acute upbeat nystagmus syndrome was induced by a paramedian stroke of the medullary brainstem. The projection of the lesion (top) onto the adequate plate XVI of the brainstem atlas of Olszewski and Baxter (1982) shows damage near the nucleus prepositus hypoglossi (Prp) in an area where neurons of the paramedian tract (PMT neurons) are located

13.2.2.6 Therapy for DBN and UBN

It is therapeutically expedient to try to treat the symptoms of persisting **DBN** with various drugs. For DBN there are prospective, randomized, placebo-controlled studies available which prove that the potassium channel blockers 3,4-diaminopyridine (Strupp et al. 2003) and 4-aminopyridine (dosage: 3 × 5–10 mg daily) (Claassen et al. 2013b) induce a significant decrease of nystagmus intensity (for review, see Strupp et al. 2017). Fampridine (Fampyra, the sustained-release form of 4-aminopyridine: 2 × 10 mg daily) is also effective (Claassen et al. 2013a) and actually recommended since this drug has official approval. In an observational case study, it was shown that chlorzoxazone, an activator of small calcium-dependent potassium channels, also reduces the intensity of DBN and is well tolerated by the patients (Feil et al. 2013).

Alternative medications are those with acetyl-DL-leucine (5 g/day), memantine (2–3 × 10–20 mg/d), or gabapentin (2–3 × 600 mg/d) (Thurtell et al. 2010; Strupp et al. 2013). The efficacy rates varied inter-individually.

Since UBN generally slowly resolves after an acute occurrence, therapy for its symptoms is often not necessary. In cases of very disturbing oscillopsia due to large amplitudes of the nystagmus or its longer duration, one can try 4-aminopyridine (3 × 5–10 mg/d) (Glasauer et al. 2005) or fampridine (2 × 10 mg/d) or memantine (2 × 10–20 mg/d) (Averbuch-Heller et al. 1997). If these are ineffective, one can try baclofen (2 × 5–10 mg/d).

13.2.2.7 Central Vestibular Syndromes in the Vertical (Roll) Plane

Perceptual deficits of gravity in the sense of pathological deviations of the SVV occur during unilateral damage along the entire VOR pathway projections and of the vestibulocerebellum. They are one of the most sensitive signs of acute brainstem lesions (in approximately 90% of cases of acute unilateral infarctions; Dieterich and Brandt 1993a; Baier and Dieterich 2009). Measurements can be performed quickly and reliably by various methods, for example, with the bucket test (◘ Fig. 3.3) or a half-spherical dome (◘ Fig. 4.7) (Dieterich and Brandt 2019). The size of SVV tilts and the restitution of SVV within 2–4 weeks is similar for unilateral peripheral vestibular and medullary brainstem lesions; the size means an average of 9.8° as opposed to 7° (Cnyrim et al. 2007).

The complete syndrome in the roll plane of the VOR is the eye-head-synkinesis called the ocular tilt reaction (OTR) (Westheimer and Blair 1975; Halmagyi et al. 1990). The OTR consists of head tilt (◘ Fig. 3.1), skew deviation (vertical deviation of the eyes with one eye up, the other down), ocular torsion of both eyes, and tilts of the SVV, all in the same direction (◘ Figs. 13.24 and 13.25). Motor signs such as head tilt and body lateropulsion—components of OTR—are typical for peripheral vestibular organ and pontomedullary lesions but less frequent in pontomesencephalic lesions. *Isolated* body lateropulsion is chiefly found in caudal lateral brainstem lesions affecting the lateral medulla. Vestibular function in the roll plane and its disorders can be mathematically modeled by an attractor model (Glasauer et al. 2018).

The pontine crossing of vestibular "graviceptive" pathways is essential for topographic diagnosis. These syndromes indicate an acute unilateral injury of the "graviceptive" vestibular pathways in the brainstem: from the vertical canals and otoliths via the *ipsilateral* (medial and superior) vestibular nuclei and the *contralateral* medial longitudinal fascicle (MLF) to the nuclei of the extraocular eye muscles and integration centers for vertical and torsional eye movements (interstitial nucleus of Cajal, INC, and rostral interstitial nucleus of the MLF, riMLF) in the rostral midbrain (Brandt and Dieterich 1994; Dieterich and Brandt 1992, 1993a).

There are distinct rules to determine the side and the site of the lesion:

- All signs in the roll plane—the complete OTR or single components (◘ Fig. 13.18)—show an *ipsiversive* tilt (ipsilateral eye undermost) in rare unilateral peripheral labyrinthine damage or in the more frequent pontomedullary lesions of the medial and/or superior vestibular nucleus below the pontine crossing (◘ Fig. 13.25).
- All signs in the roll plane (ocular motor, perceptual, postural) show a *contraversive* tilt (contralateral eye undermost) in unilateral pontomesencephalic brain-

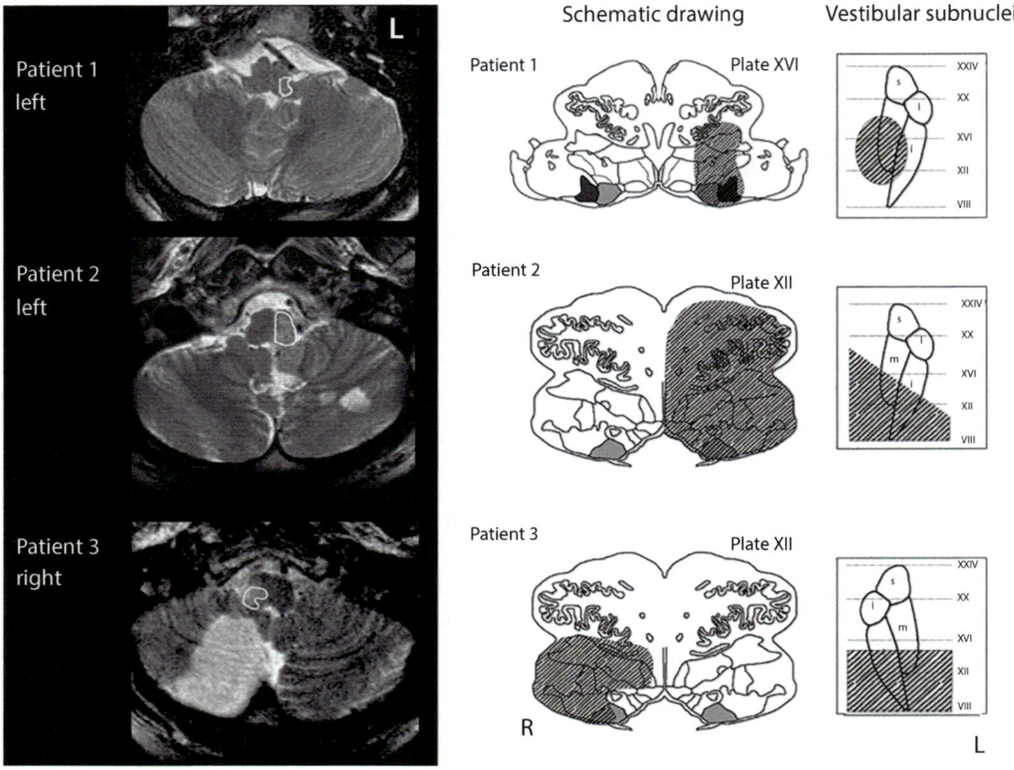

Fig. 13.24 T2-weighted MRI of three representative patients (1–3) with an acute vestibular syndrome in the roll plane of the VOR (i.e., vertical deviation of the eyes: skew deviation, ocular torsion, head and body tilt, and deviation of the subjective visual vertical in the same direction) due to an acute brainstem infarction (lesions surrounded by white lines; see left column). Projections of the lesions (striped) onto plates XII and XVI of the brainstem atlas of Olszewski and Baxter (1982) (middle column) show an affection of the vestibular nucleus which is marked in grey on both sides (light grey: medial vestibular nucleus; dark grey: inferior or spinal vestibular nucleus). Schematic drawing of the vestibular subnuclei and the lesion sites (right column)

stem lesions above the crossing of the graviceptive pathways and indicate damage to the MLF or the supranuclear INC (Fig. 13.25).

- Unilateral lesions of the vestibular nucleus due to dorsolateral pontomedullary infarctions—Wallenberg's syndrome—represent a prototype of vestibular tone imbalance in the roll plane. It manifests with lateropulsion of the eyes and the body and single components or a complete ipsilateral ocular tilt reaction (Dieterich and Brandt 1992).
- Brainstem lesions ipsilateral to the vestibular nucleus, near the ascending medial lemniscus (ipsilateral vestibulothalamic tract), also induce isolated *ipsilateral* deviations of the SVV without vertical deviation or ocular torsion (Zwergal et al. 2008).
- Unilateral lesions of the vestibulocerebellar structures (e.g., the uvula, nodulus, dentate nucleus) can also induce signs of an OTR with contraversive tilts in about 60% and ipsiversive tilts in about 25% (Baier et al. 2008; Baier and Dieterich 2009). In contraversive tilts, the affected structure is often the dentate nucleus.
- More rostrally to the midbrain, only the vestibular projection of the VOR for perception in the roll plane (determination of SVV) runs over the vestibular para-

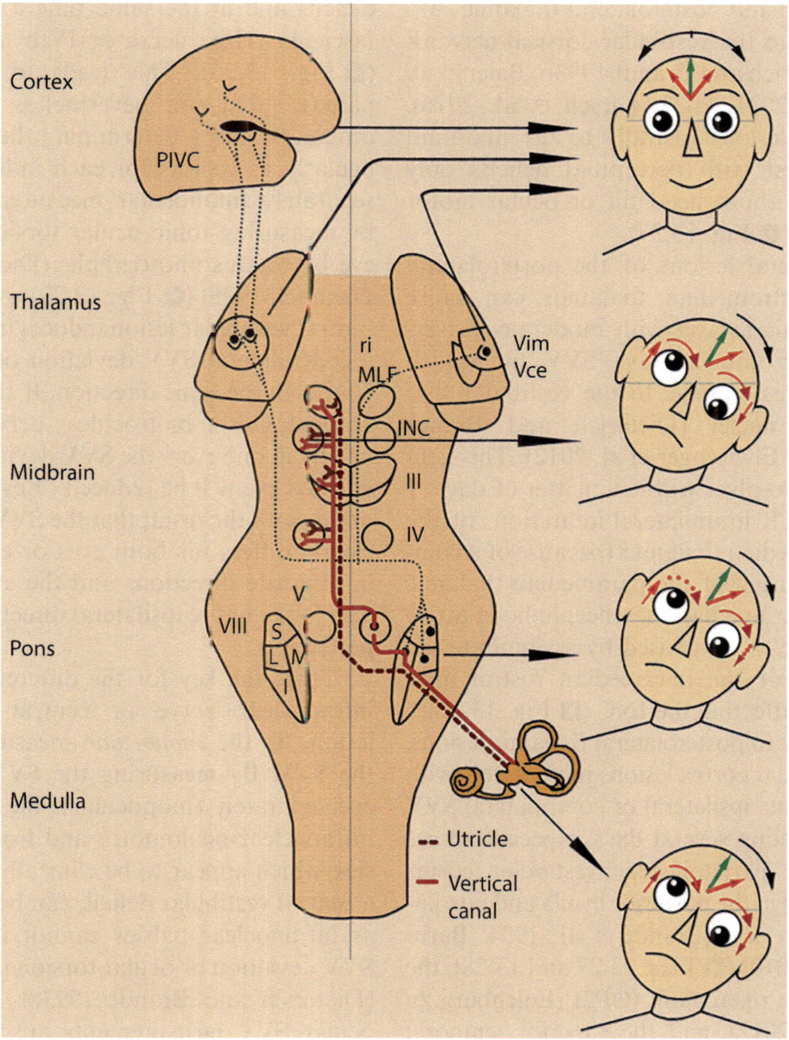

Fig. 13.25 Schematic representation of the deviation of the subjective visual vertical (SVV; arrows on the forehead) and the complete ocular tilt reaction (OTR) with head tilt, skew deviation (vertical deviation of the eyes), and ocular torsion in the same direction due to unilateral vestibular lesions from the labyrinth via the vestibular nuclei (VIII), the midbrain (ocular motor nuclei III and IV, interstitial nucleus of Cajal, INC, and rostral interstitial nucleus of the MLF, riMLF), thalamus (vestibular subnuclei Vce, Vim) to the insular-opercular vestibular cortex PIVC. A unilateral lesion of the graviceptive pathways from the otoliths (utricle) and the vertical semicircular canals causes a tone imbalance in the frontal roll plane of the VOR. The complete syndrome is the eye-head synkinesis OTR with tilts of SVV, skew deviation, ocular torsion, and head tilt in the same direction. The direction of tilts is dependent on the lesion site, i.e., ipsilateral in peripheral and pontomedullary lesions and—above the pontine crossing of vestibular pathways—contralateral in pontomesencephalic lesions. Unilateral lesions of the thalamus and cortex show only deviations of the SVV without other ocular motor signs; these deviations can be ipsilateral or contralateral. (Brandt and Dieterich 1994; Dieterich and Brandt 2019)

median and posterolateral thalamic subnuclei to the vestibular cortical network (Dieterich and Brandt 1993b; Baier et al. 2016, 2021, 2022; Kirsch et al. 2016). Thus, lesions rostrally to the midbrain manifest with perceptual deficits only (i.e., without head tilt or ocular motor signs) (◘ Fig. 13.37).

- Unilateral lesions of the posterolateral or centromedian thalamus can cause thalamic astasia with moderate ipsiversive or contraversive SVV tilt, which indicates damage to the vestibular thalamic nuclei (Dieterich and Brandt 1993b; Elwischger et al. 2012). This generally resolves within a matter of days.
- An OTR in unilateral infarctions of the paramedian thalamus (because of a common origin of the paramedian thalamic and paramedian mesencephalic in arteries in 50%) is caused by a simultaneous lesion of the paramedian rostral midbrain affecting the INC (◘ Fig. 13.26).
- Similar to posterolateral thalamic lesions, vestibular cortex lesions present only with moderate ipsilateral or contralateral SVV tilts lasting several days, especially those of the parietoinsular vestibular cortex (PIVC) in the posterior insula and retroinsular region (Brandt et al. 1994; Barra et al. 2010) (◘ Figs. 13.27 and 13.28), the parietal operculum (OP2) (Eulenburg zu et al. 2012), and the superior temporal gyrus (Baier et al. 2012b, 2021).
- If instead of a functional deficit due to a lesion, the VOR projection is stimulated on one side, the same effects will be triggered, but with signs in the opposite direction.

In midbrain lesions, complicated ocular motor syndromes are occasionally induced by the combination of a central vestibular deficit in the roll plane (e.g., due to the INC deficit) and at the same time a nuclear or fascicular IIIrd nerve or IVth nerve palsy (◘ Fig. 13.29). This leads to a "mixed pattern" that can nevertheless be clearly differentiated by determining the SVV binocularly as well as for each individual eye separately (monocular measurement), and by measuring tonic ocular torsion of each eye by fundus photographs (Dichgans and Dieterich 1995) (◘ Fig. 13.29). A unilateral central vestibular lesion induces in both eyes a contralateral SVV deviation of generally 10–20° in the same direction. If there is also an oculomotor or trochlear nerve lesion—mostly in one eye—the SVV deviation in the affected eye will be reduced or even antagonized, with the result that the SVV deviation clearly differs for both eyes or even points in opposite directions and the affected eye also looks in the ipsilateral direction (mixed pattern).

Thus, the key for the differentiation of infranuclear nerve or central vestibular lesions is the *monocular* measurement of the SVV. By measuring the SVV for each eye separately (monocular), the peripheral infranuclear oculomotor and trochlear palsies, which appear to be clinically similar to a central vestibular deficit, can be disclosed, as infranuclear palsies cannot induce any SVV deviation or ocular torsion in *both* eyes (Dieterich and Brandt 1993c). The monocular SVV measurements are important, because even the Bielschowsky head-tilt test does not allow clear differentiation between a trochlear palsy (◘ Fig. 13.30) and an OTR.

The etiology of these unilateral lesions in the roll plane is frequently an infarction as well as a hemorrhage of the brainstem or of the paramedian thalamus, which extend into the rostral midbrain (Dieterich and Brandt 1993a, b). More rarely, inflammatory, immunological, or neoplastic etiologies are found.

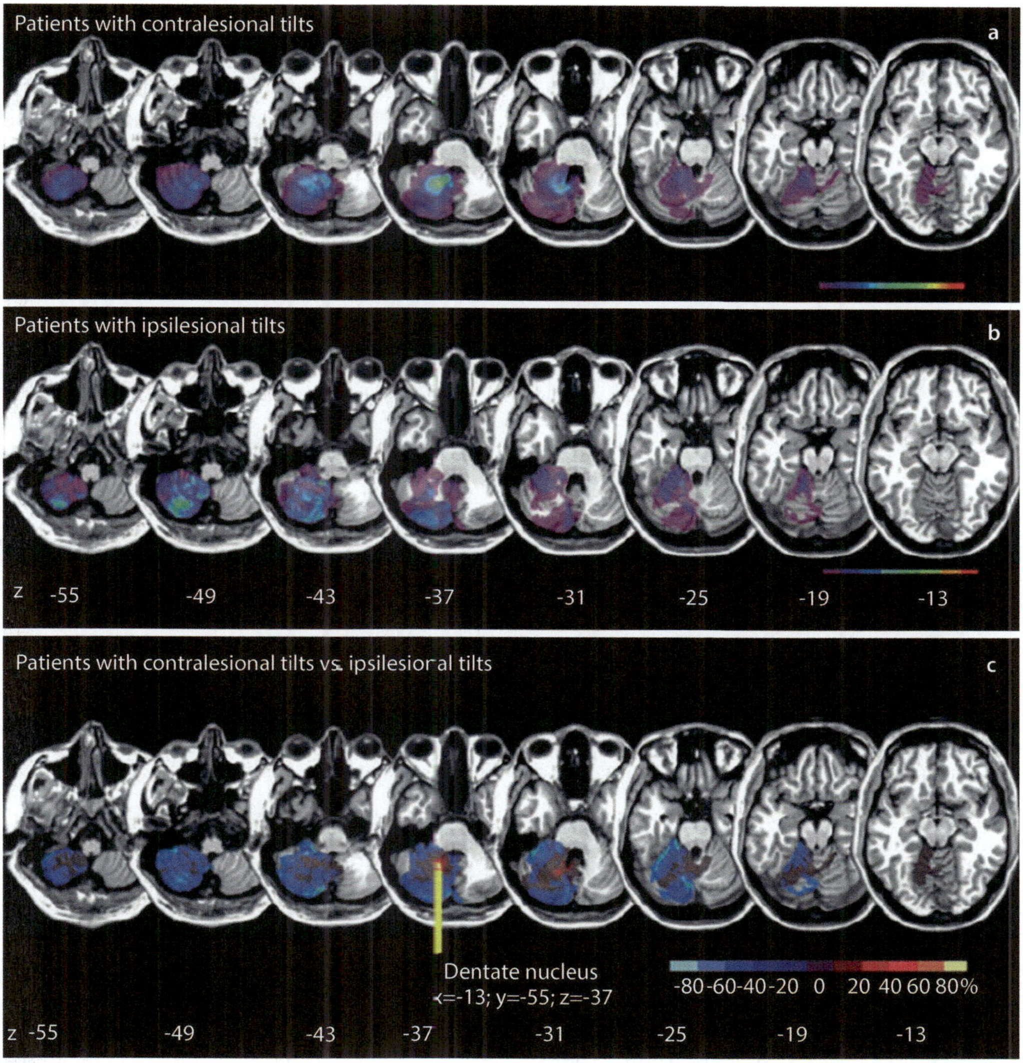

Fig. 13.26 Lesion localization in patients with acute unilateral cerebellar infarctions presenting with deviations of the subjective visual vertical (SVV). **a** Overlay lesion plot of patients with contralateral tilts of SVV (n = 23). **b** Overlay plot of the comparison group with ipsilateral tilts of SVV (n = 8). Number of overlapping lesions is illustrated by different colors coding increasing frequencies from violet (n = 1) to red (n = 8). **c** Overlay plot of the subtracted superimposed lesions of the group with contralateral SVV tilts minus the comparison group and vice versa. The percentage of overlapping lesions of the group with contralateral tilts after subtraction is illustrated by five different colors coding increasing frequencies from dark red (difference 1–20%) to white-yellow (difference 81–100%). Each color represents 20% increments. The colors from dark blue (difference −1 to −20%) to light blue (difference −81 to −100%) indicate regions damaged more frequently in the comparison group. Talairach z-coordinates of each slice are given. The anatomical area related to contralateral tilts of SVV is the dentate nucleus. (Baier et al. 2008)

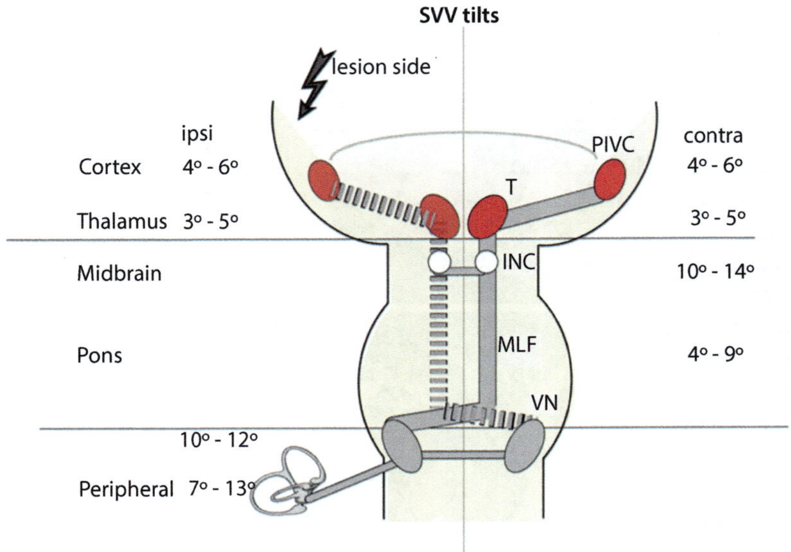

Fig. 13.27 Perceptual deviations of subjective visual vertical (SVV, in degrees) after acute unilateral lesions of the graviceptive pathways from the labyrinth via the vestibular nuclei (VN), the medial longitudinal fascicle (MLF), the interstitial nucleus of Cajal (INC), and the thalamus (T) to the multisensory vestibular cortex PIVC. Median data from 15 studies in patients with different types of vestibular lesions. Strongest SVV tilts were found in acute peripheral vestibular lesions and in brainstem lesions. Direction of tilt is ipsilateral in lesions below the crossing and contralateral in lesions above the crossing. Damage of the vestibular thalamic subnuclei or the vestibular cortical network induces either ipsilateral or contralateral tilts of mild degree. (Glasauer et al. 2018; Dieterich and Brandt 2019)

The course and prognosis here also depend on the etiology of the underlying illness. In the frequent ischemias, one can expect a significant and most often complete recovery from the symptoms in the roll plane within days to weeks due to central compensation taking place over the opposite unaffected side (Dieterich and Brandt 1992, 1993b; Cnyrim et al. 2007).

13.2.3 Central Spinning or Non-Spinning Vertigo

Clinical experience has shown that sustained rotational vertigo with spontaneous nystagmus and direction-specific falls is associated predominantly with peripheral lesions of the labyrinth and the vestibular nerve, and less frequently with lesions of the vestibular nuclei and vestibular cerebellum. Vestibular syndromes due to lesions above the level of the vestibular nuclei—that is, the midbrain, thalamus, and cortical centers—only manifest with transient rotational vertigo in exceptional cases. These syndromes generally present with to-and-fro (swaying) vertigo, disorientation, postural instability, and most often a static tone imbalance in the roll plane, as described for ocular tilt reaction (OTR) syndromes (Becker-Bense et al. 2016). In contrast to unilateral pontomedullary brainstem lesions, rotational vertigo in midbrain lesions occurred with a low frequency (14%) and transient (<1 day) course (Dieterich et al. 2018) (Figs. 13.31 and 13.32).

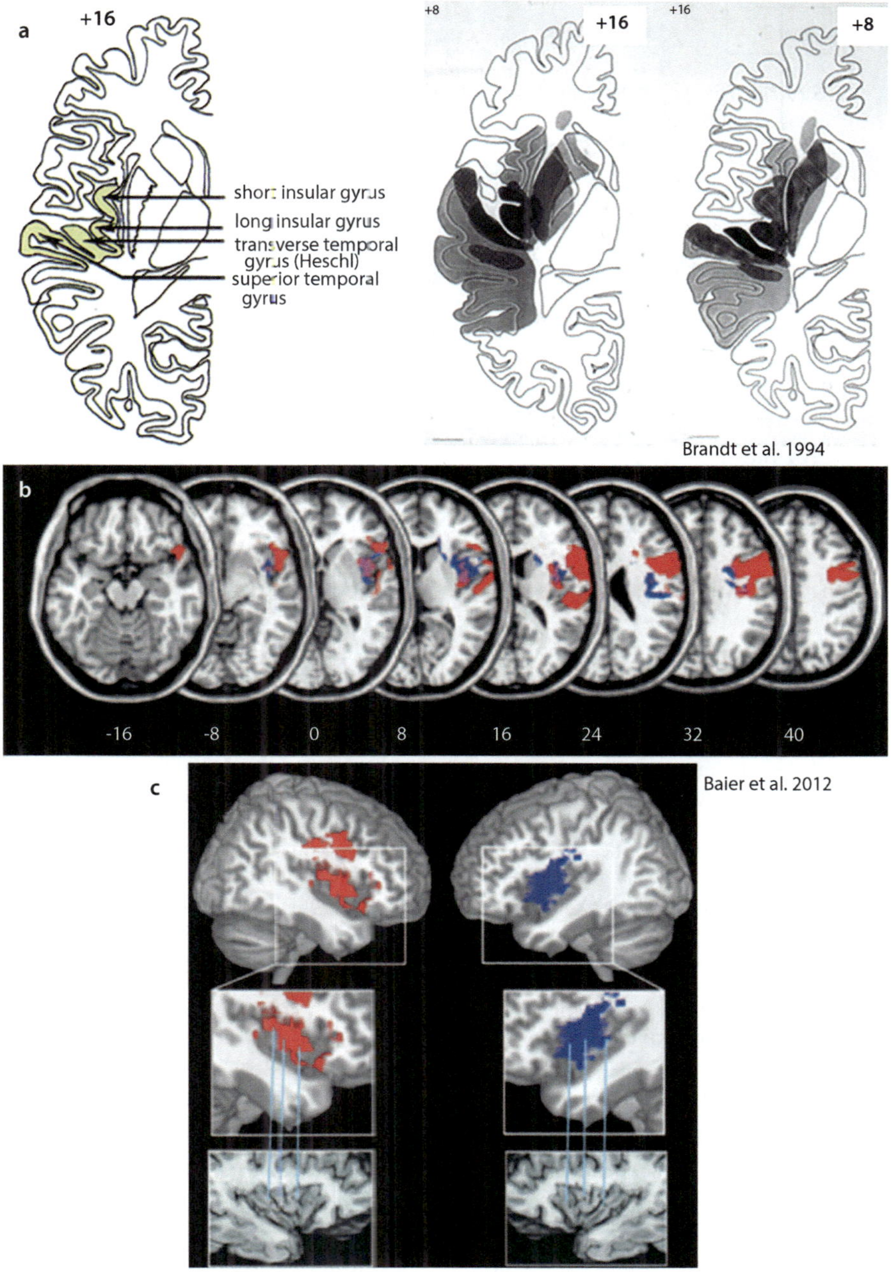

Fig. 13.28 Overlap areas of MRI lesions in patients with acute infarctions of the middle cerebral artery (MCA) and deviations of the SVV projected onto the corresponding plates of the atlas of Duvernoy. (**a**): The overlap area of 7 infarctions is located in the short and long insular gyri and the transverse temporal and superior temporal gyri (Brandt et al. 1994). (**b**): Statistical voxel-wise lesion-behavioral mapping (VLBM) with regard to the deviation of the subjective visual vertical (SVV) in 32 patients with right-sided and 22 patients with acute left-sided MCA infarctions. The overlap of the left-sided lesions (blue) is flipped to the right hemisphere; lesions of the right hemisphere are presented in red and the overlap of both hemispheres in violet. The core area of all the lesions of both hemispheres (violet) is located in the circular insular sulcus, the central insular sulcus, and the short and long insular gyri. (**c**) Insular lesion location in more detail (Baier et al. 2012b)

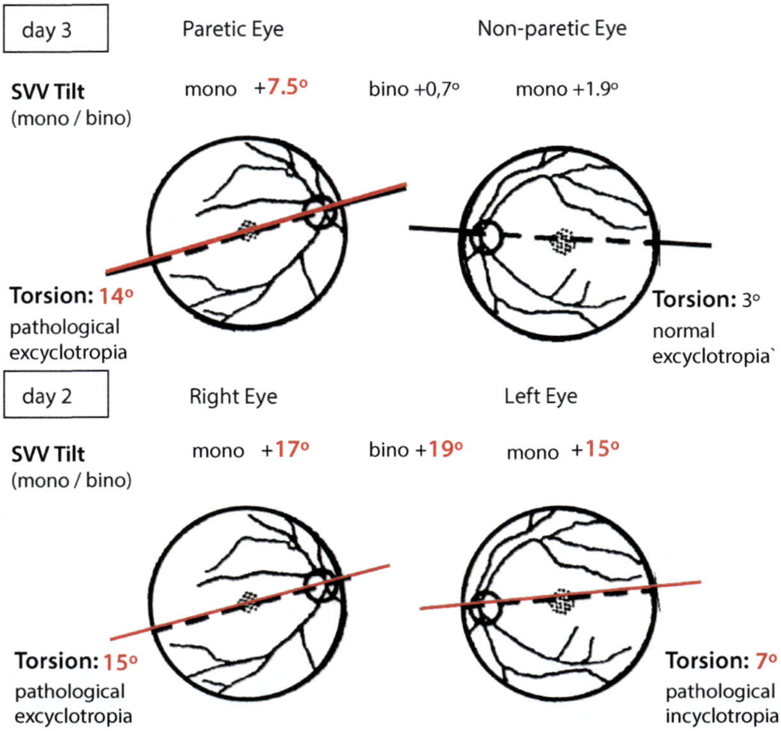

Fig. 13.29 Schematic representation of the ocular fundus to measure the eye position in the roll plane, i.e., the ocular torsion of both eyes, the data of the measurements of the subjective visual vertical (SVV) for the binocular (bino) and the monocular (mono) viewing conditions. The normal range of the SVV adjustments is 0° ± 2.5°; the normal range for the eye position in the roll plane is a mild excyclotropia of 0° to 10° bilaterally. Typical results of a peripheral infranuclear eye muscle paresis (top) in contrast to unilateral peripheral and central vestibular lesions (bottom) of the brainstem or cerebellum
Top: In an acute oculomotor palsy (day 3) the paretic eye shows a torsion, an excyclotropia of 14°, and a mild monocular deviation of the SVV of 7.5° on the affected eye only. The normal eye shows normal results with an excyclotropia of 3° and a SVV deviation of 1.9°; the binocular SVV measurement was also normal with 0.7°. Thus, a peripheral ocular motor palsy causes ocular torsion and SVV deviation in the acute phase of the paretic eye and in the chronic phase sometimes only of the non-affected eye (i.e., sensory shift when the dominant eye is initially affected).
Bottom: In an acute unilateral lesion of the brainstem or cerebellum (day 2), a binocular torsion in the same direction is the typical pattern, for example, an excyclotropia of 15° of the right eye and an incyclotropia of 7° of the left eye, combined with SVV deviations of both eyes in monocular as well as in binocular measures of 15–19°, all pointing in the same direction. Although the different patterns of SVV tilts and torsions might be difficult or confusing, they are of clinical relevance and often allow a topographic diagnosis. (Dieterich and Brandt 2019).

13

Surprisingly, acute unilateral lesions of the multiple vestibular cortex areas due to, for example, a middle cerebral artery infarction manifest primarily without vestibular symptoms such as rotational vertigo (Anagnostou et al. 2010). Only single cases have been described of patients with hemispheric strokes involving parts of the vestibular cortical network who presented with nonepileptic rotational vertigo, nystagmus, and postural imbalance which gradually improved within days (Brandt et al. 1995; Naganuma et al. 2006). The critical areas were located more often in the posterior insula (long insular gyrus IV), the adjacent retroinsular region, the transverse temporal gyrus, and in parts of the superior temporal gyrus and posterior putamen than

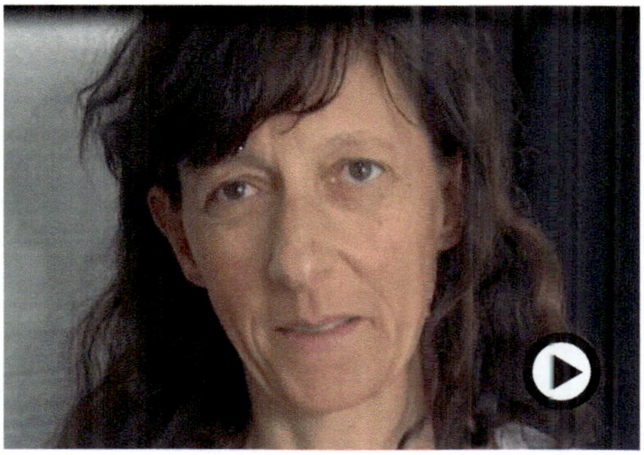

■ **Fig. 13.30** Trochlear nerve palsy on the left side (▶ https://doi.org/10.1007/000-968)

in the inferior parietal cortex preferably of the right hemisphere (Dieterich and Brandt 2015b) (■ Fig. 13.33). A loss of cortical function in one hemisphere may go undetected because the unaffected opposite hemisphere can suppress the disturbance in the affected hemisphere and determine a global percept of correct body orientation (see next paragraph). This is impossible in unilateral peripheral or brainstem failure because the vestibular tone imbalance is transmitted to both hemispheres due to the crossings in the brainstem pathways.

13.2.3.1 Cortical Versus Mesencephalic Vertigo

The rare manifestation of rotational vertigo in cases of mesencephalic brainstem, thalamic, and cortical dysfunction can be explained by the change that takes place in the neuronal coding of vestibular signals *en route* from the vestibular nuclei to the cortex: velocity perception is transformed into the perception of head position (Muir et al. 2009; Winter et al. 2015; Valerio and Taube 2016). The perception of self-motion relies on different types of neurons, that is, neurons that code self-motion velocity (head angular velocity cells) and direction (head direction cells), in cooperation with other cell types for orientation and navigation in space, such as place cells for mapping the environment and grid cells for measuring distances (Muir et al. 2009; Winter et al. 2015; Valerio and Taube 2016; Jeffery 2015; Jeffery et al. 2015). Integration from velocity to direction is necessary to update the awareness of body position in space (Brandt and Dieterich 2017). In fact, the velocity cells, which are mainly responsible for the sensation of rotation, are found primarily in the lower brainstem, whereas the head direction cell system is distributed in a network covering the anterior thalamus, hippocampal formation, and cortical areas (Dumont and Taube 2015). Because of the differences in coding, unilateral dysfunction of angular velocity cells should result in rotational vertigo, while unilateral dysfunction of head direction cells should result in non-rotational dizziness and unsteadiness (Dieterich et al. 2018; Glasauer et al. 2018) (■ Fig. 13.34). The different manifestations can be mathematically modeled by a neural network model of the head direction cell system, which predicts and confirms the clinical findings (Dieterich et al. 2018; Glasauer et al. 2018, 2019).

Furthermore, an additional concept has been proposed (Dieterich and Brandt 2015b) to explain why acute unilateral vestibular cortex lesions—for example, due to infarction of the middle cerebral artery territory—rarely manifest with transient spinning vertigo (Anagnostou et al. 2010; von Brevern et al. 2014). The idea is that a continuous visual–vestibular interactive comparison is necessary for the global perception of self-motion. Both the vestibular cortex and the visual cortex are able to sense self-motion, either via vestibular input from the semicircular canals and otoliths or via optic flow. If a vestibular mismatch exists between the two hemispheres, the hemisphere in which the vestibular and visual cortices are in agreement determines the global percept of body position and motion (Dieterich and Brandt 2015b). Thus, intact interhemispheric vestibular connections via the splenium of the corpus callosum are necessary to avoid rotational vertigo (Kirsch et al. 2016; Conrad et al. 2022a).

Rotational Vetigo

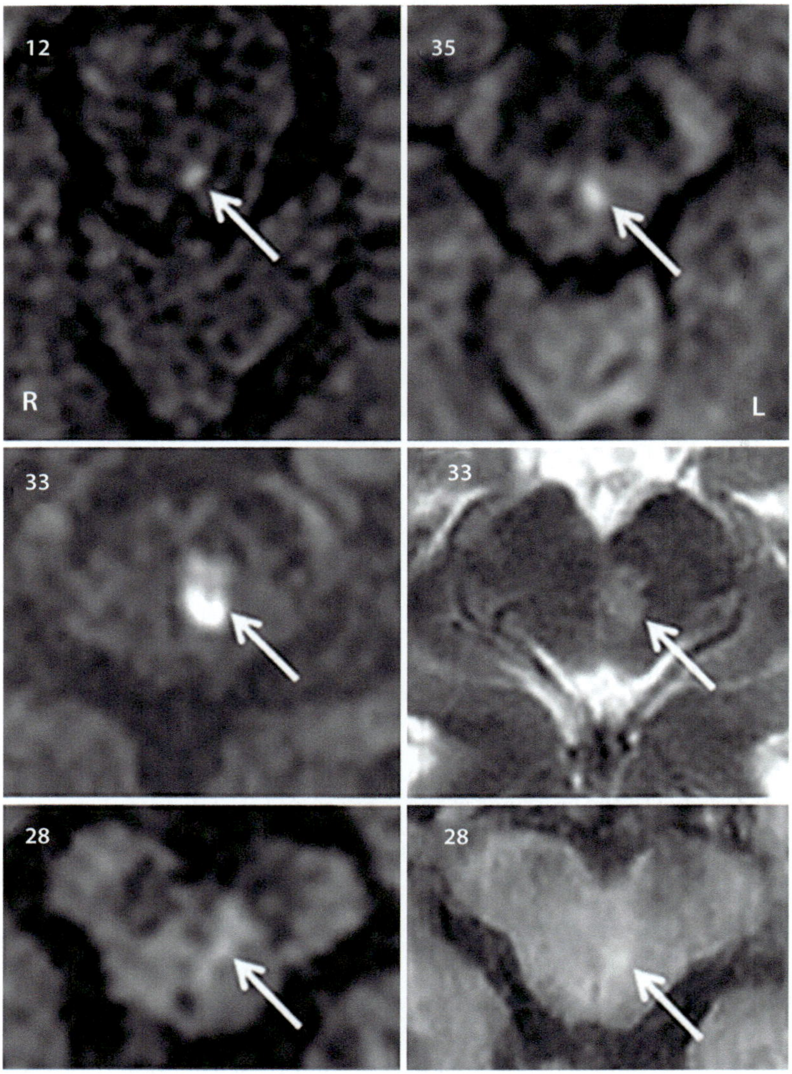

Fig. 13.31 Acute rotational vertigo in brainstem lesions. MRIs (diffusion and T2-weighted sequences) of 4 patients (no. 12, 28, 33, 35) presenting with acute transient vertigo due to unilateral midbrain strokes. Top: two transversal slices of the caudal midbrain near the pons show damage of the midbrain tegmentum affecting the MLF in which the ascending vestibular pathways are mediated. Middle and bottom: two patients with unilateral midbrain strokes near the oculomotor nucleus (Dieterich et al. 2018)

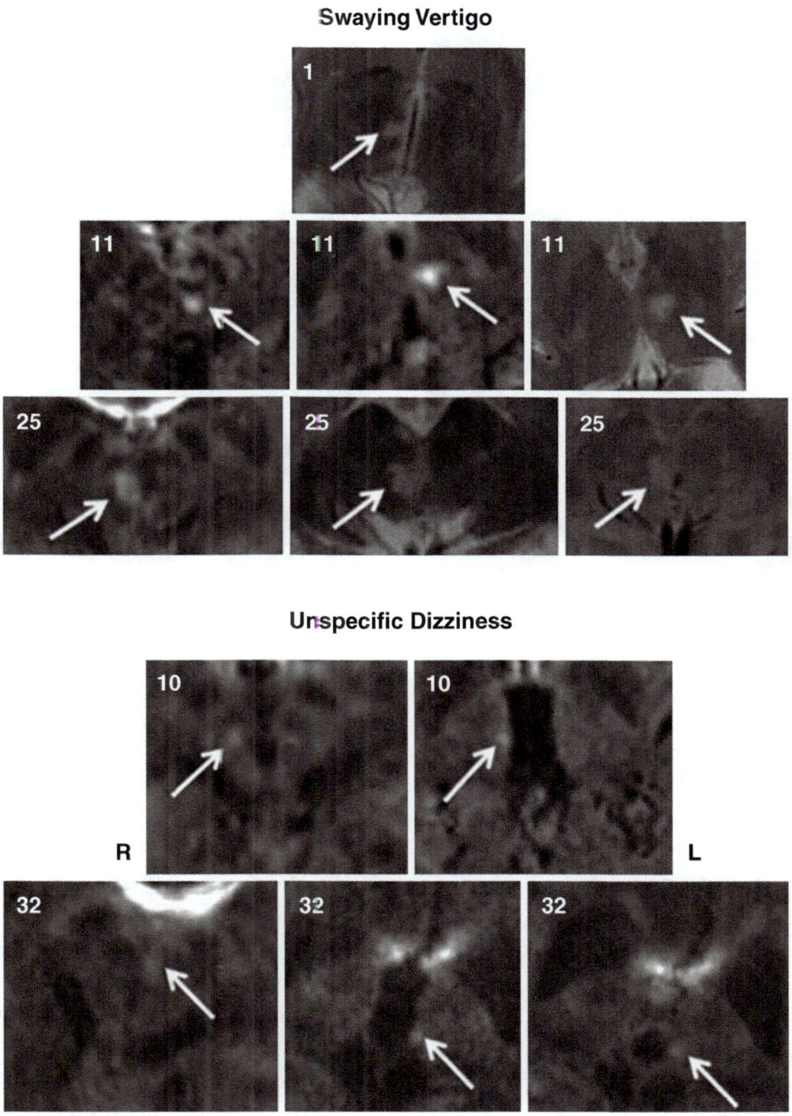

Fig. 13.32 Swaying vertigo or dizziness in midbrain lesions. MRIs of 5 patients (no. 1, 10, 11, 25, 32) with acute swaying vertigo/dizziness or unspecific dizziness due to circumscribed unilateral infarctions of the upper brainstem. The rostral midbrain lesions are located at the level of the oculomotor nucleus and the interstitial nucleus of Cajal (INC) and meso-diencephalic structures. (Dieterich et al. 2018)

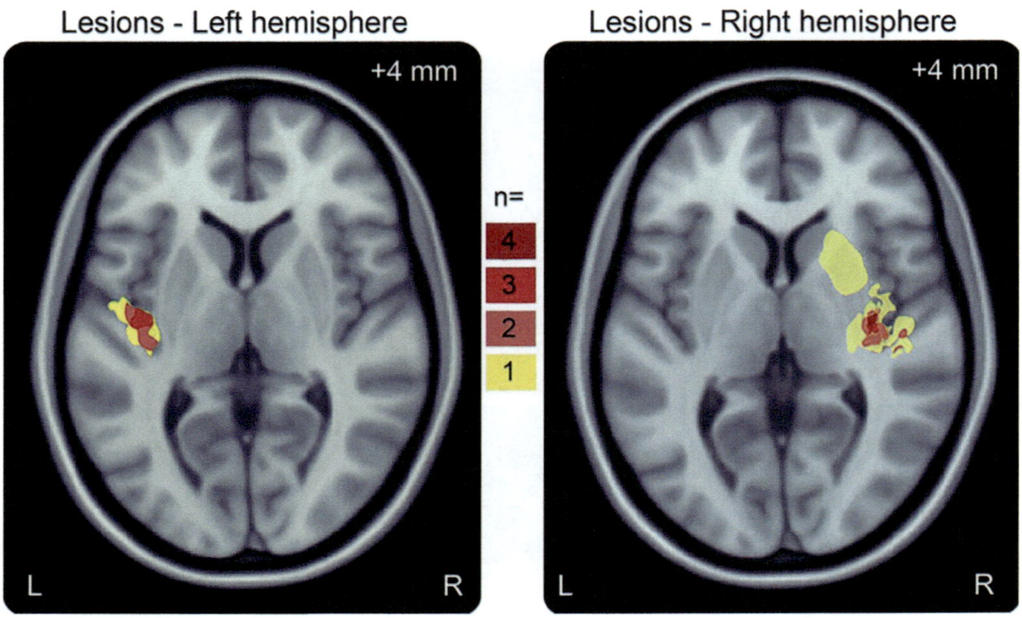

Fig. 13.33 Overlay lesion plot of 8 patients with an acute unilateral infarction of the middle cerebral artery in the temporo-insular cortex of the right ($n = 5$) and left ($n = 3$) hemisphere presenting with an acute vestibular syndrome and transient rotational vertigo, collected from different case reports. The overlap within the right hemisphere is concentrated in the posterior insula (long insular gyrus IV), the adjacent retroinsular region with the transverse temporal gyrus, and in parts of the superior temporal gyrus and posterior putamen. The lesion sites of two patients with infarctions of the parietal lobe are not depicted here. (Dieterich and Brandt 2015b)

13

13.2.4 Thalamic Astasia and Lateropulsion

Unilateral central vestibular lesions of the thalamus (Dieterich and Brandt 1993b; Baier et al. 2016) or the vestibular cortex (Brandt et al. 1994) were shown to manifest with tilts of the perceived visual vertical but without head tilt and skew torsion. These lesions can only be detected through perceptual deficits, which become apparent when the subjective visual vertical (SVV) is measured (see ▶ Chap. 3.1.1.3; ◘ Fig. 3.3). These tilts can be ipsilateral or contralateral and are thus not direction-specific as is typical for lesions of the brainstem. In the individual patient, however, the direction remains the same (Dieterich and Brandt 2019). In lesions of the posterolateral or centromedial thalamic subnuclei, postural imbalance with a transient tendency to fall can occur in the absence of motor weakness or sensory loss. This phenomenon is called *thalamic astasia* (Masdeu and Gorelick 1988; Lee et al. 2005; Elwischger et al. 2012).

In the case of medullary lesions below the vestibular nuclei, tone imbalance in the roll plane can manifest as *isolated body lateropulsion* without associated ocular motor signs or limb ataxia (Thömke et al. 2005; Kim et al. 2007; Kim et al. 2015a; Nakazato et al. 2016). This isolated lateropulsion occurs when the descending lateral vestibulospinal tract is affected (Thömke et al. 2005). If the medial or superior vestibular nucleus is affected in dorsolateral

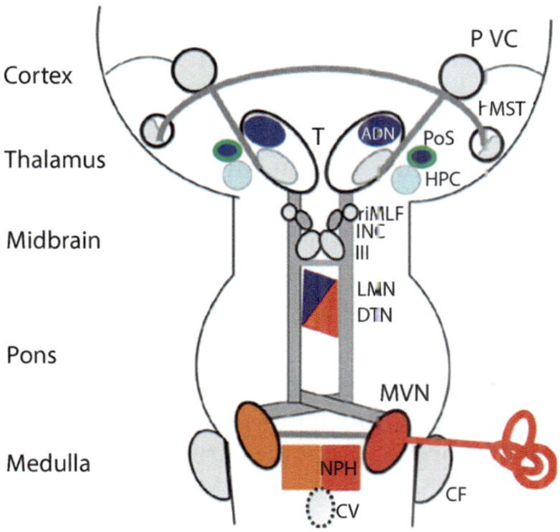

Fig. 13.34 Schematic drawing of the bilaterally organized vestibular anatomical structures from the labyrinth via the vestibular nerve and nucleus (MVN) to the multisensory vestibular cortex (parieto-insular vestibular cortex, PIVC) and the medial superior temporal area (MST) of the visual cortex with three crossings of the brainstem and two transcallosal crossings (compare to Fig. 13.5). Animal studies of rodents identified vestibular neurons with different functions, here depicted with different colors. These are head angular velocity cells (red) coding the semicircular canal signals located in the peripheral vestibular system and lower brainstem (vestibular nuclei, nucleus prepositus hypoglossi) and head direction cells (blue) located in the upper brainstem, the anterior dorsal thalamus, and cortical areas (retrosplenial cortex, postsubiculum, PoS). Place cells (light blue) in the hippocampal region (HPC) code the localization of an individual in the 3D space. Grid cells (green), responsible for the detection of distance and movement velocity, are located in the PoS. (Dieterich et al. 2018; Glasauer et al. 2018)

medullary infarcts (Wallenberg syndrome), the lateropulsion is combined with an ipsilateral OTR and transient torsional nystagmus (Brandt and Dieterich 1987; Halmagyi et al. 1990; Dieterich and Brandt 1992). Physical therapy is recommended to improve postural imbalance and gait in patients with these conditions. Lateropulsion in Wallenberg syndrome has a good prognosis (Cnyrim et al. 2007).

13.3 Higher (Cognitive) Vestibular Syndromes

The simple classification of vestibular disorders as peripheral or central disregards a third category (Fig. 13.1). In analogy to disorders of higher visual functions of the "what" and "where" pathways (De Haan and Cowey 2011), a new category, namely disorders of "higher vestibular functions," which include cognition and other non-vestibular modalities, has been proposed (Brandt et al. 2014). The hemispheric dominance of cortical activation of the vestibular network, as described above, is reflected in several supratentorial neurological disorders involving higher vestibular function. These disorders include impairment of spatial orientation, spatial attention, navigation, and balance control, and they are based on integration of multisensory—that is, visual, vestibular, and somatosensory—input. To illustrate the characteristics of disorders of higher vestibular function, we describe four conditions: hemispatial neglect, room tilt illusion, pusher syndrome, and impairment of spatial memory and navigation associated with hippocampal atrophy in peripheral bilateral vestibular loss or in degenerative brain diseases.

Further higher vestibular functions which extend into dimensions of emotion processing, social cognition (Deroualle and Lopez 2014), or distorted own-body representations (Lopez et al. 2012b, 2018; Lopez and Elzière 2018) are increasingly being investigated.

13.3.1 Hemispatial Neglect

Hemispatial neglect is a disorder caused by interrupted attention to visual stimuli within one hemifield contralateral to the acute lesion (usually of the right temporoparietal cortex) (Vallar and Perani 1986). In rare cases, transient neglect can occur after acute right or left lesions of the frontal premotor cortex (Husain and Kennard 1996). A milder form of neglect, termed visual extinction, can occur if spatial attention is less severely disturbed, or during the course of recovery from neglect.

A critical cortical lesion site that causes hemispatial neglect includes the temporo-parieto-insular cortex, which contains the key region of the multisensory vestibular network (Karnath et al. 2004; Karnath and Dieterich 2006; Karnath and Rorden 2012). The important involvement of vestibular function has been demonstrated by experimentally shifting the border of the neglect during and temporarily also after vestibular stimulation. The organization of multisensory spatial attention in each hemisphere, as well as the dominance of the right hemisphere, must be taken into account in computational modeling of the possible neuronal mechanisms of neglect (Brandt et al. 2012; Dietz et al. 2014). Specific training programs, including repetitive galvanic vestibular stimulation, have been developed to promote recovery from neglect (Volkening et al. 2018). Resting-state functional connectivity MRI in the acute phase during caloric stimulation and after recovery 6 months later (without caloric stimulation) showed similar changes of connectivity in intra- and transhemispheric visual and vestibular cortex areas (Conrad et al. 2018).

13

13.3.2 Room Tilt Illusion

The room tilt illusion is a rare disorder of paroxysmal transient upside-down vision, and it reflects cortical dysfunction of visual-vestibular interaction (Brandt 1997) (■ Fig. 13.35). Apparent inversion of vision or 90° tilts of the environment are misperceptions of verticality. The spatial orientation of the visual scene is mediated by vestibular and visual cues; both sensory systems deliver input for the adjustment of verticality in a 3D environment. As we cannot perceive two different verticals—a visual vertical and a vestibular vertical—at the same time, the two senses must match their spatial coordinates. Thus, a room tilt illusion indicates a transient mismatch of the vestibular and visual coordinate systems and is the erroneous result of an attempt to make a cortical match (Brandt 1997; Brandt et al. 2014).

The causative lesions of the room tilt illusion are mostly subcortical, located within the brainstem or even the peripheral end organ. Examples are found in bilateral vestibular failure or Menière's disease (Sierra-Hidalgo et al. 2012). As in hemispatial neglect, the cause of the disease is vestibular, but the misperception is mainly visual. The spontaneous course of episodic room tilt illusions is mostly benign (Sierra-Hidalgo et al. 2012). Therapy depends on the underlying cause; for example, carbamazepine can be used to treat neurovascular cross-compression of the vestibular nerve.

An fMRI study on the connectivity in a patient with a megalodolichobasilar artery and frequent attacks dependent on head position demonstrated increased connectivity during the attack from area V5 to the bilateral insular and opercular cortex (OP2, Ig1), while the connectivity between PIVC and V1 was diminished (Kirsch et al. 2017). A bilateral multisensory temporo-parietal region centering on the left parietal operculum, OP1, and the right Ig1 with some reservation may be engaged in resolving the visual-vestibular mismatch to restore a reliable global perception of verticality (Kirsch et al. 2017).

13.3.3 Pusher Syndrome

During acute stroke management, pusher syndrome is often under-recognized by neurologists, but physical therapists are very familiar with its signs (Pedersen et al. 1996). The syndrome is characterized by an apparent tilt of the perceived body posi-

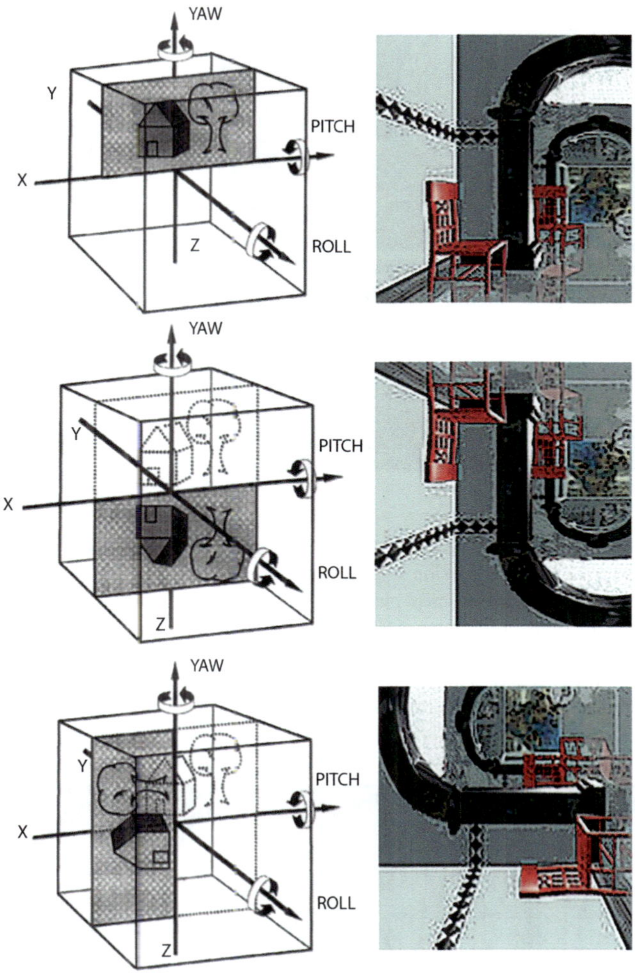

Fig. 13.35 Schematic representation of the head as a cube with the cortical matching of the vestibular and the visual 3D coordinate maps. The three major planes of action of the vestibular system are the frontal roll, the horizontal yaw, and the sagittal pitch about the *x*, *y*, and *z* axes, respectively. Top: Visual scene matched with vestibular coordinates. Middle: Room tilt illusion with 180° tilted visual scene in the pitch plane, i.e., upside-down vision. Bottom: Room tilt illusion with 90° tilt in the roll plane. (Brandt 1997, Brandt et al. 2014)

tion in space, which the patient attempts to counteract by actively pushing or tilting the body to the contralesional side. This pushing is performed by the nonparetic arm or leg (Karnath 2007; Pérennou et al. 2008). Proposed causative lesion sites include the thalamus and—perhaps more likely—the posterior part of the insula (Johannsen et al. 2006; Ticini et al. 2009; Baier et al. 2012a) (Fig. 13.36). These lesion sites contain components of the multisensory cortical vestibular network which contribute to the adjustments of subjective visual (SVV) and haptic verticality (Fig. 13.37) (Baier et al. 2021). There is a positive correlation between the extent of the pushing and the SVV deviation (Baier et al. 2012a). This occurs more frequently with lesions of the right hemisphere (42%) than with lesions of the left hemisphere (25%) and indicates a close con-

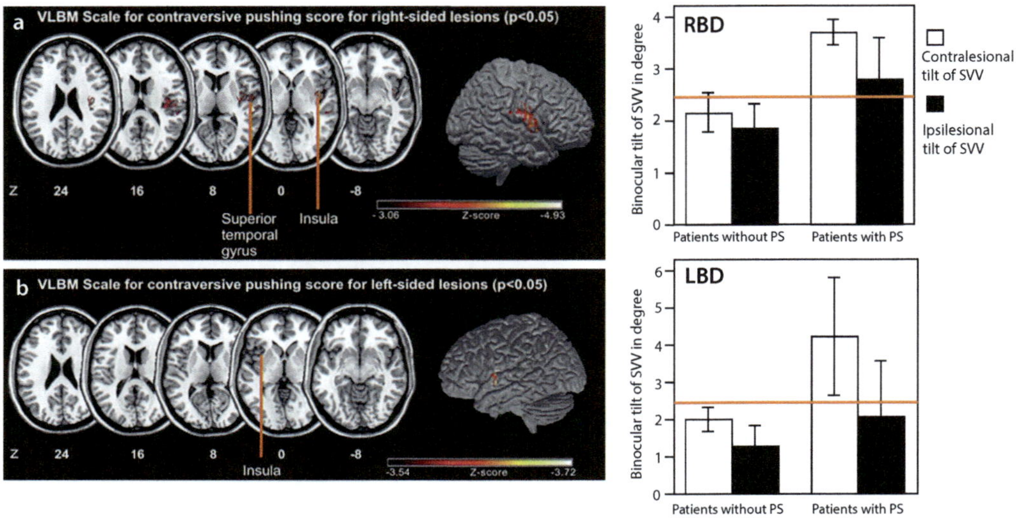

Fig. 13.36 Statistical voxel-wise lesion-behavioral mapping (VLBM) used to compare the lesion site with the amount of pushing (scale for contraversive pushing in %) in the acute phase for right-brain damage (RBD; **a**) and left-brain damage (LBD; **b**) (FDR corrected alpha threshold $p < 0.05$) (left part). The lesion areas are located in the posterior insula, the superior temporal gyrus, and the white matter. Perceptual deficits in these patients with RBD and LBD such as tilts of the subjective visual vertical (SVV; in degree) in ipsilesional and contralesional directions (right part). The yellow line indicates the normal range (+2 SD) of SVV (2.5°). (Modified after Baier et al. 2012a)

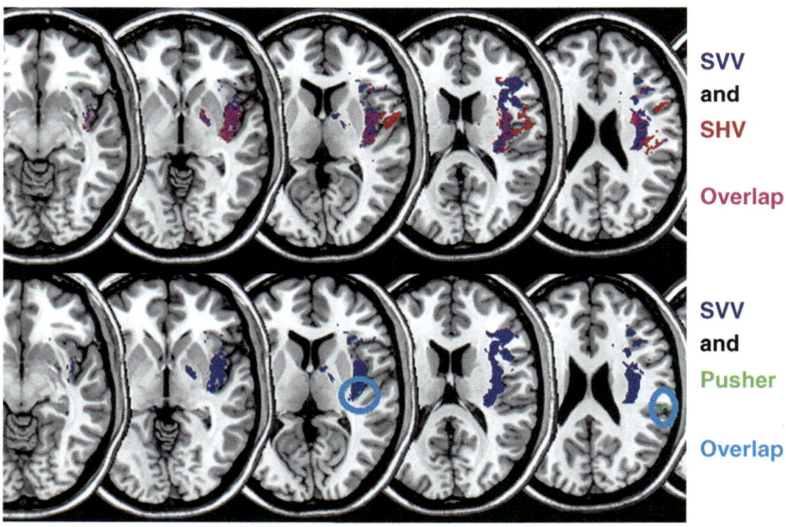

Fig. 13.37 Statistical voxel-wise lesion-behavioral mapping (VLBM) used to compare the lesion site in 82 patients with acute unilateral strokes of the right hemisphere with the deviation of the subjective visual vertical (SVV; blue), the subjective haptic vertical (SHV; red), and the amount of pushing behaviour (green) (t-test; permutation rate 5%). The overlap area for SVV and SHV is given in pink, for SVV and pusher syndrome in light blue. The main overlaps are in the insula (long insular gyrus III and IV, short insular gyrus II), the parietal operculum, inferior frontal gyrus, superior temporal gyrus, transverse temporal Gyrus Heschl, and the basal ganglia (pallidum)

nection between the control of posture and stance and the vestibular system.

The dominance of the right hemisphere of this network explains the significantly higher frequency of pushing behavior in right hemispheric strokes as compared with strokes of the left hemisphere (Abe et al. 2012). This observation is compatible with the experience of physical therapists, who find that recovery from pushing is slower after right hemispheric strokes (Abe et al. 2012).

13.3.4 Disorders of Orientation in Space and Navigation

Deficits of spatial memory, orientation, and navigation are early signs of incipient dementia in patients with *MCI and Alzheimer's disease* (Coughlan et al. 2018, 2020). Patients complain about dizziness, light-headedness, and anxiety of spatial orientation (Kremmyda et al. 2016). Testing navigation under real-world conditions was able to differentiate amyloid-positive and -negative MCI patients in amyloid-PET with more severe deficits and reduced hippocampal activity in the positive patients (Schöberl et al. 2020) (◘ Fig. 13.38).

Spatial memory and navigation are also impaired in focal *hippocampal lesions*, e.g., unilateral infarcts, and as prolonged deficits in *transient global amnesia* (Schöberl et al. 2019). However, in these disorders, it is not clear to what extent vestibular structures and functions are involved. In any case, the hippocampus is an important integration center of the large complex multisensory vestibular network.

Cognitive vestibular syndromes are not necessarily caused by central vestibular dysfunctions but peripheral vestibular disorders can also cause deficits of higher vestibular functions such as impairment of spatial memory, orientation, and navigation in chronic peripheral *bilateral vestibulopa-*

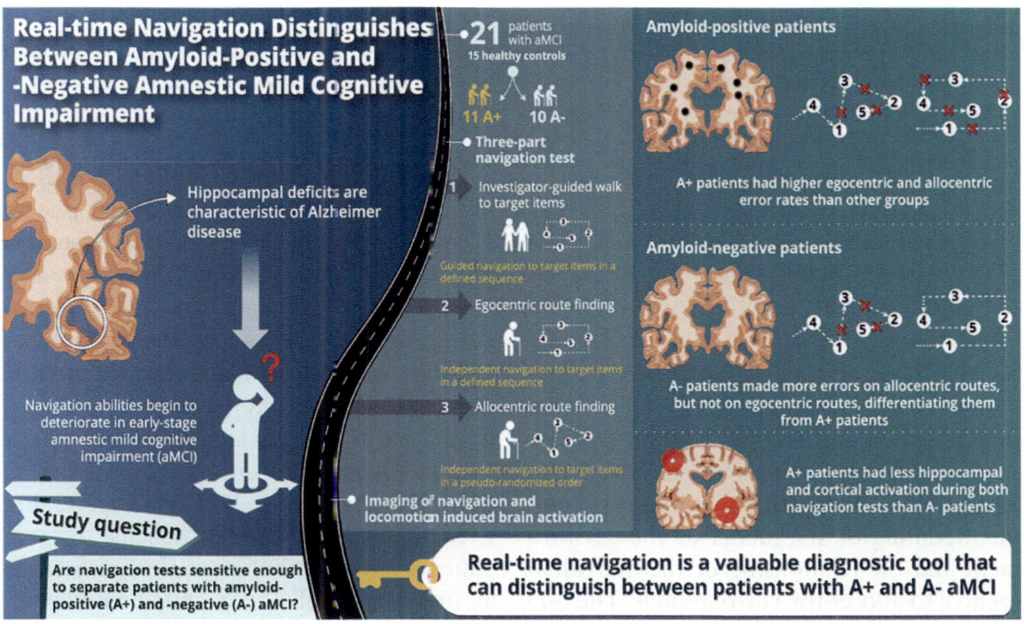

◘ **Fig. 13.38** Patients with amyloid-positive amnestic mild cognitive impairment (aMCI) perform worse in spatial orientation and navigation (egocentric and allocentric route planning) compared to amyloid-negative aMCI patients. The clinical navigation testing in real space can help to identify patients with cognitive deficits in an early stage of underlying Alzheimer's dementia. (Schöberl et al. 2020)

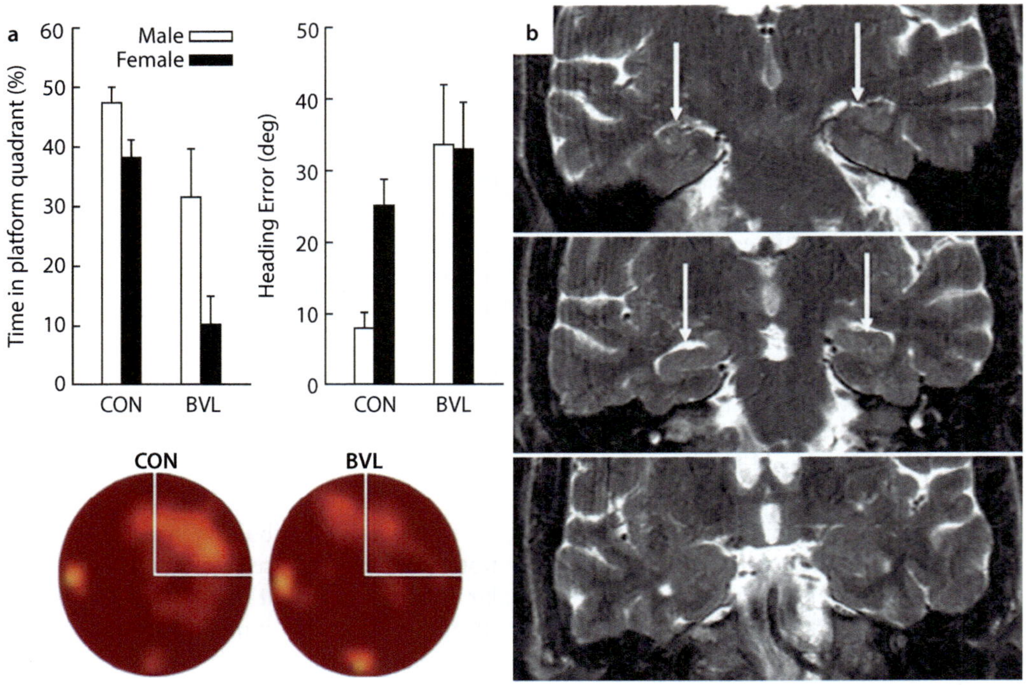

Fig. 13.39 Patients with acquired chronic bilateral vestibular loss (BVL) due to neurofibromatosis 2 (NF2) who had undergone bilateral vestibular neurectomy compared to healthy controls (CON). (**a**) When tested with a virtual variant (on a PC) of the Morris water task (left) these patients exhibited significant spatial memory and navigation deficits that closely matched the pattern of hippocampal atrophy (right). (Top left) Mean percentage of search time that each group (female and male controls and NF2 patients) spent in the platform quadrant during the no-platform probe trial of phase II. Mean initial heading error for each group during the no-platform probe trial of phase II. Error bars are ± 1 SEM. (Bottom left) Dwell time for BVL patients and controls during the no-platform probe trial. Light yellow areas indicate regions where a relatively large amount of time was spent; dark areas indicate regions where a relatively small amount of time was spent. The platform quadrant is demarcated by white lines. (**b**) In BVL patients, a 16.91% volume loss in the hippocampus (arrows) was observed in comparison to age- and sex-matched controls. Volume loss was similar for the left and right hippocampus. Analysis of variance (ANOVA) confirmed a significant difference. Shown are the examples of coronal 3 mm MRI T2-weighted images with a distance of 6 mm in a 40-year-old BVL patient. (Brandt et al. 2005)

13

thy (BVP) (Brandt et al. 2005; Previc et al. 2014). It has been shown in rodents that intact vestibular function is important for spatial memory and navigation (Smith and Zheng 2013). Navigation requires a continuous updating of the model of the environment and the relationship of the individual relative to allocentric surroundings. The 3-D coordinates rely mainly on vestibular and visual input and provide the framework for the process of updating (Brandt et al. 2005) (Fig. 13.39). It has been shown that even a chronic incomplete bilateral vestibular loss can cause an atrophy in the hippocampal formation as well as subjective and objective navigational deficits (Kremmyda et al. 2016; Dordevic et al. 2021) (Fig. 13.40). Even chronic unilateral deficits, e.g. in patients after vestibular neuritis, may cause an impairment of non-cognitive and cognitive functions that rely on vestibular input, while other cognitive functions which rely on visual input were not impaired (Dordevic et al. 2021). In some of these patients

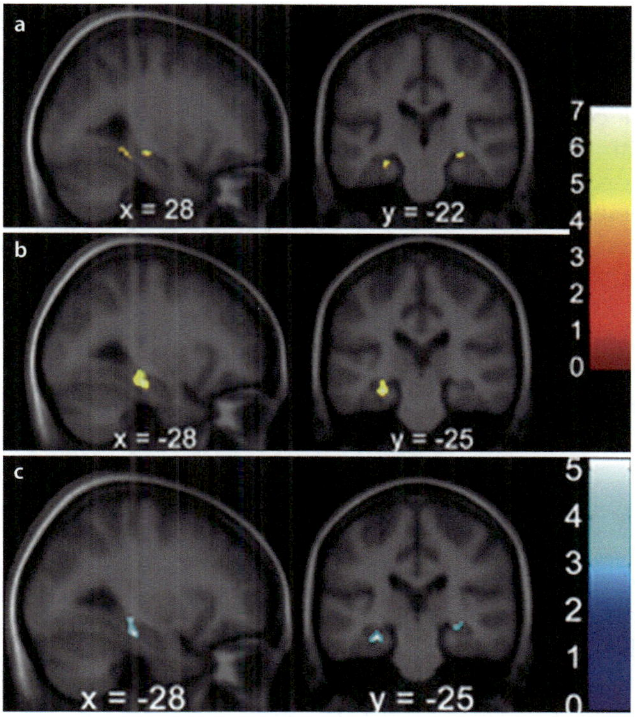

Fig. 13.40 Navigational ability and hippocampal atrophy were examined in 15 patients with bilateral vestibulopathy with residual vestibular function and a group of age- and gender-matched healthy controls. Areas of higher grey matter volume (GM): **a** Clusters of GM differences between the two groups are shown on sagittal and coronal planes through the maximum cluster in the right hemisphere and **b** left hemisphere. Clusters and significance values are from a region of interest analysis, the threshold was 3.69. **c** The wayfinding scale route strategy scores correlate negatively with the GM hippocampal volume bilaterally. Results are shown in a sagittal and coronal plane (Kremmyda et al. 2016)

a reduction of the hippocampal volume was described (Zu Eulenburg et al. 2010), whereas this was not seen in others (Dordevic et al. 2021). This is in line with a study in mice that showed transient deficits in spatial orientation after unilateral labyrinthectomy (Nguyen et al. 2021). However, whether chronic unilateral peripheral vestibular lesions cause deficits in human cognitive or non-cognitive functions (Hüfner et al. 2007a) or volume reduction of the hippocampus is still a matter of debate. In patients with BVP, other mild cognitive impairments have been described beyond deficits in spatial orientation (Popp et al. 2017). Patients with BVP profit from physical therapy (Hall et al. 2016); however, the efficacy of a specific rehabilitation for spatial memory deficits has not been tested yet.

Another aspect is a connection with the anxiety and depression networks (Hilber 2022). An example is the surprisingly low level of anxiety about falling (Decker et al. 2019) and the lack of an increasing susceptibility to develop visual height intolerance (Brandt et al. 2018), which contrast with the higher frequency of falls in BVP patients (Schniepp et al. 2017) as compared to other vestibular disorders (Brandt and Dieterich 2020). Further, room tilt illusions also occur with peripheral vestibular disorders such as Menière's disease or BVP.

Finally, it has become evident over the last years that the vestibular system is also involved in other cognitive, emotional, and psychological processes, such as own-body perception, mood, empathy, and decision-making in social cognition (Hitier et al. 2014; Lopez et al. 2018). Clinical studies have reported distressing perceptions such as increased separation of the self from the body, i.e., symptoms of depersonalization and derealization (Smith and Darlington 2013; Smith and Zheng 2013; Mast et al. 2014; Jáuregui Renaud 2015; Lopez and Elzière 2018), and dysfunction of social cognition (Deroualle and Lopez 2014).

13.4 Cerebellar Vertigo and Dizziness

Dizziness and postural imbalance due to cerebellar disorders make up about 10% of the diagnoses in a tertiary outpatient clinic (Feil et al. 2019; Zwergal et al. 2019). Mostly they manifest with swaying vertigo or dizziness, postural imbalance, and falls (Bodranghien et al. 2016; Jen and Wan 2018). Causes are degenerative hereditary cerebellar disorders, in particular, episodic ataxia type 2 (EA2) or acquired cerebellar ataxia with paraneoplastic, inflammatory, immunological, or toxic etiologies (Manto et al. 2020; Narayan et al. 2020). Ocular motor dysfunctions, including dysfunctions of saccades and pursuit, fixation suppression of the VOR, gaze-evoked, and positional nystagmus, are important for differential diagnosis. Further ocular misalignments of horizontal or vertical eye position are frequent, especially for distant fixation objects (Hüfner et al. 2015; Feil et al. 2019). In acute cerebellar disorders such as ischemic strokes, hemorrhages or inflammations, limb ataxia, dysarthria, and dysphagia may dominate. Cerebellar dysfunctions are also part of CANVAS syndrome (Szmulewicz et al. 2011; Zingler et al. 2009) (▶ Chap. 7).

The frequency of signs and symptoms of 369 patients with cerebellar vertigo and dizziness revealed (Feil et al. 2019) a persistent dizziness in 81%, episodic vertigo in 31%, and a combination of both in 21%. Of these patients, 95% presented with central ocular motor signs (saccadic pursuit, gaze-evoked nystagmus, central fixation nystagmus, and most often downbeat nystagmus). Eleven percent presented with isolated cerebellar ocular motor dysfunction and imbalance of stance and gait without limb ataxia or speech dysfunction.

Episodic ataxia type 2 (EA 2) has gained increasing clinical relevance because of several medical treatment options with varying benefit: 4-aminopyridine for EA 2, downbeat nystagmus, and cerebellar gait disorders (Strupp et al. 2004, 2011; Tsunemi et al. 2010; Schniepp et al. 2011, 2012; Muth et al. 2021). Some ataxias and cerebellar dizziness can be treated with acetyl-DL-leucine (Strupp et al. 2013; Bremova et al. 2015; reviews: Strupp et al. 2017; Kalla and Strupp 2019). In EA 2, acetazolamide can also be used.

The management is multimodal, consisting of medical treatment and physical therapy of balance and gait (Gandini et al. 2020). The therapeutic effects should be monitored by repeated posturography, gait analysis, neuroorthoptic analysis, and registrations of eye movements.

References

Abe H, Kondo T, Oouchida Y et al (2012) Prevalence and length of recovery of pusher syndrome based on cerebral hemispheric lesion side in patients with acute stroke. Stroke 43:1654–1656

Anagnostou E, Spengos K, Vassilopoulou S et al (2010) Incidence of rotational vertigo in supratentorial stroke: a prospective analysis of 112 consecutive patients. J Neurol Sci 290:33–36

Averbuch-Heller L, Tusa RJ, Fuhry L, Rottach KG, Ganser GL, Heide W, Büttner U, Leigh RJ (1997) A double-blind controlled study of gabapentin and baclofen as treatment for acquired nystagmus. Ann Neurol 41:818–825

Baier B, Dieterich M (2009) Ocular tilt reaction – a clinical sign of cerebellar infarctions? Neurology 72(6):572–573

13

Baier B, Bense S, Dieterich M (2008) Are signs of ocular tilt reaction in patients with cerebellar lesions mediated by the dentate nucleus? Brain 131:1445–1454
Baier B, Janzen J, Fechir M, Müller N, Dieterich M (2012a) Pusher syndrome – its anatomical correlate. J Neurol 259:277–283
Baier B, Suchan J, Karnath HO, Dieterich M (2012b) Neuronal correlate of verticality perception – a voxelwise lesion study. Neurology 78(10):728–735
Baier B, Conrad J, Stephan T, Kirsch V, Vogt T, Wilting J, Müller-Forell W, Dieterich M (2016) Vestibular thalamus: two distinct graviceptive pathways. Neurology 86(2):134–140
Baier B, Cuvenhaus H, Müller N, Birklein F, Dieterich M (2021) The importance of the insular cortex for vestibular and spatial syndromes. Eur J Neurol 28(5):1774–1778. https://doi.org/10.1111/ene.14660
Baier B, Cuvenhaus H, Müller N, Birklein F, Dieterich M (2022) Vestibular compensation of otolith graviceptive dysfunction in stroke patients. Eur J Neurol 29(3):905–909. https://doi.org/10.1111/ene.15193
Baloh RW, Jacobson K, Honrubia V (1993) Horizontal semicircular canal variant of benign positional vertigo. Neurology 43:2542–2549
Barra J, Marquer A, Joassin R et al (2010) Humans use internal models to construct and update sense of verticality. Brain 133:3552–3563
Becker-Bense S, Dieterich M, Buchholz H-G et al (2014) The differential effects of acute right- vs left-sided vestibular failure on brain metabolism. Brain Struct Funct 219(4):1355–1367. https://doi.org/10.1007/s00429-013-0573-z
Becker-Bense S, Buchholz HG, Baier B, Schreckenberger M, Bartenstein P, Zwergal A, Brandt T, Dieterich M (2016) Functional plasticity after unilateral vestibular midbrain infarction in human positron emission tomography. PLoS One 11(11):e0165935. https://doi.org/10.1371/journal.pone.0165935
Bense S, Stephan T, Yousry TA et al (2001) Multisensory cortical signal increases and decreases during vestibular galvanic stimulation (fMRI). J Neurophysiol 85:886–899
Bense S, Bartenstein P, Lochmann M et al (2004) Metabolic changes in vestibular and visual cortices in acute vestibular neuritis. Ann Neurol 56:624–630
Bense S, Best C, Buchholz HG, Wiener V, Schreckenberger M, Bartenstein P, Dieterich M (2006) 18F-fluorodeoxyglucose hypometabolism in cerebellar tonsil and flocculus in downbeat-nystagmus. Neuroreport 17:599–603
Bodranghien F, Bastian A, Casali C et al (2016) Consensus paper: revisiting the symptoms and signs of cerebellar syndrome. Cerebellum 15:369–391
Brandt T (1997) Cortical matching of visual and vestibular 3D coordinate maps. Ann Neurol 42(6):983–984
Brandt T (1999) Vertigo: its multisensory syndromes. Springer, London
Brandt T, Dieterich M (1987) Pathological eye-head coordination in roll: tonic ocular tilt reaction in mesencephalic and medullary lesions. Brain 110:649–666
Brandt T, Dieterich M (1988) Oscillopsia and motion perception. In: Kennard C, Clifford Rose F (eds) Physiological aspects of clinical neuro-ophthalmology. Chapman and Hall, London, pp 321–339
Brandt T, Dieterich M (1994) Vestibular syndromes in the roll plane: topographic diagnosis from brainstem to cortex. Ann Neurol 36:337–347
Brandt T, Dieterich M (1999) The vestibular cortex. Its locations, functions, and disorders. Ann N Y Acad Sci 871:293–312
Brandt T, Dieterich M (2015) Does the vestibular system determine the lateralization of brain functions? J Neurol 262:214–215
Brandt T, Dieterich M (2017) The dizzy patient: don't forget disorders of the central vestibular system. Nat Rev Neurol 13:352–362
Brandt T, Dieterich M (2018) Functional and structural benefits of separately operating right and left thalamo-cortical networks. J Neurol 265(Suppl 1):98–100
Brandt T, Dieterich M (2019) Thalamocortical network: a core structure for integrative multimodal vestibular functions. Curr Opin Neurol 32(1):154–164
Brandt T, Dieterich M (2020) 'Excess anxiety' and 'less anxiety': both depend on vestibular function. Curr Opin Neurol 33(1):136–141
Brandt T, Dieterich M, Büchele W (1986) Postural abnormalities in central vestibular brain stem lesions. In: Bles W, Brandt T (eds) Disorders of posture and gait. Elsevier, Amsterdam New York Oxford, pp 141–156
Brandt T, Dieterich M, Danek A (1994) Vestibular cortex lesions affect the perception of verticality. Ann Neurol 35:528–534
Brandt T, Bötzel K, Yousry T, Dieterich M, Schulze S (1995) Rotational vertigo in embolic stroke of the vestibular and the auditory cortex. Neurology 45:42–44
Brandt T, Bartenstein P, Danek A, Dieterich M (1998) Reciprocal inhibitory visual vestibular interaction: visual motion stimulation deactivates the parieto-insular vestibular cortex. Brain 121:1749–1758
Brandt T, Stephan T, Bense S et al (2000) Half-field visual motion stimulation: interhemispheric cross-talk (an fMRI study). Neuroreport 11:1–7

Brandt T, Schautzer F, Hamilton D et al (2005) Vestibular loss causes hippocampal atrophy and impaired spatial memory in humans. Brain 42:2732–2741

Brandt T, Dieterich M, Strupp M, Glasauer S (2012) Model approach to neurological variants of visuo-spatial neglect. Biol Cybern 259:2555–2564

Brandt T, Strupp M, Dieterich M (2014) Towards a concept of disorders of "higher vestibular function". Front Integr Neurosci 8:47. https://doi.org/10.3389/fnint.2014.00047

Brandt T, Grill E, Strupp M, Huppert D (2018) Susceptibility to fear of heights in bilateral vestibulopathy and other disorders of vertigo and balance. Front Neurol 9:406. https://doi.org/10.3389/fneur.2018.00406

Bremova T, Malinova V, Amraoui Y et al (2015) Acetyl-dl-leucine in Niemann-pick type C: a case series. Neurology 85:1368–1375

Brunetti M, Belardinelli P, Caulo M et al (2005) Human brain activation during passive listening to sounds from different locations: an fMRI and MEG study. Hum Brain Mapp 26:251–261

Chen L, Lee W, Chambers BR, Dewy HM (2011) Diagnostic accuracy of acute vestibular syndrome at the bedside in a stroke unit. J Neurol 258(5): 855–861

Choi K-D, Kim J-S (2019) Vascular vertigo. J Neurol 266:1835–1843

Claassen J, Feil K, Bardins S, Teufel et al (2013a) Dalfampridine in patients with downbeat nystagmus--an observational study. J Neurol 260: 1992–1996

Claassen J, Spiegel R, Kalla R et al (2013b) A randomised double-blind, cross-over trial of 4-aminopyridine for downbeat nystagmus–effects on slow phase eye velocity, postural stability, locomotion and symptoms. J Neurol Neurosurg Psychiatry 84:1392–1399

Cnyrim CD, Rettinger N, Mansmann U, Brandt T, Strupp M (2007) Central compensation of deviated subjective visual vertical in Wallenberg's syndrome. J Neurol Neurosurg Psychiatry 78:527–528

Cnyrim CD, Newman-Toker D, Karch C, Brandt T, Strupp M (2008) Beside differentiation of vestibular neuritis from central "vestibular pseudoneuritis". J Neurol Neurosurg Psychiatry 79(4):458–460

Coffey EBJ, Herholz SC, Chepesiuk AMP, Baillet S, Zatorre RJ (2016) Cortical contributions to the auditory frequency-following response revealed by MEG. Nat Commun 7:11070. https://doi.org/10.1038/ncomms11070

Coffey EBJ, Musacchia G, Zatorre RJ (2017) Cortical correlates of the auditory frequency-following and onset responses: EEG and fMRI evidence. J Neurosci 37(4):830–838

Conrad J, Boegle R, Ertl M et al (2018) Recovery from spatial neglect with intra- and transhemispheric functional connectivity changes in vestibular and visual cortex areas – a case study. Front Neurol 9:112

Conrad J, Habs M, Boegle R, Ertl M, Kirsch V, Stefanova-Brostek I, Eren O, Becker-Bense S, Stephan T, Wollenweber F, Duering M, Zu Eulenburg P, Dieterich M (2020) Global multisensory reorganization after vestibular brain stem stroke. Ann Clin Trans Neurol 7(10):1788–1801. https://doi.org/10.1002/acn3.51161

Conrad J, Habs M, Ruehl M, Boegle R, Ertl M, Kirsch V, Eren O, Becker-Bense S, Stephan T, Wollenweber F, Duering M, Dieterich M, zu Eulenburg P (2021) Structural reorganization of the cerebral cortex after vestibulo-cerebellar stroke. Neuroimage Clin 30:102603. https://doi.org/10.1016/j.nicl.2021.102603.

Conrad J, Habs M, Ruehl RM, Bögle R, Ertl M, Kirsch V, Eren OE, Becker-Bense S, Stephan T, Wollenweber FA, Duering M, Dieterich M, zu Eulenburg P (2022a) Reorganization of sensory networks after subcortical vestibular infarcts: A longitudinal symptom-related voxel-based morphometry study. Eur J Neurol. https://doi.org/10.1111/ene.15263

Conrad J, Boegle R, Ruehl RM, Dieterich M (2022b) Evaluating the rare cases of cortical vertigo using disconnectome mapping. Brain Struc Funct 227:3063−3073. https://doi.org/10.1007/s00429-022-02530-w

Cortese A, Simone R, Sullivan R et al (2019) Biallelic expansion of an intronic repeat in RFC1 is a common cause of late-onset ataxia. Nat Genet 51:649–658

Coughlan G, Laczo J, Hort J, Minihane A-M, Hornberger M (2018) Spatial navigation deficits – overlooked cognitive marker for preclinical Alzheimer disease? Nat Rev Neurol 14(8):496–506

Coughlan G, Puthusseryppady V, Lowry E, Gillings R, Spiers H, Minihane A-M, Hornberger M (2020) Test-retest reliability of spatial navigation in adults at-risk of Alzheimer's disease. PLoS One. https://doi.org/10.1371/journal.pone.0239077

Cox TA, Corbett JJ, Thompson S et al (1981) Upbeat nystagmus changing to downbeat nystagmus with convergence. Neurology 31:891–892

De Haan EH, Cowey A (2011) On the usefulness of 'what' and 'where' pathways in vision. Trends Cogn Sci 15(10):460–466

Decker J, Limburg K, Hennigsen P, Lahmann C, Brandt T, Dieterich M (2019) Intact vestibular function is relevant for anxiety related to vertigo. J Neurol 266(Suppl 1):89–92

Deroualle D, Lopez C (2014) Toward a vestibular contribution to social cognition. Front Integr Neurosci 14:16

Deutschländer A, Hüfner K, Kalla R et al (2008) Unilateral vestibular failure suppresses cortical visual motion processing. Brain 131:1025–1034
Dichgans M, Dieterich M (1995) Third nerve palsy with contralateral ocular torsion and binocular tilt of visual vertical, indicating a midbrain lesion. Neuro-Ophthalmol 15:315–320
Dieterich M, Brandt T (1992) Wallenberg's syndrome: lateropulsion, cyclorotation, and subjective visual vertical in thirty-six patients. Ann Neurol 31: 399–408
Dieterich M, Brandt T (1993a) Ocular torsion and tilt of subjective visual vertical are sensitive brainstem signs. Ann Neurol 33:292–299
Dieterich M, Brandt T (1993b) Thalamic infarctions: Differential effects on vestibular function in the roll plane (35 patients). Neurology 43:1732–1740
Dieterich M, Brandt T (1993c) Ocular torsion and perceived vertical in oculomotor, trochlear and abducens nerve palsies. Brain 116:1095–1104
Dieterich M, Brandt T (1995) The vestibulo-ocular reflex. Curr Opin Neurol 8(1):83–88
Dieterich M, Brandt T (2015a) The bilateral central vestibular system: its pathways, functions, and disorders. Ann N Y Acad Sci 1343:10–26
Dieterich M, Brandt T (2015b) Why acute unilateral vestibular cortex lesions mostly manifest without vertigo. Neurology 84:1680–1684
Dieterich M, Brandt T (2018a) Global orientation in space and the lateralization of brain functions. Curr Opin Neurol 31:96–104
Dieterich M, Brandt T (2018b) The parietal lobe and the vestibular system. Handb Clin Neurol 151: 119–140
Dieterich M, Brandt T (2019) Perception of verticality and vestibular disorders of balance and falls. Front Neurol 10:172. https://doi.org/10.3389/fneurol/2019.00172
Dieterich M, Büchele W (1989) MRI findings in lesions at the entry zone of the eighth nerve. Acta Otolaryngol (Stockh) Suppl.468:385–389
Dieterich M, Grünbauer M, Brandt T (1998) Direction-specific impairment of motion perception and spatial orientation in downbeat and upbeat nystagmus in humans. Neurosci Lett 245:29–32
Dieterich M, Bense S, Lutz S, Drzezga A, Stephan T, Bartenstein P, Brandt T (2003) Dominance for vestibular cortical function in the non-dominant hemisphere. Cereb Cortex 13(9):994–1007
Dieterich M, Bauermann T, Best C, Stoeter P, Schlindwein P (2007) Evidence for cortical visual substitution of chronic bilateral vestibular failure (an fMRI study). Brain 30:2108–2116
Dieterich M, Kirsch V, Brandt T (2017) Right-sided dominance of the bilateral vestibular system in the upper brainstem and thalamus. J Neurol 264(Suppl 1):55–62
Dieterich M, Glasauer S, Brandt T (2018) Why acute unilateral vestibular midbrain lesions rarely manifest with rotational vertigo: a clinical and modelling approach to head direction cell function. J Neurol 265(5):1184–1198
Dietz MJ, Friston KJ, Mattingley JB, Roepstorff A, Garrido MI (2014) Effective connectivity reveals right-hemispheric dominance in audiospatial perception: implications for models of spatial neglect. J Neurosci 34(14):5003–5011
Dordevic M, Sulzer S, Barche D, Dieterich M, Arens C, Müller NG (2021) Chronic, mild vestibulopathy leads to deficits in spatial tasks that rely on vestibular input while leaving other cognitive functions and brain volume intact. Life (Basel) 11(12):1369
Dumont JR, Taube JS (2015) The neural correlates of navigation beyond the hippocampus. Prog Brain Res 219:83–102
Elwischger K, Rommer P, Prayer D et al (2012) Thalamic astasia from isolated centromedian thalamic infarction. Neurology 78:146–147
Eulenburg zu P, Caspers S, Roski C, Eickhoff SB (2012) Meta-analytical definition and functional connectivity of the human vestibular cortex. NeuroImage 60:162–169
Feil K, Claaßen J, Bardins S, Teufel J, Krafczyk S, Schneider E, Schniepp R, Jahn K, Kalla R, Strupp M (2013) Effect of chlorzoxazone in patients with downbeat nystagmus: a pilot trial. Neurology 81(13):1152–1158
Feil K, Strobl R, Schindler A, Krafczyk S, Goldschagg N, Frenzel C, Glaser M, Schöberl F, Zwergal A, Strupp M (2019) What is behind cerebellar vertigo and dizziness? Cerebellum 18(3):320–332
Feuerecker R, Habs M, Dieterich M, Strupp M (2015) Chronic subjective dizziness: fewer symptoms in the early morning – a comparison with bilateral vestibulopathy and downbeat nystagmus syndrome. J Vestib Res 25(2):67–72
Fink GR et al (2003) Performing allocentric visuospatial judgement with induced distortion of the egocentric reference frame: an fMRI study with clinical implications. NeuroImage 20(3): 1505–1517
Gandini J, Manto M, Bremova-Ertl T, Feil K, Strupp M (2020) The neurological update: therapies for cerebellar ataxias in 2020. J Neurol 267(4): 1211–1220
Glasauer S, Hoshi M, Kempermann U, Eggert T, Büttner U (2003) Three-dimensional eye position and slow phase velocity in humans with downbeat nystagmus. J Neurophysiol 89(1):338–354
Glasauer S, Strupp M, Kalla R, Büttner U, Brandt T (2005) Effect of 4-aminopyridine on upbeat and downbeat nystagmus elucidates the mechanism of downbeat nystagmus. Ann N Y Acad Sci 1039:528–531

Glasauer S, Dieterich M, Brandt T (2018) Neuronal network-based mathematical modelling of perceived verticality in acute unilateral vestibular lesions: from nerve to thalamus and cortex. J Neurol 265(Suppl 1):101–112

Glasauer S, Dieterich M, Brandt T (2019) Computational neurology of gravity perception involving semicircular canal dysfunction in unilateral vestibular lesions. Prog Brain Res 248:303–317

Grüsser OJ, Pause M, Schreiter U (1990a) Localization and responses of neurons in the parieto-insular vestibular cortex in the awake monkeys (*Macaca fascicularis*). J Physiol 430:537–557

Grüsser OJ, Pause M, Schreiter U (1990b) Vestibular neurons in the parieto-insular vestibular cortex of monkeys (*Macaca fascicularis*): visual ans neck receptor responses. J Physiol 430:559–583

Guldin WO, Grüsser OJ (1998) Is there a vestibular cortex? Trends Neurosci 21:254–259

Hall CD, Herdman SJ, Whitney SL, Cass SP et al (2016) Vestibular rehabilitation for peripheral vestibular hypofunction: an evidence-based clinical practice guideline: from the American Physical Therapy Association Neurology Section. J Neurol Phys Ther 40(2):124–155

Halmagyi GM, Curthoys IS (1988) A clinical sign of canal paresis. Arch Neurol 45(7):737–739

Halmagyi GM, Leigh RJ (2004) Upbeat about downbeat nystagmus. Neurology 63(4):606–607

Halmagyi GM et al (1990) Tonic contraversive ocular tilt reaction due to unilateral meso-diencephalic lesion. Neurology 40:1503–1509

Hewett R, Bartolomei F (2013) Epilepsy and the cortical vestibular system: tales of dizziness and recent concepts. Front Integr Neurosci 7:73. https://doi.org/10.3389/fnint.2013.00073

13

Hewett R, Guye M, Gavaret M, Bartolomei F (2011) Benign temporo-parieto-occipital junction epilepsy with vestibular disturbance: an underrecognized form of epilepsy? Epilepsy Behav 21(4): 412–416

Hilber P (2022) The role of the cerebellar and vestibular networks in anxiety disorders and depression: the internal model hypothesis. Cerebellum 21:791–800

Hitier M, Besnard S, Smith PF (2014) Vestibular pathways involved in cognition. Front Integr Neurosci 8:59

Hodgson JC, Hirst RJ, Hudson JM (2016) Hemispheric speech lateralisation in the developing brain is related to motor praxis ability. Dev Cogn Neurosci 22:9–17

Hopf HC (1987) Vertigo and masseter paresis. A new local brain-stem syndrome probably of vascular origin. J Neurol 235:42–45

Hüfner K, Hamilton DA, Kalla R et al (2007a) Spatial memory and hippocampal volume in humans with unilateral vestibular deafferentation. Hippocampus 17:471–485

Hüfner K, Stephan T, Kalla R, Deutschländer A, Wagner J, Holtmannspötter M, Schulte-Altedorneburg G, Strupp M, Brandt T, Glasauer S (2007b) Structural and functional MRIs disclose cerebellar pathologies in idiopathic downbeat nystagmus. Neurology 69:1128–1135

Hüfner K, Frenzel C, Kremmyda O, Adrion C, Bardins S, Glasauer S, Brandt T, Strupp M (2015) Esophoria or esotropia in adulthood: a sign of cerebellar dysfunction? J Neurol 262:585–592

Husain M, Kennard C (1996) Visual neglect associated with frontal lobe infarction. J Neurol 243:652–657

Hwang K, Bertolero MA, Liu WB, D'Esposito M (2017) The human thalamus is an integrative hub for functional brain networks. J Neurosci 37: 5594–5607

Janssen JC, Larner AJ, Morris H, Bronstein AM, Farmer SF (1998) Upbeat nystagmus: clinicoanatomical correlation. J Neurol Neurosurg Psychiatry 65:380–381

Janzen J, Schlindwein P, Bense S, Bauermann T, Vucurevic G, Stoeter P, Dieterich M (2008) Neural correlates of hemispheric dominance and ipsilaterality within the vestibular system. NeuroImage 42:1508–1518

Jáuregui Renaud K (2015) Vestibular function and depersonalization/derealization symptoms. Multisens Res 28(5–6):637–651

Jeffery KJ (2015) Spatial cognition: entorhinal cortex and the hippocampal place-cell map. Curr Biol 25:R1181–R1183

Jeffery KJ, Wilson JJ, Casali G, Hayman RM (2015) Neurol encoding of large-scale three-dimensional place-properties and constraints. Front Psychol 6:927. https://doi.org/10.3389/fpsyg.2015.00927

Jen JC, Wan J (2018) Episodic ataxias. Handb Clin Neurol 155:205–215

Johannsen L, Fruhmann BM, Karnath HO (2006) Subjective visual vertical (SVV) determined in a representative sample of 15 patients with pusher syndrome. J Neurol 253:1367–1369

Kalla R, Strupp M (2019) Aminopyridines and acetyl-DL-leucine: new therapies in cerebellar disorders. Curr Neuropharmacol 17(1):7–13

Kalla R, Deutschländer A, Hüfner K et al (2006) Detection of floccular hypometabolism in downbeat nystagmus by fMRI. Neurology 66:281–283

Karnath HO (2007) Pusher syndrome – a frequent but little-known disturbance of body orientation perception. J Neurol 254:415–424

Karnath H-O, Dieterich M (2006) Spatial neglect – a vestibular disorder? Brain 129:293–305

Karnath H-O, Rorden C (2012) The anatomy of spatial neglect. Neuropsychologia 20:1010–1017

Karnath H-O, Fruhmann Berger M, Küker W, Rorden C (2004) The anatomy of cortical neglect based on voxelwise statistical analysis: a study of 140 patients. Cereb Cortex 14:1164–1172
Kattah JC, Talkad AV, Wang DZ et al (2009) HINTS to diagnose stroke in acute vestibular syndrome. Three-step bedside oculomotor examination more sensitive than early MRI diffusion-weighted imaging. Stroke 40:3504–3510
Kerber KA, Callaghan BC, Telian SA et al (2017) Dizziness symptom type prevalence and overlap: a US nationally representative survey. Am J Med 130:1465.e1–1465.e9
Kim HA, Lee H (2010) Isolated vestibular nucleus infarction mimicking acute peripheral vestibulopathy. Stroke 41:558–560
Kim HJ, Kwon HM, Huh YE, Oh MY, Lee YS (2007) Ipsilateral axial lateropulsion as an initial symptom of lateral medullary infarction: a case report. J Clin Neurol 3(4):197–199. https://doi.org/10.3988/jcn.2007.3.4.197
Kim JH, Kim S, Lee DH, Lee TK, Sung KB (2015a) Isolated axial lateropulsion with ipsilesional subjective visual vertical tilt in caudal lateral medullary infarction. J Vestib Res 25(1):41–45
Kim SH, Park SH, Kim HJ, Kim JS (2015b) Isolated central vestibular syndrome. Ann N Y Acad Sci 1343:80–89
Kirchner H, Kremmyda O, Hüfner K, Stephan T, Zingler V, Brandt T, Jahn K, Strupp M (2011) Clinical, electrophysiological, and MRI findings in patients with cerebellar ataxia and a bilaterally pathological head-impulse test. Ann N Y Acad Sci 1233:127–138
Kirsch V, Keeser D, Hergenroeder T et al (2016) Structural and functional connectivity mapping of the vestibular circuitry from human brainstem to cortex. Brain Struct Funct 221:1291–1308
Kirsch V, Keeser D, Becker-Bense S et al (2017) Vestibular and visual cortex activity during room tilt illusion. J Neurol 264(Suppl 1):70–73
Kirsch V, Boegle R, Keeser D et al (2018) Handedness-dependent functional organizational patterns within the bilateral vestibular cortical network revealed by fMRI connectivity based parcellation. NeuroImage 178:224–237
Kremmyda O, Hüfner K, Flanagin VL et al (2016) Beyond dizziness: virtual navigation, spatial anxiety and hippocampal volume in bilateral vestibulopathy. Front Hum Neurosci 10:139. https://doi.org/10.3389/fnhum.2016.00139
Laurienti PJ, Burdette JH, Wallace MT et al (2002) Deactivation of sensory-specific cortex by cross-modal stimuli. J Cogn Neurosci 14:420–429
Lee PH, Lee JH, Joo US (2005) Thalamic infarct presenting with thalamic astasia. Eur J Neurol 12:317–319
Lee H, Sohn S-I, Cho Y-W, Lee S-R, Ahn B-H, Park B-R, Baloh RW (2006) Cerebellar infarction presenting isolated vertigo. Neurology 67:1178–1183
Lee CC, Suy C, Ho HC, Hung SK, Lee MS, Chou P, Huang YS (2011) Risk of stroke in patients hospitalized for isolated vertigo. A four year follow-up study. Stroke 42:48–52
Leigh RJ, Zee DS (2016) The neurology of eye movements, 5th edn. Oxford University Press, New York Oxford
Lopez C, Elzière M (2018) Out-of-body experience in vestibular disorders – a prospective study of 210 patients with dizziness. Cortex 104:193–206
Lopez C, Blanke O, Mast FW (2012a) The vestibular cortex in the human brain revealed by coordinate-based activation likelihood estimation meta-analysis. Neuroscience 60:162–169
Lopez C, Schreyer HM, Preuss N, Mast FW (2012b) Vestibular stimulation modifies the body schema. Neuropsychologia 50(8):1830–1837
Lopez C, Nakul E, Preuss N, Elziere M, Mast FW (2018) Distorted own-body representations in patients with dizziness and during caloric vestibular stimulation. J Neurol 265(Suppl 1):S86–S94
Maihöfner C, Handwerker HO, Birklein F (2006) Functional imaging of allodynia in complex regional pain syndrome. Neurology 66(5):711–717
Manto M, Gandini J, Feil K, Strupp M (2020) Cerebellar ataxias: an update. Curr Opin Neurol 33:150–160
Mantokoudis G, Tehrani AS, Wozniak A, Eibenberger K, Kattah JC, Guede CI, Zee DS, Newman-Toker DE (2015) VOR gain by head impulse video-oculography differentiates acute vestibular neuritis from stroke. Otol Neurotol 36(3):457–465
Marti S, Straumann D, Glasauer S (2005) The origin of downbeat-nystagmus: an asymmetry in the distribution of on-directions of vertical gaze-velocity Purkinje-cells. Ann N Y Acad Sci 1039: 548–553
Masdeu JC, Gorelick PB (1988) Thalamic astasia: inability to stand after unilateral thalamic lesions. Ann Neurol 23:596–603
Mast FW, Preuss N, Hartmann M et al (2014) Spatial cognition, body representation and affective processes: the role of vestibular information beyond ocular reflexes and control of posture. Front Integr Neurosci 8:44. https://doi.org/10.3389/fnint.2014.00044
Merabet LB, Swisher JD, McMains SA et al (2007) Combined activation and deactivation of visual cortex during tactile sensory processing. J Neurophysiol 97:633–1641
Mesland BS, Finlay AL, Wertheim AH et al (1996) Object motion perception during ego-motion: patients with a complete loss of vestibular function vs. normals. Brain Res Bull 40:459–465

Migliaccio AA, Halmagyi GM, McGarvieL A, Cremer PD (2004) Cerebellar ataxia with bilateral vestibulopathy: description of a syndrome and its characteristic clinical sign. Brain 127:280–293
Mossman B, Mossman S, Purdie G, Schneider E (2015) Age dependent normal horizontal VOR gain of head impuls test measured with video-oculography. J Otolaryngol Head Neck Surg 44:29
Muir GM, Brown JE, Carey JP, Hirvonen TP, Della Santina CC, Minor LB, Taube JS (2009) Disruption of head direction cell signal after occlusion of the semicircular canals in the freely moving chinchilla. J Neurosci 29(46):14521–14533
Muth C, Teufel J, Schols L et al (2021) Fampridine and acetazolamide in EA2 and related familial EA: a prospective randomized placebo-controlled trial. Neurol Clin Pract 11:e438–e446
Naganuma M, Inatomi Y, Yonehara T, Fujioka S, Hashimoto Y, Hirano T, Uchino M (2006) Rotational vertigo associated with parietal cortical infarction. J Neurol Sci 246(1–2):159–161
Nakada T, Remler MP (1981) Primary position upbeat nystagmus. J Clin Neuroophthalmol 1:185–189
Nakazato Y, Tamura N, Ikeda K, Tanaka A, Yamamoto T (2016) Neuroanatomy of isolated body lateropulsion. Brain Nerve 68(3):263–270. https://doi.org/10.11477/mf.1416200387
Narayan RN, McKeon A, Fife TD (2020) Autoimmune vestibulocerebellar syndromes. Semin Neurol 40(1):97–115
Newman-Toker DE, Kattah JC, Alvernia JE, Wang DZ (2008) Normal head impulse test differentiates acute cerebellar strokes from vestibular neuritis. Neurology 70:2378–2385
Nguyen TT, Nam GS, Kang JJ, Han GC, Kim JS, Dieterich M, Oh SY (2021) Galvanic vestibular stimulation improves spatial cognition after unilateral labyrinthectomy in mice. Front Neurol 12:716795
Ocklenburg S, Hugdahl K, Westerhausen R (2013a) Structural white matter asymmetries in relation to functional asymmetries during speech perception and production. NeuroImage 83:1088–1097
Ocklenburg S, Beste C, Güntürkün O (2013b) Handedness: a neurogenetic shift of perspective. Neurosci Biobehav Rev 37(10 Pt 2):2788–2793
Olszewski J, Baxter D (1982) Cytoarchitecture of the human brain stem, 2nd Ed. Karger S, Basel/München/Paris/London/New York/Sydney
Pedersen PM, Wandel A, Jørgensen HS, Nakayama H, Raaschou HO, Olsen TS (1996) Ipsilateral pushing in stroke: incidence, relation to neuropsychological symptoms, and impact on rehabilitation. The Copenhagen stroke study. Arch Phys Med Rehabil 77:25–28
Pérennou DA, Mazibrada G, Chauvineau V et al (2008) Lateropulsion, pushing and verticality perception in hemisphere stroke: a causal relationship? Brain 131:2401–2413
Pierrot-Deseilligny C, Milea D (2005) Vertical nystagmus: clinical facts and hypotheses. Brain 128:1237–1246
Pierrot-Deseilligny C, Milea D, Sirmai J, Papeix C, Rivaud-Pechoux S (2005) Upbeat nystamus due to a small pontine lesion: evidence for the existence of a crossing ventral tegmental tract. Eur Neurol 54(4):186–190
Pierrot-Deseilligny C, Richeh W, Bolgert F (2007) Upbeat nystagmus due to a caudal medullary lesion influenced by gravity. J Neurol 254:120–121
Popp P, Wulff M, Finke K, Rühl M, Brandt T, Dieterich M (2017) Cognitive deficits in patients with a chronic vestibular failure. J Neurol 264(3):554–563
Pothier DD, Rutka JA, Ranalli PJ (2011) Double impairment: clinical identification of 33 cases of cerebellar ataxia with bilateral vestibulopathy. Otolaryngol Head Neck Surg 146:804–808
Previc FH, Krüger WW, Ross RA, Roman MR, Siegel G (2014) The relationship between vestibular function and topographical memory in older adults. Front Integr Neurosci. https://doi.org/10.3389/fnint.2014.00046
Rafehi H, Szmulewicz DJ, Bennett MF et al (2019) Bioinformatics-based identification of expanded repeats: a non-reference intronic pentamer expansion in RFC1 causes CANVAS. Am J Hum Genet 105:151–165
Ranalli RJ, Sharpe JA (1988) Upbeat nystagmus and the ventral tegmental pathway of the upward vestibulo-ocular reflex. Neurology 38:1329–1330
Sander T, Sprenger A, Mart S, Naumann T, Straumann D, Helmchen C (2011) Effect of 4-aminopyridine on gravity dependence and neural integrator function in patients with idiopathic downbeat nystagmus. J Neurol 258(4):618–622
Scharoun SM, Bryden PJ (2014) Hand preference, performance abilities, and hand selection in children. Front Psychol 5:1–15
Schlindwein P, Mueller M, Bauermann T, Brandt T, Stoeter P, Dieterich M (2008) Cortical representation of saccular vestibular stimulation: VEMPs in fMRI. NeuroImage 39(1):19–31
Schniepp R, Wuehr M, Ackl N et al (2011) 4-aminopyridine improves gait variability in cerebellar ataxia due to CACNA 1A mutation. J Neurol 258:1708–1711
Schniepp R, Wuehr M, Neuhaeusser M, Benecke AK, Adrion C, Brandt T, Strupp M, Jahn K et al (2012) 4-Aminopyridine and cerebellar gait: a retrospective case series. J Neurol 259(11):2491–2493

Schniepp R, Schlick C, Schenkel F, Pradhan C, Jahn K, Brandt T, Wuehr M (2017) Clinical and neurophysiological risk factors for falls in patients with bilateral vestibulopathy. J Neurol 264(2): 277–283

Schöberl F, Irving S, Pradhan C et al (2019) Prolonged allocentric navigation deficits indicate hippocampal damage in TGA. Neurology 92(3):e234–e243. https://doi.org/10.1212/WNL.0000000000006779

Schöberl F, Pradhan C, Irving S et al (2020) Real-space navigation testing differentiates between amyloid-positive and –negative aMCI. Neurology 00:1–13. https://doi.org/10.1212/WNL.0000000000008758

Shallo-Hoffmann J, Bronstein AM (2003) Visual motion detection in patients with absent vestibular function. Vis Res 43:1589–1594

Sierra-Hidalgo F, Pablo-Fernandez E, Herrero-San M et al (2012) Clinical and imaging features of the room tilt illusion. J Neurol 259:2555–2564

Smith PF, Darlington CL (2013) Personality changes in patients with vestibular dysfunction. Front Hum Neurosci 7:678

Smith PF, Zheng Y (2013) From ear to uncertainty: vestibular contributions to cognitive function. Front Integr Neurosci. https://doi.org/10.3389/fnint.2013.00084

Spiegel R, Rettinger N, Kalla R, Lehnen N et al (2009) The intensity of downbeat nystagmus during daytime. Ann N Y Acad Sci 1164:293–299

Spiegel R, Kalla R, Rettinger N, Schneider E, Straumann D et al (2010) Head position during resting modifies spontaneous daytime decrease of downbeat nystagmus. Neurology 75:1938–1932

Strupp M, Schüler O, Krafczyk S, Jahn K, Schautzer F, Büttner U, Brandt T (2003) Treatment of downbeat-nystagmus with 3,4-diaminopyridin - placebo-controlled study. Neurology 61:165–170

Strupp M, Kalla R, Dichgans M, Freilinger T, Glasauer S, Brandt T (2004) Treatment of episodic ataxia type 2 with the potassium channel blocker 4-aminopyridine. Neurology 62:1623–1625

Strupp M, Kalla R, Claassen J et al (2011) A randomized trial of 4-aminopyridine in EA2 and related familial episodic ataxias. Neurology 77:269–275

Strupp M, Teufel J, Habs M et al (2013) Effects of acetyl-DL-leucine in patients with cerebellar ataxia: a case series. J Neurol 260:2556–2561

Strupp M, Teufel J, Zwergal A, Schniepp R, Khodakhah K, Feil K (2017) Aminopyridines for the treatment of neurologic disorders. Neurol Clin Pract 7: 65–76

Szmulewicz DJ, Waterson JA, Halamgyi GM, Mossmann S, Chancellor AM, McLean CA, Storey E (2011) Sensory neuropathy as part of the cerebellar ataxia neuropathy vestibular areflexia syndrome. Neurology 76:1903–1910

Tehrani AS, Kattah JC, Kerber KA, Gold DR, Zee DS, Urrutia VC et al (2018) Diagnosing stroke in acute dizziness and vertigo: pitfalls and pearls. Stroke 49(3):788–795

Thömke F, Marx JJ, Iannetti GD, Cruccu G, Fitzek S, Urban PP, Stoeter P, Dieterich M, Hopf HC (2005) A topodiagnostic investigation on body lateropulsion in medullary infarcts. Neurology 64: 716–718

Thurtell MJ, Joshi AC, Leone AC, Tomsak RL, Kosmorsky GS, Stahl JS, Leigh RJ (2010) Cross over-trail of gabapentin and memantine as treatment for aquired nystagmus. Ann Neurol 67:676–680

Ticini LF, Klose U, Naegele T, Karnath H-O (2009) Perfusion imaging in pusher syndrome to investigate the neural substrates involved in controlling upright body position. PLoS One 4:e5737. https://doi.org/10.1371/journal.pone.0005737

Tilikete C, Milea D, Pierrot-Deseilligny C (2008) Upbeat nystagmus from a demyelinating lesion in the caudal pons. J Neuroophthalmol 28:202–206

Tsunemi T, Ishikawa K, Tsukui K, Sumi T, Kitamura K, Mizusawa H (2010) The effect of 3,4-diaminopyridine on the patients with hereditary pure cerebellar ataxia. J Neurol Sci 292:81–84

Tzourio-Mazoyer N (2016) Intra- and interhemispheric connectivity supporting hemispheric specialization. In: Kennedy H, Van Essen DC, Christen Y (eds) Micro-, meso- and macro-connectomics of the brain. Springer, Cham

Tzourio-Mazoyer N, Perrone-Bertolotti M, Jobard G, Mazoyer B, Baciu M (2017) Multi-factorial modulation of hemispheric specialization and plasticity for language in healthy and pathological conditions: a review. Cortex 86:314–339

Valerio S, Taube JS (2016) Head direction cell activity is absent in mice without the horizontal semicircular canals. J Neurosci 36(3):741–754

Vallar G, Perani D (1986) The anatomy of unilateral neglect after right hemisphere stroke lesions: a clinical CT correlation study in man. Neuropsychologia 24:609–622

Van der Ham IJ, Postma A, Laeng B (2014) Lateralization perception: the role of attention in spatial relation processing. Neurosci Biobehav Rev 45:142–148

Vanni S, Pecci R, Edlow JA et al (2015) Can emergency physicians accurately and reliably assess acute vertigo in the emergency department? Emerg Med Australas 27:126–131

Volkening K, Kerkhoff G, Keller I (2018) Effects of repetitive galvanic vestibular stimulation on spatial neglect and verticality perception-a randomised sham-controlled trial. Neuropsychol Rehabil 28(7):1179–1196

von Brevern M, Süßmilch S, Zeise D (2014) Acute vertigo due to hemispheric stroke. A case report and

comprehensive review of the literature. J Neurol Sci 339:153–156
Wagner JN, Glaser M, Brandt T, Strupp M (2008) Downbeat nystagmus: aetiology and comorbidity in 117 patients. J Neurol Neurosurg Psychiatry 79:672–677
Wenzel R, Bartenstein P, Dieterich M et al (1996) Deactivation of human visual cortex during involuntary ocular oscillations, a PET activation study. Brain 119:101–110
Westheimer G, Blair SM (1975) Synkinesis of head and eye movements evoked by brainstem stimulation in the alert monkey. Exp Brain Res 24:89–95
Winter SS, Clark BJ, Taube JS (2015) Spatial navigation. Disruption of the head direction cell network impairs the parahippocampal grid cell signal. Science 347(6224):870–874
Yacovino DA, Zanotti E, Hain TC (2019) Is Cerebellar Ataxia, Neuropathy, and Vestibular Areflexia Syndrome (CANVAS) a vestibular ganglionopathy? J Int Adv Otol 15:304–308
Zee DS, Yamazaki A, Butler PH, Gücer F (1981) Effects of ablation of flocculus and paraflocculus on eye movements in primate. J Neurophysiol 46:878–899
Zingler VC, Cnyrim C, Jahn K, Weintz E, Fernbacher J, Frenzel C, Brandt T, Strupp M (2007) Causative factors and epidemiology of bilateral vestibulopathy in 255 patients. Ann Neurol 61(6):524–532
Zingler VC, Weintz E, Jahn K, Huppert D, Cnyrim C, Brandt T, Strupp M (2009) Causative factors, epidemiology, and folow-up of bilateral vestibulopathy. Ann N Y Acad Sci 1164:505–508
Zu Eulenburg P, Stoeter P, Dieterich M (2010) Voxel-based morphometry depicts central compensation after vestibular neuritis. Ann Neurol 68(2): 241–249
Zwergal A, Dieterich M (2020) Vertigo and dizziness in the emergency room. Curr Opin Neurol 32. https://doi.org/10.1097/WCO.0000000000000769
Zwergal A, Büttner-Ennever J, Brandt T, Strupp M (2008) An ipsilateral vestibulothalamic tract adjacent to the medial lemniscus in humans. Brain 131:2928–2935
Zwergal A, Feil K, Schniepp R, Strupp M (2019) Cerebellar dizziness and vertigo: etiologies, diagnostic assessment, and treatment. Semin Neurol. https://doi.org/10.1055/s-0039-3400315

Vestibular Migraine

Contents

Supplementary Information The online version contains supplementary material available at [https://doi.org/10.1007/978-3-030-78260-3_14]. The videos can be accessed by scanning the related images with the SN More Media App.

M. Strupp et al., *Vertigo and Dizziness*, https://doi.org/10.1007/978-3-030-78260-3_14

Vestibular migraine (VM) is the most frequent cause of spontaneous episodic vertigo attacks in adults and in children (▶ Chap. 16). The term "vestibular migraine" developed during the last 20 years and dates back to a characterization of 90 patients (Dieterich and Brandt 1999). The current diagnostic criteria of the consensus document of the International Bárány Society for Neuro-Otology and the International Headache Society, ICHD, combine typical symptoms of migraine with vestibular symptoms and exclusion criteria (▶ Box 14.1):

Box 14.1 Diagnostic Criteria for Vestibular Migraine (Consensus Document of the Bárány Society and the International Headache Society) (Lempert et al. 2012a, b)

1. ***Vestibular migraine***
   (a) At least 5 episodes with vestibular symptoms of moderate or severe intensity, lasting 5 min to 72 h
   (b) Current or previous history of migraine with or without aura according to the International Classification of Headache Disorders (ICHD) (2004)
   (c) One or more migraine features with at least 50% of vestibular episodes:
   - Headache with at least 2 of the following characteristics: one-sided location, pulsating quality, moderate or severe pain intensity, aggravation by routine physical activity
   - Photophobia and phonophobia
   - Visual aura

   (d) Not better accounted for by another vestibular or ICHD diagnosis
2. ***Probable vestibular migraine***
   (a) At least 5 episodes with vestibular symptoms of moderate or severe intensity, lasting 5 min to 72 h
   (b) Only one of the criteria B and C for vestibular migraine is fulfilled (migraine history *or* migraine features during the episode)
   (c) Not better accounted for by another vestibular or ICHD diagnosis

Similar to migraine without aura, the diagnosis of VM is primarily based on the patient's history because no valid biomarkers exist so far. Although the diagnosis of VM occurs in about 7–12% of patients in an outpatient clinic for vertigo and dizziness (Brandt and Dieterich 2017) and in about 9–30% of migraine patients in an outpatient clinic for headache (Lempert and Neuhauser 2009; Lampl et al. 2019), its diagnosis is still made too rarely. When vertigo and dizziness were the key symptoms in migraine attacks in former times this was also named "migrainous vertigo" (Neuhauser et al. 2001; Neuhauser and Lempert 2004), "migraine-associated dizziness" (Cutrer and Baloh 1992; Johnson 1998; Bisdorff 2004; Brantberg et al. 2005) or "migraine-related vestibulopathy" (Cass et al. 1997).

14

The relationship between migraine with headache and VM is still not yet completely clear even after the consensus definition, since a relevant proportion of patients with vertigo and dizziness and simultaneous migraine features do not fulfill the current ICHD criteria of VM (Abouzari et al. 2020).

14.1 Patient History

The main symptoms of VM are (▪ Figs. 14.1 and ▪ 14.2):

- Recurring attacks of various combinations of vertigo, dizziness, and imbalance of stance and gait
- Visual disorders (oscillopsia or visual aura)

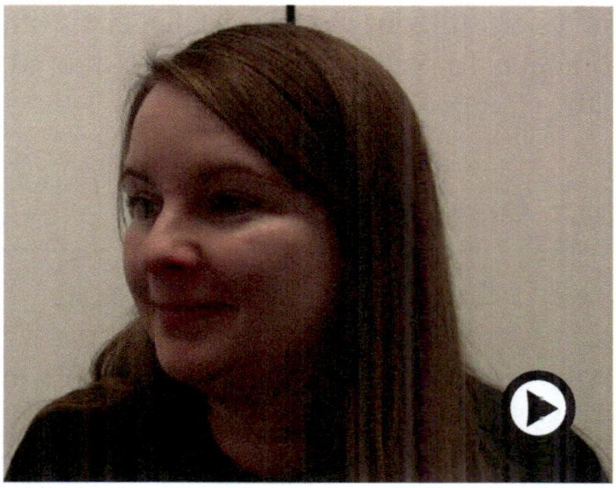

Fig. 14.1 Patient history of a patient with probable vestibular migraine (▶ https://doi.org/10.1007/000-96a)

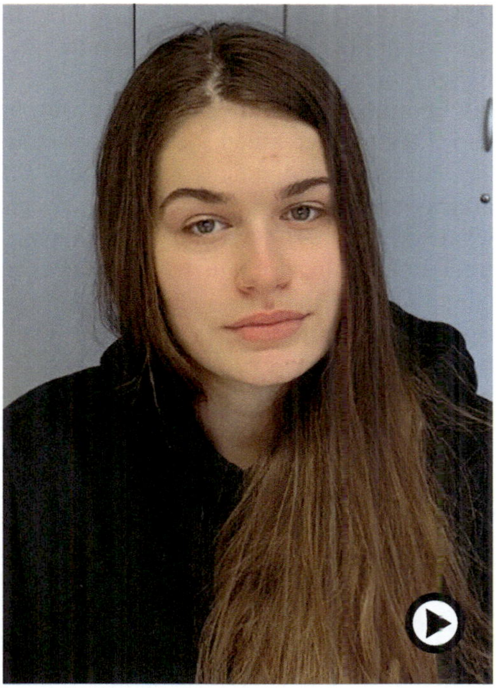

Fig. 14.2 Patient history of a patient with a vestibular migraine (▶ https://doi.org/10.1007/000-969)

- Accompanied or followed by primarily occipital head pressure or headache (more rarely unilateral localization)
- Nausea and vomiting
- Photophobia and phonophobia

As any movement increases the complaints, patients often have a need for rest. The attacks can, however, take a monosymptomatic course, manifesting with only vertigo/dizziness or also with a hearing disorder, tinnitus, or ear pressure. The audiovestibular attacks can also fulfill the diagnostic criteria of Meniere's disease. This suggests a pathophysiological connection between both diseases (Pyykkö et al. 2019), especially since patients were described with both diseases in parallel (Murofushi et al. 2018), and rare familial forms of VM showed an autosomal dominant heritage with incomplete penetrance (Gallego-Martinez et al. 2018). The monosymptomatic attacks with the main symptom of vertigo predominate in about 75% of VM patients (Dieterich and Brandt 1999; Strupp et al. 2010).

14.2 Epidemiology

Both vertigo and migraine without aura frequently occur in the population. The lifetime prevalence of vertigo is 7% and that of migraine up to 16% (4–8% male, 11.2–18.2% female) (Lipton et al. 2002; Stovner and Andree 2010). A coincidental, simultaneous occurrence of the two can be expected in 1.1%; however, epidemiological examinations have shown this occurs in 3.2% of the general population (Neuhauser et al. 2006; Lempert and Neuhauser 2009). In part this co-occurrence can be explained by the fact that patients with migraine frequently have various vertigo syndromes, e.g., BPPV, Meniere's disease (Radtke et al. 2002), or functional phobic postural dizziness (Best et al. 2009).

The 1-year prevalence of VM is 2.7% in adults in the USA, with a female share of 64.1% and a mean age of 40.9 years (Formeister et al. 2018). Migraine without aura naturally has a higher 1-year prevalence of 12–14% after puberty in women, whereas it is 7–8% in men. The relative frequency of VM in dedicated dizziness outpatient clinics is about 7–11% (Dieterich and Brandt 1999; Neuhauser et al. 2001; Strupp et al. 2010) and at least 9% in headache outpatient clinics (Lempert and Neuhauser 2009). The lifetime prevalence of VM is around 1% (Neuhauser et al. 2006). On the basis of several VM studies, women are affected 3.65 times more often than men (Dieterich and Brandt 1999; Neuhauser et al. 2001, 2006; Neff et al. 2012; Obermann et al. 2015; Cho et al. 2016; Morganti et al. 2016; Colombo et al. 2017; Muelleman et al. 2017; Formeister et al. 2018; overview in: Becker-Bense et al. 2019).

VM can manifest in every age with peaks in younger adults and between the age of 60 and 70 years (Cutrer and Baloh 1992; Cass et al. 1997; Dieterich and Brandt 1999; Neuhauser et al. 2001; Lempert and Neuhauser 2009; Strupp et al. 2010) and more often affects individuals with a history of migraine without aura (Dieterich and Brandt 1999; Neuhauser et al. 2001). The correct diagnosis in the past was mostly found about 8.4 years after the first occurrence (Thakar et al. 2001); nowadays the diagnosis is made earlier because of better knowledge of VM. At the age of menopause, attacks of migraine without aura can be replaced by attacks of isolated vertigo or dizziness (Lempert et al. 2009).

Epidemiological studies disclosed that migraine is also the most frequent cause of vertigo and dizziness in children (Batu et al. 2015; Jahn et al. 2015). If the attacks in childhood take a monosymptomatic course without headache, they cannot be differentiated clinically from "paroxysmal vertigo in childhood." The latter is considered to be equivalent to migraine, with attacks that begin between the first and fourth year of life, last only seconds to minutes, and disappear spontaneously within a few years. It corresponds to attacks of VM without headache which account for 39% of vertigo attacks in children, the most frequent form of vertigo/dizziness, followed by 21% with functional psychogenic vertigo (Batu et al. 2015) (see ▶ Chap. 16).

14.3 Diagnosis

14.3.1 Characteristics of Attacks

Attacks of VM occurred spontaneously in 21–83% (Cutrer and Baloh 1992; Cass et al. 1997; Dieterich and Brandt 1999), were dependent on the head or body position in 17–65% (Kayan and Hood 1984; Johnson 1998; Dieterich and Brandt 1999) and showed a head motion intolerance in 31–77% (Cutrer and Baloh 1992; Cass et al. 1997). In a large population-based phone interview, 67% of the participants with VM reported on spontaneous and 24% on position-dependent vertigo attacks (Neuhauser et al. 2006). Some individuals described VM attacks elicited by viewing moving objects (Waterston 2004). Accompanying symptoms in migraine patients from a headache clinic – before the introduction of the new classification criteria of VM – were instability of stance in 91%, imbalance in 82%, and rotating vertigo in 57% (Johnson 1998); this represents a high number of vestibular symptoms.

The duration of the attacks of vertigo varies greatly and lasts either only seconds to minutes or several hours to days (Cutrer and Baloh 1992; Dieterich and Brandt 1999; Neuhauser et al. 2001). The current diagnostic criteria of VM, however, require a minimum of 5 min. Attacks with a typical aura duration of 5–60 min were only found in 10–30% of the patients in earlier studies. This means that a relevant proportion of patients with VM did not fulfill the current ICHD criteria.

The association of vestibular symptoms and headache is often present, but it varies between patients and between attacks, even in the same patient. Vertigo and dizziness can precede, occur in parallel, or follow the headache (Cass et al. 1997; Neuhauser et al. 2001; Lampl et al. 2019). In an interview study on 500 headache patients, 30% reported on episodic vertigo and dizziness in relation to the headache attacks (Lampl et al. 2019). In 16%, vestibular symptoms occurred in parallel, in 10% during the preceding 2 h, and in 3% as prodromal signs during the preceding 48–72 h. Less than 59% of the VM patients reported both vertigo and headache in each attack and 6% alternating attacks with isolated vertigo or isolated headache (Neuhauser et al. 2001).

The attacks are more difficult to recognize if headache is absent (in about 30%; Dieterich and Brandt 1999). The diagnosis is simple if the attacks are generally or always accompanied by headache (or occipital head pressure) and if there is a positive family or personal history of other types of migraine (about 50%). The occurrence of migraine symptoms like light and sound hypersensitivity, need for quiet, tiredness after the attack, and urge to urinate also make diagnosis easier. Aural signs, such as hearing loss, tinnitus, and ear pressure, were found in 38% of VM patients, most often with mild and transient dysfunction (Kayan and Hood 1984; Cass et al. 1997; Johnson 1998; Neff et al. 2012).

Stress, hormone fluctuations, and sleep deficiency can trigger attacks, as in migraine without aura (Lempert et al. 2009).

14.4 Clinical Examination

14.4.1 During the Attack-Free Interval

The neurological examination during the symptom-free interval is normal, except for the ocular motor analysis. The diagnosis is aided by the fact that, contrary to other forms of migraine, 8.6–63% of persons with VM show *slight central ocular motor disorders* (Kayan and Hood 1984; Cutrer and Baloh 1992; Cass et al. 1997; Dieterich and Brandt 1999; Teggi et al. 2009; Celebisoy et al. 2008; Radtke et al. 2012; Dieterich et al. 2016) in the form of:

- Gaze-evoked nystagmus (sometimes dissociated)
- A saccadic smooth pursuit beyond age norm (especially vertical)
- A spontaneous horizontal or vertical nystagmus or fixational nystagmus (downbeat nystagmus) or
- A central positional nystagmus (Dieterich and Brandt 1999; von Brevern et al. 2005; Radtke et al. 2012; Neugebauer et al. 2013).

These mild ocular motor disturbances may increase over time. In a longitudinal study after a mean of 9 years (5.5–11 years), the frequency of central ocular motor signs increased from 8% to 28%, that of peripheral vestibular signs from 2% to 5%, and that of signs of unknown origin from 5% to 8% (Radtke et al. 2012). The dysfunction most often seen was a central positional nystagmus. Another longitudinal observation over 8 years also found an increase of central ocular motor signs (in particular of horizontal and/or vertical saccadic smooth pursuit) from 20% to 63% compared to healthy controls (Neugebauer et al. 2013). In the latter study, a successful migraine prophylaxis seemed to slow down this development.

Peripheral vestibular alterations were reported in 8–22% of VM patients as a unilateral semicircular canal dysfunction (Kayan and Hood 1984; Cutrer and Baloh 1992; Cass et al. 1997; Dieterich and Brandt 1999; Teggi et al. 2009; Celebisoy et al. 2008) or in up to 11% as a bilateral dysfunction (Kayan and Hood 1984; Cass et al. 1997; Teggi et al. 2009). Mild (!) hearing disturbances were observed too, unilaterally in 3–12% (Kayan and Hood 1984; Cass et al. 1997; Battista 2004) and bilaterally in 18% (longitudinal study over 9 years: Radtke et al. 2012). In total, in up to 52% of VM patients auditory symptoms were reported (Oh et al. 2021). More detailed audiological examinations showed hearing deficits in the lower frequency range, lower thresholds of otoacoustic emissions, and a prolonged peak V of acoustic brainstem potentials with a prolonged inter-peak latency I-V (Xue et al. 2020). These findings document that VM not only involves the peripheral but also the central auditory system.

14.4.2 During the Attack

A pathological nystagmus is frequently observed (70%) during an attack, e.g., a central positional nystagmus, which could most often be attributed to a central vestibular dysfunction (von Brevern et al. 2005). The ocular motor disturbances were of central origin in 50%, of peripheral vestibular origin in 15%, and of unknown origin in 35%. In the latter study, no hearing dysfunction was found in these VM patients. However, ear symptoms were reported in up to 38% of VM patients, including ear pressure (often bilaterally), tinnitus, and mild hearing dysfunction.

The patients are generally hypersensitive to movement and motion sickness, particularly during the migraine attack (Cutrer and Baloh 1992). Like phonophobia and photophobia during migraine attacks, this hypersensitivity to movement is possibly induced by a sensory neuron overexcitability, here, for example, of the inner-ear receptors. Such overexcitability has been included in the diagnostic criteria (Neuhauser et al. 2001). Frequencies of 31–77% were reported for head motion sensitivity.

14.5 Technical Examinations

VM is a clinical diagnosis; so far, no biomarkers exist. Neurophysiological examinations, such as posturography, VEMP, and measurements of SVV, were performed in several studies with heterogenous results. In some studies, VEMP were described as delayed, lost, or reduced in amplitude, while others reported symmetrical potentials with normal latencies and amplitudes (Dlugaiczyk et al. 2020; Dieterich et al. 2016; Baier et al. 2009b). However, cVEMP could be helpful in the differential diagnosis between VM and Menière's disease: The asymmetry ratio of cVEMP amplitudes was significantly higher for Menière's disease than for VM and higher for cVEMP than oVEMP in Menière's disease, but not in VM (Dlugaiczyk et al. 2020). SVV measurements showed normal values.

14.6 Differential Diagnosis and Clinical Problems

Occasionally it can be difficult to differentiate VM from:
- Transient ischemic attacks
- Vestibular paroxysmia and, in particular,
- Menière's disease and
- Episodic ataxia type 2.

In some cases, the diagnosis can only be established on the basis of the response to a "specific" therapy.

Transitional and mixed forms or pathophysiological combinations are currently being discussed (see above), especially for *Menière's disease* (▶ Chap. 10) and VM (◘ Fig. 14.3). Valid data are rare, in part because patients with predominantly vestibular symptoms were wrongly attributed to Menière's disease in the past. This would explain the consider-

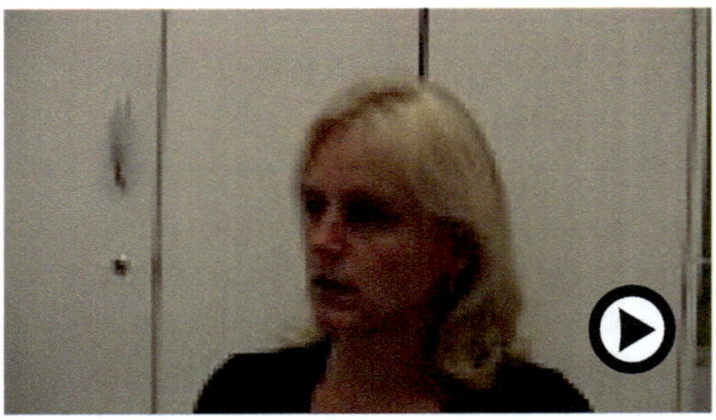

◘ **Fig. 14.3** Patient history of a patient with the combination of Menière's disease and vestibular migraine (▶ https://doi.org/10.1007/000-96b)

able difference in the prevalence of migraine in patients with "classic" Menière's disease (22%) as opposed to "vestibular" Menière's disease (81%) (Rassekh and Harker 1992). Furthermore, the clear preponderance of women vs men in some Menière's studies represents an insufficient differential diagnosis of VM in earlier times (review: Becker-Bense et al. 2019); in Menière's disease, gender distribution is equal. An interview-based study involving 78 patients with confirmed unilateral or bilateral Menière's disease determined that the lifetime prevalence of migraine with and without aura is 56% compared with 25% in an age-matched control group (Radtke et al. 2002). These figures suggest that either there is a pathophysiological link between the two diseases, or alternatively the current diagnostic criteria cannot yet differentiate between them, or both are possible.

As *BPPV* (► Chap. 9) occurs three times more frequently in migraine patients than in trauma patients according to a retrospective study (Ishiyama et al. 2000), it has been speculated that a relapsing inner ear dysfunction may be the underlying cause of the vestibular migraine attacks (e.g., in the form of a vasospasm). The pathoetiology is not yet clear. The therapy for BPPV in migraine patients is the same used to treat idiopathic BPPV, i.e., liberatory maneuvers.

Episodic ataxia type 2 (► Chap. 13) is also characterized by episodic attacks of dizziness with central ocular motor deficits, especially downbeat nystagmus, also frequent and significant during the attack-free interval (Griggs and Nutt 1995). It is an autosomal dominant disorder caused by a mutation in the calcium channel gene CACNA 1A (Ophoff et al. 1996), mainly impairing the function of cerebellar Purkinje cells. The reduced calcium current of the inhibitory Purkinje cells causes a disinhibition of cerebellar nuclei, resulting in these attacks of ataxia and ocular motor disturbances. Placebo-controlled studies showed that 4-aminopyridine (Strupp et al. 2011) as well as acetazolamide (Muth et al. 2021) are effective.

An early differential diagnosis is particularly important for VM patients because:
- They develop functional (somatoform) vertigo and dizziness significantly more often than patients with other vestibular syndromes
- Comorbidities of up to 65% occur with psychiatric disorders (anxiety and depression) (Eckhardt-Henn et al. 2008; Lahmann et al. 2015)
- They especially perceive their vestibular symptoms much more strongly and experience anxiety (Best et al. 2009; Decker et al. 2019)
- The patients often feel more impaired in their daily life

Patients with *functional dizziness* (► Chap. 15) more often describe postural or diffuse dizziness (light-headedness, feeling of emptiness in the head, unsteadiness, etc.), while at the same time they have normal findings in the neuro-otological tests. Depending on the underlying psychiatric disorder, additional symptoms will be present, for example:
- Motivation and concentration disorders
- Decline of performance
- Subjectively experienced restrictions in professional and everyday activities
- Vegetative symptoms that accompany the dizziness (tachycardia, nausea, profuse sweating, dyspnea, fear of suffocating, loss of appetite, weight loss)
- Disorders of mood
- Sleep disorders
- Symptoms of anxiety

Important differential diagnoses that must be quickly clarified are:
- Transient ischemic attacks in the vertebrobasilar system
- Basilar artery thrombosis
- Brainstem/cerebellum hemorrhage
- Basilar artery migraine

all of which can also be accompanied by headache centered primarily in the nuchal region.

Vertebrobasilar artery thrombosis and brainstem hemorrhage usually develop quite rapidly, along with:
- Vigilance disorders that can worsen until coma
- Increasing deficits of the cranial nerves
- Pareses or sensory deficits in the extremities.

A *vertebral artery dissection* can occur spontaneously or after head trauma or chiropractic maneuvers. It is associated with occipital head and nuchal pain, nuchal pressure, dizziness, and other brainstem symptoms. As smaller brainstem ischemias can be induced in the context of various mechanisms, it is especially important to consider the possibility of the more dangerous life-threatening brainstem ischemia in the differential diagnosis at the appearance of the first migraine attacks.

14.7 Course

A longitudinal study was performed in 75 patients with vestibular migraine according to the earlier criteria of Neuhauser and coworkers (2001) – very similar precursor criteria – after a follow up of 8.75 ± 1.3 years (Radtke et al. 2011). Half of the patients with possible VM developed a definite VM. In 85% of patients with definite VM, the diagnosis was confirmed; thus, the diagnosis of VM could be made with high validity on the basis of clinical criteria. Eight patients had developed a mild bilateral sensorineural hearing impairment that fulfilled formally the criteria of a bilateral Menière's disease although no typical attacks had occurred. This can complicate the differential diagnosis.

14.8 Pathophysiology and Therapeutic Principles

The basic mechanisms of vestibular dysfunction in VM are so far not clear. Different hypotheses are under discussion.

One hypothesis is based on "*a simultaneous activation of vestibular and cranial nociceptive connections*" (Balaban 2011; Balaban et al. 2011; Furman et al. 2013; Furman and Balaban 2015). In studies, the same transmitters were found in trigeminal and vestibular ganglia cells that express serotonin, capsaicin, and purinergic receptors (Balaban 2011; Ahn and Balaban 2010). Nociceptive and vestibular afferents with neurochemical similarities converge in brainstem structures such as the parabrachial nucleus, nucleus raphe, and locus coeruleus. These nuclei play an important role in the modulation of the sensitivity of nociceptive pathways. They are also related to the development of anxiety, an aspect that could explain the comorbidity of balance disorders, anxiety, and migraine (Balaban et al. 2011) (▶ Chap. 1).

Neuronal functional disorders in the brainstem are also discussed as factors in the pathophysiology of migraine without aura. Animal studies have identified the locus coeruleus in the pontine brainstem – the most important central core of the noradrenergic system – as the modulator of the cerebral blood flow in this primarily neurovascular headache syndrome, in which the trigeminovascular system along with neurogenic inflammatory reactions plays a central role (Goadsby 2000). Furthermore, the serotonergic dorsal raphe nucleus in the midbrain seems to play an important role. Positron emission tomography studies have shown that this region and that of the dorsal pons with the locus coeruleus are also activated in patients during migraine attacks without aura (Weiller et al. 1995). These brainstem nuclei are activated immediately after successful treatment of a migraine attack, but not during the symptom-free interval.

During a VM episode, a subpopulation of serotonergic and nonserotonergic dorsal raphe nucleus cells may comodulate the processing in the vestibular nuclei as well as the central amygdaloid nucleus, which also activates central vestibular processing pathways and contributes to VM (Halberstadt and

Balaban 2006). In addition, evidence continues to emerge that the trigeminal nerve plays an important role in VM and the involvement of the inner ear. It was shown that the trigeminal nerve provides a dense sensory innervation of cerebral, basilar, and meningeal blood vessels and thus of the inner ear arteries via the anterior inferior cerebellar artery (AICA). Indeed, the cochlea and the vestibular labyrinth receive trigeminal innervation via the ophthalmic branch that provides parasympathetic innervation to the basilar artery and the AICA (Vass et al. 1997, 1998). Activation of perivascular trigeminal nerve endings causes the release of substance P and calcitonin gene-related peptide (CGRP) leading to local neuroinflammation, permeability changes, vasodilatation, and edema (Moskowitz 1993; Prins et al. 1993). Thus, the trigeminal nerve directly affects neuroinflammation and blood flow of the inner ear, supporting the notion that neuroinflammatory and neurovascular effects of migraine can affect inner ear structures (Vass et al. 1997, 1998, 2001, 2004) and explain ear symptoms as well as endolymphatic hydrops.

Moreover, chronically fluctuating hydropic inner ears are less able to auto-regulate their vasculature against the changes induced by acute migraine attacks and may ultimately manifest as persisting endolymphatic hydrops (Brechtelsbauer et al. 1995; Miller et al. 1995; Vass et al. 2004; Sarna et al. 2020). Accordingly, cases have been reported with migraine-associated vascular changes that caused inner ear ischemia and endolymphatic hydrops, resulting in sensorineural hearing loss and Menière-like symptoms (Lee et al. 2000). In line with this, in a patient with migraine-associated hearing loss, but without vertigo, a severe bilateral endolymphatic hydrops was found (Liu et al. 2017b).

In brief, a transient relapsing *neuroinflammation and ischemia in the labyrinth* could explain an endolymphatic hydrops and consequently Menière-like symptoms as well as BPPV, both of which frequently occur in association with VM (Radtke et al. 2002; Lee et al. 2000). It could also explain actual data of inner ear MRIs in VM patients, in whom an endolymphatic hydrops was found (Gürkov et al. 2014; Kirsch et al. 2018; Oh et al. 2021). Variations in the hydrops degree in VM were dependent on the time interval from the last attack (Kirsch et al. 2018) (◘ Fig. 14.4). However, such an involvement of the inner ear makes the differential diagnosis between VM and Menière's disease even more difficult. While endolymphatic hydrops was rarely observed in VM patients, those with bilateral ear symptoms, patients with Meniere's disease or VM patients with concurrent MD (overlap syndrome?) frequently showed cochlear hydrops with or without vestibular hydrops (Oh et al. 2021) (◘ Fig. 14.5). This suggests that migraine pathomechanisms represent causative factors of inner ear dysfunction that lead to the common final pathway of hydrops and may be part of a continuum overlap link with MD.

With respect to the pathogenesis of VM, it is also interesting that the rare episodic ataxia type 2 (EA 2, due to a mutation of the PQ calcium channel gene on chromosome 19p13) occurs together with hemiplegic migraine in several families. The *gene for hemiplegic migraine* is also located on chromosome 19p13 (Ophoff et al. 1996). Three causative genes are now known to induce the familial forms of hemiplegic migraine (FHM): FHM1: CACNA1A, FHM2: ATP1A2, FHM3: SCN1A (De Fusco et al. 2003; Dichgans et al. 2005). Mutations in the CACNA1A-gene, which is involved in the calcium channel CaV2.1 (P/Q type), cause three calcium-related channelopathies: EA 2, familial hemiplegic migraine FHM1, and spinocerebellar ataxia type 6 (Requena et al. 2014). So far, no correlation to VM and no similar genetic defect in the same region have been found (von Brevern et al. 2006). Nevertheless, central ocular motor findings during the symptom-free interval in patients with VM, as in episodic ataxia, can point to hereditary neuronal function disorders in the brainstem nuclei (channelopathies?).

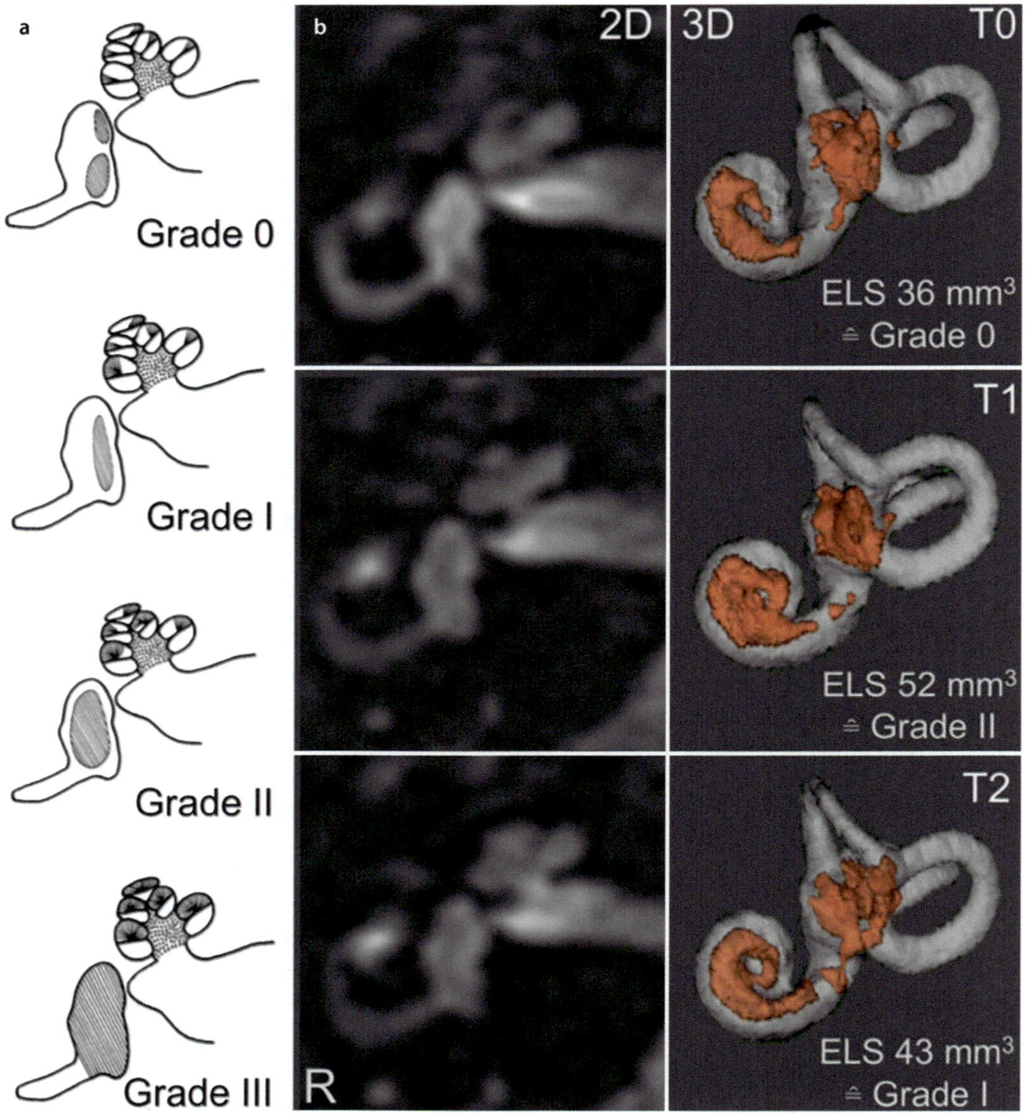

Fig. 14.4 MRI of the petrous bone showing the inner ear 4 h after i.v. administration of gadolinium contrast **b** in a patient with recurrent attacks of VM, immediately after an attack and at follow-up 3 months and 6 months later. The three-dimensional (3D) analysis of the endolymphatic space shows an endolymphatic hydrops of varying degree (**a**, schematic drawing of grade 0 to III) depending on the time interval after the last VM attack (T0 = 6 months after the attack, T1 = shortly after the attack, T2 = 3 months after the attack). (Kirsch et al. 2018)

14

Another pathogenetic approach is related to *cortical "spreading depression"* as a cause of aura. Here the vestibular symptoms were eventually classified as brainstem aura in the sense of a non-cortical spreading depression (Furman et al. 2003). This fits findings of an animal study that was able to prove a spreading depression in the brainstem of rats on the basis of changes in the local brain circulation as well as systemic blood pressure (Richter et al. 2008). Likewise, a migraine-induced ischemia in the brainstem and labyrinth could be attributed to vasospasm.

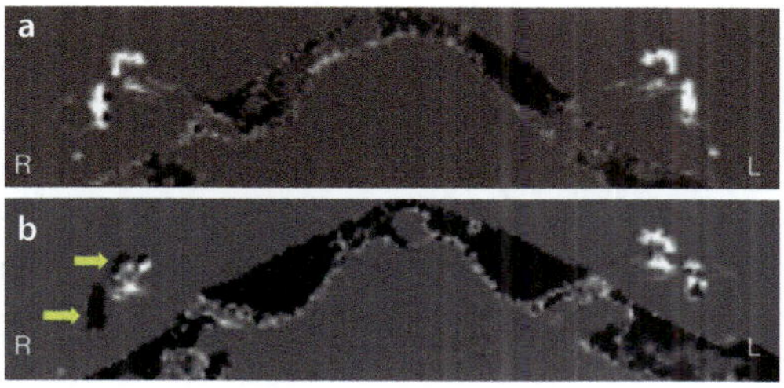

Fig. 14.5 MRI images 4 h after i.v. contrast enhancement of VM and Meniere's disease patients' inner ears. Black structures indicate endolymphatic hydrops (EH) by an absence in the perilymph space that can be identified by the contrast enhancement (white). **a** A 53-year-old female patient with pure VM. EH is not seen in the cochlea and vestibulum on both sides. **b** A 69-year-old male patient with pure Meniere's disease. The right inner ear shows severe EH in both the cochlea and the vestibulum (yellow arrows). There is no EH in the left inner ear. Area ratio of the endolymphatic space to the total fluid space constitutes 67% of the vestibulum on the right side and 13% of the vestibulum on the left side. (Oh et al. 2021)

14.8.1 Aspects From Functional and Structural Imaging

Some cortex regions activated during vestibular stimulation in human functional imaging studies include areas that are involved in nociception and pain processing, for example, the anterior insula, the orbitofrontal cortex, and the cingulum (Bucher et al. 1998; Fasold et al. 2002; Dieterich and Brandt 2008). Accordingly, imaging studies in VM patients showed a relevant overlap of the vestibular and nociceptive pathways in the brainstem, thalamus, and cortex. In these patients, a voxel-based morphometry MRI analysis disclosed a grey matter volume reduction in areas related to nociceptive, visual, and vestibular processing such as the superior, inferior, and middle temporal gyri, medial cingulum, dorsolateral prefrontal cortex, parietal and occipital cortex areas, and the insular region (Obermann et al. 2014). In line with these imaging data are neurophysiological examinations of migraine patients in whom – in contrast to healthy controls – a trigeminal stimulation induced a nystagmus. This was explained by reduced thresholds for signal transmission between both sensory systems (Marano et al. 2005). Threshold decreases were also discussed in several VM studies in which an enhanced vestibular excitability (overexcitability) was described. This includes an increased motion sensitivity up to motion sickness (Lewis et al. 2011a), a reduced suppression of otoacoustic emissions (Murdin et al. 2010), and a decreased detection threshold for dynamic head movements (Lewis et al. 2011b).

Furthermore, FDG-PET imaging in two patients during a VM attack and, for comparison, during the attack-free interval showed an increase of glucose metabolism in the attack in the thalamus and temporo-parieto-insular region bilaterally (Shin et al. 2014). This points to an activation of vestibulo-thalamo-cortical pathways. A simultaneous bilateral cerebellar activation was explained by adaptive processes aiming for a downregulation of a hyperactive vestibular system (Shin et al. 2014). A simultaneous deactivation of the bilateral occipital cortex was interpreted in line with the well-known reciprocal inhibition of the visual and vestibular systems (Brandt et al. 1998). Typically in intact sensory systems, vestibular stimulation causes an activation of multisensory vestibular cortex areas and a concurrent deactivation of visual cortex areas and vice versa (Dieterich and Brandt 2008).

The important role of the thalamus in VM was also described in an fMRI study of 12 patients (Russo et al. 2014). During vestibular caloric stimulation in the symptom-free interval, VM patients showed a normal activation pattern in the typical temporo-parietal-insular regions similar to that of patients with migraine without aura and healthy participants. However, a correlation analysis of brain activity and frequency of attacks found a positive correlation and an increased activity in the thalamus only in the patients with VM (Russo et al. 2014). An enhanced glucose activity in the antero-ventral thalamus bilaterally was also seen during a VM attack in FDG-PET (Dieterich et al. 2016). Thus, the bilateral thalamus will be an important candidate for further investigations into the pathogenesis of VM.

Structural changes in voxel-based morphometry (MRI) were found in VM patients with volume decreases in the prefrontal cortex, insular-opercular region, and the inferior parietal and supramarginal gyri, i.e., in the vestibular cortical network and the prefrontal cortex (Zhe et al. 2020). Here, the scores of the Dizziness Handicap Inventory (DHI) correlated negatively with the volume of the insular-opercular area.

14.9 Pragmatic Therapy

There are data from some smaller randomized, controlled studies on the basis of therapies performed analogously to that for migraine without aura. Here the same principles have proven valid both for treatment of the attacks of migraine and for their prophylaxis. The symptoms of dizziness and the accompanying headache can, however, react differently to the therapy or prophylaxis.

14.9.1 Treatment of the Attacks

To stop longer-lasting attacks, it is advisable to administer early a non-steroidal anti-inflammatory agent (e.g., ibuprofen, diclofenac) or an analgesic (acetylsalicylic acid as a soluble tablet or paracetamol as a suppository), possibly in combination with an antiemetic drug (e.g., metoclopramide, domperidone).

In individual cases, triptans had positive effects on attacks of vertigo, acting at the 5-$HT_{1B/1D}$ receptors of the arteries (Bikhazi et al. 1997). However, zolmitriptan, investigated in a randomized, placebo-controlled study, only had a minor effect in 10 patients with VM (Neuhauser et al. 2003): 38% of the VM group and 22% of the placebo group showed a benefit with 5 mg zolmitriptan. Another study with rizatriptan vs placebo examined the introduction of motion sensitivity and motion sickness during vestibular stimulation (Furman et al. 2011). Thirteen of 15 individuals showed a reduction of induced motion sickness after rizatriptan ($p < 0.02$); however, this was not the case for more complex stimuli.

14.9.2 Prophylactic Treatment

In a Cochrane analysis, prophylactic treatment for VM was analyzed in clinical trials (Maldonado et al. 2015): so far, none of the 558 studies fulfilled the necessary quality criteria. One double-blind, placebo-controlled, randomized trial with 95 mg metoprolol vs placebo (PROVEMIG) was closed after the inclusion of 130 VM patients because the patient inclusion was too difficult. No statistically significant effect was seen; however, the power was only around 60% (Bayer et al. 2019). A current meta-analysis was able to identify 13 publications with sufficiently standardized criteria that, however, were heterogeneously chosen and thus difficult to compare (Byun et al. 2020). Anticonvulsive drugs (topiramate, lamotrigine), calcium channel blockers, tricyclic antidepressants, beta-blockers, serotonin- and norepinephrine-reuptake inhibitors and vestibular rehabilitation had a positive evaluation for the reduction of attack frequency. This was in line with positive results of a smaller prospective multi-center study ($n = 31$) for amitriptyline, flunarizine, propanolol, and topiramate with respect to reduction of symptoms and attack frequency (Dominguez-Duran et al. 2020).

On the basis of the currently insufficient study data in VM, the official recommendation is analogous to the treatment of migraine without and with aura (von Brevern and Lempert 2020).

The treatment of first choice for migraine prophylaxis is the administration of the beta-receptor blocker metoprolol retard (95 mg/day, for example, in the evening) or propranolol (2 × 40–80 mg/day) for about 6 months.

Alternatives are topiramate (50–150 mg/day), valproic acid (600–2000 mg/day), flunarizine (5–10 mg/day in the evening), or lamotrigine (50–200 mg/day). Furthermore, antidepressants, such as amitriptyline (25–50 mg/day) or venlafaxine (37.5 mg/day), showed beneficial effects. For these medications, mostly only observations or controlled trials in a small number of VM patients have been made (Gordon et al. 1993; Lampl et al. 2005; Bisdorff 2004; Lepcha et al. 2014; Verspeelt et al. 1996; Salviz et al. 2016; Liu et al. 2017a; Byun et al. 2020).

Some drugs were effective in the reduction of both the aura and the VM attacks (Lampl et al. 2005); this points to a close pathophysiological correlation. This close connection underlines the possible role of the aura and a cortical spreading depression as a trigger for an activation within the trigeminovascular system followed by migraine headache.

In a retrospective study in 100 patients with VM, it was found that the 74 who received one of the above-mentioned drugs as migraine prophylaxis experienced a significant improvement in the duration, intensity, and frequency of their vertigo attacks as well as the associated migraine symptoms (Baier et al. 2009a).

Vestibular rehabilitation also showed positive effects in patients with VM (Vitkovic et al. 2013).

References

Abouzari M, Goshtasbi K, Moshtaghi O et al (2020) Association between vestibular migraine and migraine headache: yet to explore. Otol Neurotol 41(3):392–396

Ahn SK, Balaban CD (2010) Distribution of 5-HT1B and 5-HT1D receptors in the inner ear. Brain Res 1346:92–101

Baier B, Winkenwerder E, Dieterich M (2009a) Vestibular migraine: effects of prophylactic therapy. J Neurol 256(3):426–442

Baier B, Stieber N, Dieterich M (2009b) Vestibular-evoked myogenic potentials in "vestibular migraine". J Neurol 256(9):1447–1454

Balaban CD (2011) Migraine, vertigo and migrainous vertigo: links between vestibular and pain mechanisms. J Vestib Res 21:315–321

Balaban CD, Jacob RG, Furman JM (2011) Neurologic bases for comorbidity of balance disorders, anxiety disorders and migraine: neurotherapeutic implications. Expert Rev Neurother 11:379–394

Battista RA (2004) Audiometric findings of patients with migraine-associated dizziness. Otol Neurotol 25:987–992

Batu ED, Anlar B, Topcu M, Turanli G (2015) Vertigo in childhood: a retrospective series of 100 children. Eur J Paediatr Neurol 19:226–232

Bayer O, Adrion C, Al Tawil A, Mansmann U, Strupp M, PROVEMIG investigators (2019) Results and lessons learnt from a randomized controlled trial: prophylactic treatment of vestibular migraine with metoprolol (PROVEMIG). Trials 20(1):813

Becker-Bense S, Wittmann C, Dieterich M (2019) Balanced sex distribution in patients with Menière's disease. J Neurol 266(Suppl 1):42–46

Best C, Eckhardt-Henn A, Tschan R, Bense S, Dieterich M (2009) Psychiatric morbidity and comorbidity in different vestibular vertigo syndromes: results of a prospective longitudinal study over one year. J Neurol 256(1):58–65

Bikhazi P, Jackson C, Ruckenstein MJ (1997) Efficacy of antimigrainous therapy in the treatment of migraine-associated dizziness. Am J Otol 18(3):350–354

Bisdorff AR (2004) Treatment of migraine related vertigo with lamotrigine, an observational study. Bull Soc Sci Med Grand Duche Luxemb 2:103–108

Brandt T, Dieterich M (2017) The dizzy patient: Don't forget disorders of the central vestibular system. Nat Rev Neurol 13(6):352–362

Brandt T, Bartenstein P, Janek A, Dieterich M (1998) Reciprocal inhibitory visual-vestibular interaction: visual motion stimulation deactivates the parieto-insular vestibular cortex. Brain 121:1749–1758

Brantberg K, Trees N, Baloh RW (2005) Migraine-associated vertigo. Acta Otolaryngol 125(3):276–279

Brechtelsbauer PB, Ren TY, Miller JM, Nuttall A (1995) Autoregulation of cochlear blood flow in the hydropic Guinea pig. Hear Res 89:130–136

Bucher SF, Dieterich M, Wiesmann M, Weiss A, Zink R, Yousry TA, Brandt T (1998) Cerebral functional magnetic resonance imaging of vestibular, auditory, and nociceptive areas during galvanic stimulation. Ann Neurol 44:120–125

Byun YJ, Levy DA, Nguyen SA, Brennan E, Rizk HG (2020) Treatment of vestibular migraine: a systematic review and meta-analysis. Laryngoscope:1–9. https://doi.org/10.1002/lary.28546

Cass SP, Furman JM, Ankerstjerne K, Balaban C, Yetiser S, Aydogan B (1997) Migraine-related vestibulopathy. Ann Otol Rhinol Laryngol 106:182–189

Celebisoy N, Gökcay F, Sirin H, Bicak N (2008) Migrainous vertigo: clinical, oculographic and posturographic findings. Cephalalgia 28:72–77

Cho SJ, Kim BK, Kim BS, Kim JM, Kim SK, Moon HS, Song TJ, Cha MJ, Park KY, Sohn JH (2016)

Vestibular migraine in multicenter neurology clinics according to the appendix criteria in the third beta edition of the International Classification of Headache Disorders. Cephalalgia 36(5):454–462
Colombo B, Teggi R, NIVE Project (2017) Vestibular migraine: who is the patient? Neurol Sci 38:107–110
Cutrer FM, Baloh RW (1992) Migraine-associated dizziness. Headache 32:300–304
Decker J, Limburg K, Hennigsen P, Lahmann C, Brandt T, Dieterich M (2019) Intact vestibular function is relevant for anxiety related to vertigo. J Neurol 266(Suppl 1):89–92
De Fusco M, Marconi R, Silvestri L et al (2003) Haploinsufficiency of ATP1A2 encoding the Na+/K+ pump alpha2 subunit associated with familial hemiplegic migraine type 2. Nat Genet 33:92–196
Dichgans M, Freilinger T, Eckstein G et al (2005) Mutation in the neuronal voltage-gated sodium channel SCN1A in familial hemiplegic migraine. Lancet 366:371–377
Dieterich M, Brandt T (1999) Episodic vertigo related to migraine (90 cases): vestibular migraine? J Neurol 246:883–892
Dieterich M, Brandt T (2008) Functional brain imaging of peripheral and central vestibular disorders. Brain 131:2538–2552
Dieterich M, Obermann M, Celebisoy N (2016) Vestibular migraine: the most frequent entity of episodic vertigo. J Neurol 263(Suppl 1):82–89
Dlugaiczyk J, Habs M, Dieterich M (2020) Vestibular evoked myogenic potentials in vestibular migraine and Meniere's disease: cVEMPs make the difference. J Neurol. https://doi.org/10.1007/s00415-020-09902-4
Dominguez-Duran E, Montilla-Ibanez MA, Alvarez-Morujo de Sande MG et al (2020) Analysis of the effectiveness of the prophylaxis of vestibular migraine depending on the diagnostic category and the prescribed drug. Eur Arch Otorhinolaryngol 277(4):1013–1021
Eckhardt-Henn A, Best C, Bense S, Breuer P, Diener G, Tschan R, Dieterich M (2008) Psychiatric comorbidity in different organic vertigo syndromes. J Neurol 255(3):420–428
Fasold O, von Brevern M, Kuhberg M, Ploner CJ, Villringer A, Lempert T, Wenzel R (2002) Human vestibular cortex as identified with caloric stimulation in functional magnetic resonance imaging. Neuroimage 17:1384–1393
Formeister EJ, Rizk HG, Kohn MA, Sharon JD (2018) The epidemiology of vestibular migraine: a population-based survey study. Otol Neurotol 39(8):1037–1044
Furman JM, Balaban CD (2015) Vestibular migraine. Ann N Y Acad Sci 1343:90–96
Furman JM, Marcus DA, Balaban CD (2003) Migrainous vertigo: development of a pathogenetic model and structured diagnostic interview. Curr Opin Neurol 16:5–13
Furman JM, Marcus DA, Balaban CD (2011) Rizatriptan reduces vestibular-induced motion sickness in migraineurs. J Headache Pain 12:81–88
Furman JM, Marcus DA, Balaban CD (2013) Vestibular migraine: clinical aspects and pathophysiology. Lancet Neurol 12:706–715
Gallego-Martinez A, Espinosa-Sanchez JM, Lopez-Escamez JA (2018) Genetic contribution to vestibular diseases. J Neurol 265(Suppl 1):29–34
Goadsby PJ (2000) The pharmacology of headache. Prog Neurobiol 62:509–525
Gordon CR, Kuritzky A, Doweck I, Spitzer O, Shupak A, Hering R (1993) Vestibulo-ocular reflex in migraine patients: the effect of sodium valproate. Headache 33:129–132
Griggs RC, Nutt JG (1995) Episodic ataxias as channelopathies. Ann Neurol 37:285–287
Gürkov R, Kantner C, Strupp M, Flatz W, Krause E, Ertl-Wagner B (2014) Endolymphatic hydrops in patients with vestibular migraine and auditory symptoms. Eur Arch Otorhinolaryngol 271:2661–2667
Halberstadt AL, Balaban CD (2006) Serotonergic and nonserotonergic neurons in the dorsal raphe nucleus send collateralized projections to both the vestibular nuclei and the central amygdaloid nucleus. Neuroscience 140:1067–1077
International Headache Society (2004) ICHD, 2nd ed. Cephalalgia 24:9–160
Ishiyama A, Jacobson KM, Baloh RW (2000) Migraine and benign positional vertigo. Otol Rhinol Laryngol 109:377–380
Jahn K, Langhagen T, Heinen F (2015) Vertigo and dizziness in children. Curr Opin Neurol 28:78–82
Johnson GD (1998) Medical management of migraine-related dizziness and vertigo. Laryngoscope 108:1–28
Kayan A, Hood JD (1984) Neuro-otological manifestations of migraine. Brain 107:1123–1142
Kirsch V, Becker-Bense S, Berman A, Kierig E, Ertl-Wagner B, Dieterich M (2018) Transient endolymphatic hydrops after an attack of vestibular migraine: a longitudinal single case study. J Neurol. https://doi.org/10.1007/s00415-018-8870-3
Lahmann C, Henningsen P, Brandt T et al (2015) Psychiatric comorbidity and psychosocial impairment among patients with vertigo and dizziness. J Neurol Neurosurg Psychiatry 86:302–308
Lampl C, Katsarava Z, Diener H-C, Limmroth V (2005) Lamotrigine reduces migraine aura and migraine attacks in patients with migraine with aura. J Neurol Neurosurg Psychiatry 76:1730–1732
Lampl C, Rapoport A, Levin M, Bräutigam E (2019) Migraine and episodic vertigo: a cohort survey study of their relationship. J Headache Pain 20:33. https://doi.org/10.1186/s10194-019-0991-2

Lee H, Lopez I, Ishiyama A, Baloh RW (2000) Can migraine damage the inner ear? Arch Neurol 57:1631–1634
Lempert T, Neuhauser H (2009) Epidemiology of vertigo, migraine and vestibular migraine. J Neurol 256(3):333–338
Lempert T, Neuhauser H, Daroff RB (2009) Vertigo as a symptom of migraine. Ann N Y Acad Sci 1164:242–251
Lempert T, Olesen J, Furman J, Waterston J, Seemungal B, Carey J, Bisdorff A, Versino M, Evers S, Newman-Toker D (2012a) Vestibular migraine: diagnostic criteria. J Vestib Res 22:167–172
Lempert T, Olesen J, Furman J, Waterston J, Seemungal B, Carey J et al (2012b) Vestibular migraine: diagnostic criteria. J Vestib Res 22(4):167–172
Lepcha A, Amalanathan S, Augustine AM, Tyagi AK, Balraj A (2014) Flunarizine in the prophylaxis of migrainous vertigo: a randomized controlled trial. Eur Arch Otorhinolaryngol 271:2931–2936
Lewis RF, Priesol AJ, Nicoucar K, Lim K, Merfeld DM (2011a) Abnormal motion perception in vestibular migraine. Laryngoscope 121:1124–1125
Lewis RF, Priesol AJ, Nicoucar K, Lim K, Merfeld DM (2011b) Dynamic tilt thresholds are reduced in vestibular migraine. J Vestib Res 21:323–330
Lipton RB, Scher AI, Kolodner K, Liberman J, Steiner TJ, Stewart WF (2002) Migraine in the United States: epidemiology and patterns of health care use. Neurology 58:885–894
Liu F, Ma T, Che X, Wang Q, Yu S (2017a) The efficacy of venlafaxine, flunarizine, and valproic acid in the prophylaxis of vestibular migraine. Front Neurol 8:524
Liu IY, Ishiyama A, Sepahdari AR, Johnson K, Ishiyama G (2017b) Bilateral endolymphatic hydrops in a patient with migraine variant without vertigo: a case report. Headache 57:455–459
Maldonado FM, Birdi JS, Irving GJ, Murdin L, Kivekäs I, Strupp M (2015) Pharmacological agents for the prevention of vestibular migraine (Review). Cochrane Libr Issue 6:1–35
Marano E, Marcelli V, Di Stasio E, Bonuso S, Vacca G, Manganelli F, Marciano E, Perretti A (2005) Trigeminal stimulation elicits a peripheral vestibular imbalance in migraine patients. Headache 45:325–331
Miller JM, Ren TY, Nuttall AL (1995) Studies of inner ear blood flow in animals and human beings. Otolaryngol Head Neck Surg 112:101–113
Morganti LO, Salmito MC, Duarte JA, Bezerra KC, Simões JC, Ganança FF (2016) Vestibular migraine: clinical and epidemiological aspects. Braz J Otorhinolaryngol 82(4):397–402
Moskowitz MA (1993) Neurogenic inflammation in the pathophysiology and treatment of migraine. Neurology 43:S16–S20
Muelleman T, Shew M, Subbarayan R, Shum A, Sykes K, Staecker H, Lin J (2017) Epidemiology of dizzy patient population in a neurotology clinic and predictors of peripheral etiology. Otol Neurotol 38(6):870–875
Murdin L, Premachandra P, Davies R (2010) Sensory dysmodulation in vestibular migraine: an otoacoustic emission suppression study. Laryngoscope 120:1632–1636
Murofushi T, Tsubota M, Kitao K, Yoshimura E (2018) Simultaneous presentation of definite vestibular migraine and definite Meniere's disease: overlapping syndrome of two diseases. Front Neurol 9:749. https://doi.org/10.3389/fneur.2018.00749
Muth C, Teufel J, Schols L et al (2021) Fampridine and acetazolamide in EA2 and related familial EA: a prospective randomized placebo-controlled trial. Neurol Clin Pract 11:e438–e446
Neff BA, Staab JP, Eggers SD, Carlson ML, Schmitt WR, Van Abel KM, Worthington DK, Beatty CW, Driscoll CL, Shepard NT (2012) Auditory and vestibular symptoms and chronic subjective dizziness in patients with Ménière's disease, vestibular migraine, and Ménière's disease with concomitant vestibular migraine. Otol Neurotol 33(7):1235–1244
Neugebauer H, Adrion C, Glaser M, Strupp M (2013) Long-term changes of central ocular motor signs in patients with vestibular migraine. Eur Neurol 69(2):102–107
Neuhauser H, Lempert T (2004) Vertigo and dizziness related to migraine: a diagnostic challenge. Cephalalgia 24(2):83–91
Neuhauser H, Leopold M, von Brevern M, Arnold G, Lempert T (2001) The interrelations of migraine, vertigo and migrainous vertigo. Neurology 56:436–441
Neuhauser H, Radtke A, von Brevern M, Lempert T (2003) Zolmitriptan for treatment of migrainous vertigo: a pilot randomised placebo-controlled trial. Neurology 60:882–883
Neuhauser H, Radtke A, von Brevern M, Feldmann M, Lezius F, Ziese T, Lempert T (2006) Migrainous vertigo: prevalence and impact on quality of life. Neurology 67:1028–1033
Obermann M, Wurthmann S, Steinberg BS, Theysohn N, Diener HC, Naegel S (2014) Central vestibular system modulation in vestibular migraine. Cephalalgia 34:1053–1061
Obermann M, Bock E, Sabev N, Lehmann N, Weber R, Gerwig M, Frings M, Arweiler-Harbeck D, Lang S, Diener HC (2015) Long-term outcome of vertigo and dizziness associated disorders following treatment in specialized tertiary care: the Dizziness and Vertigo Registry (DiVeR) study. J Neurol 262(9):2083–2091
Oh S-Y, Dieterich M, Lee B, Boegle R, Kang J-J, Lee N-R, Gerb J, Hwang S-B, Kirsch V (2021) Endolymphatic hydrops in patients with vestibular migraine and concurrent Meniere's disease. Front Neurol 12. https://doi.org/10.3389/fneur.2021.594481

Ophoff RA, Terwindt GM, Vergouwe MN, van Eijk R, Oefner PJ, Hoffman SM et al (1996) Familial hemiplegic migraine and episodic ataxia type-2 are caused by mutations in the Ca2+ channel gene CACNL1A4. Cell 87:543–552

Prins M, van der Werf F, Baljet B, Otto JA (1993) Calcitonin gene-related peptide and substance P immunoreactivity in the monkey trigeminal ganglion, an electron microscopic study. Brain Res 629:315–318

Pyykkö I, Manchaiah V, Färkkilä M, Kentala E, Zou J (2019) Association between Meniere's disease and vestibular migraine. Auris Nasus Larynx 46:724–733

Radtke A, Lempert T, Gresty MA, Brookes GB, Bronstein AM, Neuhauser H (2002) Migraine and Meniere's disease. Is there a link? Neurology 59:1700–1704

Radtke A, Neuhauser H, von Brevern M et al (2011) Vestibular migraine – validity of clinical diagnostic criteria. Cephalalgia 31(8):906–913

Radtke A, von Brevern M, Neuhauser H, Hottenrott T, Lempert T (2012) Vestibular migraine: long-term follow-up of clinical symptoms and vestibulo-cochlear findings. Neurology 79:1607–1614

Rassekh CH, Harker LA (1992) The prevalence of migraine in Meniere's disease. Laryngoscope 102:135–138

Requena T, Espinosa-Sanchez JM, Lopez-Escamez JA (2014) Genetics of dizziness: cerebellar and vestibular disorders. Curr Opin Neurol 27:98–104

Richter F, Bauer R, Lehmenkühler A, Schaible HG (2008) Spreading depression in the brainstem of the adult rat: electrophysiological parameters and influences on regional brainstem blood flow. J Cereb Blood Flow Metab 28:984–994

Russo A, Marcelli V, Esposito F, Corvino V, Marcuccio L, Giannone A, Conforti R, Marciano E, Tedeschi G, Tessitore A (2014) Abnormal thalamic function in patients with vestibular migraine. Neurology 82:2120–2126

14

Salviz M, Yuce T, Acar H, Karatas A, Acikalin RM (2016) Propranolol and venlafaxine for vestibular migraine prophylaxis: a randomized controlled trial. Laryngoscope 126(1):169–174

Sarna B, Abouzari M, Lin HW, Djalilian HR (2020) A hypothetical proposal for association between migraine and Meniere's disease. Med Hypotheses 134:109430

Shin JH, Kim YK, Kim HJ, Kim JS (2014) Altered brain metabolism in vestibular migraine: comparison of interictal and ictal findings. Cephalalgia 34:58–67

Stovner LJ, Andrée C (2010) Prevalence of headache in Europe: a review for the Eurolight project. J Headache Pain 11:289–299

Strupp M, Versino M, Brandt T (2010) Vestibular migraine. Handb Clin Neurol 97:755–771

Strupp M, Kalla R, Claassen J, Adrion C, Mansmann U, Klopstock T, Freilinger T, Neugebauer H, Spiegel R, Dichgans M, Lehmann-Horn F, Jurkat-Rott K, Brandt T, Jen JC, Jahn K (2011) A randomized trial of 4-aminopyridine in EA2 and related familial episodic ataxias. Neurology 77:269–275

Teggi R, Colombo B, Bernasconi L, Bellini C, Comi G, Bussi M (2009) Migrainous vertigo: results of caloric testing and stabilometric findings. Headache 49(3):435–444

Thakar A, Anjaneyulu C, Deka RC (2001) Vertigo syndromes and mechanisms in migraine. J Laryngol Otol 115:782–787

Vass Z, Shore SE, Nuttall AL, Jancsó G, Brechtelsbauer PB, Miller JM (1997) Trigeminal ganglion innervation of the cochlea--a retrograde transport study. Neuroscience 79:605–615

Vass Z, Shore SE, Nuttall AL, Miller JM (1998) Direct evidence of trigeminal innervation of the cochlear blood vessels. Neuroscience 84:559–567

Vass Z, Steyger PS, Hordichok AJ, Trune DR, Jancsó G, Nuttall AL (2001) Capsaicin stimulation of the cochlea and electric stimulation of the trigeminal ganglion mediate vascular permeability in cochlear and vertebro-basilar arteries: a potential cause of inner ear dysfunction in headache. Neuroscience 103:189–201

Vass Z, Dai CF, Steyger PS, Jancsó G, Trune DR, Nuttall AL (2004) Co-localization of the vanilloid capsaicin receptor and substance P in sensory nerve fibers innervating cochlear and vertebro-basilar arteries. Neuroscience 124:919–927

Verspeelt J, De Locht P, Amery WK (1996) Postmarketing study of the use of flunarizine in vestibular vertigo and in migraine. Eur J Clin Pharmacol 51:15–22

Vitkovic J, Winoto A, Rance G, Dowell R, Paine M (2013) Vestibular rehabilitation outcomes in patients with and without vestibular migraine. J Neurol 260:3039–3048

von Brevern M, Lempert T (2020) Vestibular migraine: treatment and prognosis. Semin Neurol 40(19):83–86

von Brevern M, Zeise D, Neuhauser H, Clarke AH, Lempert T (2005) Acute migrainous vertigo: clinical and oculographic findings. Brain 128:365–374

von Brevern M, Ta N, Shankar A, Wiste A, Siegel A, Radtke A, Sander T, Escayg A (2006) Migrainous vertigo: mutation analysis of the candidate genes CACNA1A, ATP1A2, SCN1A, and CACNB4. Headache 46(7):1136–1141

Waterston J (2004) Chronic migrainous vertigo. J Clin Neurosci 11:384–388

Weiller C, May A, Limmroth V, Jüpter M, Kaube H, van Schayck R, Coenen HH, Diener HC (1995) Brain stem activation in spontaneous human migraine attacks. Nat Med 1:658–660

Xue J, Ma X, Lin Y et al (2020) Audiological findings in patients with vestibular migraine and migraine: history of migraine may be a cause of low-tone sudden sensorineural hearing loss. Audiol Neurootol 20:1–6

Zhe X, Gao J, Chen L et al (2020) Altered structure of the vestibular cortex in patients with vestibular migraine. Brain Behav 10:e01572

Functional Dizziness and Vertigo

Contents

Supplementary Information The online version contains supplementary material available at [https://doi.org/10.1007/978-3-030-78260-3_15]. The videos can be accessed by scanning the related images with the SN More Media App.

M. Strupp et al., *Vertigo and Dizziness*, https://doi.org/10.1007/978-3-030-78260-3_15

15.1 Current Classification

Functional dizziness is the current term for vertigo and dizziness syndromes that manifest with one or more vestibular symptoms such as vertigo or dizziness, unsteadiness, or imbalance of stance and gait but without a causative organic etiology. These syndromes were formerly named somatoform or psychogenic vertigo and dizziness (◘ Fig. 15.1). In the International Classification of Diseases (ICD-11; WHO 2015), "vestibular symptoms" are now used independently from their origin in organic, psychiatric, and functional vertigo and dizziness syndromes.

The committee for the International Classification of Vestibular Disorders (ICVD) of the Bárány Society – the International Society of Neurootology – during the last years elaborated a consensus document on the definition of functional vertigo and dizziness with the new term "persistent postural-perceptual dizziness" (PPPD or 3PD) (Staab et al. 2017; Staab 2020). The core features of this disorder are based on the long-lasting experiences and several common findings in syndromes such as phobic postural vertigo (PPV; Brandt and Dieterich 1986; Brandt 1996), space-motion discomfort (SMD; Jacob et al. 1989; 1993; 2009), visual vertigo (VV; Bronstein 1995a, b, 2004), and chronic subjective dizziness (CSD; Staab et al. 2004; Staab and Ruckenstein 2007). Studies of PPV, VV, SMD, and CSD identified a number of functional alterations in balance mechanisms associated with these clinical entities (Querner et al. 2000; Querner et al. 2002; Krafczyk et al. 2006; Holmberg et al. 2006; Wühr et al. 2013; Schniepp et al. 2014; Indovina et al. 2015) and additional investigations separated them from primary psychiatric disorders (Brandt and Dieterich 1986; Kapfhammer et al. 1997; Staab 2012). These findings appeared largely applicable to PPPD, indicating that it is a functional, not a structural or psychiatric, vestibular disorder (Dieterich et al. 2016; Dieterich and Staab 2017; Staab et al. 2017).

It is important for the clinician and for the patient that functional dizziness can and has to be diagnosed *positively* by typical symptom constellations and not only negatively by the exclusion of a structural/organic lesion.

"Persistent postural-perceptual dizziness" (PPPD or 3PD) is defined as a chronic vestibular disorder according to criteria A–E, all of which have to be fulfilled to make the diagnosis (Staab et al. 2017) ▶ Box 15.1:

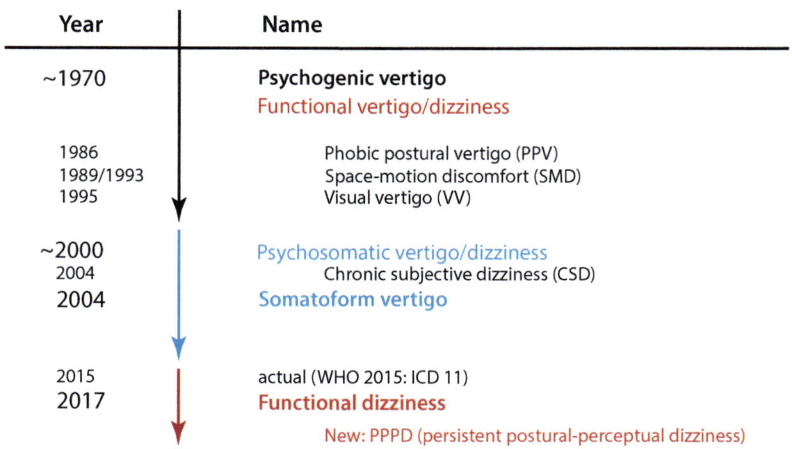

◘ **Fig. 15.1** Changes in terminology of functional dizziness during the last 50 years. From psychogenic or functional vertigo to functional dizziness; from phobic postural vertigo and chronic subjective dizziness to persistent postural-perceptual dizziness (PPPD)

Box 15.1 Diagnostic Criteria of Persistent Postural-Perceptual Dizziness (PPPD or 3PD) (Staab et al. 2017)

1. One or more symptoms of dizziness, unsteadiness, or non-spinning vertigo are present on most days for 3 months or more. Symptoms may be present for hours but not during the whole day, nearly every day (for more than 15 of 30 days), and tend to increase over the day.
2. Persistent symptoms occur spontaneously without provocation but are exacerbated by 3 factors: (1) upright posture, (2) active or passive motion without regard to direction or position, and (3) exposure to moving visual stimuli or complex visual patterns.
3. The disorder is precipitated by conditions that cause vertigo, unsteadiness, dizziness, or problems with balance including acute, episodic, or chronic vestibular syndromes, other neurological or medical illness, or psychological distress.
4. Symptoms cause significant distress or functional impairment.
5. Symptoms are not better accounted for by another disease or disorder.

Functional dizziness is the cause of a large proportion of the complex forms of vertigo and dizziness syndromes in a specialized outpatient clinic for vertigo and balance disorders (Table 1.1 and Fig. 1.3). Two forms are differentiated:

- *Primary* functional dizziness and vertigo syndromes
- *Secondary* functional dizziness and vertigo syndromes that develop after acute structural vestibular vertigo, another neurological or medical illness, or psychological distress (Huppert et al. 1995; Eckhardt-Henn et al. 2009) (Fig. 15.2)

In the course of their functional dizziness, about 70% of these patients still complain about symptoms, even after several years, and are more impaired in their professional and daily activities than patients with structural organic forms of dizziness (Furman and Jacob 1997; Yardley and Redfern 2001;

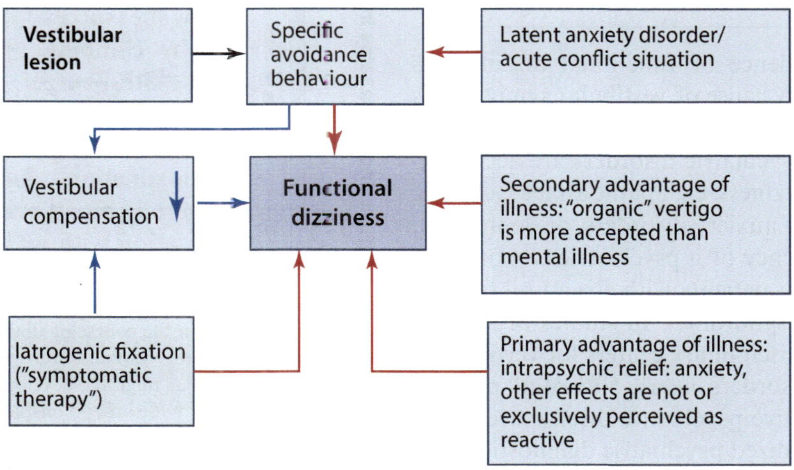

Fig. 15.2 Pathogenetic model of secondary functional dizziness/vertigo, triggered by structural organic vertigo. (Modified from Dieterich and Eckhardt-Henn 2006). Red arrows indicate a facilitating influence, blue arrows an inhibiting influence

Eckhardt-Henn et al. 2003). The most frequent associated psychiatric disorders are:
- Anxiety and phobic disorders
- Depressive disorders
- Dissociative disorders (conversion syndrome)
- Somatoform disorders (ICD-10: F45)
- Depersonalization /derealization syndromes (more seldom)

There is a high comorbidity between these psychiatric disorders and several organic vertigo syndromes. Structured interviews and various psychometric tests have found evidence of a psychiatric comorbidity in 65% of patients with vestibular migraine, 57% of patients with Menière's disease, and 51% of patients with vestibular paroxysmia (Eckhardt-Henn et al. 2008; Best et al. 2009a, b; Lahmann et al. 2015a). In contrast, the comorbidity in patients with BPPV is only 15% and in patients with vestibular neuritis 22%, which is equivalent to the level of 20% found in normal control groups (Eckhardt-Henn et al. 2008).

15.1.1 Epidemiology and Psychiatric Comorbidity

The prevalence of functional dizziness as the primary cause of vestibular symptoms is estimated to be 8–10% (Staab 2013). Several primary psychiatric disorders are accompanied by dizziness, e.g., panic attacks, chronic fluctuating anxiety disorders, or depression. The frequency of a psychiatric comorbidity is higher in patients with structural organic vestibular syndromes. In studies of specialized interdisciplinary centers for vertigo and balance disorders, nearly 50% of all patients had an active psychiatric disease according to standardized psychiatric diagnostic interviews (SCID-I) (Hanel et al. 2009; Best et al. 2009a, b; Lahmann et al. 2015a). However, the prevalence of psychiatric disorders was not equally distributed between all organic vestibular syndromes but showed particularly high rates in vestibular migraine (49%) and vestibular paroxysmia (51%) (Lahmann et al. 2015a).

Similar findings for psychiatric morbidity and comorbidity have also been reported in a prospective psychometric follow-up study conducted over 1 year in different groups of patients with organic vestibular vertigo syndromes. While the patients with BPPV, vestibular neuritis, and Menière's disease exhibited normal or normalizing values, it was conspicuous that only the patients with vestibular migraine had a persistent, clearly elevated incidence of psychiatric disorders (Best et al. 2009a; ◘ Fig. 15.3). They also felt themselves more hindered in their daily life by dizziness, experienced the vestibular symptoms as being stronger, and had more anxiety than all other vertigo patients (Best et al. 2009b; Tschan et al. 2011). Moreover, patients with a prehistory of a mental illness were at a clearly higher risk of becoming ill with another psychiatric disorder following a an organic vertigo syndrome (◘ Fig. 15.4).

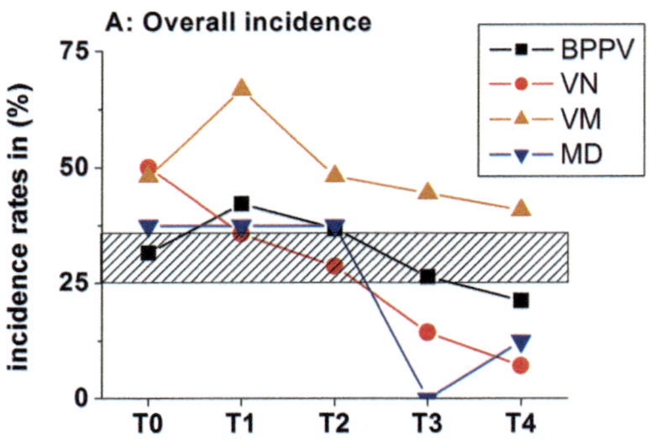

◘ **Fig. 15.3** Prospective longitudinal analysis of the incidence (in %) of the development of a somatoform/psychiatric disorder in the course of illness in patients with various structural vestibular vertigo syndromes. Patients with vestibular migraine develop a secondary functional/somatoform disorder conspicuously more often (BPPV benign paroxysmal positioning vertigo, VN vestibular neuritis, VM vestibular migraine, MD Menière's disease; T0 = time of the diagnosis of the illness, T1 = 6 weeks, T2 = 3 months, T3 = 6 months, T4 = 1 year later)

15

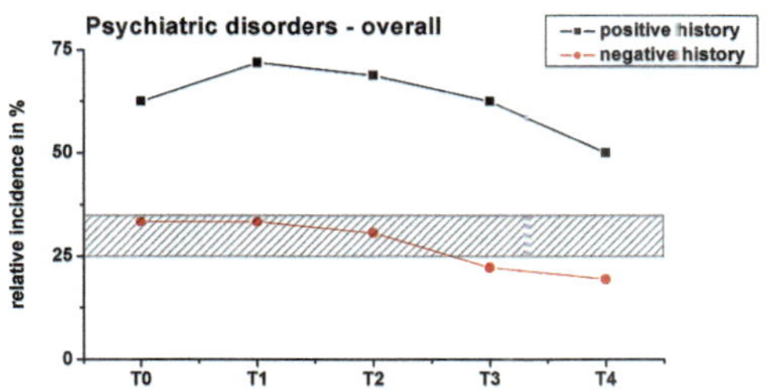

Fig. 15.4 Relative incidence of a patient becoming ill with a psychiatric disorder after having had a structural vestibular vertigo syndrome dependent on his/her prehistory of psychiatric disorders

The extent of vestibular damage or vestibular dysfunction, however, had no influence on the further course of the psychiatric stress (Best et al. 2006, 2009a; Lahmann et al. 2015a). Only the degree of the initially experienced vertigo, not that of the vestibular function disorder, had a predictive value in patients with vestibular neuritis, but not in patients with BPPV for the development of a functional (somatoform) vertigo in the course of the disorder (Heinrichs et al. 2007). Even a persistent anxiety about a renewed episode of vertigo had predictive value for the later occurrence of a panic or functional/somatoform disorder in patients with vestibular neuritis (Godemann et al. 2006).

Since primarily patients with vestibular migraine are at a particularly high risk of developing a functional (somatoform) dizziness, this possibility should be considered early in the therapeutic deliberations.

Comorbidities for anxiety disorders and depression do not only exist in patients with organic vestibular syndromes but also in patients with functional dizziness. Of course, phobic postural vertigo (PPV) and chronic subjective dizziness (CSD) did also occur without psychiatric comorbidities. In patients with CSD, 60% had clinically relevant symptoms of an anxiety disorder and 45% of a depression, but 25% showed no psychiatric comorbidity (Staab 2012). In patients with functional dizziness and concomitant vestibular migraine or Meniere's disease, the acute attacks of structural vestibular dysfunction overlay a persisting basal unsteadiness, swaying dizziness, or light-headedness (Neff et al. 2012).

15.1.2 Diagnosis

15.1.2.1 History

Since functional dizziness first seems to occur without psychopathological symptoms, as a rule this causes the patients to go to ENT doctors, neurologists or internists. The patients describe experiencing frequent (Figs. 15.5 and 15.6):

- Postural imbalance or a diffuse feeling of dizziness
- Light-headedness
- An emptiness in the head
- Unsteadiness when walking
- A feeling of toppling over or of losing touch with the ground
- Very rarely rotatory vertigo with accompanying vegetative symptoms and nausea

Depending on the underlying psychiatric disease (see above), the following additional symptoms can be present:

- Disorders of motivation and concentration
- Decline in performance
- Subjectively experienced restrictions in professional and daily activities
- Vegetative symptoms that accompany the dizziness (accelerated heart rate, nausea, sweats, apnea, fear of suffocating, loss of appetite, weight loss)
- Emotional and mood disorders
- Sleep disturbances
- Symptoms of anxiety

Typically all of these symptoms are experienced and described as reactive; i.e., the patients believe that the symptoms are triggered and induced by the dizziness. Patients

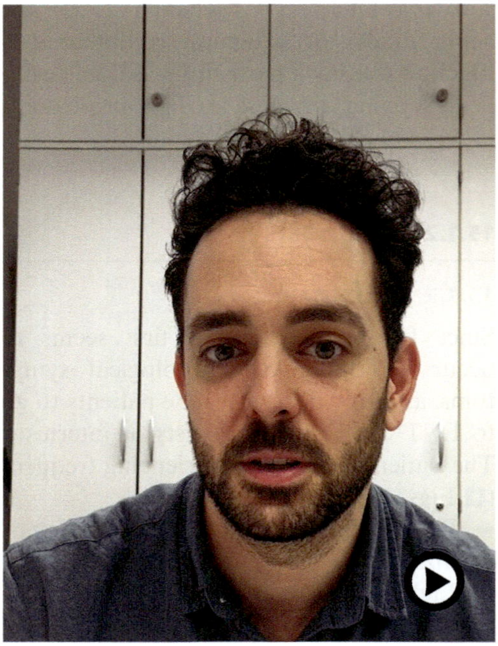

Fig. 15.5 Functional dizziness: patient history (► https://doi.org/10.1007/000-96d)

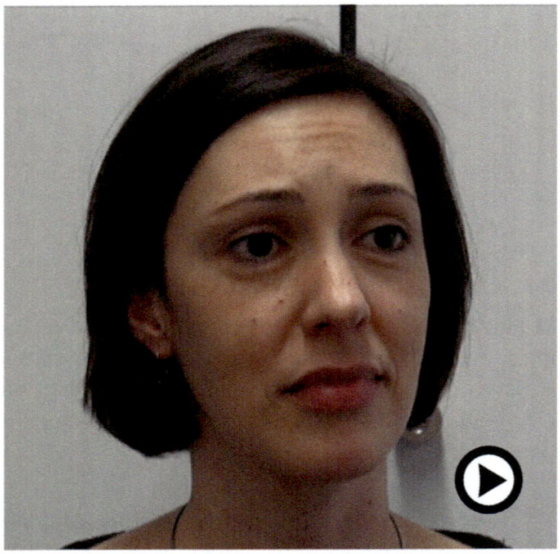

Fig. 15.6 Functional dizziness: patient history (► https://doi.org/10.1007/000-96c)

seldom spontaneously report conflict and stress situations that can function as triggers of vertigo and dizziness; often they are initially totally unaware of them. This makes it difficult to establish the diagnosis and has firstly to be worked out together with the patient.

The following key symptoms and *positive* characteristics of *functional phobic postural dizziness* quickly help to establish the diagnosis (Brandt and Dieterich 1986; Brandt 1996):

- *Dizziness, unsteadiness or light-headedness*:

  Dizziness is most often described as postural dizziness or light-headedness with fluctuating degrees of unsteadiness of stance and gait, in part combined with an attack-like fear of falling without real falls, in part also involuntary body swaying of short duration.
- *Dissociation between complaints and objective findings:*

  Patients complain of dizziness and subjective unsteadiness of stance and gait (e.g., with fear of falls) without signs and symptoms of gait instability, without falls (Schlick et al. 2016) and with normal results in neurotological testing.
- *Situational triggers or enhancement*:

  Symptoms often occur or are enhanced in typical situations known to be external triggers of other phobic syndromes (e.g., bridges, driving a car, large empty rooms, long corridors, tight spaces, crowded places, large crowds in a store or restaurant, cinema), or during visual stimulation (e.g., cinema, television, store).
- *Improvement during distraction (dual task)*:

  Dizziness improves or resolves during sport activities (bicycling, tennis), during more complicated balance conditions, and during distraction (conversation with friends, entertainment), while it increases again at rest or under simpler conditions (e.g., standing after bicycling).
- *Fewer complaints in the morning, increasing over day* (Feuerecker et al. 2015).
- *Generalization and chronification*:

  During the course of the illness, the patient begins to generalize the symptoms and increasingly to avoid the triggering stimuli.

- *Vegetative disturbances and anxiety*:
  During or shortly after the attacks or phases of enhanced symptoms (frequently mentioned only when asked), patients report vegetative disturbances and anxiety; most also report attacks of dizziness without anxiety.
- *Relaxation effect*:
  If asked, patients usually report that their symptoms improve after imbibing a little alcohol or dosage of tranquilizers.
- *Precipitants*:
  Initially there is often an organic vestibular illness, e.g., resolved vestibular neuritis, BPPV (Huppert et al. 1995), other medical illness in the individuum or the family, or special psychosocial stress situations (Kapfhammer et al. 1997).
- *Personality traits*:
  Patients with functional phobic postural dizziness often exhibit obsessive–compulsive and perfectionistic personality traits and reactive–depressive symptoms during the course of the disease.

Here it is important to determine these so-called "positive" criteria of the symptoms and not only exclude other illnesses.

15.2 Clinical and Technical Examinations

A detailed neurological, neurotological, and neuroophthalmological examination as well as technical vestibular testing is necessary to exclude important structural differential diagnoses and disclose a *secondary* functional dizziness. Moreover, careful examination is the most important therapeutic measure to relieve at first the patient of his fear of having an organic illness and then explain some underlying mechanisms ("increased self-observation" in the context of the corresponding primary personality structure). This increased self-observation leads to a change of postural strategy that can easily be identified by *posturography* (Krafczyk et al. 2006; Brandt et al. 2012; Wühr et al. 2013, 2017) and is helpful to establish the diagnosis (see below ► Sect. 15.4.2).

15.3 Further Clinical Aspects and Course of the Illness

Functional dizziness in the adult can manifest in every age. Functional phobic postural dizziness is most common in the second and fifth decade (here the most frequent form of vertigo and dizziness) without a preference of females or males (Strupp et al. 2003).

The combination of postural vertigo with subjective instability of stance and gait in patients with normal neurological findings in vestibular and balance test results (otoneurological examination, videooculography including caloric irrigation, imaging) (► Chaps. 3 and 4) or disorders that cannot explain the symptoms, and a compulsive personality structure are characteristic. The monosymptomatic subjective disorder of balance is connected with standing or walking, and manifests with attack-like worsening that occurs with or without recognizable triggers and with or without accompanying anxiety. The absence of recognizable triggers or vertigo without accompanying anxiety causes many patients and occasionally the doctor treating them to doubt the diagnosis of a functional disorder. If functional dizziness remains untreated, the symptoms worsen, generalization develops, and avoidance behavior increases until the patient is unable to leave his/her own apartment without help.

Patients with functional dizziness generally have a tendency to intensified introspection and the need "to keep everything under control" due to a compulsive primary personality (in the sense of "pronounced personality traits"). They are more likely to be ambitious and place high demands on themselves and are often easily irritated and fearful (Kapfhammer et al. 1997; Staab et al.

2014). Personality traits measured with the NEO Personality Inventory-Revised (NEO-PI-R) were examined and showed that CSD patients had higher trait anxiety, but lower NEO-PI-R extraversion, warmth, positive emotions, openness to feelings, and trust ($p < 0.05$). They were more likely to have a composite temperament of high trait anxiety plus low warmth or excitement seeking (Staab et al. 2014). Even in an MRI study of healthy volunteers, it could be shown that personality traits modulate subcortical and cortical vestibular and anxiety responses to sound-evoked vestibular stimulation (Indovina et al. 2014). The authors concluded from these data that the combination of high neuroticism and low extraversion represents a risk for developing a functional dizziness syndrome by a higher connectivity of visual-vestibular and anxiety networks which may lead to a lower level of controlling mechanisms of posture (Indovina et al. 2014). Furthermore, personality traits and individual differences predict threat-induced changes in postural control (Zaback et al. 2015).

Psychological traumatization and adverse life events were equally distributed between patients with organic and functional vestibular syndromes (Radziej et al. 2015). Thus, they alone do not favor the development of a functional disorder.

Such patients rarely go to a psychiatrist first; they tend to see the "specialist" for their symptom, especially as they feel themselves to be organically sick. Therefore, the illness often lasts quite a long time before a final diagnosis is made, previously, 3 years on average (Huppert et al. 1995). The diagnosis is often established only after a number of visits to different specialists, superfluous laboratory examinations, and erroneous classifications such as "cervicogenic vertigo," "vestibular paroxysmia," or – no longer in use – "recurrent vertebrobasilar ischemia", with correspondingly unsuccessful treatment attempts.

A longitudinal follow-up study (5–16 years) on 106 patients showed an improvement rate of 75% after careful examination and detailed explanation of the mechanisms (Huppert et al. 2005). In none of these patients did the diagnosis have to be revised. Similar results were described in a psychoeducative cognitive behavioral therapy with an improvement of 78% at follow-up 32 months after therapy (Schaaf and Hesse 2015). Also a prospective study comparing patients with functional dizziness at baseline, after therapy and 12 months later following either "integrative psychotherapy" (manualized intervention containing elements of education, cognitive behavior therapy and psychodynamic therapy), or a moderated self-help group showed a significant improvement in both groups of this larger sample (81 vs 78 patients) (Limburg et al. 2021).

15.3.1 Differential Diagnosis

The differential diagnosis of functional dizziness includes psychiatric syndromes as well as vestibular and non-vestibular organic syndromes. The most important organic vestibular and non-vestibular syndromes include:

- Bilateral vestibulopathy (▶ Chap. 7)
- Hemodynamic orthostatic dizziness (Kim et al. 2019)
- Vestibular paroxysmia (▶ Chap. 11)
- Syndrome of a third mobile windows (▶ Chap. 12)
- Vestibular migraine (▶ Chap. 14)
- Cerebellar dizziness and episodic ataxia type 2 (▶ Chap. 13.4)
- Orthostatic tremor with a pathognomonic frequency peak of 13–18 Hz in electromyography and posturography (Gerschlager and Brown 2011)

The most important psychiatric syndromes besides the types of functional dizziness in anxiety, depression, dissociative, and somatoform disorders in a narrower sense (ICD10: F45) include the following:

- Panic disorder with or without agoraphobia
- Space phobia (Marks 1981)
- Mal-de-Debarquement syndrome (▶ Chap. 20), for which heterogeneous pathoetiologies are discussed (Murphy 1993; Cohen et al. 2018; Mucci et al. 2018; review: Saha and Cha 2020)

In contrast to the long list of possible differential diagnoses, the combination of traits connected with the complaints, normal physical neurootological findings, and primary personality type are so characteristic that there is seldom any doubt as to the diagnosis after the first detailed examination.

15.4 Pathophysiology and Therapeutic Principles

Currently two pathogenetic mechanisms of functional dizziness are differentiated:

- ***Primary*** functional (somatoform) vertigo and dizziness syndromes: They occur without preceding structural/ organic vertigo syndromes and may have similar pathogenetic mechanisms like those of psychiatric disorders (anxiety or phobic, depressive, dissociative, or somatoform disorders). They should be differentiated from psychiatric vestibular syndromes.
- ***Secondary*** functional (somatoform) vertigo and dizziness syndromes: They occur during or after a structural organic vertigo syndrome, another neurological or medical illness, or psychological distress (◘ Fig. 15.2).

In certain predisposed patients, a feedback loop between a bodily sensation (e.g., lightheadedness, swaying dizziness) and a physical symptom of illness (e.g., rotatory vertigo in vestibular neuritis) results in a cognitive-catastrophizing interpretation (◘ Fig. 15.2). This means that the bodily symptom is seen as a danger, as an expression of a basically severe or life-threatening physical illness (Eckhardt-Henn et al. 2009). Subsequently, anxiety and panic reactions can escalate in intensity. A similar pathogenetic model was proposed by J. Staab in chronic subjective dizziness, CSD (Staab 2013). Such somatosensory amplification is based on the *efference-copy model*, first described by Von Holst and Mittelstaedt (1950), that is nowadays also an established model of somatoform disorders (Barsky and Wyshak 1990; Lahmann et al. 2010; Henningsen et al. 2018).

15.4.1 Efference-Copy Model

The illusory perception of postural dizziness and instability of stance can be explained by a disturbance of space constancy, which results from a partial decoupling of the actual re-afference from the efference-copy signal for active head and body movements (Brandt and Dieterich 1986; Brandt 1996). This partial decoupling is based on a change from an “open loop” strategy (healthy volunteers) to a “closed loop” strategy of body posture that was documented and disclosed in patients with functional phobic postural dizziness (PPV; Wühr et al. 2013) and can be easily used for diagnosis.

Under normal conditions, we do not perceive self-generated, slight body sway or head movements as accelerations during upright stance. The environment also appears to be stationary during these active movements, although there are shifts of retinal images caused by these relative movements. “Space constancy” seems to be maintained by the simultaneous occurrence of a voluntary impulse to initiate a movement and the delivery of adequate information in parallel to identify self-motion (◘ Fig. 15.7). According to Von Holst and Mittelstaedt (1950), this so-called “efference copy” may provide a sensory pattern of expectation based on earlier

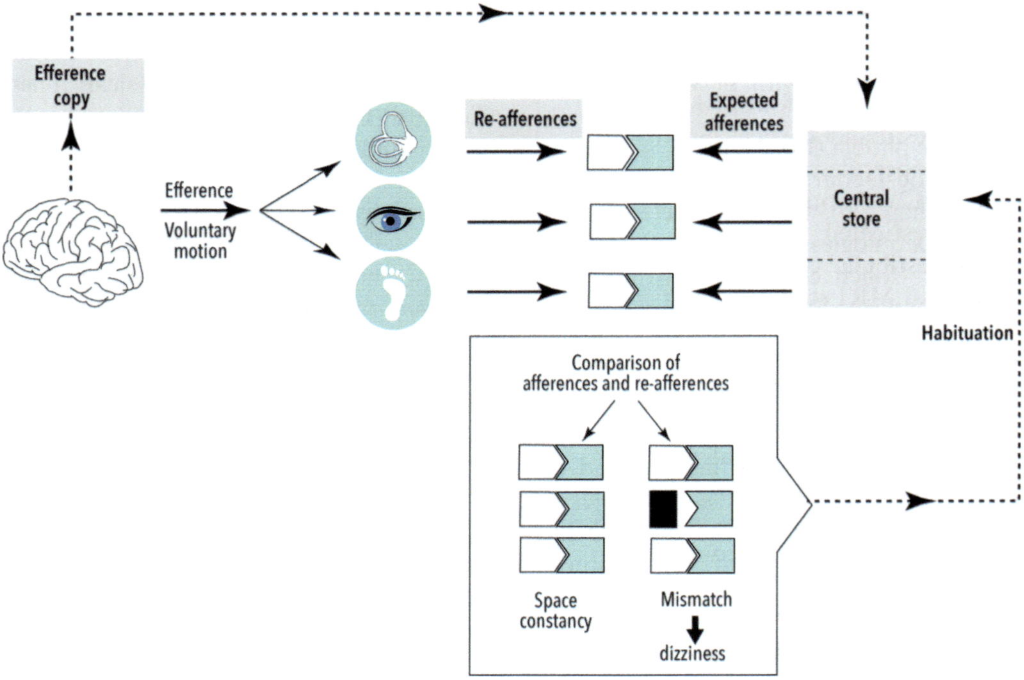

Fig. 15.7 Schematic drawing showing how vertigo/dizziness develops due to a disturbance of the space-constancy mechanism during active motion. (Modified from Brandt 1996). Voluntary head movements lead to stimulation of the vestibular, visual, and somatosensory sensory organs. Their messages are compared with a multisensory pattern of expectation provided by an internal model that was calibrated by earlier experience of motion. The expected pattern is prepared simultaneously by the efference-copy signal, which is sent in parallel with the voluntary movement impulse. If the concurrent sensory stimulation and the pattern of expectation are in agreement, the self-motion is perceived and "space constancy" is maintained. However, if there is an incongruence between the incoming and the expected pattern due to a partial "decoupling" of the efference-copy signal and the re-afference, a sensorimotor mismatch, then vertigo, dizziness, and imbalance develop. The subject no longer experiences a voluntary head movement in a stationary surrounding, but rather a threatening disorientation with exogenic head acceleration and a concurrent illusory movement of the surrounding

experience (internal model), which by means of the movement-triggered actual sensory information is then so interpreted that self-motion can be differentiated from the motion of the environment. If this efference copy is missing, e.g., if we move the eyeball with a finger on the eyelid, illusory movements of the environment occur, i.e., oscillopsia. The sensation of dizziness and vertigo described by these patients (involving involuntary body sway and the occasional perception of individual head movements as disturbing external perturbations with simultaneous illusional movements of the surroundings) can be explained by a transient decoupling of efference-copy and re-afference; i.e., a mismatch occurs between the anticipated and the actual motion (Brandt et al. 2012).

Healthy persons can experience similar mild sensations of vertigo without simultaneous anxiety during a state of total exhaustion, when the difference between voluntary head movements and involuntary sway becomes blurred. In patients with functional phobic postural dizziness, this partial decoupling may be caused by their constant preoccupation with anxious monitoring and checking of balance (Brandt 1996). This leads to the perception of sensorimotor adjustments that would otherwise be made unconsciously by means of learned (and reflex-like) muscle activation programs called up to maintain upright posture. This explanation based on the efference-copy model is nowadays often used for functional (somatoform) disorders (Barsky and Wyshak 1990; Lahmann et al. 2010). It is also the basis for current neuropsycho-behavioral models and computational psychosomatics and computational psychiatry using, for example, Bayesian models (Petzschner et al. 2017; Henningsen et al. 2018).

15.4.2 Analysis of Stance and Gait

Precise posturographic analyses show that these patients with functional dizziness increase their postural sway during normal stance by co-contracting the flexor and extensor muscles of the foot. This is an expression of an unnecessary fearful strategy to control stance. Subjective imbalance in functional dizziness is associated with characteristic changes in the coordination of open- and closed-loop mechanisms of postural control by which sensory feedback is used inadequately during undisturbed stance (PPV; Wühr et al. 2013). Healthy subjects use this strategy only when in real danger of falling. During difficult balancing tasks, such as tandem stance with eyes closed, the posturographic data of the patients do not differ from those of healthy subjects, i.e., the more difficult the demands of balance, the more "healthy" the balance performance of the patients with functional dizziness (PPV; Querner et al. 2000; ◘ Fig. 15.8). These patients often report that unsteadiness especially increases when looking at moving

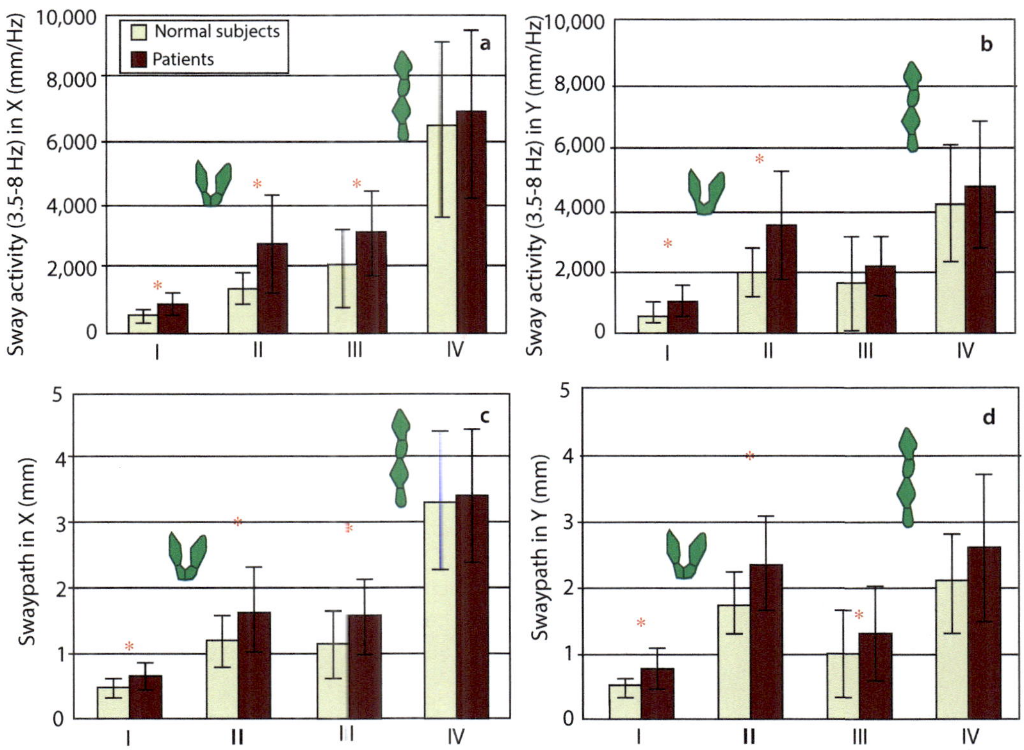

◘ **Fig. 15.8** **a–d** Body sway parameters revealed by a posturographic examination of healthy subjects and patients with functional phobic postural dizziness during different conditions of stance of increasing difficulty (I: normal stance with eyes open; II: normal stance with eyes closed; III: tandem stance with eyes open; IV: tandem stance with eyes closed). The more difficult the conditions, the more normal the performance of patients with functional dizziness. (Modified from Querner et al. 2000)

visual scenes. When exposed to large-field visual motion stimulation in the roll plane, body sway did not exhibit any increased risk of falling, but – in contrast to healthy volunteers – the stimulation-induced body sway was suppressed early (Querner et al. 2002) (◘ Fig. 15.9).

The use of automatized analysis of sway patterns in posturography (▶ Sect. 4.5) under various conditions (e.g., with eyes open or closed, standing on firm ground or on foam rubber) together with a neuronal network allows in many cases a decision as to whether, for example, the pattern of a

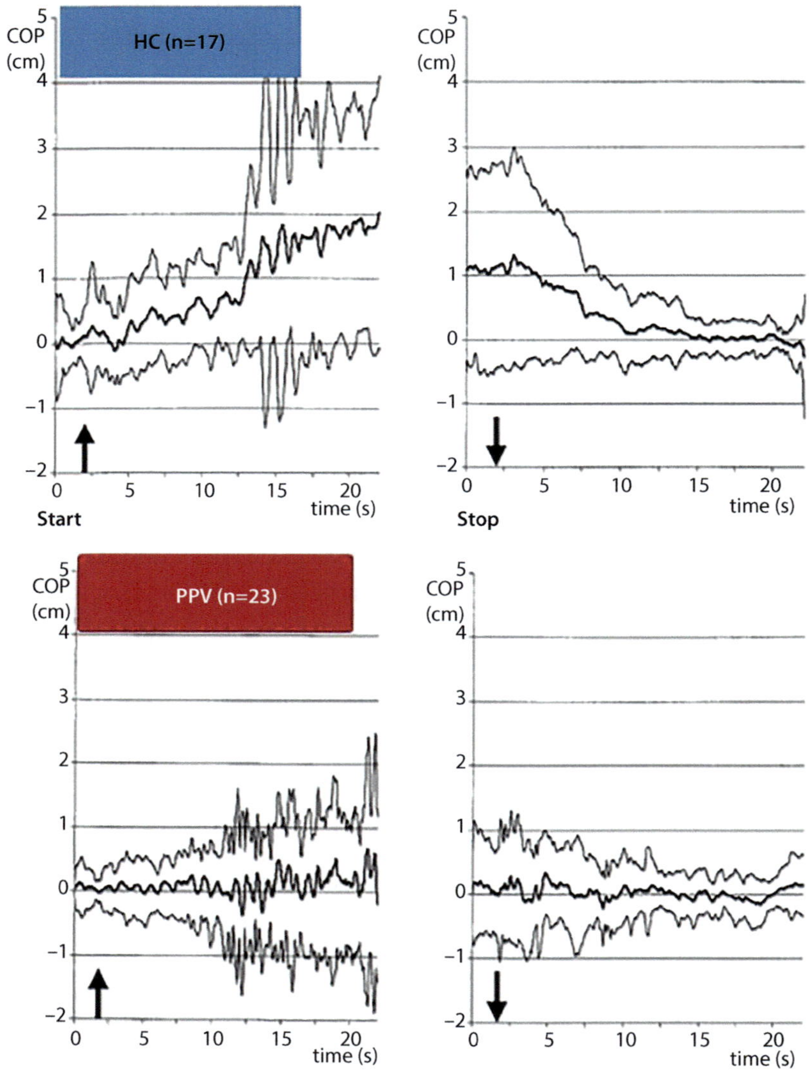

◘ **Fig. 15.9** Body sway during visual stimulation. Body sway (COP, center of pressure, in cm) of posturography in healthy volunteers (top) and in patients with functional phobic postural vertigo (PPV, bottom) while standing on the platform with the head in front of a half-spherical dome with random dots on the surface. Measures were performed before, during, and after dome rotation clockwise (observer's view). Healthy volunteers showed a lateral body sway, while patients suppressed this early (i.e., smaller sway amplitudes during stimulation, note COP scales). Arrows indicate start and stop of visual stimulation. (From Querner et al. 2002)

15

functional phobic postural dizziness is present or other important differential diagnoses (e.g., bilateral vestibulopathy, orthostatic tremor, or cerebellar syndrome) (Krafczyk et al. 2006; Brandt et al. 2012). The typical pattern of a body sway reduction during more difficult stance conditions was also seen in the gait analysis (► Sect. 4.5) with three different speeds: slow, preferred, and fast (Schniepp et al. 2014; Wühr et al. 2017). In patients with functional dizziness, less variability of gait parameters was found during slow and preferred speed compared to healthy participants and an improvement to normalization during fast speed. Absent visual feedback led to more pronounced gait deteriorations indicating a higher reliance of the patients on visual information during walking (Schniepp et al. 2014). These findings support the view that the gait characteristics of patients with functional dizziness can be attributed to an inadequate, cautious gait control. In particular, distracting attention (by e.g. sensory or sensorimotor dual task) normalized leg muscle activity and balance parameters (PPV; Wühr et al. 2017) (◘ Fig. 15.10). Thus, distraction can be included in a therapeutic concept.

In summary, recording body sway parameters (posturography) under different sensory conditions as well as gait analysis in patients with functional dizziness document – similar to people with height vertigo – a stronger anxious control of stance and gait with a co-contraction of antagonistic leg muscles (◘ Fig. 15.11). This results in the transition of a normal automated control of stance (open loop) to a continuous voluntary regulation (closed loop), a strategy that healthy subjects use during difficult conditions of stance and gait such as walking on ice. The enhanced body control again leads to a subjective sensation of swaying which exacerbates the vicious circle (Brandt and Huppert 2014, Brandt et al. 2015). In individuals with fear of heights or anxiety the enhanced body control can even influence eye movements (Staab 2014) and freeze gaze to the horizon (Kugler et al. 2014).

15.4.3 Brain Imaging

The mechanisms of enhanced control with co-contraction of leg muscles during simple conditions of stance and gait are reflected in several brain imaging studies. A multimodal MRI study in 44 patients with functional dizziness showed a volume reduction of gray matter in the cerebellum and concurrent volume increase in the bilateral thalamus and motor cortex (PPV; Popp et al. 2018). This can be explained by a reduced automated sensorimotor control (cerebellum) on the one hand and an enhanced voluntary motor control (cortex) on the other. In parallel, functional connectivity between brain areas changed and showed a reduction of fibers from the prefrontal cortex to the cerebellum bilaterally and a strong increase of fibers to the thalamus, anterior insula, parahippocampus, amygdala, and anterior cingulum (Popp et al. 2018) (◘ Fig. 15.12). These areas with enhanced connectivity belong to the network of emotions, anxiety, and depression, which also presented with a stronger connectivity in depression and anxiety disorders (Feldker et al. 2016; Heitmann et al. 2016). This is in line with the finding that the data of the Beck-Depression-Inventory (BDI) were positively correlated with the gray volume increase of several prefrontal cortex areas and the precentral gyrus but negatively correlated (volume decrease) with cerebellar areas and the middle occipital gyrus (Popp et al. 2018; Huber et al. 2020). Furthermore, analysis of

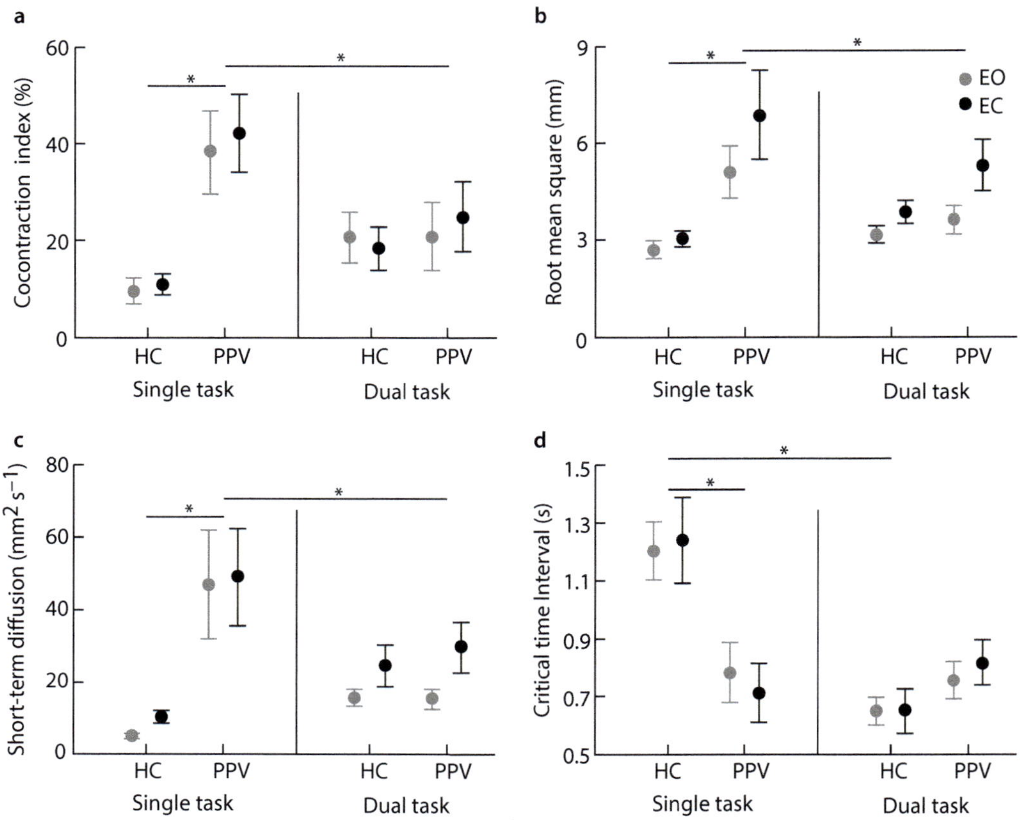

Fig. 15.10 Cocontraction of antigravity leg muscles and analysis of body sway behavior. **a** Cocontraction indexes of the examined leg muscle pair (i.e., tibialis anterior and soleus muscles) and **b** root mean square of postural sway, **c** short-term (open-loop) diffusion coefficients, and **d** critical time intervals in healthy controls (HC) and patients with functional phobic postural vertigo (PPV) for the 4 stance conditions: single task, standing with eyes open (EO; grey dots) vs standing with eyes closed (EC; black dots) and dual task standing with EO vs standing with EC while performing a cognitive dual task. During a single task, patients exhibited an inadequate neuromuscular regulation of balance, characterized by enhanced cocontractions of antigravity leg muscles, increased root mean square of postural sway, and short-term diffusion activity (indicating abnormal open-loop control), as well as a shortened critical time interval (implying that the primary sensory feedback threshold of the postural control system is lowered). Balance regulation normalized when patients were distracted by performing a cognitive dual task (*significant difference). (From Wühr et al. 2017)

15

cortical thickness revealed greater values in healthy controls compared to the patients for the ventromedial prefrontal cortex, the insular sulcus, and the lingual gyrus in the left hemisphere, and a region bordering the anterior cingulate gyrus and the cuneus in the right hemisphere (Fig. 15.13).

Accordingly, in other studies an increased cognitive processing of body position, stance, and gait was found during body movements in patients with PPPD (Popkirov et al. 2018) and an altered functional brain connectivity between the cerebellum and the thalamus (visually induced dizziness;

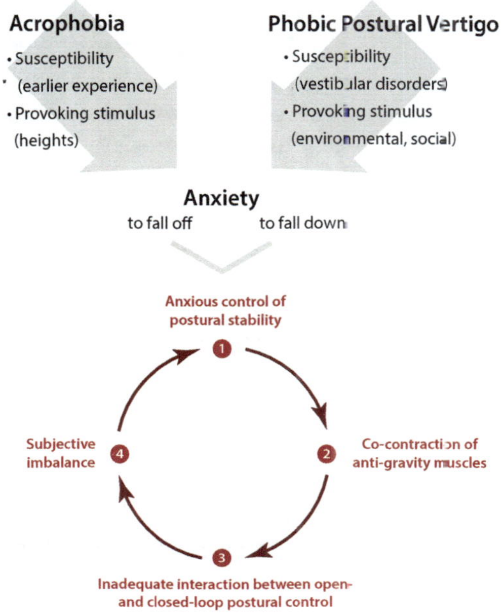

Fig. 15.11 Hypothesized circular cascade of symptom emergence in functional dizziness. Arrow lines indicate the direction of the causal chain. (1) A conscious concentration on control of postural stability might trigger (2) cocontraction of antigravity muscles, thereby causing (3) an inadequate mode of interaction between open- and closed-loop mechanisms within the postural control systems. This might lead to (4) subjective imbalance, which in turn would enhance (1) conscious control of posture. (From Wühr et al. 2013)

Van Ombergen et al. 2017). Patients with PPPD further showed decreased connectivity between the left hippocampus and right inferior frontal gyrus, bilateral temporal lobes, bilateral insular and parietal opercular cortices, bilateral occipital lobes, and cerebellum (Lee et al. 2018). Thus, patients with functional dizziness had reduced connectivity among areas involved in multisensory vestibular processing and spatial cognition, but increased connectivity in networks linking visual and emotional processing (Lee et al. 2018). A dysfunction of precuneus and cuneus in the resting state with altered intra- and inter-network functional connectivity was further described in PPPD patients (Li et al. 2019, 2020). The authors suggested that the spontaneous functional activity of cuneus and precuneus could potentially lead to an abnormal integration of visual and vestibular information and abnormalities in external environment monitoring.

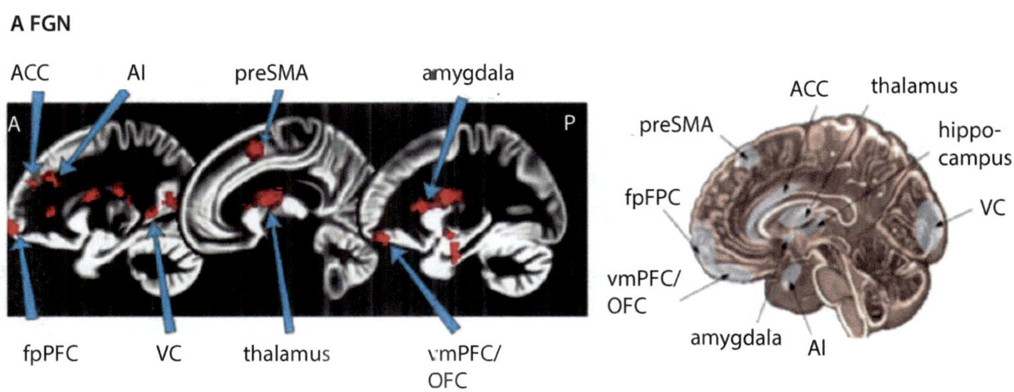

Fig. 15.12 Altered functional connectivity networks in functional phobic postural vertigo patients (PPV) compared to healthy controls, here the fear-generation network. $P < 0.05$ was set after FDR correction with a critical cluster size of 50. Patients showed higher functional connectivity than HCs between fpPFC and thalamus, anterior insula, parahippocampal gyrus, ACC, amygdala, and posterior medial frontal gyrus (ACC anterior cingulate cortex, AI anterior insula, FGN fear-generation network, fpPFC frontopolar prefrontal cortex, OFC orbitofrontal cortex, preSMA pre-supplementary motor area, vmPFC ventromedial prefrontal cortex, VC visual cortex). (From Popp et al. 2018)

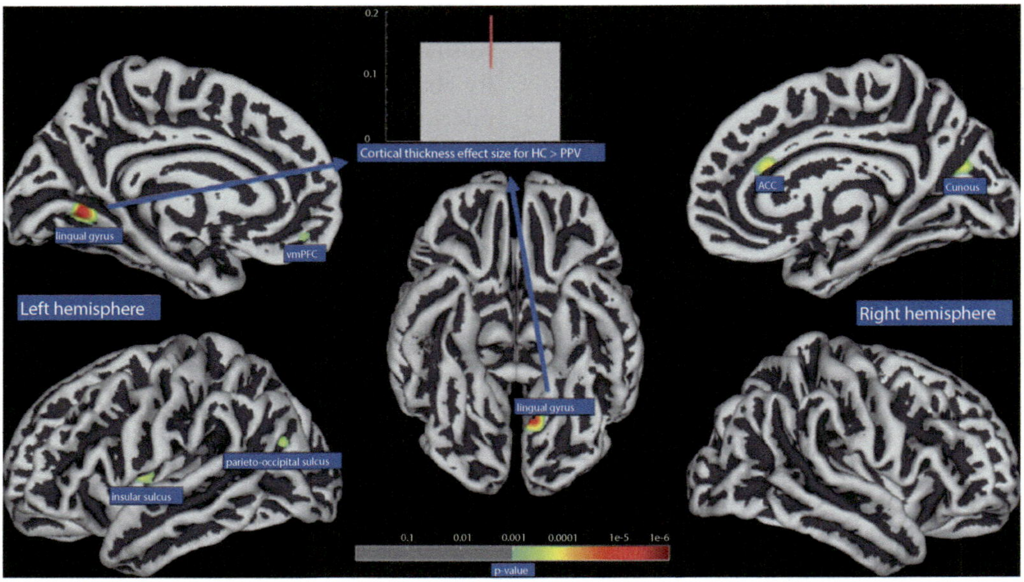

Fig. 15.13 Differences in cortical thickness in patients with functional phobic postural vertigo (PPV) compared to healthy controls (HC). All results shown reflect regions where patients had a lesser cortical thickness: vmPFC, insular sulcus, parieto-occipital sulcus, ACC, lingual gyrus, and cuneus. Exemplary effect size illustrated for the finding in the lingual gyrus of the left hemisphere (ACC anterior cingulate cortex, vmPCF ventromedial prefrontal cortex). (From Popp et al. 2018)

15.5 Therapy

A basic requirement, and the most important therapeutic measure, is to relieve the patient of his fear of having an organic illness by carefully examining him. Then a detailed explanation is necessary on the underlying mechanism, which is an "increased self-observation" and body control in the context of the corresponding primary personality structure. The patient needs the understanding to be ready to change his behavior, for example, with the help of relaxation techniques (yoga, thai chi, chi gong, autogenous training), regular physical training, and possibly vestibular rehabilitation with balance exercises. The latter may have, however, a worsening effect due to a too strong concentration on balance control, for example, during monotonic walking on a treadmill. In some cases, desensitization by exposure to the causative situations should follow; i.e., the patient should not avoid such situations but, on the contrary, seek them out. Regular exercise is most important; it has proven to be helpful to give the patient confidence in his/her own sense of balance.

This procedure in follow-up studies showed an improvement of dizziness symptoms in up to 70% of patients with functional phobic dizziness (Brandt et al. 1994; Huppert et al. 2005). More recently, psychoeducational and psychotherapeutic interventions were developed that in first pilot studies showed beneficial effects on dizziness and dysfunctional illness representations (Tschan et al. 2012; Schaaf and Hesse 2015; Lahmann et al. 2015b) as well as an improvement of postural strategies (Best et al. 2015).

Cognitive and behavioral therapy in combination with vestibular rehabilitation was shown to significantly improve symptoms in controlled studies with small groups of patients (PPV; Andersson et al. 2006; Holmberg et al. 2006). However, a follow-up examination after 1 year in a group of the treated patients determined that the positive effect was not maintained (Holmberg et al. 2007). In summary, systematic analyses of previous therapy studies were able to prove the efficacy of psychotherapeutic-psychosomatic treatment approaches (Schmid et al. 2011; Edelman et al. 2012; Mahoney et al. 2013). Since balance training also leads to an improvement (Thompson et al. 2015; Kristiansen et al. 2019), a combination of the following is suitable:

- Cognitive-psychoeducational and behavioral therapy.
- Pharmacotherapy (especially selective serotonin-reuptake inhibitors) (Staab 2013), such as 5–10 mg escitalopram or, e.g., paroxetine, citalopram, fluvoxamine, or sertraline. Depending on the psychiatric comorbidity tri-/tetracyclic antidepressants such as opipramol or alternatively in concurrent sleep disorders amitriptyline and mirtazapine are possible.
- Regular exercises

  which might be necessary for some months to improve and stabilize the situation for a longer time. This can be combined with optokinetic stimulation (Choi et al. 2021).

An integrated concept of psychoeducational-behavioral therapy and vestibular rehabilitation showed longer lasting positive effects for the dizziness symptoms as well as the accompanying psychiatric dysfunction like anxiety and depression (Lahmann et al. 2015b; Limburg et al. 2021). Similar positive effects were, however, also seen in a self-help group monitored by a psychologist (Limburg et al. 2021). This finding underlines the importance of a thorough diagnostic testing and a detailed explanation of pathomechanisms in functional dizziness to reduce the fear of an organic illness and improve postural strategies.

The indication for therapy depends on the clinical findings and the underlying conflict or stress situation in the individual patient. Long-term techniques should be selected according to the underlying conflict situation (e.g., psychodynamic therapy or psychoanalysis) and comorbidity. For subjects with a strongly pronounced disorder and considerable suffering, we recommend a combination of psychotherapy, therapy with a psychoactive drug and balance training.

References

Andersson G, Asmundson GJ, Denev J, Nilsson J, Larsen HC (2006) A controlled trial of cognitive behavior therapy combined with vestibular rehabilitation in the treatment of dizziness. Behav Res Ther 44:1265–1273

Barsky AJ, Wyshak GL (1990) Hypochondriasis and somatosensory amplification. Br J Psychiatry 157:404–409

Best C, Eckhardt-Henn A, Diener G, Bense S, Breuer P, Dieterich M (2006) Interaction of somatoform and vestibular disorders. J Neurol Neurosurg Psychiatry 77:658–664

Best C, Eckhardt-Henn A, Tschan R, Bense S, Dieterich M (2009a) Psychiatric morbidity and comorbidity in different vestibular vertigo syndrome: results of a prospective longitudinal study over one year. J Neurol 256(1):58–65

Best C, Eckhardt-Henn A, Tschan R, Dieterich M (2009b) Who is a risk for psychiatric distressed after vestibular disorder? – results from a prospective one-year follow-up. Neuroscience 164(4): 1579–1587

Best C, Tschan R, Stieber N et al (2015) STEADFAST: psychotherapeutic intervention improves postural strategy of somatoform vertigo and dizziness. Behav Neurol 2015:456850

Brandt T (1996) Phobic postural vertigo. Neurology 46:1515–1519

Brandt T, Dieterich M (1986) Phobischer Attacken-Schwankschwindel, ein neues Syndrom. Münch Med Wochenschr 128:247–250

Brandt T, Huppert D (2014) Fear of heights and visual height intolerance. Curr Opin Neurol 27(1): 111–117

Brandt T, Huppert D, Dieterich M (1994) Phobic postural vertigo: a first follow-up. J Neurol 241: 191–195

Brandt T, Strupp M, Novozhilov S, Krafczyk S (2012) Artificial neural network posturography detects the transition of vestibular neuritis to phobic postural vertigo. J Neurol 259:182–184

Brandt T, Kugler G, Schniepp R et al (2015) Acrophobia impairs visual exploration and balance during standing and walking. Ann N Y Acad Sci 1343:37–48

Bronstein AM (1995a) The visual vertigo syndrome. Acta Otolaryngol (Stockh) 520:45–48

Bronstein AM (1995b) Visual vertigo syndrome. Clinical and posturography findings. J Neurol Neurosurg Psychiatry 59:182–184

Bronstein AM (2004) Vision and vertigo: some visual aspects of vestibular disorders. J Neurol 251: 381–387

Choi SY, Choi JH, Oh EH, Oh SJ, Choi KD (2021) Effect of vestibular exercise and optokinetic stimulation using virtual reality in persistent postural-perceptual dizziness. Sci Rep 11(1):14437

Cohen B, Yakushin SB, Cho C (2018) Hypothesis: the vestibular and cerebellar basis of the mal de debarquement syndrome. Front Neurol 9:28. https://doi.org/10.3389/fneur.2018.00028

Decker J, Limburg K, Hennigsen P, Lahmann C, Brandt T, Dieterich M (2019) Intact vestibular function is relevant for anxiety related to vertigo. J Neurol 266(Suppl 1):89–92

Dieterich M, Eckhardt-Henn A (2006) Neurologische und somatoforme Schwindelsyndrome. In: Henningsen P, Gündel H, Ceballos-Baumann A (eds) Neuro-Psychosomatik. Grundlagen und Klinik neurologischer Psychosomatik. Schattauer, Stuttgart, pp 253–265

Dieterich M, Staab J (2017) Functional dizziness: from phobic postural vertigo and chronic subjective dizziness to persistent postural-perceptual dizziness. Curr Opin Neurol 139:447–468

Dieterich M, Staab JP, Brandt T (2016) Functional (psychogenic) dizziness. Chap. 37. In: Carson A, Hallett M, Stone J (eds) Handbook of clinical neurology, Vol., 138 (3rd series): functional neurologic, disorders. Elsevier, pp 447–468

Eckhardt-Henn A, Breuer P, Thomalske C, Hoffmann SO, Hopf HC (2003) Anxiety disorders and other psychiatric subgroups in patients complaining of dizziness. J Anxiety Disord 431: 1–20

Eckhardt-Henn A, Best C, Bense S, Breuer P, Diener G, Tschan R, Dieterich M (2008) Psychiatric comorbidity in different organic vertigo syndromes. J Neurol 255(3):420–428

Eckhardt-Henn A, Tschan R, Best C, Dieterich M (2009) Somatoforme Schwindelsyndrome. Nervenarzt 80:909–917

Edelman S, Mahoney AE, Cremer PD (2012) Cognitive behavior therapy for chronic subjective dizziness: a randomized, controlled trial. Am J Otolaryngol 33:395–401

Feldker K, Heitmann CY, Neumeister P, Bruchmann M et al (2016) Brain responses to disorder-related visual threat in panic disorder. Hum Brain Mapp 37(12):4439–4453

Feuerecker R, Habs M, Dieterich M, Strupp M (2015) Chronic subjective dizziness: fewer symptoms in the early morning--a comparison with bilateral vestibulopathy and downbeat nystagmus syndrome. J Vestib Res 25:67–72

Furman JM, Jacob RG (1997) Psychiatric dizziness. Neurology 48:1161–1166

Gerschlager W, Brown P (2011) Orthostatic tremor - a review. Handb Clin Neurol 100:457–462

Godemann F, Schabowska A, Naetebusch B, Heinz A, Ströhle A (2006) The impact of cognitions on the development of panic and somatoform disorders: a prospective study in patients with vestibular neuritis. Psychol Med 36:99–108

Hanel G, Henningsen P, Herzog W, Sauer N, Schaefert R, Szecsenyi J, Löwe B (2009) Depression, anxiety, and somatoform disorders: vague or distinct categories in primary care? Results from a large cross-sectional study. J Psychosom Res 67(3):189–197

Heinrichs N, Edler C, Eskens S, Mielczarek MM, Moschner C (2007) Predicting continued dizziness after an acute peripheral vestibular disorder. Psychosom Med 69:700–707

Heitmann CY, Feldker K, Neumeister P et al (2016) Abnormal brain activation and connectivity to standardized disorder-related visual scenes in social anxiety disorder. Hum Brain Mapp 37(4):1559–1572

Henningsen P, Gundel H, Kop WJ, Lowe B, Martin A, Rief W, Van den Bergh O (2018) Persistent physical symptoms as perceptual dysregulation: a neuropsychobehavioral model and its clinical implications. Psychosom Med 80(5):422–431

Holmberg J, Karlberg M, Harlacher U, Rivano-Fischer M, Magnusson M (2006) Treatment of phobic postural vertigo. A controlled study of cognitive-behavioral therapy and self-controlled desensitization. J Neurol 253:500–506

Holmberg J, Karlberg M, Harlacher U, Magnusson M (2007) One-year follow-up of cognitive behavioral therapy for phobic postural vertigo. J Neurol 254:1189–1192

Huber J, Flanagin VL, Popp P, zu Eulenburg P, Dieterich M (2020) Network property changes during visual motion stimulation in patients with phobic postural vertigo. Brain Behav 18:e01622

Huppert D, Kunihiro T, Brandt T (1995) Phobic postural vertigo (154 patients): its association with vestibular disorders. J Audiol 4:97–103

Huppert D, Strupp M, Rettinger N, Hecht J, Brandt T (2005) Phobic postural vertigo – a long-term follow-up (5 to 15 years) of 106 patients. J Neurol 252:564–569

Indovina I, Ricelli R, Staab JP et al (2014) Personality traits modulate subcortical and cortical vestibular and anxiety responses to sound-evoked otolithic receptor stimulation. J Psychosom Res 77:391–400

Indovina I, Ricelli R, Chiarella G et al (2015) Role of the insula and vestibular system in patients with chronic subjective dizziness: an fMRI study using sound-evoked vestibular stimulation. Front Behav Neurosci 9;9:334

Jacob RG, Lilienfeld SO, Furman JM, Durrant JD, Turner SM (1989) Panic disorder with vestibular dysfunction: further clinical observation and description of space and motion phobic stimuli. J Anxiety Disord 3:117–130

Jacob RG, Woody SR, Clark DB, Lilienfeld SO, Hirsch BE, Kucera GD, Furman JM, Durrant JD (1993) Discomfort with space and motion: a possible marker of vestibular dysfunction assessed by the Situational Characteristics Questionnaire. J Psychopathol Behav Assess 15:299–324

Jacob RG, Redfern MS, Furman JM (2009) Space and motion discomfort and abnormal balance control in patients with anxiety disorders. J Neurol Neurosurg Psychiatry 80:74–78

Kapfhammer HP, Mayer C, Hock U, Huppert D, Dieterich M, Brandt T (1997) Course of illness in phobic postural vertigo. Acta Neurol Scand 95:23–28

Kim HA, Bisdorff A, Bronstein A et al (2019) Hemodynamic orthostatic dizziness/vertigo: diagnostic criteria. J Vestib Res 29:45–56

Krafczyk S, Tietze S, Swoboda W, Valkovic P, Brandt T (2006) Artificial neural network: a new diagnostic posturographic tool for disorders of stance. Clin Neurophysiol 117:1692–1698

Kristiansen L, Magnussen LH, Juul-Kristensen B, Mæland S et al (2019) Feasibility of integrating vestibular rehabilitation and cognitive behaviour therapy for people with persistent dizziness. Pilot Feasibility Studies 5(1):69

Kugler G, Huppert D, Schneider E et al (2014) Fear of heights freezes gaze to the horizon. J Vestib Res 24:433–441

Lahmann C, Henningsen P, Dinkel A (2010) Somatoforme und funktionelle Störungen. Nervenarzt 81:1383–1396

Lahmann C, Henningsen P, Brandt T et al (2015a) Psychiatric comorbidity and psychosocial impairment among patients with vertigo and dizziness. J Neurol Neurosurg Psychiatry 86:302–308

Lahmann C, Henningsen P, Dieterich M, Radziej K, Schmid G (2015b) Tailored care for somatoform vertigo/dizziness: study protocol for a randomised controlled trial evaluating integrative group psychotherapy. J Neurol 262(8):1867–1875

Lee JO, Lee ES, Kim JS, Lee YB, Jeong Y, Choi BS, Staab JP (2018) Altered brain function in persistent postural perceptual dizziness: a study on resting state functional connectivity. Hum Brain Mapp 39(8):3340–3353

Li K, Si L, Cui B, Ling X, Shen B, Yang X (2019) Altered spontaneous functional activity of the right precuneus and cuneus in patients with persistent postural-perceptual dizziness. Brain Imaging Behav. https://doi.org/10.1007/s11682-019-00168-7

Li K, Si L, Cui B, Ling X, Shen B, Yang X (2020) Altered intra- and inter-network functional connectivity in patients with persistent postural-perceptual dizziness. NeuroImage Clin 26:102216

Limburg K, Radziej K, Sattel H, Henningsen P, Dieterich M, Lahmann C (2021) Tailored care for patients with functional vertigo and dizziness: a randomised controlled trial evaluating integrative group psychotherapy compared to self-help groups. J Clin Med 10(10):2215

Mahoney AEJ, Edelman S, Cremer PD (2013) Cognitive behavior therapy for chronic subjective dizziness: longer-term gains and predictors of disability. Am J Otolaryngol 34:115–120

Marks JM (1981) Space "phobia": a pseudo-agoraphobic syndrome. J Neurol Neurosurg Psychiatry 48:729–735

Mucci V, Jacquemyn Y, Van Ombergen A, Van de Heyning PH, Browne CJ (2018) A new theory on GABA and calcitonin gene-related peptide involvement in Mal de Debarquement Syndrome predisposition factors and pathophysiology. Med Hypotheses 120:128–134

Murphy TP (1993) Mal de debarquement syndrome: a forgotten entity? Otolaryngol Head Neck Surg 109:10–13

Neff BA, Staab JP, Eggers SD et al (2012) Auditory and vestibular symptoms and chronic subjective dizziness in patients with Meniere's disease, vestibular migraine, and Meniere's disease with concomitant vestibular migraine. Otol Neurotol 33:1235–1244

Petzschner FH, Weber LAE, Gard T, Stephan KE (2017) Computational psychosomatics and computational psychiatry: toward a joint framework for differential diagnosis. Biol Psychiatry 82(6):421–430

Popkirov S, Staab JP, Stone J (2018) Persistent postural-perceptual dizziness (PPPD): a common, characteristic and treatable cause of chronic dizziness. Pract Neurol 18(1):5–13

Popp P, zu Eulenburg P, Stephan T, Bögle R, Habs M, Henningsen P, Feuerecker R, Dieterich M (2018) Cortical alterations in phobic postural vertigo–a multimodal imaging approach. Ann Clin Transl Neurol 5(6):717–729. https://doi.org/10.1002/acn3.570

Querner V, Krafczyk S, Dieterich M, Brandt T (2000) Patients with somatoform phobic postural vertigo: the more difficult the balance task, the better the balance performance. Neurosci Lett 285: 21–24

Querner V, Krafczyk S, Dieterich M, Brandt T (2002) Phobic postural vertigo. Body sway during visually induced roll vection. Exp Brain Res 143(3):269–275. https://doi.org/10.1007/s00221-001-0955-y

Radziej K, Schmid G, Dinkel A et al (2015) Psychological traumatization and adverse life events in patients with organic and functional vestibular symptoms. J Psychosom Res 79:123–129

Saha, K, Cha YH (2020) Mal de Debarquement Syndrome. Semin Neurol 40(1):160–164

Schaaf H, Hesse G (2015) Patients with long-lasting dizziness: a follow-up after neurotological and psychotherapeutic in patient treatment after a period of at least 1 year. Eur Arch Otorhinolaryngol 272:1529–1535

Schlick C, Schniepp R, Loidl V et al (2016) Falls and fear of falling in vertigo and balance disorders: a controlled cross sectional study. J Vestib Res 25:241–251

Schmid G, Henningsen P, Dieterich M, Sattel H, Lahmann C (2011) Psychotherapy in vertigo – a systematic review. J Neurol Neurosurg Psychiatry 82(6):601–606

Schniepp R, Wühr M, Huth S et al (2014) Gait characteristics of patients with phobic postural vertigo: effects of fear of falling, attention, and visual input. J Neurol 261(4):738–746

Staab JP (2012) Chronic subjective dizziness. Continuum (Minneap Minn) 18:1118–1141

Staab JP (2013) Behavioural neuro-otology. In: Bronstein AM (ed) Oxford textbook of vertigo and imbalance. Oxford University Press, Oxford, UK, pp 333–346

Staab JP (2014) The influence of anxiety on ocular motor control and gaze. Curr Opin Neurol 27:118–124

Staab JP (2020) Persistent postural-perceptual dizziness. Semin Neurol 40(1):130–137

Staab JP, Ruckenstein MJ (2007) Expanding the differential diagnosis of dizziness. Arch Otolaryngol Head Neck Surg 133:170–176

Staab JP, Ruckenstein MJ, Amsterdam JD (2004) A prospective trial of sertraline for chronic subjective dizziness. Laryngoscope 114:1637–1641

Staab JP, Rohe DE, Eggers SD, Shepard NT (2014) Anxious, introverted personality traits in patients with chronic subjective dizziness. J Psychosom Res 76:80–83

Staab JP, Eckhardt-Henn A, Horii A et al (2017) Diagnostic criteria for persistent postural-perceptual dizziness (PPPD): consensus document of the Committee for the Classification of Vestibular Disorders of the Barany Society. J Vestib Res 27(4):191–208

Strupp M, Glaser M, Karch C, Rettinger N, Dieterich M, Brandt T (2003) The most common form of dizziness in middle age: phobic postural vertigo. Nervenarzt 74:911–914

Thompson KJ, Goetting JC, Staab JP et al (2015) Retrospective review and telephone follow-up to evaluate a physical therapy protocol for treating persistent postural-perceptual dizziness: a pilot study. J Vestib Res 25:97–104

Tschan R, Best C, Beutel M et al (2011) Patients' psychological well-being and resilient coping protect from secondary somatoform vertigo and dizziness (SVD) one year after vestibular disease. J Neurol 258:104–112

Tschan R, Eckhardt-Henn A, Scheurich V, Best C, Dieterich M, Beutel M (2012) Steadfast-effectiveness of a cognitive behavioral self-management program of patients with somatoform vertigo and dizziness. Psychother Psychosom Med Psychol 62(3–4):111–119

Van Ombergen A, Heine L, Jillings S, Roberts RE, Jeurissen B, Van Rompaey V, Wuyts FL (2017) Altered functional brain connectivity in patients with visually induced dizziness. Neuroimage Clin 14: 538–545

Von Holst E, Mittelstaedt H (1950) Das Reafferenzierungsprinzip (Wechselwirkungen zwischen Zentralnervensystem und Peripherie). Naturwissenschaften 37(20):461–476

WHO. International Classification of Diseases, 11th edition, beta draft. Persistent postural-perceptual dizziness. 2015. Available at: http://id.who.int/icd/entity/2005792829

Wühr M, Pradhan C, Novozhilov S et al (2013) Inadequate interaction between open- and closed-loop postural control in phobic postural vertigo. J Neurol 260:1314–1323

Wühr M, Brandt T, Schniepp R (2017) Distracting attention in phobic postural vertigo normalizes leg muscle activity and balance. Neurology 88(3):284–288. https://doi.org/10.1212/WNL.0000000000003516

Yardley L, Redfern MS (2001) Psychological factors influencing recovery from balance disorders. J Anxiety Disord 15:107–119

Zaback M, Cleworth TW, Carpenter MG, Adkin AL (2015) Personality traits and individual differences predict threat-induced changes in postural control. Hum Mov Sci 40:393–409

Vertigo and Dizziness in Childhood

Contents

Supplementary Information The online version contains supplementary material available at [https://doi.org/10.1007/978-3-030-78260-3_16]. The videos can be accessed by scanning the related images with the SN More Media App.

M. Strupp et al., *Vertigo and Dizziness*, https://doi.org/10.1007/978-3-030-78260-3_16

16.1 Clinical Aspects

Most forms of vertigo and dizziness and vestibular syndromes of adulthood can also appear in childhood (◘ Table 16.1). For this reason, we will restrict ourselves in this chapter to the essential features of an indicative patient history and specific clinical aspects. Children describe their complaints – depending on their age – less precisely and with

◘ **Table 16.1** Vertigo and disturbance of vestibular function in childhood

Labyrinth/nerve	**Central vestibular origin**
Hereditary/congenital	
Labyrinthine malformation	Familial episodic ataxias especially EA2
Syndrome of the third mobile windows/Perilymph fistulas	Cerebellar ataxias Downbeat nystagmus syndrome
Embryopathic malformations (rubella, cytomegalovirus)	
Toxic agents	
Various hereditary audiovestibular syndromes	
Familial bilateral vestibulopathy	
Syphilitic labyrinthitis	
Positive family history of migraine	
Recurrent vertigo of childhood	
Vestibular migraine of childhood Basilar-type migraine	
Acquired	
Labyrinthitis with vestibulopathy (viral, bacterial)	Infratentorial tumors (medulloblastoma, astrocytoma, epidermoid cysts, meningioma)
Syndrome of the third mobile windows/perilymph fistulas	Epileptic aura, vestibular epilepsy
Trauma (transverse petrous bone fracture, benign paroxysmal positioning vertigo)	Trauma (brainstem or vestibulocerebellar contusion)
Menière's disease	Encephalitis
Acute unilateral vestibulopathy/labyrintitis/otitis media	Toxic agents (e.g., upbeat/downbeat nystagmus when on anticonvulsants)
Herpes zoster oticus	
Cholesteatoma	
Ototoxic drugs	
Cogan's syndrome, other inner-ear autoimmune disorders	

less relevance for therapy than do adults. Moreover, the examination results for balance and ocular motor functions (Devaraja 2018) depend more on their concerted cooperation.

16.1.1 Epidemiology

The widespread and, to some extent, contradictory data of epidemiological studies on vertigo and dizziness in childhood are due to the varying approaches of questioning, methods (questionnaires, interviews, physical investigations), and – most importantly – the medical specialization of the head of the study. In a large National Health Interview Survey on children aged 3–17 years, dizziness or imbalance was reported in 3.5 million patients (5.6%) with a mean age of 11.5 years (dizziness: 1.5 million patients; balance impairment: 2.3 million patients) without any preference of sex (Brodsky et al. 2019). In this study, the most common diagnoses for dizziness were depression or child psychiatric disorders, side effects from medication, head/neck injury or concussion, and developmental motor coordination disorders. In an earlier study, the prevalence of at least one vertigo attack in the last year was reported in 15% of children of school age (Russell and Abu-Arafeh 1999). The frequency of vertigo or dizziness attacks assessed by a questionnaire in adolescence (mean age 14.5 years) revealed that 72% had experienced episodic vertigo or dizziness during the last 3 months which in most cases was associated with orthostatic complaints (Langhagen et al. 2015).

A review of 2726 cases on the differential diagnoses of vertigo in children concluded that the top four diagnoses were vestibular migraine (23.8%), benign paroxysmal vertigo of childhood (13.7%), idiopathic or no identified association (11.7%), and labyrinthitis/acute vestibular syndrome (8.47%), thus accounting for 57% of cases (Davitt et al. 2017). In another study, vestibular migraine accounted for 39% of vertigo attacks in children as the most frequent form of vertigo/dizziness, followed by 21% with functional psychogenic vertigo (Batu et al. 2015).

Several established risk factors in adults could also be found by asking 1482 schoolchildren between the age of 12 and 19 years to fill out a questionnaire on different types of vertigo/dizziness and related potential independent risk factors, namely, gender, stress, muscular pain in the neck and shoulder region, sleep duration, and migraine (Filippopulos et al. 2017). A functional vestibular impairment was found in 36.5% of 2528 children with the key symptom of balance or hearing disorders (Wiener-Vacher et al. 2018). A population-based epidemiological survey revealed a prevalence of peripheral vestibular disorders of 15.16 per 100,000 individuals. The most frequent were benign paroxysmal positional vertigo (10.21), followed by an acute vestibular syndrome (3.5) and Menière's disease (1.54) (Hülse et al. 2019). It is striking that these authors do not report on vestibular migraine, which in other studies is the most frequent cause of vertigo in children. As expected, chronic or episodic vertigo syndromes affect physical well-being assessed as health-related quality of life, which was not related to gender and vertigo types but appeared to be higher in children aged 12–18 suffering from vertigo as compared to children aged 8–11 years (Deissler et al. 2017). In a cross-sectional analysis using the 2008 National Health Interview Survey, which included a balance and dizziness supplement, an association was found in adults with an increased risk of cognitive and psychiatric comorbidity such as depression and anxiety disorders (Bigelow et al. 2019). The same authors confirmed this in another National Health Interview Survey for children aged 3–17 years (with a 1-year prevalence of vertigo of 1.56%). The children had significantly higher odds of attention deficit disorders, learning disability, developmental delay, and intellectual disability, which made utilization of special education services more likely as compared to other children (Bigelow et al. 2019). Ocular motor disorders may also lead to dizziness in childhood, e.g., disorders of convergence; special orthoptic therapies may be effective (Wiener-Vacher et al. 2019).

16.1.2 Clinical Synopsis

Episodic vertigo syndromes in childhood are associated with migraine in about 50% of the cases (Jahn et al. 2009, 2011). Formerly it was termed benign paroxysmal vertigo of childhood (Basser 1964), but is now called "vestibular migraine of childhood" (Batu et al. 2015) (▶ Chap. 14) and "recurrent vertigo of childhood" (see below). Benign paroxysmal positional vertigo, acute peripheral vestibular syndrome due to viral or bacterial inflammations of the ear, vestibular paroxysmia, syndrome of the third mobile windows of a semicircular canal, episodic ataxias, or vestibular epilepsy occur more rarely. Predisposing factors for vertigo or dizziness in childhood are recurrent bouts of otitis, traumatic brain injury, and a positive family history of migraine (Niemensivu et al. 2007).

16.1.2.1 Vestibular Migraine of Childhood and "Recurrent Vertigo of Childhood"

16

In children with recurrent vertigo, migraine plays an important role (Abu-Arafeh and Russell 1995; Basser 1964; Batu et al. 2015; Jahn et al. 2015; Devaraja 2018). The leading symptoms are recurrent spontaneous attacks of vertigo or dizziness with different duration and different accompanying symptoms such as vomiting, pallor, fearfulness, postural imbalance, ataxia, and/or nystagmus in otherwise healthy children. For its description, different terms have been used which has caused some confusion. Therefore, a new classification with three categories "vestibular migraine of childhood," "probable vestibular migraine of childhood," and "recurrent vertigo of childhood" was elaborated (van de Berg et al. 2021); the details and the clinical features of the different types are described below.

16.1.2.2 Benign Paroxysmal Positional Vertigo (BPPV)

BPPV (▶ Chap. 9) in children is generally caused by trauma (Brodsky et al. 2018b, c). The most frequently affected semicircular canal is the posterior (Yao et al. 2019); in two thirds of patients, several canals are affected. The typical treatment by positioning maneuvers in the plane of the affected canal is effective; however, children with a history of a vestibular migraine or recurrent paroxysmal vertigo of childhood have significantly higher rates of relapses (Brodsky et al. 2018a, b).

16.1.2.3 Vestibular Paroxysmia

Vestibular paroxysmia due to neurovascular compression of the eighth nerve causes frequent short episodes of vertigo in adults and rarely in children (see ▶ Chap. 11). The attacks usually cease after low-dose carbamazepine administration (2–4 mg/kg daily; Lehnen et al. 2015). Operative decompression should only be considered as a last resort ratio since vascular, brain, and bone structures grow at different speeds in children, so that compression syndromes in our experience mostly resolve spontaneously (Huppert et al. 2017).

16.1.2.4 Syndrome of the Third Mobile Windows

There is also a unilateral (Lee et al. 2011) or bilateral (Kanaan et al. 2011) bony dehiscence of the superior semicircular canal syndrome in childhood. It differs from that in adults in manifesting primarily with auditory symptoms (autophonia, tinnitus, and hearing disorders). Initial experience has shown that conservative treatment should be given first (Lee et al. 2011; van Bulck et al. 2019).

16.1.2.5 Acute Peripheral Vestibular Syndrome

Sustained spinning vertigo can be the main symptom of an acute vestibular syndrome, e.g., caused by a viral (▶ Chap. 8) or bacterial inflammation or otitis media which requires otoscopy and depending on the findings imaging of the temporal bone with antiviral/antibiotic treatment or a head trauma (▶ Chap. 18).

16.1.2.6 Vertigo and Dizziness Following a Traumatic Head/Brain Injury

In childhood and adolescence, traumatic head/brain injuries may cause peripheral vestibular dysfunctions in about 25%, especially post-traumatic benign paroxysmal positional vertigo or a vestibular deficit by a fracture of the petrous bone (Brodsky et al. 2018b, c). In most cases, the type of dizziness is described as numbness or lightheadedness (Heyer et al. 2018). In most cases, e.g., athletes after a head trauma, the complaints were not attributable to one main type of dysfunction, even after special tests of the vestibular and ocular motor system (Reneker et al. 2018).

16.1.2.7 Bilateral Vestibulopathy

Swaying vertigo and postural imbalance worsening in darkness and on uneven ground as well as oscillopsia with active or passive head movements are typical for bilateral vestibulopathy also in childhood (▶ Chap. 7). In children, it can be caused by malformation of the labyrinth, viral or bacterial inflammation, or ototoxic antibiotics.

16.1.2.8 Functional Dizziness

Functional dizziness (see ▶ Chap. 15) may also occur in children and there are several reports on the comorbidity of postural imbalance with anxiety disorders (Erez et al. 2004; Skirbekk et al. 2012). The fraction of functional ("somatoform") vertigo and dizziness in childhood was reported to be 5–21% (Erbek et al. 2006; Riina et al. 2005; Jahn et al. 2015; Batu et al. 2015).

16.1.2.9 Central Vertigo/Dizziness Syndromes

If dizziness occurs with slowly increasing central vestibular and ocular motor dysfunctions, an MRI investigation is mandatory because of a relative frequency of brainstem and cerebellar tumors in childhood (Jahn et al. 2009).

16.1.3 Differential Diagnoses of Vertigo, Dizziness, and Balance Disorders

The following three key symptoms (with or without accompanying clinical findings) are helpful for the differential diagnosis of childhood forms of vertigo:

16.1.4 Attacks of Vertigo

- *Episodic vertigo without pathological findings in the attack-free interval*: vestibular migraine/recurrent paroxysmal vertigo of childhood, vestibular paroxysmia, epileptic aura or vestibular epilepsy, orthostatic dysregulation, functional or psychogenic vertigo
- *Episodic vertigo with inner-ear hypoacusis*: syndrome of a third mobile window/superior canal dehiscence syndrome/perilymph fistula, Menière's disease, vestibular paroxysmia
- *Episodic vertigo with ocular motor abnormalities in the attack-free interval*: vestibular migraine, familial episodic ataxia type 2
- *Episodic vertigo followed in the course of the disease by oscillopsia during head movements and imbalance that worsens in darkness*: development of bilateral vestibular failure (also with familial vestibulopathy)

- *Paroxysmal, short (<1 min) attacks of spinning vertigo during changes in head position relative to gravity*: BPPV (post-traumatic)

16.1.5 Sustained Vertigo (Lasting Days or a Few Weeks)

- *Sustained vertigo without hearing loss*: acute vestibular syndrome (former vestibular neuritis) or bacterial inflammation
- *Sustained vertigo with hearing loss*: labyrinthitis, inner-ear autoimmune disease
- *Post-traumatic sustained vertigo*: transverse petrous bone fracture, labyrinthine contusion

16.1.6 Stance and Gait Imbalance With and Without Oscillopsia

- *Delayed stance and gait development with or without hearing loss*: congenital bilateral vestibulopathy
- *Stance and gait instability with oscillopsia during walking and head movements*: congenital or early acquired bilateral vestibulopathy, perilymph fistula, post-traumatic otolithic vertigo
- *Slowly increasing stance and gait instability as well as oscillopsia during head movements*: various hereditary and congenital disorders causing progressive audio-vestibular loss
- *Progressive ataxia, balance, and ocular motor disorders*: infratentorial tumors with lesions of vestibulocerebellar and/or pontomedullary brainstem structures, spinocerebellar ataxias with or without downbeat nystagmus

We now discuss in detail four special forms of vertigo/dizziness syndromes in childhood.

16

16.2 Vestibular Migraine of Childhood and Recurrent Vertigo of Childhood

Vestibular migraine of childhood – formerly called recurrent paroxysmal vertigo of childhood – is the most frequent form of spontaneous episodic vertigo in children with a prevalence ranging from 2.6% to 39% (Abu-Arafeh and Russell 1995; Batu et al. 2015; Jahn et al. 2015; Devaraja 2018). It is characterized by sudden brief attacks of vertigo associated with nystagmus. It normally begins between ages 1 and 4 years, and can remit spontaneously within a few years. The course of the disease is, however, not homogeneous. The current diagnostic criteria for the three forms are as follows (van de Berg et al. 2021):

Vestibular migraine of childhood

A. At least five episodes with vestibular symptoms of moderate or severe intensity, lasting between 5 min and 72 h
B. A current or past history of migraine with or without aura
C. At least half of episodes are associated with at least one of the following three migraine features:
   1. Headache with at least two of the following four characteristics:
      (a) One-sided location
      (b) Pulsating quality
      (c) Moderate or severe pain intensity
      (d) Aggravation by routine physical activity
   2. Photophobia and phonophobia
   3. Visual aura
D. Age < 18 years
E. Not better accounted for by another headache disorder, vestibular disorder, or other condition

Probable vestibular migraine of childhood

A. At least three episodes with vestibular symptoms of moderate or severe intensity, lasting between 5 min and 72 h
B. Only one of the criteria B and C for vestibular migraine of childhood
C. Age < 18 years
D. Not better accounted for by another headache disorder, vestibular disorder, or other condition

Recurrent vertigo of childhood

A. At least three episodes with vestibular symptoms of moderate or severe intensity, lasting between 1 min and 72 h
B. None of the criteria B and C for vestibular migraine of childhood
C. Age < 18 years
D. Not better accounted for by another headache disorder, vestibular disorder, or other condition

In a long-term follow-up study, five of ten children older than 11 years of age reported that their dizziness attacks had stopped (Krams et al. 2011). Frequently, there are transitions to other forms of migraine with and without aura (Lanzi et al. 1994; Zhang et al. 2012). Similar transitions have also been described for the benign paroxysmal torticollis of childhood, which spontaneously wears off to manifest later as vestibular migraine/recurrent paroxysmal vertigo (Brodsky et al. 2018a). About 50% of dizzy children also complain about headache (Balatsouras et al. 2007). Episodic ataxia type 2 can clinically mimic vestibular migraine in childhood/recurrent paroxysmal vertigo (Bertholon et al. 2010; Strupp et al. 2010).

It has been repeatedly pointed out that reliable prospective studies on the efficacy of medical treatment in children are still missing (Langhagen et al. 2016; Jahn et al. 2015). The therapy of choice for frequent attacks of vestibular migraine/recurrent paroxysmal vertigo of childhood is the analogous migraine prophylaxis administered to adults with migraine (Byun et al. 2020). It is our experience that children may benefit from magnesium 300–600 mg per day in particular. Non-pharmacologic prophylaxis is still generally recommended in accordance with the guidelines of the American Academy of Neurology (Lewis et al. 2004). Recommended non-pharmacological measures include physical exercise, sleep hygiene, avoidance of triggering food items, and behavioral therapy (Gelfand 2013; Kacperski 2015; Devaraja 2018).

16.3 Episodic Ataxias

So far, nine forms of episodic ataxia (EA) have been described (Jen and Wan 2018; Piarroux et al. 2020). They are mostly autosomal dominant ion-channel diseases. The main symptom is recurrent attacks with ataxia in combination with cerebellar and/or vestibular disorders even in the attack-free interval. EA2 is clearly the most frequent form, whereas EA1 is very rare. The other forms have been described in only a few families.

EA2 is the clinically most relevant subtype and is an important differential diagnosis for vestibular migraine (Strupp et al. 2010; Brandt and Strupp 1997; Jen and Wan 2018; Jen 2008) (▶ see Chap. 14). As a rule, EA2 manifests in late childhood or in early adulthood. The attacks generally last for hours or up to one day (◘ Fig. 16.1). They can occur spontaneously but typical triggers are exercise, stress, coffee, or alcohol. Similar to vestibular migraine, about 90% of patients with EA2 present with central cerebellar ocular motor disorders, such as saccadic pursuit, gaze-evoked nystagmus, impaired fixation suppression of the vestibulo-ocular reflex, and especially

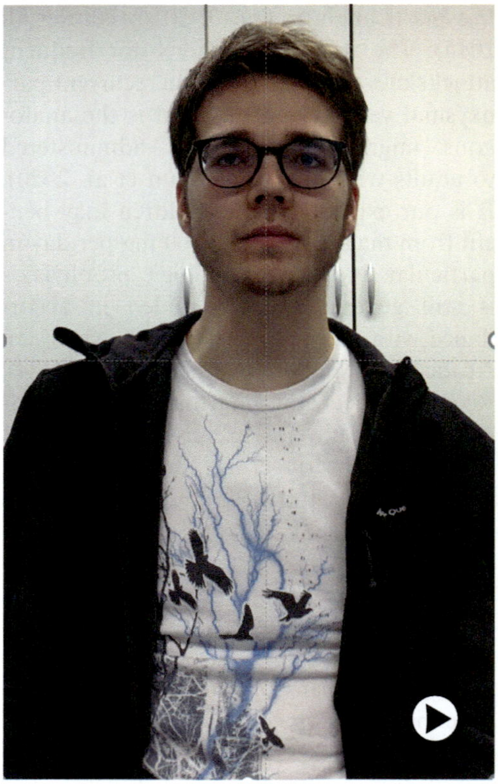

■ Fig. 16.1 Patient history of a patient with episodic ataxia type 2 (▶ https://doi.org/10.1007/000-96f)

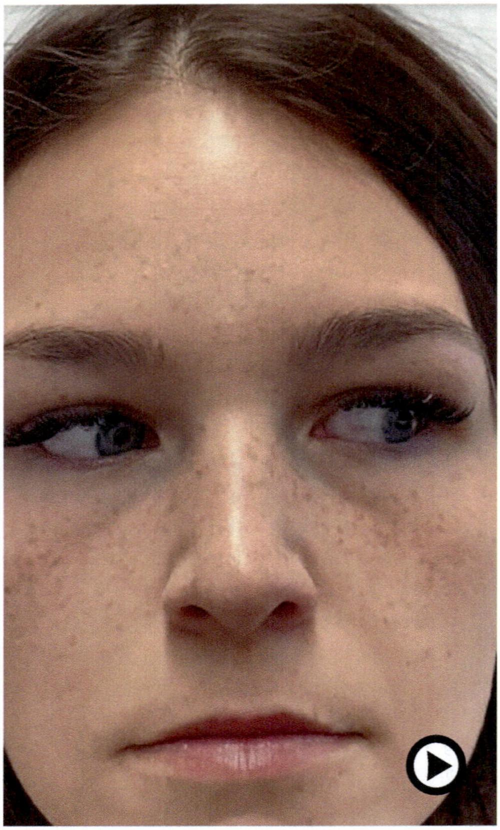

■ Fig. 16.2 Downbeat nystagmus syndrome in a patient with episodic ataxia type 2 (▶ https://doi.org/10.1007/000-96e)

downbeat-nystagmus (Strupp et al. 2007) (■ Fig. 16.2). EA2 is caused by mutations in the so-called PQ-calcium channel gene on chromosome 19p13; this is found in only 60–70% of all clinically confirmed diagnoses (Jen et al. 2004; Jen and Wan 2018). Attacks are prevented by avoiding physical exertion, emotional stress, and alcohol.

Acetazolamide (Griggs et al. 1978; Griggs and Nutt 1995) and increasingly the prolonged-release form of 4-aminopyridine are used for prophylaxis. A placebo-controlled cross-over study revealed a significant effect of both acetazolamide in a dose of 750 mg daily and the prolonged-release form of 4-aminopyridine (details below) (Muth et al. 2021). The effectiveness of acetazolamide frequently decreases after 1–2 years or the treatment must be discontinued because of adverse side effects such as nephrolithiasis.

In an open trial, a positive effect was seen with the potassium channel blocker 4-aminopyridine (Strupp et al. 2004). A placebo-controlled double-blind cross-over study showed that 4-aminopyridine (3 × 5 mg daily) significantly reduced the attack frequency and improved quality of life (Strupp et al. 2011). The mechanism was also investigated in animal mod-

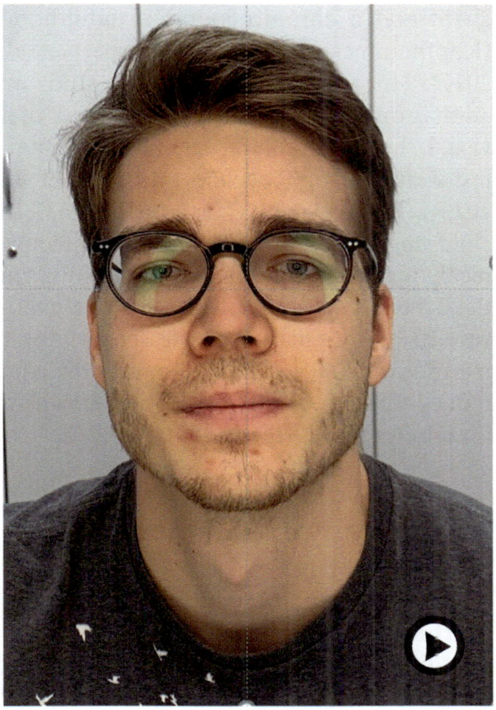

Fig. 16.3 Therapy efficacy of 4-aminopyridine in patients with episodic ataxia type 2 (▶ https://doi.org/10.1007/000-96g)

els in which 4-aminopyridine normalized the irregular depolarization of Purkinje-cells in mutant mice models (Alvina and Khodakhah 2010). Usually the treatment with 4-aminopyridine is well tolerated in low dosages. Electrocardiograms are recommended before and after administration of a test dosage; the QTc-time should not be elongated. The current choice of therapy in adults is 4-aminopyridine in its sustained release form, fampridine, 2 × 10 mg per day (Fig. 16.3) (Claassen et al. 2013; Strupp et al. 2017; Muth et al. 2021).

The other type of episodic ataxia, EA1, is characterized by recurrent attacks with ataxia and interictal neuro-myokymia. It is based on mutations of the potassium channel. The neuro-myokymia and in part even the attacks can be successfully treated with potassium channel blockers like phenytoin or carbamazepine. In addition, acetazolamide can be administered in daily doses of 62.5–1000 mg to avoid attacks (see Jen and Wan 2018). The effect of acetazolamide is probably due to an alteration of the pH value, in terms of an acidosis, which leads, for example, to reduced potassium conductivity.

16.4 Motion Sickness

Motion sickness is elicited by real or virtual motion stimulation mostly during passive transportation in vehicles. It occurs with unfamiliar (non-habitual) motion stimuli, particularly when there is a visual-vestibular intersensory mismatch. Such a mismatch occurs when passengers in a car or bus try to read while travelling. Then vision does not sense a motion, while the accelerations caused by the vehicle stimulate the vestibular system. Children below the age of 1 year are highly resistant to motion sickness probably because they only use the visual system to a limited extent for self-motion perception and, therefore, are less subject to visual-vestibular conflicts (Brandt et al. 1976; Huppert et al. 2017). Motion sickness susceptibility was investigated in two representative, cross-sectional, population-based surveys: One was targeted at parents with children aged 6 months to 18 years and the other at parents with children aged 3 months to 5 years approaching 7569 and 12,720 households, respectively (Huppert et al. 2019). The main findings in the first survey were that 9.2% were susceptible to motion sickness with a slight female preponderance and in the second study only 1.2% were susceptible. Motion sickness below the age of 1 year was exceptionally rare. The frequency of susceptibility was highest in the range between the age of 4 and 13 years, and declined in postpubertal children and adolescents. This course of the frequency of motion sickness susceptibility from infancy to adolescence is characterized by an inverse U-shaped curve: Phase 1 has high resistance in the first year of life when infants may be less subject to visual-vestibular mismatch; phase 2 has a prepubertal peak possibly due to an oversensitivity to a visual-vestibular mismatch; phase 3 has a postpubertal decline best explained by habituation through repetitive motion stimulation during various kinds of vehicle transportation (Huppert et al. 2019). In an earlier study on children between 9 and 18 years old, no differences were found with respect to susceptibility, gender, age, type of transportation, or physical activity (Dobie et al. 2001).

16.5 Visual Height Intolerance and Acrophobia

There is a large amount of literature on psychiatric epidemiological surveys on the susceptibility of children to various anxiety disorders and specific phobias, which we will not discuss here. Visual height intolerance, including the specific phobia fear of heights (acrophobia), has a life-time prevalence in adults of 28% (females = 32%, males = 25%) (Huppert et al. 2013). A study on the frequency and phenomenology of visual height intolerance in prepubertal children (8–10 years) reported that the prevalence rate was higher than in adults and there was no gender preponderance as in adults (Huppert and Brandt 2015). Since about 50% of the afflicted children reported a spontaneous improvement or remission by the age of 8–10 years, two types of courses must be assumed: a favorable, spontaneous course in childhood (Huppert and Brandt 2015) and a chronic course in adulthood (Kapfhammer et al. 2016; Huppert et al. 2017). This view is supported by a study on adults, only 4.5% of whom reported that visual height intolerance initially manifested in the first decade (Huppert et al. 2013). Teleologically, "fear of heights" in children can be interpreted as a protective mechanism to avoid catastrophic falls. On the other hand, controlled repetitive exposure to heights may promote sensorimotor maturation of outdoor locomotion and reduce inappropriate avoidance behavior (Sandseter and Kennair 2011).

16

16.6 Therapy of Childhood Forms of Vertigo

The treatment of these various forms of vertigo/dizziness corresponds to that in adults; however, a pediatrician should be closely consulted. There are no specific studies available on the therapy of most forms of vertigo in childhood. Consequently, the treatment recommendations are similar to those made for adults but with adjusted dosages.

References

Abu-Arafeh I, Russel G (1995) Paroxysmal vertigo as a migraine equivalent in children: a population-based study. Cephalagia 15:22–25

Alvina K, Khodakhah K (2010) The therapeutic mode of action of 4-aminopyridine in cerebellar ataxia. J Neurosci 30:7258–7268

Balatsouras DG, Kaberos A, Assimakopoulos D, Katotomichelakis M, Economou NC, Korres SG (2007) Etiology of vertigo in children. Int J Pediatr Otorhinolaryngol 71:487–494

Basser LS (1964) Benign paroxysmal vertigo of childhood. A variety of vestibular neuronitis. Brain 87:141–152

Batu ED, Anlar B, Topcu M, Turanli G (2015) Vertigo in childhood: a retrospective series of 100 children. Eur J Paediatr Neurol 19:226–232

Bertholon P, Chabrier S, Riant F, Tournier-Lasserve E, Peyron R (2010) Episodic ataxia type 2: unusual aspects in clinical and genetic presentation. Special emphasis in childhood. J Neurol Neurosurg Psychiatry 80:1289–1292

Bigelow RT, Semenov YR, Hoffman HJ, Agrawal Y (2019) Association between vertigo, cognitive and psychiatric conditions in US children: 2012 National Health Interview Survey. Int J Pediatr Otorhinolaryngol 28(130):109802. https://doi.org/10.1016/j.ijporl.2019

Brandt T, Strupp M (1997) Episodic ataxia type 1 and 2 (familial periodic ataxia/vertigo). Audiol Neurootol 2:373–383

Brandt T, Wenzel D, Dichgans J (1976) Die Entwicklung der visuellen Stabilisation des aufrechten Standes beim Kind: Ein Reifezeichen in der Kinderneurologie. Arch Psychiatr Nervenkr 223:1–13

Brodsky J, Kaur K, Shoshany T, Lipson S, Zhou G (2018a) Benign paroxysmal migraine variants of infancy and childhood: transitions and clinical features. Eur J Paediatr Neurol 22:667–673

Brodsky JR, Lipson S, Wilber J, Zhou G (2018b) Benign paroxysmal positional vertigo (BPPV) in children and adolescents: clinical features and response to therapy in 110 pediatric patients. Otol Neurotol 39:344–350

Brodsky JR, Shoshany TN, Lipson S, Zhou G (2018c) Peripheral vestibular disorders in children and adolescents with concussion. Otolaryngol Head Neck Surg 159:365–370

Brodsky JR, Lipson S, Bhattacharyya N (2019) Prevalence of pediatric dizziness and imbalance in the United States. Otolaryngol Head Neck Surg:194599819887375. https://doi.org/10.1177/0194599819887375

Byun YJ, Levy DA, Nguyen SA, Brennan E, Rizk HG (2020) Treatment of vestibular migraine: a systematic review and meta-analysis. Laryngoscope 0:1–9. Doi: https://doi.org/10.1002/lary.28546

Claassen J, Teufel J, Kalla R, Spiegel R, Strupp M (2013) Effects of dalfampridine on attacks of patients with episodic ataxia type 2: an observation study. J Neurol 260:668–669

Davitt M, Delvecchio MT, Aronoff SC (2017) The differential diagnosis of vertigo in children a systematic review of 2726 cases. Pediatr Emerg Care. https://doi.org/10.1097/PEC.0000000000001281

Deissler A, Albers L, von Kries R, Weinberger R, Langhagen T, Gerstl L, Heinen F, Jahn K, Schröder AS (2017) Health-related quality of life of children/adolescents with vertigo: retrospective study from the German Center of Vertigo and Balance Disorders. Neuropediatrics 48:91–97

Devaraja K (2018) Vertigo in children; a narrative review of the various causes and their management. Int J Pediatr Otorhinolaryngol 111:32–38

Dobie T, McBride D, Dopie T Jr, May J (2001) The effects of age and sex on susceptibility to motion sickness. Aviat Space Environ Med 72:13–20

Erbek SH, Erbek SS, Yilmaz I, Topal O, Ozgirgin N, Ozluoglu LN et al (2006) Vertigo in childhood: a clinical experience. Int J Pediatr Otorhinolaryngol 70:1547–1554

Erez O, Gordon CR, Sever J, Sadeh A, Mintz M (2004) Balance dysfunction in childhood anxiety: findings and theoretical approach. J Anxiety Disord 18:341–356

Filippopulos FM, Albers L, Straube A, Gerstl L, Blum B, Langhagen T, Jahn K, Heinen F, von Kries R, Landgraf MN (2017) Vertigo and dizziness in adolescents: risk factors and their population attributable risk. PLoS One 13(12):e0187819. https://doi.org/10.1371/journalpone.0187819

Gelfand AA (2013) Migraine and childhood periodic syndromes in children and adolescents. Curr Opin Neurol 26:262–268

Griggs RC, Nutt JG (1995) Episodic ataxias as channelopathies. Ann Neurol 37:285–287

Griggs RC, Moxley RT, Lafrance RA, McQuillen J (1978) Hereditary paroxysmal ataxia: response to acetazolamide. Neurology 28:1259–1264

Heyer GL, Young JA, Fischer AN (2018) Lightheadedness after concussion: not all dizziness is vertigo. Clin J Sport Med 28:272–277

Hülse R, Warken C, Biesdorf A, Erhart M, Rotter N, Hörmann K, Wenzel A (2019) Prevalence of peripheral vestibular diseases in children in Germany. HNO 10. https://doi.org/10.1007/s00106-019-00747-6

Huppert D, Brandt T (2015) Fear of heights and visual height intolerance in children 8-10 years. J Child Adolesc Behav 3:4

Huppert D, Langhagen T, Brandt T (2017) Benign course of episodic dizziness disorders in childhood. J Neurol 264(Suppl 1):4–6

Huppert D, Grill E, Brandt T (2013) Down on heights? One in three has visual height intolerance. J Neurol 260: 597–604

Huppert D, Grill E, Brandt T (2019) Survey of motion sickness susceptibility in children and adolescents aged 3 months to 18 years. J Neurol 266(Suppl 1):65–73

Jahn K, Zwergal A, Strupp M, Brandt T (2009) Schwindel im Kindesalter. Nervenheilkunde 28:47–52
Jahn K, Langhagen T, Schroeder AS, Heinen F (2011) Vertigo and dizziness in childhood – update on diagnosis and treatment. Neuropediatrics 42: 129–134
Jahn K, Langhagen T, Heinen F (2015) Vertigo and dizziness in children. Curr Opin Neurol 28:78–82
Jen JC (2008) Hereditary episodic ataxias. Ann N Y Acad Sci 1142:250–253
Jen JC, Wan J (2018) Episodic ataxias. Handb Clin Neurol 155:205–215
Jen J, Kim GW, Baloh RW (2004) Clinical spectrum of episodic ataxia type 2. Neurology 62:17–22
Jen JC, Graves TD, Hess EJ, Hanna MG, Griggs RC, Baloh RW (2007) Primary episodic ataxias: diagnosis, pathogenesis and treatment. Brain 130: 2484–2493
Kacperski J (2015) Prophylaxis of migraine in children and adolescents. Paediatr Drugs 17:217–226
Kanaan AA, Raad RA, Hourani RG, Zaytoun GM (2011) Bilateral superior semicircular canal dehiscence in a child with sensorineural hearing loss and without vestibular symptoms. Int J Pediatr Otorhinolaryngol 75:877–879
Kapfhammer HP, Fitz W, Huppert D, Grill E, Brandt T (2016) Visual height intolerance and acrophobia: distressing partners for life. J Neurol 263: 1946–1953
Krams B, Echenne B, Leydet J, Rivier F, Roubertie A (2011) Benign paroxysmal vertigo of childhood: long-term outcome. Cephalalgia 31:439–443
Langhagen T, Albers L, Heinen F, Straube A, Filippopulos F, Landgraf MN, Gerstl L, Jahn K, von Kries R (2015) Period prevalence of dizziness and vertigo in adolescents. PLoS One 10(9):e0136512. https://doi.org/10.1371/journal-pone.0136512
Langhagen T, Landgraf MN, Huppert D, Heinen F, Jahn K (2016) Vestibular migraine in children and adolescents. Curr Pain Headache Rep 20(12):67
Lanzi G, Balottin U, Fazzi E, Tagliasacchi M, Manfrin M, Mira E (1994) Benign paroxysmal vertigo of childhood: a long-term follow-up. Cephalalgia 14:458–460
Lee GS, Zhou G, Poe D, Kenna M, Amin M, Ohlms L, Gopen Q (2011) Clinical experience in diagnosis and management of superior semicircular canal dehiscence in children. Laryngoscope 121: 2256–2261
Lehnen N, Langhagen T, Heinen F, Huppert D, Brandt T, Jahn K (2015) Vestibular paroxysmia in children: a treatable cause of short vertigo attacks. Dev Med Child Neurol 57:393–396
Lewis D, Ashwal S, Hershey A, Hirtz D, Yonker M, Silberstein S et al (2004) Practice parameter: pharmacological treatment of migraine headache in children and adolescents: report of the American Academy of Neurology quality standards subcommittee and the practice committee of the Child Neurology Society. Neurology 63:2215–2224
Muth C, Teufel J, Schöls L, Synofcik M, Franke C, Timmann D, et al. (2021) Fampridine and Acetazolamide in EA2 and related Familial EA: a prospective randomized placebo-controlled trial. Neurol Clin Pract e438–446
Niemensivu R, Kentala E, Wiener-Vacher S, Pyykko I (2007) Evaluation of vertiginous children. Eur Arch Otorhinolaryngol 264:1129–1135
Piarroux J, Riant F, Humbertclaude V, Remerand G, Hadjadj J, Rejou F, Coubes C, Pinson L, Meyer P, Roubertie A (2020) FG14-related episodic ataxia: delineating the phenotype of Episodic Ataxia type 9. Ann Clin Transl Neurol. https://doi.org/10.1002/acn3.51005
Reneker JC, Cheruvu VK, Yang J, James MA, Cook CE (2018) Physical examination of dizziness in athletes after a concussion: a descriptive study. Musculoskelet Sci Pract 34:8–13
Riina N, Ilmari P, Kentala E (2005) Vertigo and imbalance in children: a retrospective study in a Helsinki University otorhinolaryngology clinic. Arch Otolaryngol Head Neck Surg 131:996–1000
Russel G, Abu-Arafeh I (1999) Paroxysmal vertigo in children- an epidemiological study. Int J Pediatr Otorhinolaryngol 49(1):105–107
Sandseter EB, Kennair LE (2011) Children's risky play from an evolutionary perspective: the anti-phobic effects of thrilling experiences. Evol Psychol 9: 257–284
Skirbekk B, Hansen BH, Overbeck B, Wentzel-Larsen T, Kristensen H (2012) Motor impairment in children with anxiety disorders. Psychiatry Res 198:135–139
Strupp M, Kalla R, Dichgans M, Freilinger T, Glasauer S, Brandt T (2004) Treatment of episodic ataxia type 2 with the potassium channel blocker 4-aminopyridine. Neurology 62:1623–1625
Strupp M, Zwergal A, Brandt T (2007) Episodic ataxia type 2. Neurotherapeutics 4:267–273
Strupp M, Versino M, Brandt T (2010) Vestibular migraine. Handb Clin Neurol 97:755–771
Strupp M, Kalla R, Claassen J, Adrion C, Mansmann U, Klopstock T, Freilinger T, Neugebauer H, Spiegel R, Dichgans M, Lehmann-Horn F, Jurkat-Rott K, Brandt T, Jen JC, Jahn K (2011) A randomized trial of 4-aminopyridine in EA2 and related familial episodic ataxias. Neurology 77:269–275

Strupp M, Teufel J, Zwergal A, Schniepp R, Khodakhah K, Feil K (2017) Aminopyridines for the treatment of neurologic disorders. Neurol Clin Pract 7:65–76

Van Bulck P, Leupe PJ, Forton GEJ (2019) Children with posterior semicircular canal dehiscence: a case series. Int J Pediatr Otorhinolaryngol 123:51–56

Van de Berg, R, Widdershoven, J, Bisdorff, A Evers S, Wiener-Vacher S, Cushing, SL, Mack KJ, Kim JS, Jahn K Strupp M, Lempert T (2021) Vestibular migraine of childhood and recurrent vertigo of childhood: diagnostic criteria consensus document of the Committee for the Classification of Vestibular Disorders of the Bárány Society and the International Headache Society. J Vest Res 31:(1)1−9

Wiener-Vacher SR, Quarez J, Priol AL (2018) Epidemiology of vestibular impairments in a pediatric population. Semin Hear 39:229–242

Wiener-Vacher SR, Wiener SI, Ajrezo L et al (2019) Dizziness and convergence insufficiency in children: screening and management. Front Integr Neurosci 13:25

Yao Q, Song Q, Wang H, Shi H, Yu D (2019) Benign paroxysmal positional vertigo in children. Clin Otolaryngol 44:21–25

Zhang D, Fan Z, Han Y, Wang M, Xu L, Luo J, Ai Y, Wang H (2012) Benign paroxysmal vertigo of childhood: diagnostic value of vestibular test and high stimulus rate auditory brainstem response test. Int J Pediatr Otorhinolaryngol 76:107–110

Medication-Related Dizziness

Content

M. Strupp et al., *Vertigo and Dizziness*, https://doi.org/10.1007/978-3-030-78260-3_17

Dizziness and imbalance can also be caused by medicine, a possibility that is often overlooked (Rascol et al. 1995; Borup Johansen et al. 2013; Chimirri et al. 2013; Hornibrook and Smith 2014; Moreno-Rius 2019) (◘ Table 17.1). However, it is more often overestimated because it is mentioned as a side effect for many drugs. The key to diagnosis of such cases is a carefully taken patient history. The temporal relationship between the onset of the respective drug treatment and the occurrence of symptoms is especially important (if suspected, try drug elimination). If this is not the case, one should, of course, look for a different underlying cause of the symptoms. As the complaints and the clinical picture greatly differ and the underlying mode of action of many drugs that induce dizziness is unclear, there is still no satisfactory classification of drug-induced dizziness/vertigo.

- On the one hand, certain drugs are known to have ototoxic effects, such as aminoglycosides, which cause direct (practically selective) damage of the vestibular hair cells (see ► Chap. 10).
- On the other hand, drugs such as anticonvulsants (e.g., carbamazepine and diphenylhydantoin) cause pronounced central (dose-dependent) ocular motor disorders. Although, according to their principal mode of action, they affect all neurons of the central nervous system (overview in Rascol et al. 1995; Cianfrone et al. 2011), the latter mostly cause cerebellar dysfunctions (Esser and Brandt 1983; Moreno-Rius 2019).

Clinical neurological investigations frequently reveal saccadic pursuit of eye movements and a gaze-holding deficit in all directions (see ► Chap. 3). Ocular motor

◘ **Table 17.1** Drug groups that can cause dizziness as a side effect

Nervous and musculoskeletal systems	**Heart, blood vessels, blood**
Anticonvulsants	Beta-receptor blockers
Analgesics	Anti-arrhythmics
Tranquilizers	Vasodilators/vasoconstrictors
Muscle relaxants	Anticoagulants
Hypnotics	**Kidneys and bladder**
Antiemetics	Diuretics
Antidepressants	Spasmolytics
Anticholinergics	**Respiratory organs**
Dopamine agonists	Expectorants
Antiphlogistics	Antitussives
Local anesthetics	Bronchospasm relaxants
Hormones	Mucus dissolvents
Corticosteroids	**Miscellaneous**
Antidiabetics	Antiallergics
Gonadal hormones	Prostaglandins
Oral contraceptives	X-ray contrast media
Inflammations	
Antibiotics	
Tuberculostatics	
Antihelminitics	
Antifungals	

dysfunctions, which indicate adverse drug effects or intoxication, are primarily found after intake of hydantoins, barbituates, carbamazepine, benzodiazepines, amitriptyline, and alcohol. These different substances may be analogous or distinct in their site of action within the labyrinths, brainstem, and cerebellum. Ocular motor disorders, such as positional, downbeat, gaze-evoked nystagmus, slowing down of saccades, alteration of the vestibular ocular reflex, or its suppression by fixation and ophthalmoplegia, are described in correlation to drug uptake or serum levels. Most of the ocular motor disturbances are possibly due to a pharmacologically induced transient dysfunction of the vestibulo-cerebellar flocculus loop (Esser and Brandt 1983).

Antihypertensives and diuretics are also relevant, as they can lead to orthostatic dizziness: many patients experience this dysregulation as a brief, temporary postural dizziness when they stand up (Kim et al. 2019); it can lead to dangerous falls (overview in Tinetti 2002). The diagnosis can be supported by measuring the blood pressure in different body positions. ◘ Table 17.1 presents a selection of drug groups that elicit the undesired side effect of dizziness.

Above all, the elderly can have dizziness and light-headedness as a side effect of drugs, especially cardiovascular drugs or medication that acts on the central nervous system (Shoair et al. 2011).

References

Borup Johansen N, Ayadipanah M, Sonnenschein ES, Christensen HR, Jürgens G (2013) Dizziness as a side effect of pharmacological therapy. Ugeskr Laeger 175:2720–2725

Chimirri S, Aiello R, Mazzitello C, Mumoli L, Palleria C, Altomonte M, Citraro R, De Sarro G (2013) Vertigo/dizziness as a drug's adverse reaction. J Pharmacol Pharmacother 4(Suppl1):104–109

Cianfrone G, Pentangelo D, Cianfrone E, Mazzei F, Turchetta R, Orlando MP, Altissimi G (2011) Pharmacological drugs inducing ototoxicity, vestibular symptoms and tinnitus: a reasoned and update guide. Eur Rev Med Pharmacol Sci 15:601–636

Esser J, Brandt T (1983) Pharmakologisch verursachte Augenbewegungsstörungen – Differentialdiagnose und Wirkungsmechanismus. Fortschr Neurol Psychiat 51:41–56

Hornibrook J, Smith PF (2014) Dizziness caused by medications. N Z Med J 127:84–85

Kim HA, Bisdorff A, Bronstein AM, Lempert T, Rossi-Izquierdo M, Staab JP, Strupp M, Kim JS (2019) Hemodynamic orthostatic dizziness/vertigo: diagnostic criteria. J Vestib Res 29:45–56

Moreno-Rius J (2019) Opiod addiction and the cerebellum. Neurosci Behav Rev 107:238–251

Rascol O, Hain TC, Brefel C, Benazet M, Clanet M, Montastruc JL (1995) Antivertigo medications and drug-induced vertigo. Pharmacol Rev Drugs 50:777–791

Shoair OA, Nyandege AN, Slattum PW (2011) Medication-related dizziness in the older adult. Otolaryngol Clin North Am 44:455–471

Tinetti ME (2002) Preventing falls in elderly persons. N Engl J Med 348:42–49

Traumatic Forms of Vertigo and Dizziness

Contents

M. Strupp et al., *Vertigo and Dizziness*, https://doi.org/10.1007/978-3-030-78260-3_18

After head and neck pain, dizziness is the most frequent chronic complication of a mild head trauma (Friedman 2004; Kashluba et al. 2006; Schütze et al. 2008; Akin et al. 2017; Mucha et al. 2018; Marcus et al. 2019) or of a whiplash injury (Ernst et al. 2005). If radiological methods do not reveal a petrous bone fracture with hemotympanum or the presence of air in the labyrinth (pneumo-labyrinth) or a brainstem contusion cannot be clinically confirmed, the first questions to ask are the following:

- Is this dizziness organic or functional (Staab 2006)?
- What is the underlying mechanism of the dizziness (peripheral or central vestibular or functional)?

The following post-traumatic forms of vertigo and dizziness are well known:

- BPPV
- Unilateral or bilateral peripheral vestibular disorder culminating in labyrinthine failure (e.g., due to a labyrinth contusion or a petrous bone fracture)
- Syndrome of the third mobile windows (e.g., perilymph fistula that leads to a pathological transfer of pressure)
- Barotrauma-induced vertigo with various manifestations
- Acute central vestibular syndrome due to traumatic dissection of the vertebral artery or brainstem contusion with central signs and symptoms

Frequently a false diagnosis of "cervical vertigo and dizziness" is made to explain dizziness following a whiplash injury. It is still a subject of controversy whether this form of vertigo exists at all and, if so, what its pathomechanism could be (see below). However, it is probable that in many cases of a whiplash injury or head trauma, a loosening of otoconia (even without BPPV) takes place, resulting in a post-traumatic otolithic vertigo in the form of a transient gait and postural instability over days (not over weeks, not chronic).

The therapy should, in most cases, include physical therapy with vestibular training after a detailed explanation of the type of symptoms and their origin. Here specific etiologies, such as BPPV, damage of the VOR, or central vestibular lesions with disorders of stance and gait, have to be taken into account (Eagle et al. 2021, 2022; Hoffer et al. 2004; Herdman and Clendaniel 2014).

18.1 Traumatic Peripheral Vestibular Forms of Vertigo

18.1.1 Post-traumatic BPPV

The most frequent peripheral labyrinthine form of vertigo is BPPV (▶ Chap. 9). It is characterized by short attacks of spinning vertigo and typical vertical-torsional crescendo–decrescendo nystagmus, which is triggered by positioning the head toward the affected ear or tilting it backward and resolves within seconds. Spinning vertigo and nystagmus occur after positioning with a short latency of seconds and cease temporarily after repeated positioning maneuvers.

The frequency of traumatic BPPV differs considerably in various studies, ranging between 5% and 57%, with a median of about 25–28% (Davies and Luxon 1995; Hoffer et al. 2004; Gordon et al. 2004; Motin et al. 2005; Luryi et al. 2018). Compared to the idiopathic form of BPPV, it is more frequently bilateral and asymmetrical (32% vs 19%) and occurs more often in younger patients (mean age 40–61 years) and more often in males (40% vs 27%) (Haripriya et al. 2018; Luryi et al. 2018). Occasionally it is also found in children. In two-thirds of the cases, the posterior canal is affected; in one-third, the horizontal canal (Ahn et al. 2011).

The interval between the actual head trauma or whiplash injury and its manifestation as BPPV can last from days up to several weeks. It is possible that the otoconia become detached from the macula bed in two steps or in the first phase remain in the endolymphatic space of the utricle and only reach the canal later, at which time they induce the typical positioning vertigo. This delay can be important in situations requiring expert witness evidence. Immediately after the trauma the patients occasionally complain of unsteadiness of gait (like walking on a mattress), probably due to a traumatic "otolithic vertigo," before subsequently the typical symptoms of BPPV appear. Traumatic BPPV has been frequently reported after neurosurgical, maxillary, and ENT operations of the skull (Chiarella et al. 2007) as well as dental surgery (Chang et al. 2016).

The pathophysiology and treatment of post-traumatic BPPV correspond to those of idiopathic BPPV (▶ Chap. 9). The therapy phase is significantly longer, in part because it frequently occurs bilaterally, and liberatory maneuvers have to be repeated, beginning with the treatment of the more-affected ear until the patient is symptom-free (Ahn et al. 2011). The efficiency is the same for idiopathic and post-traumatic BPPV (Suarez et al. 2011; Luryi et al. 2018) and the recurrence rate similar (Ahn et al. 2011; Brandt et al. 2006, 2010; Suarez et al. 2011; Luryi et al. 2018).

The different types of liberatory maneuvers (Semont, Epley) are successfully used for a canalolithiasis of the posterior canal (review: Bhattacharyya et al. 2017) (▶ Chap. 9). Generally, more than 90% of patients are asymptomatic after 1 week of treatment (von Brevern et al. 2006; Mandala et al. 2012, 2020). Cases of the more rarely affected horizontal canal are treated with a "barbecue" maneuver, a 12-h period of lying on the healthy ear (Fife et al. 2008), or by the Gufoni maneuver (Kim et al. 2012a, b). Therapy failures are very rare (<1%).

18.1.2 Traumatic Vestibulopathy

A unilateral hemorrhage or a petrous bone fracture (vestibulocochlear disorders occur more frequently with transverse than with longitudinal fractures) can lead to direct injury of the vestibular nerve or the labyrinth. This causes:

- Violent spinning vertigo, which continues for days
- Horizontal torsional nystagmus to the unaffected side
- Posture and gait instability with deviation to the affected side
- Nausea and vomiting

The clinical symptoms are similar to those of acute unilateral vestibulopathy (▶ Chap. 8).

Three forms of petrous bone fractures can be differentiated: mixed, longitudinal, and transverse (Rafferty et al. 2006; Gladwell and Viozzi 2008):

- Longitudinal petrous bone fractures (◘ Fig. 18.1) are more frequent; they cause injury to the middle ear and bleeding from the ear
- Transverse petrous bone fractures (◘ Fig. 18.2) with labyrinthine lesion and resulting spinning vertigo and hearing loss, as well as possible injury to the facial nerve occur more rarely

If there is a direct trauma of the petrous bone and corresponding symptoms of spinning vertigo and hearing loss, but the injury cannot be confirmed either macroscopically or by X-ray, one speaks of a labyrinthine contusion.

The first phase of manifest dysfunction is characterized by a strong feeling of illness with continuous spinning vertigo, nausea, and vomiting. These symptoms slowly dissipate over 2–3 weeks. Bed rest and antivertiginous drugs (e.g., dimenhydrinate) should be prescribed only within the first days for severe nausea and vomiting, similar to the therapy in acute vestibulopathy, as

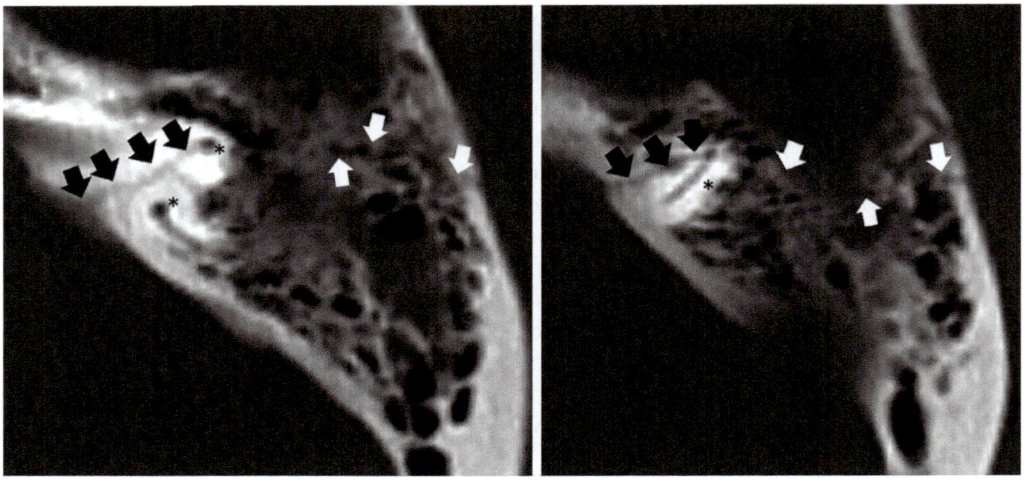

Fig. 18.1 Longitudinal petrous bone fracture left (black and white arrows) through the superior* semicircular canal

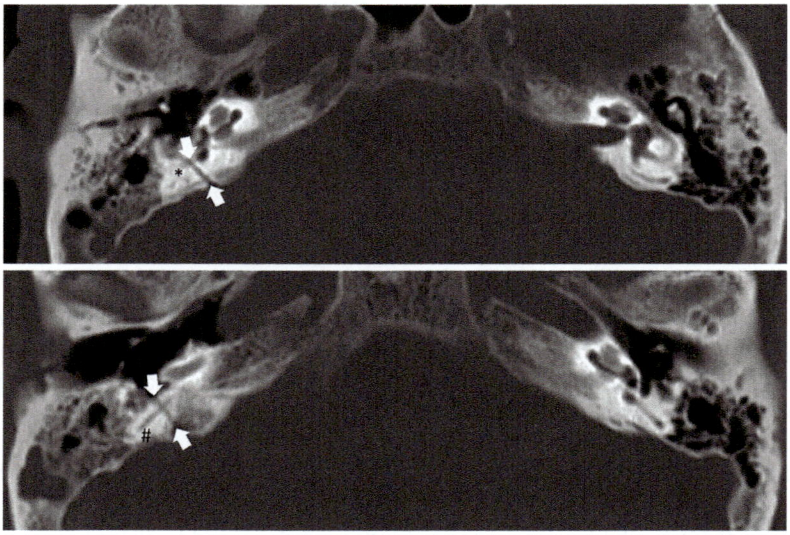

Fig. 18.2 Transverse petrous bone fracture right (arrows) through the horizontal* and posterior # semicircular canal

these drugs delay central compensation. The patient should begin a vestibular training and rehabilitation program as soon as possible to accelerate and improve central compensation (review: Sulway and Whitney 2019; Tjernstrom et al. 2016). Similarly, treatment with corticosteroids (methylprednisolone) is also indicated for a few days, in most cases because of trauma-induced edema.

Vertigo, dizziness with or without oscillopsia, and/or hearing loss are also frequent complications of traumas due to military or terrorist blasts (Scherer et al. 2007). They can take a progressive course (Hoffer et al. 2010).

A distinction can be made between traumatic vestibulopathy and "mild" traumatic brain injuries, in which pathological vestibular findings were reported in 3%–21% for the caloric testing of the horizontal semicircular canals (Zhou and Brodsky 2015), but not for the horizontal video-HIT (Alshehri et al. 2016). Otolithic dysfunction was found in 29% (Scherer et al. 2011) to 52% (Akin et al. 2017) presenting with pathological cVEMP in 25–32% (Ernst et al. 2005; Lee et al. 2011). Sports-related contusions in children and adolescents were accompanied by abnormal results in detailed neurootological testing of the otoliths in 18% for the cVEMP and in 13% for the SVV adjustments (Zhou and Brodsky 2015).

18.1.3 Traumatic Syndrome of the Third Mobile Windows: Superior Semicircular Dehiscence Syndrome and the rare Perilymph Fistula

Frequent traumatic causes of syndromes of a third mobile window (▶ Chap. 12) are moderate-to-severe direct brain injuries with temporal bone fractures or barotraumas (Maitland 2001; Mucha et al. 2018). Usually the air in the middle ear is of normal atmospheric pressure, since the air supply via the nasopharynx passes through the Eustachian tube. In disorders of air supply to the Eustachian tube, painful pressure gradients occur on the eardrum and in the middle ear. During head trauma, extreme increases in pressure can occur in the middle ear and cause a defect at the round and oval windows or more rarely a luxation of the stapes footplate in the direction of the inner ear with pathological transfer of pressure to the perilymphatic space or with a pneumolabyrinth (Sarac et al. 2006; Hatano et al. 2009). The changes in pressure can also lead to a dehiscence of the superior (i.e., anterior) semicircular canal (superior canal dehiscence syndrome, SCDS) (review: Ward et al. 2017). The consequences are:

- Attacks of dizziness, in part with oscillopsia, generally due to pressure changes (from coughing, pressing, sneezing, lifting heavy weights, or loud sounds).
- Fluctuating hearing loss.
- Seldom autophonia, i.e., sounds within the body, are heard by the affected ear due to an enhanced bone conduction.
- Ear pressure.
- Tinnitus, often pulsatile.

The complaints can depend on the position of the head or on movement as in other syndromes of a third mobile window (Maitland 2001; Bourgeois et al. 2005; Young et al. 2019) (▶ Chap. 12) (DVD). Generally, a high-resolution CT of the inner ear can prove the etiology, e.g., a bony defect of the superior semicircular canal. The presence of air in the labyrinth (pneumo-labyrinth) following a trauma indicates the traumatic etiology (Tsubota et al. 2009).

Clinically, dizziness can be classified as either a canal type with spinning vertigo and nystagmus or an otolithic type with postural vertigo and unsteadiness of stance and gait, especially during linear head acceleration (when standing up or walking). The otolithic type of dizziness can also be caused by luxation of the stapes footplate without resulting in continuous perilymph leakage; this happens when the luxated stapes footplate via the peri/endolymph fluid pressure stimulates the otoliths during the acoustically induced stapedial reflex (otolithic Tullio phenomenon). In this case, loud sounds of certain frequencies induce paroxysmal excitations of the superior semicircular canal via a bony dehiscence due to an SCDS (vertical torsional nystagmus, oscillopsia, instability of stance) or otolithic symptoms (head tilt and postural instability in Tullio phenomenon).

For clinical practice, it is important to note that the term "perilymph fistula" reflects a direct connection of the perilymphatic space with another space, resulting in a loss of perilymph fluid. This diagnosis or misdiagnosis was made too often in the past and continues to be made too often, and is furthermore under discussion (Deveze et al. 2018). The current classification is given in Box 12.3. Besides the aforementioned tests of a third mobile window syndrome, the measurement of cochlin-tomoprotein was found helpful to prove the discharge of perilymph fluid (Ikezono et al. 2018).

An initially conservative therapy of several days of bed rest with the head elevated, perhaps mild sedation and the administration of laxatives, results in recovery in the majority of cases. If such conservative therapy fails, and hearing loss or vestibular symptoms increase, then an exploratory tympanotomy or in cases of a dehiscence of the superior canal surgical canal plugging or capping is indicated (▶ Chap. 12).

18.1.4 Alternobaric Vertigo

Rapid changes of pressure in the middle ear – primarily during the decompression experienced by divers (Klingmann et al. 2006) or by pilots and aircrews during flights (Subtil et al. 2007) – can cause a transient spinning vertigo that is called alternobaric vertigo. At the very beginning of the spinning vertigo and nystagmus, which spontaneously resolves after seconds or hours, there is a feeling of fullness in the ear. Acute spinning vertigo indicates an inadequate stimulation of a semicircular canal, which is triggered by an asymmetrical, excessive acute pressure on the round and oval windows in the middle ear (Molvaer and Albrektsen 1988). The same mechanism underlies the syndrome of the third mobile windows (formerly called: perilymph fistulas).

Dysfunctions of the Eustachean tube are a special risk factor for developing alternobaric vertigo (Uzun 2005). Women appear to be at a higher risk of developing alternobaric vertigo during scuba diving than men (Klingmann et al. 2006), but retrospective studies do not show that this vertigo leads to life-threatening situations under water.

18.1.5 Otolithic Dizziness

Traumatic otolithic dizziness and postural imbalance probably occurs more often than is generally assumed (Brandt and Daroff 1980; Ernst et al. 2005). Immediately after a head trauma or after a latency, patients often report having experienced:

- Postural imbalance that is exacerbated by head movements
- Oscillopsia during head movements
- Gait instability that is like walking on a water bed

These are typical disorders of otolithic function. As shown in animal studies, the traumatic accelerations probably cause loosening of the otoconia, which leads to unequal otolithic masses on the two sides. The different otolithic weights on the two sides can result in a temporary disturbance of spatial orientation.

Systematic testing of otolith function, by measurements of c/oVEMP or SVV, has been done only rarely. After explosion trauma, 29–52% of patients showed otolith dysfunctions (Scherer et al. 2011; Akin et al. 2017). In 25–32% of patients with blunt cranial trauma, pathological cVEMP were found (Ernst et al. 2005; Lee et al. 2011).

Within days or weeks, however, central compensation corrects for the otolithic imbalance, and the postural instability during head movements and gait ataxia abate. If complaints persist, a differential diagnosis must be made which takes into account the possibility of a secondary functional (somatoform) vertigo (Dieterich and Staab 2017).

One should keep in mind that a traumatic brain injury may also lead to disorders of the autonomic nervous system (Esterov and Greenwald 2017) resulting in a vagal dysfunction of the heart (La Fountaine et al. 2011) and the circulation (Dobson et al. 2017). This may contribute to transient posttraumatic dizziness. To complicate matters, neuronal networks for emotions (in particular anxiety) overlap with those of autonomic and vestibular functions (Balaban and Thayer 2001).

18.2 Traumatic Central Vestibular Syndromes

The various central vestibular syndromes are triggered by disorders of brainstem or cerebellar function in connection with a contusion or hemorrhage or, indirectly, due to a traumatic vertebral dissection. In principle, parts of the brainstem and cerebellum, the midbrain and thalamus, the pons to the medulla oblongata and cerebellum, can be affected; the mesencephalon is affected relatively often. The individual central syndromes are described in ▶ Chap. 13.

Post-traumatic central ocular motor disorders were often seen in combination with peripheral vestibular dysfunctions. During the acute phase after trauma (up to day 4), the frequency was 5% to 45% (Tuohimaa 1978; Ernst et al. 2005), after 5 months and later, it was 3–8% (Berman and Fredrickson 1975; Tuohimaa 1978; Davies and Luxon 1995). Typical signs were gaze-evoked nystagmus, impaired fixation suppression of the VOR, saccadic pursuit and disturbances of antisaccades and predictive saccades (Balaban et al. 2016; Szczupak et al. 2016).

MRI scans of the brain only rarely show abnormalities after a mild traumatic brain injury (Useche and Bermudez 2018). However, functional imaging methods (using diffusion tensor imaging) were able to demonstrate microstructural axon damage in the patients with a loss of consciousness (Hayes et al. 2015) and after sports-related concussion in adolescents (Borich et al. 2013). Furthermore, in patients with mild head trauma and loss of consciousness, white matter lesions (Kraus et al. 2007; Hayes et al. 2015), cerebral microbleedings, and axonal damage in combination with peripheral vestibular deficits (Gattu et al. 2016) were observed. The patients with vestibular signs and symptoms had a lower fiber density within the cerebellum and fusiform gyrus compared to those without ($p < 0.05$; Alhilali et al. 2014).

18.3 Traumatic Cervical Vertigo and Dizziness

The question of whether there is a medical entity "cervical vertigo and dizziness" is still a subject of controversy (see ▶ Chap. 22). The neck afferents not only take part in coordinating eyes, head, and body; but they are also involved in the orientation of the body in space and the control of posture. This means that in principle a stimulation or lesion of these structures could trigger vertigo. It has been shown in animal experiments in primates (Macaca) that a unilateral local anesthesia or cutting of the superior cervical roots induces a tendency to fall due to a temporary increase of tone of the extensor muscles on the ipsilateral side and a decrease on the contralateral side, as well as ipsiversive past-pointing. Positional nystagmus, however, is elicited only in certain species and to different degrees (most pronounced in rabbits, less in cats) but not at all in Rhesus monkeys (De Jong et al. 1977). This type of positional nystagmus that derives from an imbalance in tone of the superior cervical roots has not been proven to exist in humans. Patients with C2 root blockades (for cervical headache) exhibit a slight instability of gait with minor ipsilateral deviation of gait and past-pointing without ocular motor disorders (Dieterich et al. 1993); this corresponds to findings in the animal experiments with macaques. One would expect similar symptoms such as instability of gait in "cervicogenic vertigo," always in connection with cervico-vertebrogenic pain and movement restriction of the cervical vertebrae but not with spinning vertigo or spontaneous, positional, or provocation-induced nystagmus.

In line with these neurophysiological findings, a few patients were described who presented with very short, head-motion induced attacks of vertigo and postural imbalance for seconds that occurred for a few days in association with acute unilaterally accentuated neck pain and constraints of head rotations (Brandt and Huppert 2016). No patient had a history of an initial head or neck injury; neurological and otoneurological examinations revealed no deficits.

Unfortunately, there are still no useful tests to confirm "cervical vertigo and dizziness" (gait instability), as the tests available use passive head turns while the trunk is fixed and trigger the same amount of nystagmus with the same frequency in healthy subjects (Holtmann et al. 1993). These tests are still in use in some places nowadays, but they fail to give meaningful results. For this reason, the differential diagnosis must always include careful otoneurological diagnostics (Ernst et al. 2005), especially if complaints are not initially present but appear only in the course of the disorder. In such a case, a secondary functional (psychogenic) vertigo must be considered, since it can appear in up to ca. 50% of patients with a primarily organic vertigo syndrome, depending on the comorbidity (Eckhardt-Henn et al. 2008; Dieterich and Staab 2017).

18.4 Post-traumatic Functional Dizziness

If vertigo persists for a long time after a head trauma or a whiplash injury and no otoneurological or ocular motor deficits can be determined, this can indicate a functional (psychogenic) vertigo and dizziness. The diagnosis of functional dizziness can, however, only be made when "positive" diagnostic criteria are found (▶ Chap. 15).

18

Functional dizziness is the most frequent cause of chronic vertigo and dizziness to date in specialized centers and in neurological patients. It often occurs secondary to organic forms of vertigo, e.g., following a traumatic brain injury (Huppert et al. 1995; Eckhardt-Henn et al. 2008). A clear increase in the cases of functional phobic postural dizziness was observed in Georgia after a strong earthquake (Tevzadze and Shakarishvili 2007). In cases of chronic, long-term complaints, the desire to retire must also be considered in the differential diagnosis.

References

Ahn SK, Jeon SY, Kim JP, Park JJ, Hur DG, Kim DW, Woo SH, Kwon OJ, Kim JY (2011) Clinical characteristics and treatment of benign paroxysmal positional vertigo after traumatic brain injury. J Trauma 70:442–446

Akin FW, Murnane OD, Hall CD et al (2017) Vestibular consequences of mild traumatic brain injury and blast exposure: a review. Brain Inj 31:1188–1194

Alhilali LM, Yaeger K, Collins M, Fakhran S (2014) Detection of central white matter injury underlying vestibulopathy after mild traumatic brain injury. Radiology 272(1):224–232

Alshehri MM, Sparto PJ, Furmann JM, Fedor S, Mucha A, Henry LC, Whitney SL (2016) The usefulness of the video head impuls test in children and adults post-concussion. J Vest Res 26(5–6):439–446

Balaban CD, Thayer JF (2001) Neurological bases for balance-anxiety links. J Anxiety Disord 15:53–79

Balaban CD, Hoffer ME, Szczupak M et al (2016) Oculomotor, vestibular, and reaction time tests in mild traumatic brain injury. PLoS One 11:e0162168

Berman JM, Fredrickson JM (1975) Vertigo after head injury: a five-year follow-up. J Otolaryngol 7(3):237–245

Bhattacharyya N, Gubbels SP, Schwartz SR et al (2017) Clinical practice guideline: benign paroxysmal positional vertigo (Update). Otolaryngol Head Neck Surg Mar 156:S1–S47

Borich M, Makan N, Boyd L et al (2013) Combining whole-brain voxel-wise analysis with in vivo tractography of diffusion behavior after sports-related concussion in adolescents: a preliminary report. J Neurotrauma 30:1243–1249

Bourgeois B, Ferron CH, Bordure P, Beauvillain de Montreuil C, Legent F (2005) Exploratory tympanotomy for suspected traumatic perilymphatic fistula. Ann Otolaryngol Chir Cervicofac 122: 181–186

Brandt T, Daroff RB (1980) The multisensory physiological and pathological vertigo syndromes. Ann Neurol 7:195–203
Brandt T, Huppert D (2016) A new type of cervical vertigo: head motion-induced spells in acute neck pain. Neurology 86:974–975
Brandt T, Huppert D, Hecht J, Karch C, Strupp M (2006) Benign paroxysmal positioning vertigo: a long-term follow up (6:17 years) of 125 patients. Acta Otolaryngol 126:160–163
Brandt T, Huppert D, Hüfner K, Zingler VC, Dieterich M, Strupp M (2010) Long-term course and relapses of vestibular and balance disorders. Restor Neurol Neurosci 28:69–82
Chang T-P, Lin Y-W, Sung P-Y, Chuang H-Y, Chung H-Y, Liao W-L (2016) Benign paroxysmal positional vertigo after dental procedures: a population-based case-control study. Plos One 11(4):e0153092
Chiarella G, Leopardi G, De Fazio L, Chiarella R, Cassandro C, Cassandro E (2007) Iatrogenic benign paroxysmal positional vertigo: review and personal experience in dental and maxillo-facial surgery. Acta Otorhinolaryngol Ital 27:126–128
Davies RA, Luxon LM (1995) Dizziness following head injury: a neurological study. J Neurol 242:222–230
De Jong PTVM, de Jong JMBV, Cohen D, Jongkees LDW (1977) Ataxia and nystagmus induced by injection of local anesthetics in the neck. Ann Neurol 1:240–246
Deveze A, Matsuda H, Elziere M, Ikezono T (2018) Diagnosis and treatment of perilymphatic fistula. Adv Otorhinolaryngol 81:133–145
Dieterich M, Staab JP (2017) Functional dizziness: from phobic postural vertigo and chronic subjective dizziness to persistent postural-perceptual dizziness. Curr Opin Neurol 30:107–113
Dieterich M, Pöllmann W, Pfaffenrath V (1993) Cervicogenic headache: electronystagmography, perception of verticality, and posturography in patients before and after C2-blockade. Cephalalgia 13:285–288
Dobson JL, Yarbrough MB, Perez J et al (2017) Sport-related concussion induces transient cardiovascular autonomic dysfunction. Am J Physiol Regul Integr Comp Physiol 312:R575–R584
Eagle SR, Kontos AP, Collins MW, Mucha A et al (2021) Targeted intervention improves symptoms and impairments in patients with mild traumatic brain injury with chronic symptom: a prospective, multiple interventional resaerach trial. J Spec Oper Med 21(2):61–66
Eagle SR, Feder A, Manderino LM, Mucha A et al (2022) Concurrent validity of vestibular/ocular motor screening (VOMS) tool with dizziness handicap inventory (DHI) among adolescents with vestibular symptoms/impairment following concussion. Phys Ther Sport 53:34–39. https://doi.org/10.1016/j.ptsp.2021.11.003
Eckhardt-Henn A, Best C, Bense S, Breuer P, Diener G, Tschan R et al (2008) Psychiatric comorbidity in different organic vertigo syndromes. J Neurol 255:420–428
Ernst A, Basta D, Seidl RO, Todt I, Scherer H, Clarke A (2005) Management of posttraumatic vertigo. Otolaryngol Head Neck Surg 132:554–558
Esterov D, Greenwald BD (2017) Autonomic dysfunction after mild traumatic brain injury. Brain Sci 7:100
Fife TD, Iverson DJ, Lempert T et al (2008) Practice parameter: therapies for benign paroxysmal positional vertigo (an evidence-based review): report of the Quality Standards Subcommittee of the American Academy of Neurology. Neurology 70:2067–2074
Friedman JM (2004) Post-traumatic vertigo. Med Health 87:296–300
Gattu R, Akin FW, Cacace AT, Hall CD, Murnane OD, Haacke EM (2016) Vestibular, balance, microvascular, and white matter neuroimaging characteristics of blast injuries and mild traumatic brain injury: four case reports. Brain Inj 30(12):1501–1514
Gladwell M, Viozzi C (2008) Temporal bone fractures: a review for the oral and maxillofacial surgeon. J Oral Maxillofac Surg 66:513–522
Gordon CR, Levite R, Joffe V, Gadoth N (2004) Is posttraumatic benign paroxysmal positional vertigo different from the idiopathic form? Arch Neurol 61:1590–1593
Haripriya GR, Mary P, Dominic M, Goyal R, Sahadevan A (2018) Incidence and treatment outcomes of posttraumatic BPPV in traumatic brain injury patients. Indian J Otolaryngol Head Neck Surg 70(3):337–341
Hatano A, Rikitake M, Komori M, Irie T, Moriyama H (2009) Traumatic perilymph fistula with the luxation of the stapes into the vestibule. Auris Nasus Larynx 36:474–478
Hayes JP, Miller DR, Lafleche G, Salat DH, Verfaellie M (2015) The nature of white matter abnormalities in blast-related mild traumatic brain injury. NeuroImage Clin 9:148–156
Herdman S, Clendaniel RA (2014) Vestibular rehabilitation. FA Davis, Philadelphia
Hoffer ME, Gottshal KR, Moore R, Balough BJ, Wester E (2004) Characterizing and treating dizziness after mild head trauma. Otol Neurotol 25:135–138
Hoffer ME, Balaban C, Gottshall K, Balough BJ, Maddox MR, Penta JR (2010) Blast exposure: vestibular consequences and associated characteristics. Otol Neurotol 31:232–236

Holtmann S, Reiman V, Schöps P (1993) Clinical significance of cervico-ocular reactions. Laryngorhinootologie 72:306–310
Huppert D, Kunihiro T, Brandt T (1995) Phobic postural vertigo (154 patients): its association with vestibular disorders. J Audiol 4:97–103
Ikezono T, Matsumura T, Matsuda, et al (2018) The diagnostic performance of a novel ELISA for human CTP (Cochlin-tomoprotein) to detect perilymph leakage. PLoS One 13(1):e0191498.
Kashluba S, Casey JE, Paniak C (2006) Evaluating the utility of ICD-10 diagnostic criteria for postconcussion syndrome following mild traumatic brain injury. J Int Neuropsychol Soc 12:111–118
Kim JS, Oh SY, Lee Sh et al (2012a) Randomized clinical trial for geotropic horizontal canal benign paroxysmal positional vertigo. Neurology 79(7):700–707
Kim JS, Oh SY, Lee SH et al (2012b) Randomized clinical trial for apogeotropic horizontal canal benign paroxysmal positional vertigo. Neurology 78(3):159–166
Klingmann C, Knauth M, Praetorius M, Plinkert PK (2006) Alternobaric vertigo – really a hazard? Otol Neurotol 27:1120–1125
Kraus MF, Susmaras T, Caughlin BP, Walker CJ, Sweeney JA, Little DM (2007) White matter integrity and cognition in chronic traumatic brain injury: a diffusion tensor imaging study. Brain 130:2508–2519
La Fountaine MF, Gossett JD, De Meersman RE et al (2011) Increased QT interval variability in 3 recently concussed athletes: an exploratory observation. J Athl Train 46:230–233
Lee JD, Park MK, Lee BD et al (2011) Otolith function in patients with head trauma. Eur Arch Otorhinolaryngol 268:1427–1430
Luryi AL, LaRouere M, Babu S, Bojrab DI, Zappia J, Sargent EW, Schutt CA (2018) Traumatic versus idiopathic benign positional vertigo: analysis of disease, treatment, and outcome characteristics. Otolaryngol Head Neck Surg 160(19:131–136
Maitland CG (2001) Perilymphatic fistula. Curr Neurol Neurosci Rep 1:486–491
Mandala M, Santoro GP, Asprella LG et al (2012) Double-blind randomized trial on short-term efficacy of Semont maneuver for the treatment of posterior canal benign paroxysmal positional vertigo. J Neurol 259(5):882–885
Mandala M, Califano L, Casani AP et al (2020) Double-blind randomized trial on the efficacy of the forced prolonged position for treatment of lateral canal benign paroxysmal positional vertigo. Laryngoscope 131:E1296
Marcus HJ, Paine H, Sargeant M, Wolstenholme S et al (2019) Vestibular dysfunction in acute traumatic brain injury. J Neurol 266:2430–2433
Molvaer OI, Albrektsen G (1988) Alternobaric vertigo in professional divers. Undersea Biomed Res 15:271–282
Motin M, Keren O, Groswasser Z, Gordon CR (2005) Benign paroxysmal positional vertigo as the cause of dizziness in patients after severe traumatic brain injury: diagnosis and treatment. Brain Inj 19: 693–697
Mucha A, Fedor S, Demarco D (2018) Vestibular dysfunction and concussion. Handb Clin Neurol 158:135–144
Rafferty MA, McConn Walsh R, Walsh MA (2006) A comparison of temporal bone fracture classification systems. Clin Otolaryngol 31:287–291
Sarac S, Cengel S, Sennaroglu L (2006) Pneumolabyrinth following traumatic luxation of the stapes into the vestibule. Int J Pediatr Otorhinolaryngol 70: 159–161
Scherer MR, Burrows H, Pinto R, Somrack E (2007) Characterizing self-reported dizziness and otovestibular impairment among blast-injured traumatic amputees: a pilot study. Mil Med 172:731–737
Scherer MR, Burrows H, Pinto R et al (2011) Evidence of central and peripheral vestibular pathology in blast-related traumatic brain injury. Otol Neurotol 32:571–580
Schütze M, Kundt G, Buchholz K, Piek J (2008) Which factors are predictive for long-term complaints after mild traumatic brain injuries? Versicherungsmedizin 60:78–83
Staab JP (2006) Chronic dizziness: the interface between psychiatry and neuro-otology. Curr Opin Neurol 19:41–48
Suarez H, Alonso R, Arocena M, Suarez A, Geisinger D (2011) Clinical characteristics of positional vertigo after mild head trauma. Acta Otolaryngol 131:377–381
Subtil J, Varandas J, Galrão F, Dos Santos A (2007) Alternobaric vertigo: prevalence in Portuguese Air Force pilots. Acta Otolaryngol 127:843–846
Sulway S, Whitney SL (2019) Advances in vestibular rehabilitation. Adv Otorhinolaryngol 82: 164–169
Szczupak M, Hoffer ME, Murphy S, Balaban CD (2016) Posttraumatic dizziness and vertigo. Handb Clin Neurol 137:295–300
Tevzadze N, Shakarishvili R (2007) Vertigo syndromes associated with earthquake in Georgia. Georgian Med News 148–149:36–39
Tjernstrom F, Zur O, Jahn K (2016) Current concepts and future approaches to vestibular rehabilitation. J Neurol 263(Suppl 1):S65–S70

Tsubota M, Shojaku H, Watanabe Y (2009) Prognosis of inner ear function in pneumolabyrinth: case report and literature review. Am J Otolaryngol 30:423–426

Tuohimaa P (1978) Vestibular disturbances after acute mild head injury. Acta Otolaryngol Suppl. 359: 3–67.

Useche JN, Bermudez S (2018) Conventional computer tomography and magnetic resonance in brain concussion. Neuroimaging Clin N Am 28(1):15–29

Uzun C (2005) Evaluation of predive parameters related to eustachian tube dysfunction for symptomatic middle ear barotrauma in divers. Otol Neurotol 26:59–64

Von Brevern M, Seelig T, Radtke A, Tiel-Wilck K, Neuhauser H (2006) Long-term efficacy of Epley's manoeuvre: a double-blind randomized trial. J Neurol Neurosurg Psychiatry 77:980–982

Ward BK, Carey JP, Minor LB (2017) Superior canal dehiscence syndrome: lessons from the first 20 years. Front Neurol 8:177

Young AS, McMonagle B, Pohl DV, Magnussen J, Welgampola MS (2019) Superior semicircular canal dehiscence presenting with recurrent positional vertigo. Neurology 93:1070–1072

Zhou G, Brodsky JR (2015) Objective vestibular testing of children with dizziness and balance complaints following sports-related concussions. Otolaryngol Head Neck Surg 152:1133–1139

Motion Sickness

Contents

M. Strupp et al., *Vertigo and Dizziness*, https://doi.org/10.1007/978-3-030-78260-3_19

19.1 Clinical Aspects and Pathogenesis

Acute motion sickness arises during passive transportation in motor vehicles; it resolves spontaneously within 1 day at the most after the disappearance of the inducing stimulus. The full picture of acute severe motion sickness evolves with initial symptoms of:

- Light-headedness or foggy head
- Physical discomfort
- Tiredness
- Periodic yawning
- Pallor
- Light dizziness with apparent surround-motion and self-motion

An increase in facial pallor is followed by cold sweats, increased salivation, hypersensitivity to smells, occipital head pain, and feelings of pressure in the upper abdomen. Finally, the central symptoms of nausea, retching, and vomiting develop with motor incoordination, loss of drive and concentration, apathy, and fear of impending doom (Money 1970; Brandt 1976; Golding 2016; Zhang et al. 2016). Motion sickness on land, but particularly seasickness and its triggers, symptoms, and preventive measures were well known in Greek, Roman, and Chinese antiquity (Huppert et al. 2017; see ► Chap. 23).

Motion sickness is not caused by vestibular "over-stimulation" during strong accelerations of the body, but by unfamiliar (i.e. non-adapted) motion stimuli and particularly by intersensory perceptual incongruences among the visual, vestibular, and somatosensory systems. The most important concept explaining the pathogenesis of motion sickness is the so-called mismatch theory (Reason 1978; Dichgans and Brandt 1978; Brandt 1976; Zhang et al. 2016) (◘ Fig. 15.5). According to this theory, the decisive trigger is the incongruence of the signals of motion from various sensory channels or the incongruence between expected and actual sensory stimulation.

19

Furthermore, other hypothetical mechanisms are also discussed (Bertolini and Straumann 2016), e.g., based on experiments suggesting that the spatial orientation of the velocity storage of the vestibulo-ocular reflex plays a role in the generation of motion sickness due to head movements (Dai et al. 2007).

Well-known varieties of motion sickness are:

- Car sickness (visual-vestibular conflict of stimuli)
- Sea sickness (unfamiliar, complex linear, and angular accelerations of low frequency, below 1 Hz)
- Vehicle simulator or virtual reality sickness (optokinetic motion sickness)
- Space sickness (incongruent sensory stimuli of the otoliths, semicircular canals, and the visual system during active head movements in microgravity)

Epidemiological studies have found a statistically significant association of migraine and susceptibility to motion sickness (Neuhauser and Lempert 2004; Evans et al. 2007; Cuomo-Granston and Drummond 2010), above all in vestibular migraine patients (Boldingh et al. 2011). The prevalence of motion sickness is higher in patients with some vestibular disorders, but lower in bilateral vestibulopathy, probably because in the latter the visuo-vestibular mismatch is less effective (Takahashi et al. 1997; Paillard et al. 2013; Murdin et al. 2015; Golding 2016; Golding and Patel 2017). A relevant comorbidity of most vestibular disorders with an increased susceptibility to motion sickness was confirmed in a prospective epidemiological study (Strupp et al. 2018). In this study, similar to that of Murdin et al. (2015), patients with bilateral vestibulopathy were not immune to motion sickness but more resistant. Pregnant women are particularly susceptible (Takov and Tadi 2019). The frequency of motion sickness susceptibility from infancy to adolescence is characterized by three phases, a high resistance in the first year of life, a prepubertal peak of oversensitivity, and a postpubertal decline (Huppert et al. 2019; see ▶ Chap. 16).

19.2 Course and Therapeutic Principles

Despite considerable interindividual variation in resistance, every healthy individual can experience motion sickness when exposed to extreme acceleration stimuli (e.g., cross-coupled accelerations like Coriolis effects) (◘ Fig. 19.1). Figures on the incidence of motion sickness in different motor vehicles vary between 1% and 90%. During the first days of an Atlantic crossing with moderate turbulence, about 25–30% of ship passengers experience motion sickness, whereas 80% of subjects on small life rafts or adrift with flotation vests become severely seasick. The latter's survival chances are reduced by the additional loss of water and electrolytes.

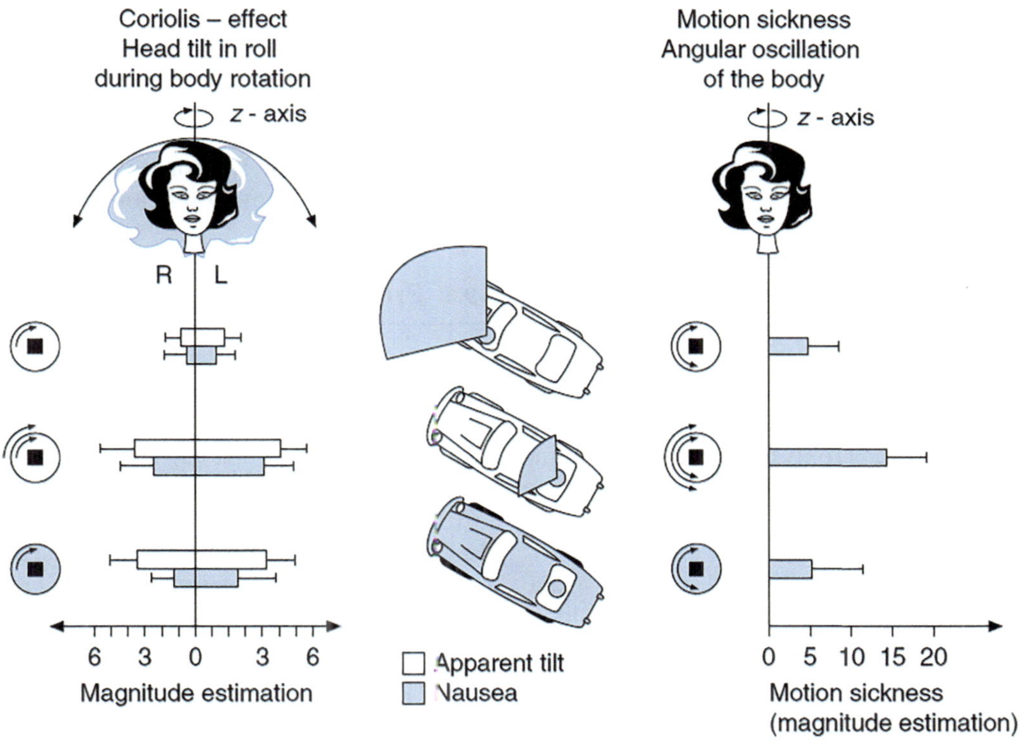

◘ **Fig. 19.1** Visual influences during body acceleration in a combined drum and chair system and their effects on vertigo and motion sickness. Left: magnitude estimations of apparent tilt and nausea induced by sideward tilts of the head during simultaneous body rotation while sitting. Coriolis effects are induced in the process by the cross-coupled accelerations (left). Magnitude estimation of motion sickness induced by 15 min of sinusoidal angular oscillation of the body on a rotatory chair with a frequency of 0.02 Hz and peak velocity of 100°/s (right). The three visual conditions were eyes open (top), rotary chair and drum movements mechanically coupled (middle), and eyes open in complete darkness (bottom). The experimentally induced nausea was greatest when the vestibular and visual information on movement was contradictory (combined movement of chair and drum). This corresponds to the experience in moving vehicles. Motion sickness is least pronounced when vision can simultaneously check body acceleration (in the driver's seat); conversely, motion sickness is greatest when the vestibular acceleration apparently contradicts visual information (in the back seat with predominantly stationary contrasts in the visual field or when reading). (Reproduced with permission from Brandt et al. (1976))

Women are more susceptible than men, and children and young adults are more susceptible than the aged. Newborns and infants up to the age of 1 year are extremely resistant to motion sickness, apparently because they use the visual system for dynamic space orientation only after they have learned to stand alone and walk. They obviously do not experience a provoking visual-vestibular conflict of self-motion perception while being transported in a vehicle (Brandt et al. 1976). Loss of labyrinthine function causes higher resistance to motion sickness (Strupp et al. 2018), whereas eye closure on a ship does not prevent sea sickness.

Motion sickness is an acute clinical syndrome. Nausea and vomiting develop within minutes to hours, and the symptoms show spontaneous remission within hours to 1 day after the stimulus ceases. If the stimulus continues (ship or space travel), relief occurs via centrally mediated adaptation (habituation) within 3 days (Koch et al. 2018).

The most effective physical means of prevention of motion sickness is adaptation (habituation) by intermittent exposure to the stimulus (Koch et al. 2018). This adaptation, however, is only temporary and specific for each type of acceleration; i.e., resistance to sea-sickness does not protect against flight sickness.

If "vestibular training" does not make the subject resistant, his/her head should be kept still during the stimulus, and additional accelerations that are complexly coupled with the vehicle motion should be avoided. Susceptibility is less when lying than when sitting (Golding et al., 1995) and less for the person in the front passenger seat than for someone sitting in the back seat (Takov and Tadi 2019).

Motion sickness develops above all in closed vehicles or while reading on the back seat of a car, when the body is being accelerated but a stationary environment is being viewed, which contradicts the labyrinthine stimuli. By maintaining adequate visual control of the vehicle movement, one can significantly reduce motion sickness from that experienced under eyes-closed conditions. Conversely, susceptibility is significantly increased if primarily stationary contrasts fill the field of vision (Dichgans and Brandt 1973; Probst et al. 1982).

Antivertiginous drugs such as dimenhydrinate (dramamine®) or scopolamine (transderm scop®) can inhibit the spontaneous activity of the vestibular nuclei neurons as well as the neuronal frequency modulation during body acceleration, thus reducing the susceptibility to motion sickness.

19.3 Pragmatic Therapy

The possibilities of physical prevention and pharmacological measures (Bles et al. 2000; Shupak and Gordon 2006; Spinks et al. 2011; Huppert et al. 2011; Murdin et al. 2011; Golding 2016; Leung and Hon 2019) are listed in ◘ Tables 19.1 and 19.2. As a transdermal therapeutic system (TTS), scopolamine is the preferred drug for prophylaxis. If applied in patch form, it must be stuck to the skin (e.g., behind the ear) 4–8 h before travelling because of the delayed release of the active agent. Low-dose transnasal scopolamine was also very effective without relevant sedative side effects (Simmons et al. 2010). Scopolamine is more effective than cinnarizine (Gil et al. 2012), promethazine, or dimenhydrinate. Second-

Table 19.1 Physical maneuvers to prevent motion sickness

Measure	Goal
Before	
"Vestibular training" by repeated exposure to stimulus and active head movements	Movement-specific central habituation
Vehicle simulator training	Utilization of the visual-vestibular transfer of habituation
Acute	
Fixation of the head	Avoidance of additional accelerations, which are complexly coupled with vehicle acceleration (e.g., Coriolis effect)
Head position (toward the vector of gravitation). Ship: supine; car: supine with head in the direction of movement; helicopter: sitting position	Utilization of the head-axis-specific difference in resistance to the acceleration; acceleration along the z-axis most favorable
Possible counter-regulation of the body motion induced by vehicle acceleration (e.g., inclining toward the curve)	
Visual control of the vehicle movement; if not possible, then close the eyes	Avoidance of a visual-vestibular conflict (mismatch) of perception

Table 19.2 Drug prophylaxis for motion sickness

Drugs	Side effects
Antihistamine 50–100 mg dimenhydrinate (Dramamine)	Sedation, reduced reactions and concentration, dryness of the mouth, blurred vision, light-headedness
Belladonna alkaloids 0.5 mg scopolamine as transdermal therapeutic system (Transderm Scop) 4–6 h before trip onset, effective up to 72 h	

generation antihistamines (e.g. cetirizine) are less sedative but also less effective (Leung and Hon 2019). Doubling the usual single doses (100 mg dimenhydrinate; 0.6 mg scopolamine) clearly increases the central sedating side effects without causing any essential improvement in resistance to motion sickness (Wood et al. 1966). A combination of scopolamine with a sympathicomimetic drug, such as ephedrine or dextroamphetamine, increases the efficacy with simultaneous reduction of sedative adverse effects (Wood and Graybiel 1970; Golding 2016). Because of the dependence caused by dextroamphetamine, a combination with this substance is not generally recommended but reserved for exceptional cases, e.g., during military flight missions (Leung and Hon 2019). Phenytoin was also tested for efficacy against motion sickness (Knox et al. 1994); however, in view of its side effects, it is also not recommended (Murdin et al. 2011).

References

Bertolini G, Straumann D (2016) Moving in a moving world: a review on vestibular motion sickness. Front Neurol 7:14

Bles W, Bos JE, Kruit H (2000) Motion sickness. Curr Opin Neurol 13:19–25

Boldingh MI, Ljostad U, Mygland A, Monstad P (2011) Vestibular sensitivity in vestibular migraine: VEMP's and motion sickness susceptibility. Cephalalgia 31:1211–1219

Brandt T (1976) Optisch-vestibuläre Bewegungskrankheit, Höhenschwindel und klinische Schwindelformen. Fortschr Med 94:177–1188

Brandt T, Wenzel D, Dichgans J (1976) Die Entwicklung der visuellen Stabilisation des aufrechten Standes beim Kind: Ein Reifezeichen in der Kinderneurologie. Arch Psychiat Nervenkr 223:1–13

Cuomo-Granston A, Drummond PD (2010) Migraine and motion sickness: what is the link? Prog Neurobiol 91:300–312

Dai M, Raphan T, Cohen B (2007) Labyrinthine lesions and motion sickness susceptibility. Exp Brain Res 1748:477–487

Dichgans J, Brandt T (1973) Optokinetic motion-sickness and pseudo-Coriolis effects induced by moving visual stimuli. Acta Otolaryngol 76: 339–348

Dichgans J, Brandt T (1978) Visual-vestibular interaction: effects of self-motion perception and postural control. In: Held R, Leibowitz HW, Teuber HL (eds) Handbook of Sensory Physiology, Vol VIII Perception. Springer, Berlin Heidelberg New York, pp 755–804

Evans RW, Marcus D, Furman JM (2007) Motion sickness and migraine. Headache 47:607–610

Gil A, Nachum Z, Tal D, Shupak A (2012) A comparison of cinnarizine and transdermal scopolamine for the prevention of seasickness in a naval crew: a double-blind, randomized, crossover study. Clin Neuropharmacol 35:37–39

Golding JF (2016) Motion sickness. Handb Clin Neurol 137:371–390

Golding JF, Patel M (2017) Menières, migraine, and motion sickness. Acta Otolaryngol 137:495–502

Golding JF, Markey HM, Stott IR (1995) The effects of motion direction, body axis, and posture on motion sickness induced by low frequency linear oscillation. Aviat Space Environm Med 66:1046–1051

Huppert D, Strupp M, Mückter H, Brandt T (2011) Which medication do I need to manage dizzy patients? Acta Otolaryngol 131:228–241

Huppert D, Benson J, Brandt T (2017) A historical view of motion sickness – a plague at sea and on land, also with military impact. Front Neurol 8:114

Huppert D, Grill E, Brandt T (2019) Survey of motion sickness susceptibility in children and adolescents aged 3 months to 18 years. J Neurol 266(Suppl 1):65–73

Knox GW, Woodard D, Chelen W, Ferguson R, Johnson L (1994) Phenytoin for motion sickness: clinical evaluation. Laryngoscope 1994:935–939

Koch A, Cascorbi I, Westhofen M, Dafotakis M, Klapa S, Kuhtz-Buschbeck JP (2018) The neurophysiology and treatment of motion sickness. Dtsch Arztebl Int 115:687–696

Leung AKC, Hon KL (2019) Motion sickness: an overview. Drugs Context 8:2019-9-4. https://doi.org/10.7573/dic.2019-9-4

Money KE (1970) Motion sickness. Physiol Rev 50: 1–39

Murdin L, Golding J, Bronstein A (2011) Managing motion sickness. BMJ 343:d7430

Murdin L, Chamberlain F, Cheema S, Ashad Q, Gresty MA, Golding JF, Bronstein A (2015) Motion sickness in migraine and vestibular disorders. J Neurol Neurosurg Psychiatry 86:585–587

Neuhauser H, Lempert T (2004) Vertigo and dizziness related to migraine: a diagnostic challenge. Cephalalgia 24:83–91

Paillard AC, Quarck G, Paolino F, Denise P, Paolino M, Golding JF, Ghulyan-Bedikian V (2013) Motion sickness susceptibility in healthy subjects and vestibular patients: effects of gender, age, and trait-anxiety. J Vestib Res 23:203–209

Probst T, Krafczyk S, Büchele W, Brandt T (1982) Visuelle Prävention der Bewegungskrankheit im Auto. Arch Psychiat Nervenkr 231:409–421

Reason JT (1978) Motion sickness adaptation: a neural mismatch model. J Roy Soc Med 71:819–829

Shupak A, Gordon CR (2006) Motion sickness: advances in pathogenesis, prediction, prevention, and treatment. Aviat Space Environ Med 77: 1213–1223

Simmons RG, Phillips JB, Lojewski RA et al (2010) The efficiency of low-dose transnasal scoloamine for motion sickness. Aviat Space Environ Med 81(4):405–412

Spinks AB, Wasiak J (2011) Scopolamine (hyoscine) for preventing and treating motion sickness. Cochrane Database Syst Rev (6):CD002851

Strupp M, Brandt T, Huppert D, Grill E (2018) Prevalence of motion sickness in various vestibular disorders: a study on 749 patients. J Neurol 265(Suppl 1):S95–S97

Takahashi M, Ogata M, Miura M (1997) The significance of motion sickness in the vestibular system. J Vestib Res 7:179–187

Takov V, Tadi P (2019) Motion sickness. In: StatPearls [internet]. StatPearls Publishing, Trasure Island. PMID: 30969528

Wood CD, Graybiel A (1970) Evaluation of antimotion sickness drugs: a new effective remedy revealed. Aerospace Med 41:932–933

Wood CD, Graybiel A, Kennedy RS (1966) Comparison of effectiveness of some antimotion sickness drugs using recommended and larger than recommended doses as tested in the slow rotation room. Aerospace Med 37:259–262

Zhang LL, Wang JQ, Qi RR, Pan LL, Li M, Cai YL (2016) Motion sickness: current knowledge and recent advantage. CNS Neurosci Ther 22:15–24

Mal de Débarquement Syndrome

Contents

M. Strupp et al., *Vertigo and Dizziness*, https://doi.org/10.1007/978-3-030-78260-3_20

Mal de Débarquement Syndrome (MdDS) mostly occurs after disembarquement following a long sea voyage and is characterized by a distressing perception on land of seemingly enduring low-frequency rocking, bobbing, or swaying sensations of the body or the ground with subjective unsteadiness (Brown and Baloh 1987; Murphy 1993; Cha 2009). Weaker and transient forms of MdDS-like symptoms – also termed "sea legs" or "land sickness" – are occasionally experienced by the majority of healthy individuals after such exposure (Hain and Cherchi 2016; van Ombergen et al. 2016; Schepermann et al. 2019). Although MdDS typically develops after long sea voyages, it has also been reported to occur after prolonged exposure to passive motion on land or during air travel. In rare cases, these complaints last for months or years and require medical therapy often without a convincing treatment-specific efficacy (Van Ombergen et al. 2016; Canceri et al. 2018; Saha and Cha 2020).

The Classification Committee of the Bárány Society compiled a consensus-document with the following diagnostic criteria (Cha et al. 2020) (▶ Box 20.1):

Box 20.1 Criteria for the Diagnosis of Mal de Débarquement Syndrome (Cha et al. 2020)

1. Non-spinning vertigo characterized by an oscillatory sensation present continuously or for most of the day.
2. Onset occurs within 48 h after the end of exposure to passive motion.
3. Symptoms temporarily reduce with exposure to passive motion.
4. Symptoms continue for >48 h
   (a) In evolution (>48 h, when observation time < 1 month)
   (b) Transient MdDS (>48 h – ≤ 1 month)
   (c) Persistent MdDS (>1 month).
5. Symptoms not better accounted for by another disease or disorder.

Mal de Débarquement syndrome is called persistent if it lasts longer than a month. Affected individuals may develop associated symptoms, such as spatial disorientation, motion intolerance, fatigue, headache, or anxiety. Differential diagnoses or misdiagnoses may be episodic or oscillating dizziness without preceding body motion, e.g., functional dizziness (▶ Chap. 15), or similar bodily symptoms elicited by stress, anxiety, or depressive disorders (Mucci et al. 2018). Epidemiologically there is a female preponderance for susceptibility to MdDS and a high comorbidity with migraine (Cha et al. 2018). Historically, MdDS is a long-known condition with descriptions of analogous symptoms dating back to Erasmus von Darwin (1796) and even to ancient Greek and Roman authors (Huppert et al. 2016).

20.1 Pathophysiology

Attempts to explain the pathophysiological mechanisms of MdDS are manifold and consequently not particularly convincing. They include a specific functional disturbance of the ocular motor velocity storage mechanism and the vestibulo-cerebellar nodulus (Cohen 2019), hypothetical "pseudo-hallucinations" of the vestibular memory system, as well as more general approaches of an abnormal synchronization of sensorimotor networks (Moeller and Lempert 2007; Van Ombergen et al. 2016; Schepermann et al. 2019; Clark et al. 2013), or just functional (somatoform) disorders.

The natural average motion profile of oceanliners mainly comprises the low frequency range of 0.1–0.4 Hz (Wawrzynski and Krata 2016) that closely matches the predominant frequency (0.2–0.3 Hz) of inner rocking sensations and bodily oscillations in patients with MdDS (Dai et al. 2014; Cohen et al. 2018). In an experimental model to elicit symptoms of MdDS in healthy subjects, motion stimulation consistently evoked rocking sensations and postural alterations most pronounced in the anterior-posterior dimension during standing with eyes closed which were primarily characterized by a distinct peak in the low-frequency sway spectrum close to the stimulation frequency (Schepermann et al. 2019). A comparison of such aftereffects of body sway dependent on various oscillatory motion stimuli in the frontal roll or sagittal pitch-plane revealed that the most effective motion stimuli were not the sinusoidal movements about a single axis but rather unpredictable low-frequency multidirectional motion stimuli as generated by a motor-driven multidirectional motion platform (Hexapod, ◘ Fig. 20.1). This contradicts the hypothesis by Cohen et al. (2018) that MdDS represents a distinct functional disturbance of the vestibulo-cerebellar system in the roll-plane activated by the velocity storage of the vestibular neuronal circuitry.

Brain imaging comprising structural MRI, resting-state functional MRI, and FDG-PET scans is compatible with the view that motion-induced changes in visuo-vestibular cortical networks in combination with an increased activity within the prefrontal cortex and a simultaneous decrease of activity in the vestibulo-cerebellum (Jeon et al. 2020) are very similar to those changes seen in anxiety disorders (Duval et al. 2015) and (somatoform) functional phobic postural vertigo (Popp et al. 2018; Huber et al. 2020).

The symptoms and course of MdDS remind the experienced clinician of other chronical syndromes, such as functional diz-

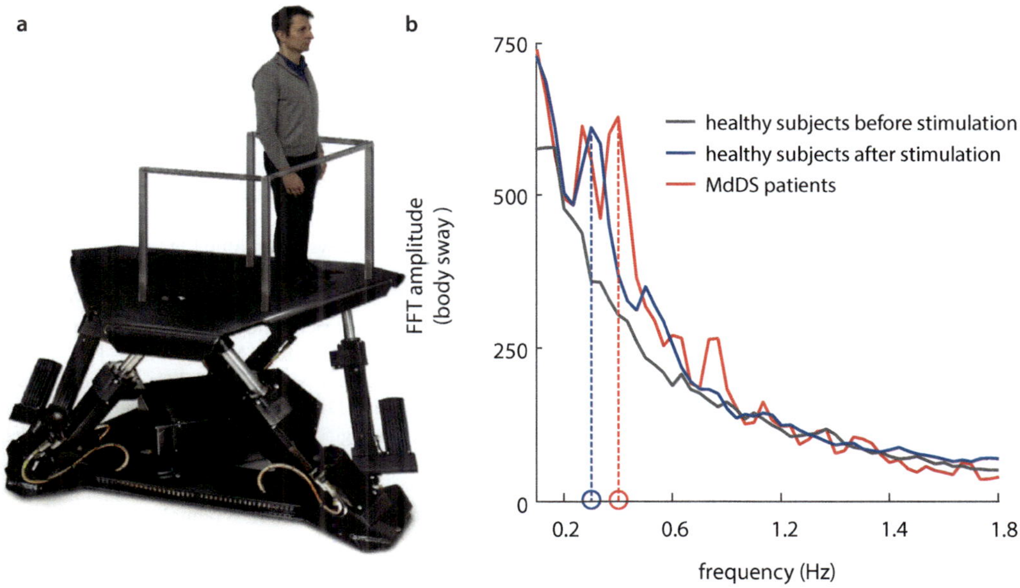

◘ **Fig. 20.1** Motor-driven motion platform (Hexapod) for simultaneous 6 degrees-of-freedom motion stimulation, by which motion can be generated along all 3 rotatory (yaw, pitch, roll) and translational axes (left). Comparison of the anterior-posterior body sway of patients with MdDS with those of healthy volunteers before (HS pre) and 5 min after (HS post) a 30-min stimulation (right). Corresponding Fourier transformed (FFT) amplitude spectrum indicates the distinct peak in the low-frequency spectrum in body sway of HS post-stimulation and patients (blue and red circles). Shortly after motion stimulation, sway behavior of HS assimilates to that of patients and in particular exhibits a distinct peak in the low-frequency spectrum of AP-sway close to the supplied motion stimulation frequency. Thus, pathological and experimentally elicited abnormal body sway coincide for patients and controls. (Modified from Scheperman et al. 2019)

ziness (▶ Chap. 15), tinnitus, tension headache, or neuropathic pain, all of which may share some common mechanisms.

20.2 Therapy

Various therapeutical measures have been recommended depending on the different pathophysiological hypotheses. They include medical compounds, such as antidepressants (specially SSRI) or the transient use of tranquilizers, visual/vestibular motion stimulation programs, and non-invasive transcranial magnetic stimulation, as well as experimental adjustments of the vestibulo-ocular reflex (Nachum et al. 2004; Cha and Baloh 2013; van Ombergen et al. 2016, Canceri et al. 2018; Cha et al. 2019, Cohen 2019). As long as there are no convincing, controlled, prospective therapeutic studies, the old clinical rule applies: "The more widespread the therapeutic offers, the more doubtful and insecure the efficacy."

We think that the best management of MdDS patients is based on a careful medical history and neurootological investigation to exclude other disorders mimicking MdDS. In a second step, informing the patient about the non-threatening character of the condition is essential, along with encouraging the patient to maintain a normal lifestyle with regular exercise to overcome avoidance behavior. This is analogous to the management of secondary functional dizziness, especially as both conditions are very similar.

References

Brown JJ, Baloh RW (1987) Persistent mal de Débarquement syndrome: a motion-induced subjective disorder of balance. Am J Otolaryngol 8:219–222

Canceri JM, Brown R, Watson SR, Browne CJ (2018) Examination of current treatments and symptom management strategies used by patients with mal de Débarquement syndrome. Front Neurol 9:943

Cha YH (2009) Mal de Débarquement. Semin Neurol 29:520–527

Cha YH, Cui YY, Baloh R (2013) Repetitive transcranial magnetic stimulation for mal de Débarquement-syndrome. Otol Neurootol 34:175–179

Cha YH, Cui YY, Baloh RW (2018) Comprehensive clinical profile of mal de Débarquement syndrome. Front Neurol 9:261

Cha YH, Gleghorn D, Doudican B (2019) Occipital and cerebellar theta burst stimulation for mal de Débarquement syndrome. Otol Neurotol 40:e928–e937

Cha YH, Baloh R, Cho C, Magnusson M, Song JJ, Strupp M, Wuyts F, Staab JP (2020) Mal de Débarquement syndrome: diagnostic criteria consensus document of the classification committee of the Bárány Society. J Vestib Res 30:285–293

Clark BC, LePorte A, Clark S, Hoffman RL, Quick A, Wilson TE, Thomas JS (2013) Effects of persistent mal de Débarquement syndrom on balance, psychological traits, and motor cortex excitability. J Clin Neurosci 20:446–450

Cohen B (2019) Dedication to Mingjia Dai, Ph.D. for discovery of the first successful treatment of the mal de Débarquement syndrome. Front Neurol 10:1196

Cohen B, Yakushin SB, Cho C (2018) Hypothesis: the vestibular and cerebellar basis of the mal de Débarquement syndrome. Front Neurol 9:28

Dai M, Cohen B, Smouha E, Cho C (2014) Readaptation of the mal de Débarquement syndrome: a 1-year follow-up. Front Neurol 5:124

Darwin E (1796) Why after voyage ideas of vibratory motions are perceived on shore. In: Zoonomia or the laws of organic life, vol 1. J. Johnson, London

Duval ER, Javanbakht A, Liberzon I (2015) Neural circuits in anxiety and stress disorders: a focused review. Ther Clin Risk Manag 11:115–126

Hain TC, Cherchi M (2016) Mal de Débarquement-syndrome. Handb Clin Neurol 137:391–395

Huber J, Flanagin VL, Popp P, zu Eulenburg P, Dieterich M (2020) Network changes in phobic postural vertigo. Brain Behav 10(6):e01622

Huppert D, Oldelehr H, Krammling B, Benson J, Brandt T (2016) What the ancient Greeks and Romans knew (and did not know) about seasickness. Neurology 86:560–565

Jeon S-H, Park Y-H, Oh S-Y et al (2020) Neural correlates of Mal de Débarquement syndrome: neuropsychological and imaging data. Front Neurol 11:585

Moeller L, Lempert T (2007) Mal de Débarquement: pseudo-hallucinations from vestibular memory? J Neurol 254:813–815

Mucci V, Canceri JM, Brown R, Dai M, Yakushin S, Watson S, Van Ombergen A, Topsakal V, Van de

Heyning PH, Wuyts FL, Browne CJ (2018) Mal de Débarquement syndrome: a survey on subtypes, misdiagnoses, onset and associated psychological features. J Neurol 265:486–499

Murphy TP (1993) Mal de Débarquement syndrome: a forgotten entity? Otolaryngol Head Neck Surg 109:10–13

Nachum Z, Shupak A, Letichevsky V, Ben-David J, Tal D, Tamir A, Talmon Y, Gordon CR, Luntz M (2004) Mal de Débarquement and posture: reduced reliance on vestibular and visual cues. Laryngoscope 114:581–586

Popp P, zu Eulenburg P, Stephan T, Bögle R, Habs M, Henningsen P, Feuerecker R, Dieterich M (2018) Cortical alterations in phobic postural vertigo–a multimodal imaging approach. Ann Clin Translat Neurol 5:717–729

Saha K, Cha YH (2020) Mal de Débarquement-syndrome. Semin Neurol 40(1):160–164

Schepermann A, Bardins S, Penkava J, Brandt T, Huppert D, Wuehr M (2019) Approach to an experimental model of mal de Débarquement syndrome. J Neurol 266(Suppl 1):74–79

Van Ombergen A, Van Rompaey V, Maes LK, Van de Heyning PH, Wuyts FL (2016) Mal de Débarquement syndrome: a systematic review. J Neurol 263:843–854

Wawrzynski W, Krata P (2016) On ship roll resonance frequency. Ocean Eng 126:92–114

Visual Height Intolerance and Acrophobia

Contents

M. Strupp et al., *Vertigo and Dizziness*, https://doi.org/10.1007/978-3-030-78260-3_21

Physiological height vertigo is a visually induced destabilization of stance and locomotion accompanied by individually varying levels of strong anxiety and vegetative symptoms at the sight of towers, ladders, buildings, a cliff, or a mountain ridge. In Anglo-American countries, the term "height vertigo" is unusual; instead "fear of heights" or "acrophobia" is used, which in psychiatric nomenclature are classified as a variant of specific phobias in accordance with the criteria of the "Diagnostic and Statistical Manual of Mental Disorders". These language-specific terms require a clear definition for medical and scientific use with respect to the susceptibility and the severity of the condition.

21.1 Definitions and Grading of Susceptibility

Teleologically, visual height intolerance with avoidance behavior when exposed to heights is beneficial to prevent anxiety and panic attacks as well as catastrophic falls. Many animal species and humans have a largely gene-based fear and avoidance behavior when visually approaching a cliff or an abyss ("visual cliff" phenomenon; Walk et al. 1957). Visual height intolerance is thus physiological and must be differentiated from pathological acrophobia. Subjective visual height intolerance develops within several seconds after a glance into an abyss, but once the inducing situation disappears, it rapidly resolves. Although height vertigo has so far been considered mainly a phobia, there is a physiological explanation for the postural instability and vertigo caused by optical stimuli at the sight of freestanding buildings (Bles et al. 1980; Brandt et al. 1980) (◘ Fig. 21.1). Physiological visual height intolerance is rather a "distance vertigo" caused by "visual destabilization" of upright posture, when the distance between the observer's eye and the nearest visible stationary contrasts within the field of vision becomes critically large. Then head and body sway can no longer be corrected by vision, since the movements cannot be registered by the sensors due to the sub-threshold smallness of the retinal shift. The vestibular and somatosensory signals of a shifting of the body's center of gravity over the standing surface contradict the visual information of preserved body stability. Under such stimulus conditions, the body sway is measurably increased, and above all the visual postural reflexes to the disturbing input are so impaired that there is real danger of an accident or fall. The critical stimulus parameters of the trigger and practical pointers for prophylaxis can be derived from this physiological mechanism (◘ Table 21.1).

Psychiatrists use the term "acrophobia" to define a specific phobia according to the classification schemes of ICD 10 (International Classification of Diseases) and DSM-V (Diagnostic and Statistical Manual of Mental Disorders) which requires therapy (World Health Organisation 1993). The nonmedical Anglo-American community, however, uses the same term to refer to a less pronounced visual height intolerance that does not fulfil the criteria of a specific phobia.

To overcome this conceptual confusion and to clearly distinguish between physiological and psychopathological mechanisms at heights, the following three terms have been proposed to define the different states of responses to height exposure (◘ Table 21.2) (Brandt et al. 2012a, b; Brandt and Huppert 2014; Huppert et al. 2020):

1. A *physiological height imbalance* of posture that results from an impaired visual control of stance and gait when the distance to stationary surroundings becomes too large for visual detection and counteraction of body movements (Brandt et al. 1980).
2. A *more or less distressing, stimulus-dependent visual height intolerance*, which causes the apprehension of losing balance or falling, but does not meet the criteria of a specific phobia.

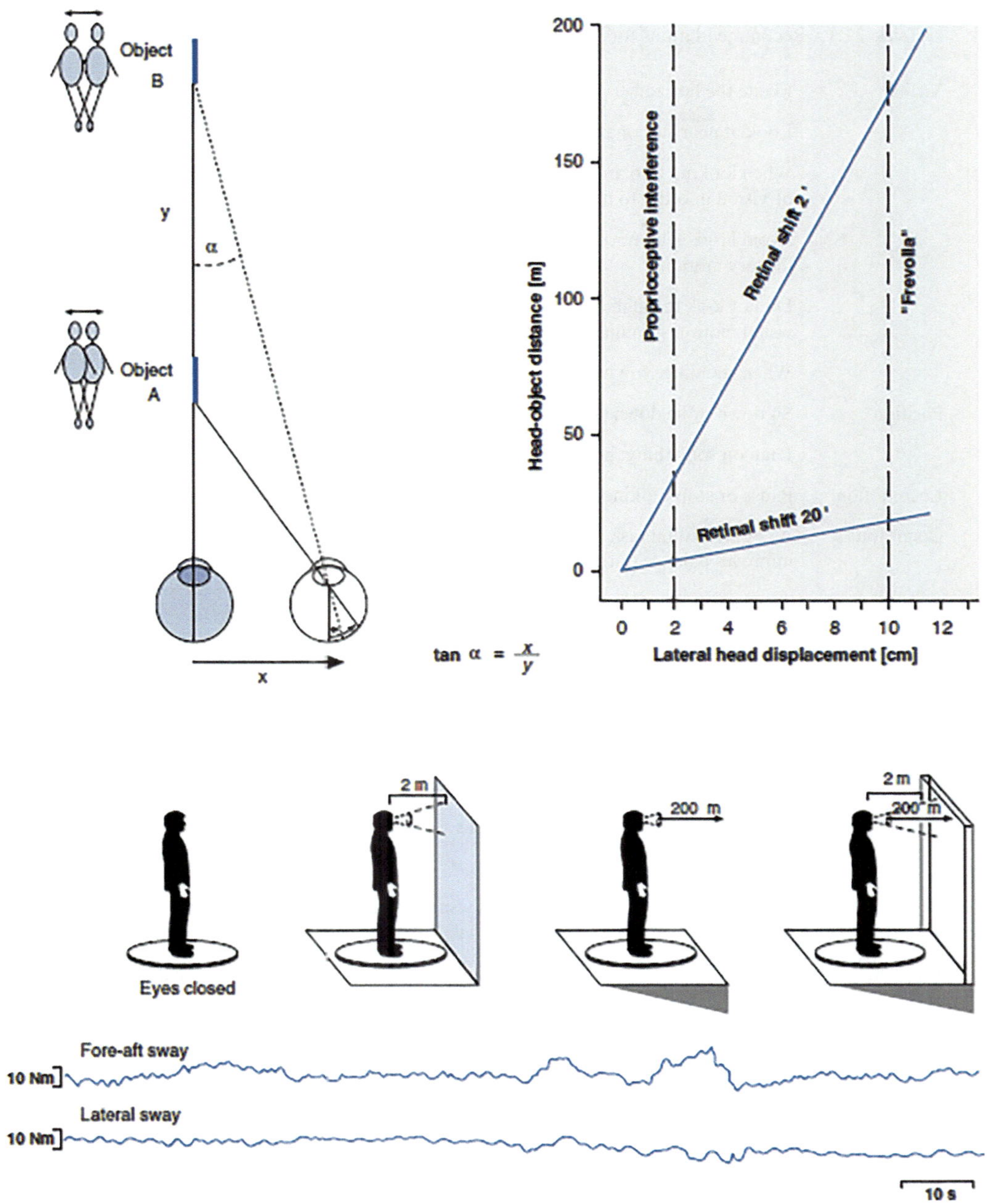

Fig. 21.1 Physiological visual height imbalance of posture. Geometrical analysis indicates that head sway with respect to the surroundings is visually detected with more difficulty if the distance between the eyes and surrounding contrasts increases. When objects are fixated, the same geometric relationship pertains for efferent and re-afferent perception of the eye movements triggered by the head sway. Actually, there is a reinforcement of the posturographically measurable body sway under such visual conditions (below). Fore–aft and lateral body sway is minimal with eyes open 2 meters in front of a structured wall, and maximal when looking into the distance without nearby contrasts. As soon as nearby stationary contrasts appear in the visual field periphery while gazing in the distance, they are used for the visual stabilization of stance. (From Brandt et al. 1980)

Table 21.1 Recommendations for behavioral coping strategies for visual height intolerance

Vision	Fixate the horizon
	Look at near stationary contrasts.
	When looking into an abyss, keep near stationary objects in sight in the peripheral field of vision in order to maintain visual control of posture.
	Avoid large-field motion stimuli (for example, clouds) that can lead to visually induced illusory motion.
	Do not look through binoculars without some kind of support/stabilization (misleading visual motion stimulus).
	When standing, you may close your eyes for a while (to reduce anxiety).
Position	Sit down or lie down (symptoms maximal when standing, minimal when lying).
	Lean on something; hold tight to something.
Locomotion	Pause or stop walking (symptoms increase with locomotion at heights).
Cognition	A cognitive dual task (e.g., naming items from a given category) reduces anxiety and improves balance during stance and locomotion.
	Try to overcome any avoidance behavior.

Modified from Brandt et al. (2015)

Table 21.2 Forms of physiological and psychopathological conditions active during exposure to visual heights

Term	Prevalence	Mechanism	Clinical relevance
Physiological visual height imbalance	100%	Impaired visual control of postural balance	None
Visual height intolerance	28%	Distress and anxiety when exposed to heights	50% of those afflicted
Acrophobia (fear of heights)	3–6%	Specific phobia	100% (requires psychotherapy)

Modified from Brandt and Huppert (2014)

3. *Fear of heights or acrophobia*, a specific phobia representing the severest end of the spectrum.

Common questionnaires to validate susceptibility to fear of heights either compare self-reports and overt-behavioral procedures (Cohen 1977) or measure height-relevant interpretation biases to assess the relationship between biased interpretations and symptoms of acrophobia (Steinman and Teachman 2011). On the basis of various epidemiological and phenomenological studies, a short questionnaire was developed and validated that allows (1) a continuous quantification of the severity of visual height intolerance within a metric interval scale from 0 to 13 and (2) differentiation of the diagnosis of acrophobia by including two additional questions (Huppert et al. 2017).

21.2 Epidemiology and Susceptibility Across Lifespan

First historical descriptions of fear of heights can be found in Roman and Greek antique texts. (▶ Chap. 23) (Bauer et al. 2012; Huppert et al. 2013a; Huppert and Brandt 2018; Huppert et al. 2020). Most available epidemiological studies focus on symptoms of fear of heights (acrophobia) mainly based on features of panic attacks. Acrophobia has a lifetime prevalence of 3.1–6.4% (Agras et al. 1969; Curtis et al. 1998; Becker et al. 2007; Stinson et al. 2007; Depla et al. 2008; Oosterink et al. 2009; LeBeau et al. 2010; Kapfhammer et al. 2015). In two representative Germany-wide epidemiological studies ($n = 3517$, $n = 2012$), the major results were (Huppert et al. 2013b; Kapfhammer et al. 2016):

- The lifetime prevalence of the more broadly defined visual height intolerance was 28% in adults and slightly higher in women (32%) than in men (25%).
- The risk of developing visual height intolerance is higher in those individuals with a positive family history of such, an intolerance with additional illnesses such as liability to motion sickness, Menière's disease (9%), anxiety disorders, or migraine (21%).
- The majority of susceptible individuals experience a chronic unfavorable course of illness, which is particularly associated with the presence of coexisting major depression, chronic fatigue, panic attacks, initial traumatic trigger, social phobia, other specific phobic fears, and female sex (Kapfhammer et al. 2016).
- Visual height intolerance can develop throughout the lifespan but most often (30%) occurs for the first time during the second decade of life. The main symptoms during height exposure in predisposed persons include anxiety; to-and-fro vertigo; unsteadiness and gait insecurity; weak knees; inner agitation; and vegetative symptoms such as rapid heartbeat, sweating, drowsiness, and tremor.
- The most common trigger situations are looking down from towers, followed by hiking and mountaineering, climbing ladders, walking over a bridge, and looking down from a high-rise window. For about half of affected individuals the trigger situations generalize in the further course of susceptibility (57%).
- A coping strategy for over half of those affected is to avoid triggering situations, which leads to restrictions in daily activities and reduced quality of life (Huppert et al. 2013a; Schäffler et al. 2014).

Psychiatric evaluations revealed that in 22.5% of susceptible individuals symptoms may from time to time worsen to the intensity of panic attacks. There is a high level of comorbidity with anxiety disorders (16.7%) and depressive syndromes (26.1%), but not with other somatoform disorders (Kapfhammer et al. 2016). The same psychiatric comorbidity was reported for almost half of patients with a few other structural vertigo/dizziness syndromes, for example, vestibular migraine or Menière's disease (Best et al. 2009a, b; Lahmann et al. 2015). In another study, the prevalence of susceptibility to visual height intolerance and fear of heights was found to be increased in various groups of vestibular diseases, including functional phobic postural dizziness (64%), vestibular migraine (61%,), vestibular paroxysmia (56%), benign paroxysmal positional vertigo (54%), unilateral vestibulopathy (49%), and Menière's disease (48%), but was normal compared to the general population in patients with bilateral vestibulopathy (29%) (Brandt et al. 2018). A possible explanation for the latter observation is that patients with bilateral vestibulopathy may expose themselves less frequently to heights because of their inherent postural instability (Brandt et al. 2018). An alternative explanation is the finding that patients with bilateral vestibulopathy have less anxiety (which is the major cause of fear of heights) than patients with other vestibular disorders (Decker et al. 2019; Brandt and Dieterich 2020).

Associations are known to exist between anxiety disorders and alcohol drinking behavior (Morris et al. 2005; Blumenthal et al. 2010; Schneier et al. 2010; Buckner and Matthews 2012). This kind of comorbidity was also shown for specific phobias in a large representative epidemiological survey in the United States (Stinson et al. 2007) with varying frequencies among the subtypes of specific phobias (LeBeau et al. 2010; MacDonald et al. 2011): it was higher for animal, situational, and blood/injury subtypes as compared to environmental subtypes (Becker et al. 2007; Depla et al. 2008). In contrast, there is no evidence that visual height intolerance and fear of heights are significantly associated with alcohol misuse (Huppert et al. 2013a). With respect to self-efficacy, a cross-sectional survey revealed a lower level of general self-confidence in susceptible individuals, in particular in those who do not actively seek help or expose themselves to height situations (Grill et al. 2014).

Finally, a survey among pre-pubertal children aged 8–10 years on the frequency and phenomenology of visual height intolerance and fear of heights revealed a prevalence of 34% with no gender preponderance (Huppert and Brandt 2015; see ▶ Chap. 16).

21.3 Stance, Gait, and Visual Exploration Under Real Height Stimulation

Increased postural threat, for instance, while walking on a modestly elevated support surface in the laboratory, causes gait changes especially in older people. These changes are characterized by a reduced speed of walking, shorter steps, decreased cadence, and longer times in double support (Brown et al. 2002; Delbaere et al. 2009; Tersteeg et al. 2012). Analogously, standing on elevated surfaces in the laboratory alters static postural control, in particular with a musculoskeletal stiffening of the postural control apparatus (Carpenter et al. 2001). These postural alterations are accompanied by changes in vestibulospinal balance reflexes in terms of a greater coupling between vestibular inputs and body sway responses (Horslen et al. 2014). This threat-induced modulation of vestibulospinal reflexes is presumably closely related to postural stiffening by anti-gravity muscle co-contraction (see also ▶ Chap. 15 for comparison). An analogous modulation of sensorimotor balance reflexes can be observed while standing on the ground when balance is threatened by unpredictable tilts of the support surface (Lim et al. 2017). This finding suggests that alterations in sensorimotor balance control at heights are primarily elicited by fear and anxiety rather than by the visual height stimulus alone. Correspondingly, personality traits measured by questionnaires on anxiety and willingness to take physical risks are associated with postural alterations when standing at the edge of an elevated platform (Zaback et al. 2015). Moreover, acrophobic individuals have a poorer postural performance in static and dynamic balance tasks (Boffino et al. 2009).

The above-described studies were performed preferably in the laboratory and tested balance function under threat conditions in healthy subjects. Neurophysiological studies on sensorimotor control in individuals with more or less severe visual height intolerance including acrophobia have been conducted during real exposure to heights (◘ Fig. 21.2). These experiments were performed on

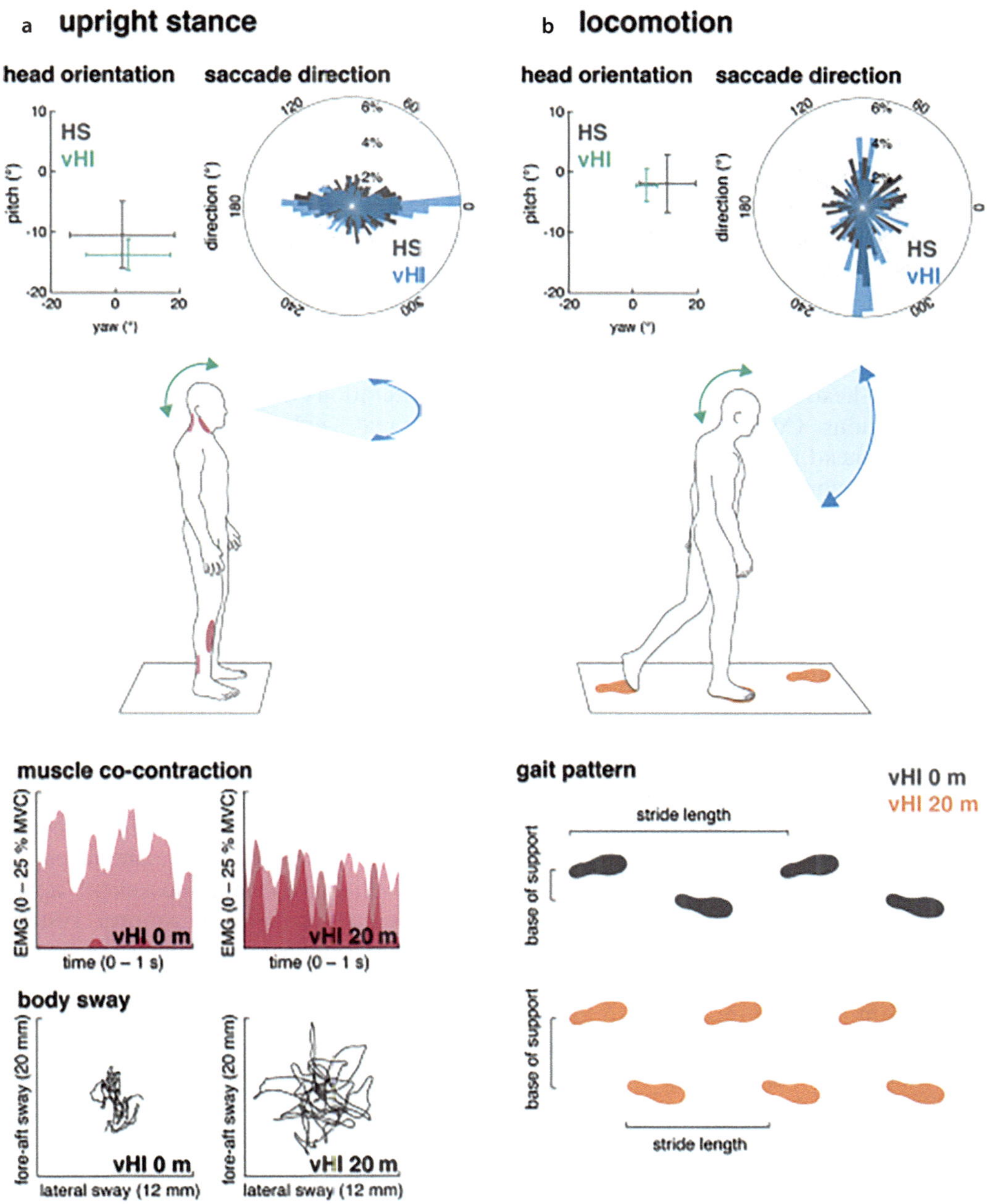

Fig. 21.2 Overview of height-induced alterations of visual exploration, postural and locomotion control in individuals with visual height intolerance (vHI), and healthy insusceptible subjects (HS) while being exposed to heights on an emergency balcony 20 meters above ground. **a** Behavioral alterations during quiet upright stance. **b** Behavioral alterations during locomotion. Top panel: group means and interquartile ranges of head orientation and histograms of the direction of corresponding saccadic eye movements. During both standing and walking, individuals with vHI show considerably reduced head movements. Saccadic eye movements during stance in individuals with vHI are preferably directed along the horizontal plane. In contrast, during locomotion, they perform saccades primarily along the vertical plane. Bottom panel: During height exposure, postural control in individuals with vHI is characterized by increased co-contraction of anti-gravity muscles and increased body sway amplitudes. Locomotion is characterized by a slow and cautious mode of walking, with a reduced stride length and a broadened base of support (Huppert et al. 2020)

an open escape balcony at a height of 20 meters above ground level with a focus on either visual exploration behavior by the use of mobile infrared eye-tracking goggles with integrated inertial sensors for monitoring of head movements (Kugler et al. 2014a, b), or on kinematics and muscle activation patterns during stance and gait behavior (Wühr et al. 2014; Schniepp et al. 2014). These experiments demonstrated that susceptible individuals standing on the balcony exhibit fewer and amplitude-limited eye-in-head saccades with longer fixation durations. Corresponding reductions in angular head movements were observed in all dimensions, i.e., yaw, pitch, and roll plane (◘ Fig. 21.2, upper panel). Total gaze-in-space behavior was considerably restricted to a smaller area as compared to non-susceptible controls who freely explored the entire visual field including the abyss (Wühr et al. 2014). Thus, visual exploration in susceptible individuals confines itself along the horizon or toward a centered position at the horizon. In other words, fear of heights appears to freeze the gaze to the horizon. Finally, experiments revealed an activity-dependent anisotropy of visual exploration in susceptible individuals. In contrast to quiet stance where gaze primarily stays in the horizontal dimension, gaze-in-space behavior during locomotion is mainly restricted to the vertical dimension. This exploration pattern is focused on the "vertical strip" in the heading direction and may augment visual control of balance and avoidance of obstacles in precarious locomotion contexts (Kugler et al. 2014b).

With respect to static postural control in susceptible individuals, the relationship between alterations in body sway and muscle activity measures with subjective estimates of fear at heights was examined. Body sway alterations as well as leg and neck muscle co-contraction increased with increasing subjective anxiety (Wühr et al. 2014) (◘ Fig. 21.2, left lower panel). In accordance with the above-described laboratory-based findings in healthy controls, this observation was explained as a fear-induced lowering of the threshold for sensorimotor balance reflexes accompanied by an increased stiffening of the complete postural control apparatus. Analogously, gait alterations of susceptible individuals during real height exposure resemble those seen in healthy subjects when walking on modestly elevated support surfaces, in particular a reduction of walking speed and stride length and increased double support phases. These are typical features of cautious gait control, a strategy, which, however, is overridden during walking at fast speeds (Schniepp et al. 2014) (◘ Fig. 21.2, right lower panel).

Taken together, experimental evidence on behavioral changes of gaze, balance, and locomotion control in susceptible individuals during exposure to real heights reveals a stiffening strategy that encompasses the whole anti-gravity musculoskeletal apparatus, including the ocular-motor system. This threat-induced stiffening is associated with a sensitization of sensorimotor balance reflexes, a cautious mode of voluntary motion, and an activity-dependent restriction of visual exploration (Brandt et al. 2015). These alterations can best be described by the common expression of being "scared stiff" by fear of heights – a behavioral response that results in tonic immobility. This motor response of a tonic stiffening of eye, head, and body movements may represent an atavistic motor reaction resembling feigning death, a primitive reflex observed throughout the entire animal world (Brandt et al. 2015). Feigning death was first described in snakes by Kilpatrick (1893). Accordingly, anxiety appears to be the critical psychopathological symptom that causes the typical, but not specific eye and body motor responses to height exposure in subjects with visual height intolerance.

21.4 Irrational Anxiety of Falling Rather Than Perception of Height is Causative

Behavioral responses at heights could be triggered by anxiety and/or the visual perception of depth. Tersteeg et al. (2012) directly addressed the question of differential contributions to postural alterations at heights in an experiment on healthy subjects who were walking on a 3.5-meter-high narrow walkway while the sight of the drop could be temporarily replaced by a visual surround comparable to ground level. Interestingly, they observed that the mere postural threat by the knowledge of danger rather than the actual perception of height was responsible for the switch to a cautious gait pattern. This is in line with the observation that the sensitization of vestibulospinal reflexes at height exposure appears to be primarily driven by anxiety and fear of falling rather than the mere visual perception of depth (Horslen et al. 2014; Lim et al. 2017). Further, changes in balance control and locomotion in individuals susceptible to visual height intolerance were shown to scale with the severity of subjectively perceived anxiety (Wühr et al. 2014; Schniepp et al. 2014). In contrast, withdrawal of visual depth perception by eye closure or upward gaze only mildly modulates behavioral alterations at heights in these individuals. A study in a comprehensive cohort of individuals with different degrees of susceptibility (insusceptible or susceptible up to acrophobic according to the Visual Height Intolerance Scale – VHISS; Huppert et al. 2017) further suggests that the intensity of perceived anxiety at heights and the extent of corresponding behavioral alterations is directly proportional (Wühr et al. 2019). Accordingly, the magnitude of postural responses scaled with both the subjectively felt anxiety during exposure and the severity of individual susceptibility to height intolerance.

Based on this evidence, a hypothetical cascade on emergence of symptoms during height exposure has been proposed (Brandt et al. 2015; Wühr et al. 2019). Accordingly, (1) anxiety about falling off or falling down at heights triggers a vicious circle with (2) a co-contraction of anti-gravity muscles that results in (3) increased sensitivity of sensorimotor balance reflexes and a rigid regulation of body sway, which (4) aggravates subjective imbalance and in turn intensifies the initial anxiety (■ Fig. 21.3). In line with this proposed symptom-cascade, postural changes during height exposure are linked to an increased self-awareness of body sway (Cleworth et al. 2019). There is growing evidence that the vestibular system – by means of reciprocal interconnections within a multilocal anxiety system – influences both cognition and emotional regulation in animal models and humans (Hilber et al. 2019). This raises the question whether preserved vestibular function is relevant for distressing anxiety and whether loss of vestibular function reduces general liability to anxious behavior (Brandt and Dieterich 2020). Indeed, patients with bilateral vestibulopathy – as

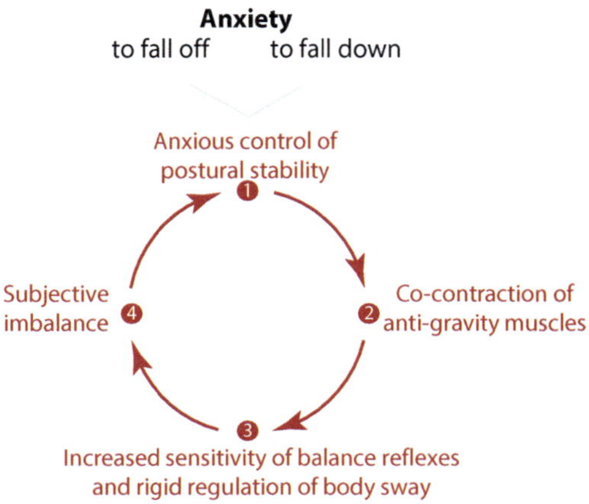

Fig. 21.3 Symptom cascade in persons susceptible to acrophobia and visual height intolerance, the vicious circle. Anxious concentration on control of postural stability triggers co-contraction of the anti-gravity muscles, thereby causing an increased sensitivity of sensorimotor balance reflexes and a rigid regulation of body sway. This leads to subjective imbalance, which in turn enhances anxious control of posture. (Modified from Brandt et al. 2015 and Huppert et al. 2020)

distinct from other vestibular disorders – have no increased susceptibility to visual height intolerance compared to the general population (Brandt et al. 2018). In line with this finding, patients with bilateral vestibulopathy do not report anxiety about falling despite having an increased risk of falling (Decker et al. 2019; Schlick et al. 2015).

These findings strongly support the impact of anxiety as a trigger and pathophysiological factor of visual height intolerance and acrophobia. However, the severity of anxiety does not always parallel the severity of the neurophysiological parameters of stance and gait, as found in a study on the influence of the absolute height above ground on various bodily parameters (Wühr et al. 2019).

21.5 The Role of Absolute Height Above Ground on the Magnitude of Visual Height Intolerance and Acrophobia

In psychophysical magnitude estimations, the influence of the net altitude was determined under real conditions on a high building under construction (Brandt et al. 1980). For most subjects, fear of height was already reported to be highest on the fourth floor and seemingly saturated at a height of about 20 meters. Accordingly, there were no significant differences among the intensities of subjective fear of height experienced at altitudes of 20, 50, or 100 meters, although some individuals reported increased fear on the 20th floor. This initial observation was later re-examined in more detail by means of virtual reality technology in a comprehensive cohort of individuals with different degrees of susceptibility (insusceptible or susceptible up to acrophobic as differentiated by the Visual Height Intolerance Severity Scale (VHISS) (Huppert et al. 2017; Wühr et al. 2019). Virtual height exposure at seven discrete elevation levels between 0.5 and 100 meters provoked similar changes in postural and autonomic measures (Wühr et al. 2019) as observed during real in vivo stimulation (Cleworth et al. 2012). Body sway and musculoskeletal stiffening linearly increased with increasing height up to 20 meters above ground, beyond which the intensity of postural responses saturated. In contrast, anxiety was found to further increase with height and only saturated above 40 meters in non-acrophobic and 70 meters in acrophobic participants (Wühr et al. 2019) (Fig. 21.4). This difference in

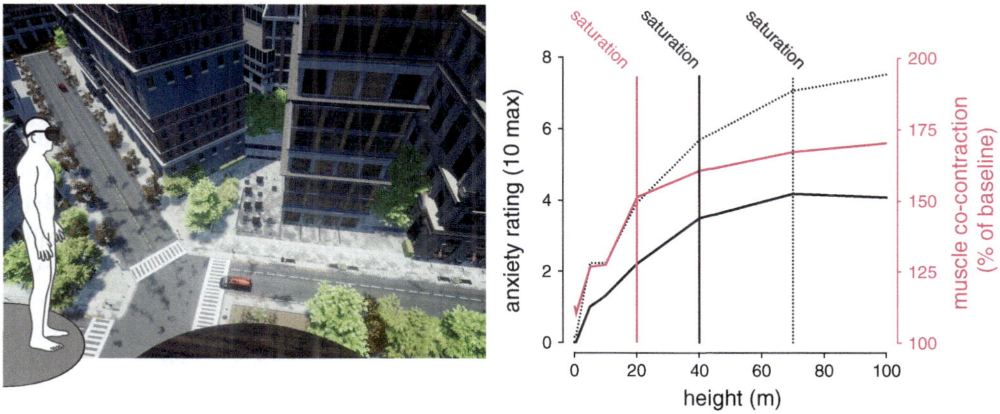

Fig. 21.4 The dependency of anxiety and postural responses on absolute height above ground as studied by using virtual reality technology. Left panel: exemplary view of the virtual scene at 40 meters above ground. Subjects were exposed to virtual heights ranging from 0 to 100 meters via a head-mounted display. Right panel: anxiety ratings (gray solid line: non-acrophobic individuals; gray dotted line: acrophobic individuals) initially increase with increasing height above ground but saturate for heights above 40 meters in non-acrophobic and heights above 70 meters in acrophobic individuals. In contrast, bodily responses, e.g., muscle co-contraction (pink solid line) saturate already for heights above 20 meters in both acrophobic and non-acrophobic individuals. (Modified from Wühr et al. 2019)

height dependency suggests a dissociation between sensorimotor and emotional reactions when confronted with heights.

21.6 Behavioral Recommendations for Prevention and Therapy of Visual Height Intolerance

Visual height intolerance and acrophobia are characterized by a dissociation between subjective fear and objective danger of falling. Although the affected individuals are able to recognize this discrepancy, they can typically overcome inappropriate avoidance behavior only with difficulty. The above-discussed experiments allow recommendation guidelines for coping strategies to avoid or minimize visual height intolerance and acrophobia under natural stimulus height conditions (Table 21.1). The recommendations for visual and positional behavior are based on the stimulus characteristics required for optimal visual and somatosensory contribution to postural balance (Brandt et al. 1980). The efficacy of cognitive dual tasking has been revealed in susceptible individuals during height exposure (Schniepp et al. 2014; Wühr et al. 2014). Attentional distraction was also shown to improve performance of postural balance in non-susceptible individuals (Johnson et al. 2020). With respect to psychotherapy, most studies and reviews emphasize that behavioral therapy and its sub-form cognitive behavioral therapy can be effective in the treatment of specific phobias such as acrophobia (Brandt and Huppert 2014). In particular, exposure therapy approaches for fear of heights are based on the assumption that anxiety and behavioral responses to fear-related stimuli will attenuate within the course of repeated exposures (Abelson and Curtis 1989).

Psychotherapy for acrophobia and also for agoraphobia is dominated by behavioral therapy approaches, which can be classified as either systematic or in vivo desensibilization strategies; "virtual reality" exposure is also used (Pull 2005). The method of systematic desensibilization (Wolpe 1958) is based on the creation of a graduated hierarchy of visual scenes that cause anxiety. These scenes are then presented to the patients during a period of calm after they have "absolved a training phase of muscle relaxation." In vivo desensibilization procedures, in which anxiety is supposed to be reduced during provoking situations that are close to life and not imagined, are, however, more effective. The stepwise approach ("successive approximation") to the fear-inducing situation is supported by instructions and reinforcement. So-called contact desensibilization (Ritter 1969) especially stresses the advantages of the therapist's participation and physical nearness, which serves as a model for the patient ("participant modelling") during the graduated approach to situations triggering height vertigo. An alternative method is the patient's in vivo confrontation with the strongest provoking situation for as long as possible, so-called flooding. There are first indications that glucocorticoids can improve psychotherapy for "fear removal" in cases of acrophobia (de Quervain et al. 2011). Cumulative histories of anxiety neurosis patients with phobias show that even without psychotherapy, most childhood phobias and 40–60% of adult phobias improve spontaneously or resolve after an interval of 5–6 years (Agras et al. 1972; Noyes et al. 1980).

A behavioral treatment approach is in line with therapeutic approaches already used by J.W. von Goethe (1771) in the 18th century. In the ninth book of the "Straßburger Tischgesellschaft, Selbsterziehung," he describes how he successfully treated his acrophobia by climbing up daily to the top of the "Straßburger Münster." His technique can be defined as a self-controlled in vivo desensibilization between "successive approximation" and "flooding." Whereas there is broad evidence that repeated confrontation with real or virtual fear-inducing height stimuli can result in a rapid remission of anxiety and autonomic responses in afflicted individuals, recent studies indicate that threat-induced changes in balance regulation may largely persist across repeated exposures to heights (Arroll et al. 2017; Wühr et al. 2019). Finally, while a wide range of therapies have been proven effective in the short-term, therapeutic improvements do not persist in the long-term in most cases (Wang 1997; Vervliet et al. 2013).

References

Abelson JL, Curtis GC (1989) Cardiac and neuroendocrine responses to exposure therapy in height phobics: desynchrony within the "physiological response system". Behav Res Ther 27:561–567

Agras WS, Sylvester D, Oliveau DC (1969) The epidemiology of common fears and phobia. Compr Psychiatry 10:151–156

Agras WS, Chapin HN, Oliveau DC (1972) The natural history of phobia. Arch Gen Psychiatry 26: 315–317

Arroll B, Wallace HB, Mount V, Humm SP, Kingsford D (2017) A systematic review and meta-analysis of treatment for acrophobia. Med J Aust 206:263–267

Bauer M, Huppert D, Brandt T (2012) Fear of heights in ancient China. J Neurol 259:2223–2225

Becker ES, Rinck M, Türke V, Kause P, Goodwin R, Neumer S, Markgraf J (2007) Epidemiology of specific phobia subtypes: findings from the Dresden mental health study. Eur Psychiatry 22:69–74

Best C, Eckhardt-Henn A, Tschan R, Bense S, Dieterich M (2009a) Psychiatric morbidity and comorbidity in different vestibular vertigo syndrome: results of a prospective longitudinal study over one year. J Neurol 256(1):58–65

Best C, Eckhardt-Henn A, Tschan R, Dieterich M (2009b) Who is a risk for psychiatric distressed after vestibular disorder? – results from a prospective one-year follow-up. Neuroscience 164(4):1579–1587

Bles W, Kapteyn TS, Brandt T, Arnold F (1980) the mechanism of physiological height vertigo: II. Posturography. Acta Otolaryngol (Stockh) 89:534–540

Blumenthal H, Leen-Feldner EW, Frala JL, Badour CL, Ham LS (2010) Social anxiety and motives for alcohol use among adolescents. Psychol Addict Behav 24:529–534

Boffino CC, Cardoso de Sá CS, Gorenstein C, Brown RG, Basile LFH, Ramos RT (2009) Fear of heights: cognitive performance and postural control. Eur Arch Psychiatry Clin Neurosci 259:114–119

Brandt T, Dieterich M (2020) “Excess anxiety” and “less anxiety”: both depend on vestibular function. Curr Opin Neurol 33:136–141

Brandt T, Huppert D (2014) Fear of heights and visual height intolerance. Curr Opin Neurol 27:111–117

Brandt T, Arnold F, Bles W, Kapteyn TS (1980) The mechanism of physiological height vertigo: I theoretical approach and psychophysics. Acta Otolaryngol (Stockh) 89:513–523

Brandt T, Strupp M, Huppert D (2012a) Height intolerance – an underrated threat. J Neuro 259:759–760

Brandt T, Benson J, Huppert D (2012b) What to call “non-phobic” fear of heights? Br J Psychiatry 190:81

Brandt T, Kugler G, Schniepp R, Wuehr M, Huppert D (2015) Acrophobia impairs visual exploration and balance during standing and walking. Ann N Y Acad Sci 1343:37–48

Brandt T, Grill E, Strupp M, Huppert D (2018) Susceptibility of fear of heights in bilateral vestibulopathy and other disorders of vertigo and balance. Front Neurol 9:406

Brown LA, Gage WH, Ploych MA, Sleik RJ, Winder TR (2002) Central set influences on gait. Exp Brain Res 145:286–296

Buckner JD, Matthews RA (2012) Social impressions while drinking account for the relationship between alcohol-related problems and social anxiety. Addict Behav 37:533–536

Carpenter MG, Frank JS, Silcher CP, Peysar GW (2001) The influence of postural threat on the control of upright stance. Exp Brain Res 138:210–218

Cleworth TW, Horslen BC, Carpenter MG (2012) Influence of real and virtual heights on standing balance. Gait Posture 36:172–176

Cleworth TW, Adkin AL, Allum JHJ, Inglis JT, Chua R, Carpenter MG (2019) Postural threat modulates perceptions of balance-related movement during support surface rotations. Neuroscience 404:413–422

Cohen DC (1977) Comparison of self-report and overt-behavioral procedures for assessing acrophobia. Behav Ther 8:17–23

Curtis GC, Magee WJ, Eaton WW, Wittchen HU (1998) Specific fears and phobias. Epidemiology and classification. Br J Psychiatry 173:212–217

De Quervain DJ, Bentz D, Michael T, Bolt OC, Wiederhold BK, Margraf J, Wilhelm FH (2011) Glucocorticoids enhance extinction-based psychotherapy. Proc Natl Acad Sci 108:6621–6625

Decker J, Limburg K, Henningsen P, Lahmann C, Brandt T, Dieterich M (2019) Intact vestibular function is relevant for anxiety related vertigo. J Neurol 266:S89–S92

Delbaere K, Sturnieks DL, Crombez G, Lord SR (2009) Concern about falls elicits changes in gait parameters in conditions of postural threat in older people. J Gerontol A Biol Sci Med Sci 64: 237–242

Depla MF, ten Have ML, van Balkom AJ, de Graaf R (2008) Specific fears and phobias in the general population: results from the Netherlands mental health survey and incidence study (NEMESIS). Soc Psychiatry Psychiatr Epidemiol 43:200–208

Grill E, Schäffler F, Huppert D, Müller M, Kapfhammer HP, Brandt T (2014) Self-efficacy beliefs are associated with visual height intolerance: a cross-sectional survey. PLoS One 9(12):e116220

Hilber P, Cendelin J, Le Gall L, Machado ML, Tuma J, Besnard S (2019) Cooperation of the vestibular and cerebellar networks in anxiety disorders and depression. Prog Neuropsycholpharmacol Biol Psychiatry 89:310–321

Horslen BC, Dakin CJ, Inglis JT, Blouin JS, Carpenter MG (2014) Modulation of human vestibular reflexes with increased postural threat. J Physiol 592:3671–3685

Huppert D, Brandt T (2015) Fear of heights and visual height intolerance in children 8 to 10 years. J Child Adolesc Behav 3:219

Huppert D, Brandt T (2018) Dizziness and vertigo syndromes viewed with a historical eye. J Neurol 265:127–133

Huppert DK, Grill E, Kapfhammer HP, Brandt T (2013a) Fear of heights and mild visual height intolerance independent of alcohol consumption. Brain Behav 3:596–601

Huppert D, Grill E, Brandt T (2013b) Down on heights? One in three has visual height intolerance. J Neurol 260:597–604

Huppert D, Benson J, Krammling B, Brandt T (2013c) Fear of heights in Roman antiquity and mythology. J Neurol 260:2430–2432

Huppert D, Grill E, Brandt T (2017) A new questionnaire for estimating the severity of visual height intolerance and acrophobia by a metric interval scale. Front Neurol 8:211

Huppert D, Wuehr M, Brandt T (2020) Acrophobia and visual height intolerance: advances in epidemiology and mechanisms. J Neurol 267 (Suppl 1): 231–240

Johnson KJ, Watson AM, Tokuno CD, Carpenter MG, Adkin AL (2020) The effects of distraction on threat-related changes in standing balance control. Neurosci Lett 716:134635

Kapfhammer HP, Huppert D, Grill E, Fitz W, Brandt T (2015) Visual height intolerance and acrophobia: clinical characteristics and comorbidity patterns. Eur Arch Psychiatry Clin Neurosci 265:375–385

Kapfhammer HP, Fitz W, Huppert D, Grill E, Brandt T (2016) Visual height intolerance and acrophobia: distressing partners for life. J Neurol 263: 1946–1953

Kilpatrick JW (1893) Feigned death in snakes. Science 22:208–209

Kugler G, Huppert D, Schneider E, Brandt T (2014a) Fear of heights freezes gaze to the horizon. J Vestib Res 24:433–441

Kugler G, Huppert D, Eckl M, Schneider E, Brandt T (2014b) Visual exploration during locomotion limited by fear of heights. PLoS One 9(8):e105906

Lahmann C, Henningsen P, Brandt T, Strupp M, Jahn K, Dieterich M, Eckhardt-Henn A, Feuerecker R, Dinkel A, Schmid G (2015) Psychiatric comorbidity and psychosocial impairment among patients with vertigo and dizziness. J Neurol Neurosurg Psychiatry 86:302–308

LeBeau RT, Glenn D, Liao B, Wittchen HU, Beesdo-Baum K, Ollendick T, Craske MG (2010) Specific phobia: a review of DSM-IV specific phobia and preliminary recommendations for DSM-V. Depress Anxiety 27:148–167

Lim SB, Cleworth TW, Horslen BC, Blouin JS, Inglis JT, Carpenter MG (2017) Postural threat influences vestibular-evoked muscular responses. J Neurophysiol 117:604–611

MacDonald R, Crum RM, Storr CL, Schuster A, Bienvenu OJ (2011) Sub-clinical anxiety and the onset of alcohol use disorders: longitudinal associations from the Baltimore ECA follow-up, 1981–2004. J Addict Dis 30:45–53

Morris EP, Stewart SH, Ham LS (2005) The relationship between social anxiety disorder and alcohol use disorders: a critical review. Clin Psychol Rev 25:734–760

Noyes R, Clancy J, Hoenk PR, Slymen DJ (1980) The prognosis of anxiety neurosis of anxiety neurosis. Arch Gen Psychiatry 37:173–178

Oosterink F, de Jongh A, Hoogstraten J (2009) Prevalence of dental fear and phobia relative to other fear and phobia types. Eur J Oral Sci 117:135–143

Pull CB (2005) Current status of virtual reality exposure therapy in anxiety disorders: editorial review. Curr Opin Psychiatry 18:7–14

Ritter B (1969) Treatment of acrophobia with contact desensibilisation. Behav Res Ther 7:41–45

Schäffler F, Müller M, Huppert D, Brandt T, Tiffe T, Grill E (2014) Consequences of visual height intolerance for quality of life: a qualitative study. Qual Life Res 23:697–705

Schlick C, Schniepp R, Loidl V, Wuehr M, Hesselbarth K, Jahn K (2015) Falls and fear of falling in vertigo and balance disorders: a controlled cross-sectional study. J Vestib Res 25:241–251

Schneier FR, Foose TE, Hasin DS, Heimberg RG, Liu SM, Grant BF, Blanco C (2010) Social anxiety disorder and alcohol use disorder co-morbidity in the National Epidemiologic Survey on alcohol and related conditions. Psychol Med 40:977–988

Schniepp R, Kugler G, Wuehr M, Eckl M, Huppert D, Pradhan C, Huth S, Jahn K, Brandt T (2014) Quantification of gait changes in subjects with visual height intolerance when exposed to heights. Front Hum Neurosci 8:963

Steinman SA, Teachman BA (2011) Cognitive processing and acrophobia: validating the heights interpretation questionnaire. J Anxiety Disord 25: 896–902

Stinson FS, Dawson DA, Patricia Chou S, Smith S, Goldstein RB, June Ruan W, Grant BF (2007) The epidemiology of DSM-IV specific phobia in the USA: result from the National Epidemiology Survey on alcohol and related conditions. Psychol Med 37:1047–1059

Tersteeg MC, Marple-Horvat DE, Loram ID (2012) Cautious gait in relation to knowledge and vision of height: is altered visual information the dominant influence? J Neurophysiol 107:2686–2691

Vervliet B, Craske MG, Hermans D (2013) Fear extinction and relapse: state of the art. Annu Rev Clin Psychol 9:215–248

von Goethe JW (1771) In: Selbstbiographische Schriften, Dichtung und Wahrheit. 9. Buch der Straßburger Tischgesellschaft, Selbsterziehung

Walk RD, Gibson EJ, Tighe TJ (1957) Behaviour of light- and dark-raised rats on a visual cliff. Science 126:80–81

Wang H (ed) (1997) Huangdi neijing yanjiu dacheng (the great compendium of the research on the Huangdi Neijing). Beijing chubanshe, Beijing

Wolpe J (1958) Psychotherapy by reciprocal inhibition. Stanford University Press, Stanford

World Health Organisation (1993) The ICD-10 classification of mental and behavioral disorders, clinical description and diagnostic guidelines. WHO, Geneva

Wühr M, Kugler G, Schniepp R, Eckl M, Pradhan C, Jahn K, Huppert D, Brandt T (2014) Balance control and anti-gravity muscle activity during the experience of fear at heights. Physiol Rep 2(2):e00232

Wühr M, Breitkopf K, Decker J, Ibarra G, Huppert D, Brandt T (2019) Fear of heights in virtual reality saturates 20 to 40 m above ground. J Neurol 266:80–87

Zaback M, Cleworth TW, Carpenter MG, Adkin AL (2015) Personality traits and individual differences predict threat-induced changes in postural control. Hum Mov Sci 40:393–409

Cervical Dizziness

Contents

M. Strupp et al., *Vertigo and Dizziness*, https://doi.org/10.1007/978-3-030-78260-3_22

Cervical vertigo (or better: dizziness since it is not a spinning vertigo) is the subject of long-standing interdisciplinary debate, in particular concerning its various forms and pathomechanisms (Brandt 1996; Brandt and Bronstein 2001; Hain 2015; Li and Peng 2015; Knapstad et al. 2019; Reiley et al. 2017; Seemungal et al. 2022). Many definitions have been given for cervical vertigo/dizziness, some of which require pain and some of which do not.

It is well recognized that somatosensory signals from musculotendinous receptors in the neck provide accurate kinesthetic feedback of head movements. These signals contribute to the perception of head motion and self-motion during active locomotion by converging with vestibular and visual input.

The difficulty of clinical evaluation is based on:

- Insufficient pathophysiological knowledge of function and multimodal interaction of the sensory signals from the neck afference
- The existing confusion about the concept of so-called cervical vertigo

The neural connections between the neck receptors and the central vestibular system – the cervico-ocular reflex and the neck reflexes for postural control – have been investigated experimentally in animals (Igarashi et al. 1972; de Jong et al. 1977), however, so far without convincing clinical relevance (Peng 2018). Unilateral surgical deafferentation of C1 to C3 in the squirrel monkey and in the cat and local suboccipital anesthesia in the rhesus monkey (Cohen 1961) resulted in a locomotor ataxia. Local anesthesia of posturolateral neck tissue in humans elicited an increased ipsilateral and decreased contralateral extensor muscle tone; the subjects showed a tendency to fall, gait deviation, and past pointing toward the anesthetized side (Barre 1926; Hinoki and Kurosawa 1964; de Jong et al. 1977). These findings were confirmed in patients with cervical headache after unilateral therapeutic anesthetic C2 neck blockades: no specific abnormalities could be established in these patients by posturographic tests, subjective visual vertical measurements, or eye movement recordings (Dieterich et al. 1993). The only small and transient disturbances of ipsilateral gait deviation can be due to the minor contribution of the cervico-ocular reflex in subjects with an intact peripheral vestibular system (with a gain of 0.1–0.2 as compared to 1.0 of the vestibulo-ocular reflex). However, when vestibular sensitivity decreases, as in patients with bilateral vestibulopathy, the cervico-ocular reflex becomes more sensitive and more important to compensate for the vestibular loss.

It is difficult to apply these findings to patients with occipital neck/head pain who complain about postural and gait imbalance, because the diagnosis cannot yet be confirmed. The earlier recommended neck-turning test alone with the examination of the static cervico-ocular reflex or Romberg's test of stance while the patient leans his head backward is non-specific and insufficiently standardized (de Jong and Bles 1986). It was shown, for example, that turning the trunk under the fixed head induces nystagmus in patients with a cervical syndrome as often as it does in healthy controls (Holtmann et al. 1993). Optimistic reports that cannot be confirmed by the current literature on the frequency of cervical vertigo and the "fantastic" successes achieved by chiropractic treatment must be carefully assessed. They may, for instance, represent a liberatory maneuver in patients with BPPV.

Somatosensors in the muscles, joints, and skin can also induce sensations of self-motion and trigger nystagmus. Vision satisfactorily substitutes for sensory loss caused by disorders such as polyneuropathy, bilateral vestibular loss, or spinal cord diseases, and thus ensures spatial orientation and postural control in the day time; however, in darkness or under poor visual conditions, disturbed proprioception typically causes postural dizziness. There is, therefore, also a somatosensory dizziness which may manifest with a distressing perception of swaying, dizziness, postural and gait imbalance, and instability.

The mostly controversial debate about the reality or fiction of cervical dizziness resembles a "war between believers and doubters," lacking any corresponding practical significance. The cervical syndrome is treated by drugs and physical therapy, and once other causes and a bilateral vestibulopathy (▶ Chap. 7) are excluded, the hypothetical neurophysiological explanation mentioned above is still mainly only of theoretical significance (Brandt and Bronstein 2001).

22.1 Head Motion-Induced Cervical Split-Second Vertigo

The above scientific discourse focused on the missing clinical or experimental relevance of an acute neck pain syndrome associated with a longer-lasting spinning vertigo or balance disorder. In the initial phase, however, of an acute cervical syndrome with a restricted mobility of head vs. trunk movements, rapid voluntary head movements often elicit spells of cervical vertigo/dizziness or seemingly body pushes sometimes causing postural instability for fractions of a second (Brandt and Huppert 2016). Their clinical relevance is moderate; they require no particular treatment since there is a spontaneous remission within days. Some patients spontaneously complain of this kind of "cervical split-second vertigo," but it is often only reported after the physician has asked specifically about it. The symptoms are described as apparently involuntary body perturbations or tilts, or apparent movements of the surroundings only elicited by rapid – not by slow – head movements that are hindered by a painful blocking of head rotations.

The sensorimotor mechanism for the perception of space constancy during active movements described by von Holst and Mittelstaedt (1950) may serve as a hypothetical mechanism of this type of cervical vertigo/dizziness: the efference copy and the reafference principle. This led to many theoretical and experimental publications of the so-called internal model theory (Wolpert et al. 1995; Blakemore et al. 2002). If one applies this principle to our patients, the expected reafference of an intended head rotation may fail to correspond to the pattern of sensory input calibrated by earlier experience of head motions (◘ Fig. 22.1). This mismatch occurs when the actual movement falls shorter than the expected movement because of the painful neck muscle stiffness (Brandt and Huppert 2016). Either the attacks remit spontaneously when the patient recovers from the neck pain syndrome or, if the syndrome becomes chronic, then the actual and expected head motion-induced reafferent input is gradually readjusted.

22.2 Vertebral Artery Compression/Occlusion Syndrome

There is a rare but clinically most relevant and well-defined vascular form of cervical vertigo in which head rotation causes a symptomatic compression or even occlusion of the dominant vertebral artery: vertebral compression/occlusion syndrome, also known as Bow Hunter's syndrome (Kuether et al. 1997; Vilela et al. 2005; Brandt and Baloh 2005; Kim et al. 2022). Despite its rareness, there are three good reasons to address this syndrome within a separate section:

1. The initial manifestation is characterized by spinning vertigo and nystagmus elicited by head rotation to one side in the yaw plane.
2. There is a danger of impending, life-threatening vertebrobasilar infarcts.

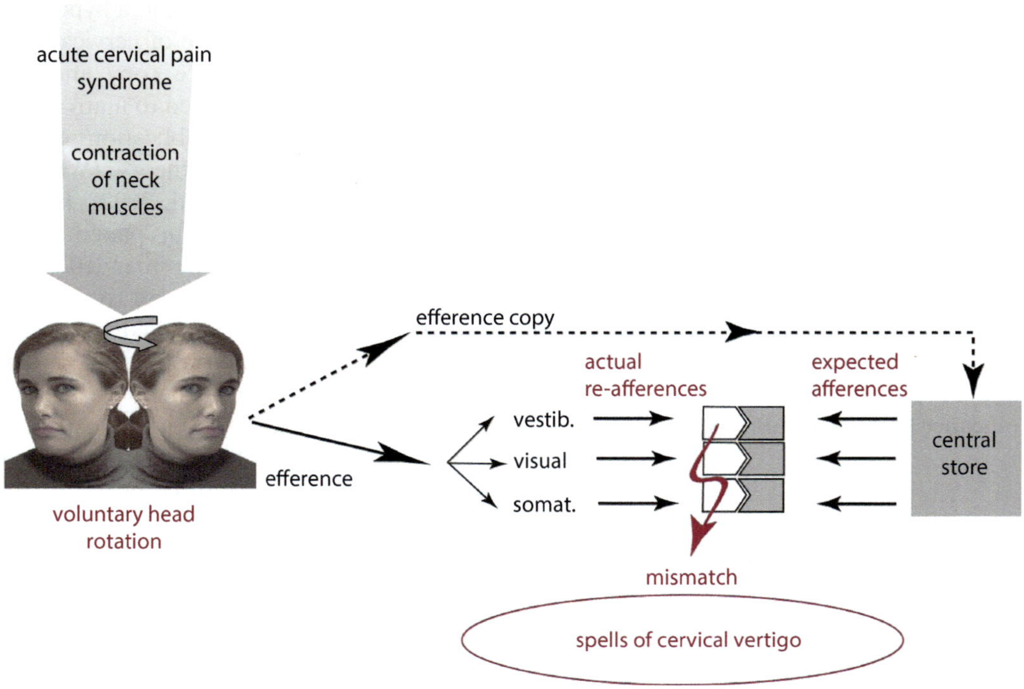

Fig. 22.1 Pathophysiological model of head motion-induced cervical vertigo push. Schematic diagram showing how neck muscle stiffness can cause a sensorimotor disarrangement with dizzy spells of apparent body motion and instability (bottom). In a "neural mismatch concept," cervical vertigo is caused by a mismatch of the efference-copy signal about the intended head rotation and the actual reafference. Active head rotation leads to stimulation of musculotendinous neck receptors, the messages of which correspond with the pattern of expected somatosensory visual and vestibular signals because of earlier sensorimotor experience of head movements (central store or internal model). The pattern of sensory expectation is released by the efference-copy signal. The efference-copy signal is emitted simultaneously with the efference signal to the neck muscles for the intended movement impulse. If the head movement is smaller than intended due to stiffness of the neck muscles, the reafference signal is smaller than required, resulting in a sensorimotor mismatch. Then head movements may be erroneously perceived as external perturbations causing a distressing short push of postural imbalance. Somat. somatosensory, Vestib. vestibular. (From Brandt and Huppert 2016)

3. It can be efficiently cured by surgical decompression in the majority of cases (Rastogi et al. 2015; Duan et al. 2016; Strickland et al. 2017).

Most patients afflicted with this condition exhibit a stenosis or vessel malformation (e.g., hypoplasia or termination in the posterior inferior cerebellar artery) of the vertebral artery on the same side as the precipitating horizontal head rotation. Thus, the major blood supply of the vertebrobasilar territory depends on the "dominant" contralateral vertebral artery. A head rotation in the yaw plane toward the nondominant artery can then compress the dominant vertebral artery usually at the atlantoaxial C1 - C2 level (Rastogi et al. 2015; Duan et al. 2016). The most frequent causes of a susceptibility of vertebral arteries to become mechanically compressed during head rotation are due to muscular and tendinous insertions, osteophytes, and degenerative changes resulting from cervical spondylosis, particularly at the atlantoaxial joint, but also less frequently at other levels of the cervical column (Duan et al. 2016), or vascular reasons such as aneurysms or arterial dissections (Rastogi et al. 2015; Xue et al. 2020). The key symptom is a severe rotational vertigo elicited by a prolonged horizontal head rotation which rapidly abates when the head is rotated back to its normal position. During the vertigo attack, a downbeating nystagmus has been repeatedly observed, which is the reason why an ischemic dysfunction of the brainstem (Rosengart et al. 1993) or of caudal cerebellar midline structures (Iida et al. 2018) was assumed. More accurate analyses of the nystagmus in the attack disclosed a mixed spinning-linear downbeat nystagmus with an initial horizontal component toward the compressed vertebral artery which reversed its direction with maintenance of the precipitating head rotation (Strupp et al. 2000; Choi et al. 2005). The direction of the initial nystagmus and its directional reversal are best explained by a transient ischemia of the labyrinth on the side of the compressed artery, in particular the anterior and horizontal semicircular canals, and the cochlea with an associated tinnitus. The initial signs and symptoms reflect an excitation by depolarization (causing transient hyperexcitability with ectopic discharges). If the ischemia lasts longer, the membrane potential depolarizes further, and the axonal membrane can no longer be excited (Strupp et al. 2000). This kind of pathophysiological sequence of events is typical but not specific for the syndrome (Strupp et al. 2000; Choi et al. 2005; Brandt and Baloh 2005), and in severe cases, ischemia of the brainstem will certainly cause other additional central signs and symptoms.

Although a tentative diagnosis of vertebral artery compression can be made by transcranial Doppler sonography, digital dynamic angiography is still the gold standard to secure the diagnosis (Rastogi et al. 2015; Duan et al. 2016). Depending on the severity and in particular the cause, therapy comprises conservative, surgical, or endovascular interventions (Duan et al. 2016). Surgical decompression is the primary treatment approach for patients with a bony compression of the vertebral artery (Rastogi et al. 2015). Different surgical approaches, anterior vs. posterior decompressions with or without fusions of the vertebrae, have been described, but proof that one is the superior method is still lacking (Strickland et al. 2017); the risk of injury to the vertebral artery is possibly lower in anterior decompressions (Schunemann et al. 2018).

References

Barre JA (1926) Sur une syndrome sympathique cervical posterieur et sa cause frequente: l'arthrte cervicale. Rev Neurol 45:1246–1253

Blakemore SJ, Wolpert DM, Frith CD (2002) Abnormalities in the awareness of action. Trends Cogn Sci 6:237–242

Brandt T (1996) Cervical vertigo – reality or fiction? Audiol Neurootol 1:187–196

Brandt T, Baloh RW (2005) Rotational vertebral artery occlusion. A clinical entity or various syndromes? Neurology 65:1156–1157

Brandt T, Bronstein AM (2001) Cervical vertigo. J Neurol Neurosurg Psychiatry 71:8–12

Brandt T, Huppert D (2016) A new type of cervical vertigo: head motion-induced spells in acute neck pain. Neurology 86:974–975

Choi KD, Shin HY, Kim JS et al (2005) Rotational vertebral artery syndrome: oculographic analysis of nystagmus. Neurology 65:1287–1290

Cohen LA (1961) Role of eye and neck proprioceptive mechanisms in body orientation and motor coordination. J Neurophysiol 24:1–11

De Jong JMBV, Bles W (1986) Cervical dizziness and ataxia. In: Bles W, Brandt T (eds) Disorders of posture and gait. Elsevier, Amsterdam, New York, Oxford, pp 185–206

De Jong PTVM, de Jong JMBV, Cohen B, Jongkees LBW (1977) Ataxia and nystagmus induced by injection of local anesthetics in the neck. Ann Neurol 1:240–246

Dieterich M, Pöllmann W, Pfaffenrath V (1993) Cervicogenic headache: electronystagmography, perception of verticality and posturography in patients before and after C2-blockade. Cephalalgia 13:285–288

Duan G, Xu J, Shi J, Cao Y (2016) Advances in the pathogenesis, diagnosis and treatment of Bow Hunter's syndrome: a comprehensive review of the literature. Intervent Neurol 5:29–38

Hain TC (2015) Cervicogenic causes of vertigo. Curr Opin Neurol 28:69–73

Hinoki M, Kurosawa R (1964) Studies on vertigo provoked by neck and nape muscles. Notes on vertigo of cervical origin Some observations on vertiginous attacks caused by injection of procaine solution into neck and nape muscles in man. Oto Rhino Laryngol Clin (Kyoto) 57:10–20

Holtmann S, Reiman V, Schöps P (1993) Clinical significance of cervico-ocular reactions. Laryngorhinootologie 72:306–310

Igarashi M, Miyata H, Alford BR, Wright WK (1972) Nystagmus after experimental cervical lesions. Laryngoscope 82(9):1609–1621

Iida Y, Murata H, Johkura K, Higashida T, Tanaka T, Tateishi K (2018) Bow Hunter's syndrome by nondominant vertebral artery compression: a case report, literature review, and significance of downbeat nystagmus as the diagnostic clue. World Neurosurg 111:367–372

Kim JS, Newman-Toker DE, Kerber KA, Jahn K, Bertholon P, Waterston J, Lee H, Bisdorff A, Strupp M (2022) Vascular vertigo and dizziness: Diagnostic criteria. J Vestib Res 32:(3)205−222

Knapstad MK, Nordahl SHG, Goplen FK (2019) Clinical characteristics in patients with cervicogenic dizziness: a systematic review. Health Sci Rep 2(9):e134

Kuether T, Nesbit GM, Clark WM, Barnwell SL (1997) Rotational vertebral artery occlusion: a mechanism of vertebrobasilar insufficiency. Neurosurgery 41:427–432

Li Y, Peng B (2015) Pathogenesis, diagnosis, and treatment of cervical vertigo. Pain Physician 18:E583–E595

Peng B (2018) Cervical vertigo: historical reviews and advances. World Neurosurg 109:347–350

Rastogi V, Rawls A, Moore O, Victoria B, Khan S, Saravanapavan P, Midivelli S, Raviraj P, Khanna A, Bidari S, Hedna VS (2015) Rare etiology of Bow Hunter's syndrome and systematic review of literature. J Vasc Interv Neurol 8:7–16

Reiley AS, Vickory FM, Funderburg SE, Cesario RA, Clendanial RA (2017) How to diagnose cervicogenic dizziness. Arch Physiother 7:12. https://doi.org/10.1186/s40945-017-0040-x

Rosengart A, Hedges TR, Teal PA et al (1993) Intermittent downbeat nystagmus due to vertebral artery compression. Neurology 43:216–218

Schunemann V, Kim J, Dornbos D 3rd, Nimjee SM (2018) C2-C3 anterior cervical arthrodesis in the treatment of Bow Hunter's syndrome: case report and review of the literature. World Neurosurg 118:284–289

Seemungal BM, Agrawal Y, Bisdorff A, Bronstein A, Cullen KE, Goadsby PJ, Lempert T, Kothari S, Lim PB, Magnusson M, Marcus HJ, Strupp M, Whitney SL (2022) The Barany Society position on 'Cervical Dizziness'. J Vestib Res 32(6):487−499

Strickland BA, Pham MH, Bakhsheshian J, Russin JJ, Mack WJ, Acosta FL (2017) Bow Hunter's syndrome: surgical management (video) and review of the literature. World Neurosurg 103:953.e7–953.e12. https://doi.org/10.1016/j.wneu.2017.04.101

Strupp M, Planck JH, Arbusow V, Steiger H-J, Brückmann H, Brandt T (2000) Rotational vertebral artery occlusion syndrome with vertigo due to "labyrinthine excitation". Neurology 54:1376–1379

Vilela MD, Goodkin R, Lundin DA, Newll DW (2005) Rotational vertebrobasilar ischemia: hemodynamic assessment and surgical treatment. Neurosurgery 56:36–45

von Holst E, Mittelstaedt H (1950) Das Reafferenzprinzip (Wechselwirkung zwischen Zentralnervensystem und Peripherie). Naturwissenschaften 37:464–476

Wolpert DM, Ghahramani Z, Jordan MI (1995) An internal model for sensorimotor integration. Science 269:1880–1882

Xue S, Shi H, Du X, Ma X (2020) Bow Hunter's syndrome combined with ipsilateral vertebral artery dissection/pseudoaneurysm: case study and literature review. Br J Neurosurg. https://doi.org/10.1080/02688697.2020.1718604

A Historical View of Vertigo, Dizziness, and Balance Disorders

Contents

M. Strupp et al., *Vertigo and Dizziness*, https://doi.org/10.1007/978-3-030-78260-3_23

23.1 Synopsis

This chapter deals with etymological aspects of various terms and definitions of dizziness and vertigo and some probably first descriptions of symptoms, syndromes, and disorders. Looking to history discloses linguistic, cultural, and medical details which fascinate and illuminate our current understanding of vertigo, dizziness, and balance disorders, a major medical complaint on all continents since antiquity (Huppert and Brandt 2018).

Seasickness, fear of heights, and adverse effects of alcohol were the major areas where descriptions of vertigo and dizziness were found in Roman, Greek, and Chinese texts from about 730 BC to 600 AD. A few detailed accounts were suggestive of specific vestibular disorders such as Menière's attacks (*Huangdi Neijing, the Yellow Thearch's Classic of Internal Medicine*) or vestibular migraine (Aretaeus of Cappadocia). Further, the etymological and metaphorical meanings of the terms and their symptoms provide fascinating historical insights, e.g., Vespasian's feelings of dizzy exultations when becoming emperor (69 AD) after Nero's suicide or the figurative meaning of German "Schwindel" (vertigo) derived from English "swindle" to express "financial fraud" in the eighteenth century (Huppert and Brandt 2018).

The growth of knowledge of the vestibular system and its functions began primarily in the nineteenth century. Erasmus Darwin, however, was ahead of his times. His work *Zoonomia, or the Laws of Organic Life*, in 1794 described new dizziness syndromes and concepts of sensorimotor control, including the mechanism of fear of heights, and made early observations on positional alcohol vertigo. The latter is beautifully illustrated by the German poet and cartoonist Wilhelm Busch (1832–1908), who also documented the alleviating effect of the "morning after drink" (Fig. 23.3). The mechanism underlying positional alcohol vertigo, i.e., the differential gravities of alcohol and endolymph, was discovered later in the nineteenth century. The first textbook on Neurology (*Lehrbuch der Nervenkrankheiten des Menschen*, 1840) by Moritz Romberg contained general descriptions of signs and symptoms of various conditions with the key symptom of vertigo, but no definition of vestibular disorders. Our current knowledge of vestibular function and disorders dates back to the seminal work of a group of nineteenth-century scientists, e.g., Jan Evangelista Purkinje, Ernst Mach, Josef Breuer, Hermann Helmholtz, and Alexander Crum-Brown (Henn and Young 1975; Cohen 1984; Brandt 1991; Wade and Tatler 2005).

When searching historical texts dating from antiquity for the terms vertigo and dizziness, it is necessary and useful to consider their etymological meanings.

23.2 Etymology

Latin, for example, has at least two source words to describe the condition vertigo. "Vertigo" in Latin refers to turning, spinning, and rotating, and is derived from the verb "vertere," meaning to turn. Another word "caligo" means darkening of the eyes, funereal crepe, and dizziness. It and not the word "vertigo" appears in ancient text passages referring to heights ("altitudo") and symptoms of fear of heights (Georges 2010; Huppert et al. 2013). The word "caligo" was also used metaphorically for dizziness arising from feelings of exultation or for being overwhelmed and losing one's grip on reality. For example, Tacitus in his work *Historiae* describes how Vespasian wanted to become Emperor himself after Nero's suicide: he is said to have felt dizzy when the soldiers addressed him as "Emperor" and used other high-ranking titles (Huppert et al. 2013; Brandt and Huppert 2014).

The Germanic languages also provide fascinating etymologies for words used to describe symptoms of dizziness. The word giddy is believed to be derived from the Old English word "gidig," meaning insane or, literally, possessed by a god. The *Oxford Dictionary of English* (Stevenson 2010) defines the word dizzy as "having or involving a sensation of spinning around and losing one's balance." It is said to originate in the Old English word "dysig," meaning foolish, and is thought to be related to Low German "dusig," meaning giddy, and Old High German "tusic," which translates as foolish or weak (Stapleton 2007). From the Proto-Germanic root "swimen," meaning to move to and fro, the various Indo-European languages developed words for the concepts: for example, Low German = "swajen" meaning to move to and fro as with the wind and Middle High German = "swimen" meaning to sway about; Old Norse = "svimi" meaning to swoon; Norwegian = "svime; svima" meaning to stagger; Dutch zwaaien = to sway about.

The development in English took an unexpected turn: from Old English = "swima" meaning "Schwindel" or from Old English "swäman" meaning "zwerven" to Middle English = "sweigh, sweye" meaning a sweeping or swinging motion. Modern English has derived "sway." Two Indo-European roots led to the development of two meanings in English: to sway and to swindle. In German, the original meaning led to the medical term "Schwindel." Apparently the second figurative meaning of "Betrug" (in English 'fraud') arose gradually from the sixteenth century on and was derived from the English "swindler" first appearing in the eighteenth century when German Jews in England began using the term "schwindel" (German pronunciation for English 'swindle') to express the concept of "financial fraud." By the nineteenth century, the meaning of "Betrug" for "Schwindel" was in use in German (Grimm and Grimm 1854; Kluge and Seebold 2002; Janz et al. 2003; Duden 2017; Huppert and Brandt 2018).

23.3 Definitions

The current medical definitions of vertigo, dizziness, and imbalance are based on the recommendations made by the Classification Committee of the International Bárány Society for Neuro-Otology. "Vertigo is the sensation of self-motion when no self-motion is occurring; dizziness is the sensation of disturbed or impaired spatial orientation without a false or distorted sense of motion; and imbalance or unsteadiness is the feeling of being unstable while sitting, standing, or walking without a particular directional preference" (Bisdorff et al. 2009). All three sensations can occur in peripheral, central, and higher vestibular disorders (Brandt and Dieterich 2017).

23.4 Seasickness/Motion Sickness

The ancient Romans/Greeks and Chinese were quite familiar with seasickness as witnessed by numerous descriptions of seasickness, its triggers, symptoms, and measures to prevent it. Body movements caused by waves were known to be the critical stimuli. Especially Greek and Roman texts evoke the roughness of seas and the unpleasantness of odors as major triggers, as well as symptoms of nausea, emesis, vertigo, anorexia, faintness, apathy, headache and impending doom. It was also widely known that other illnesses, a person's current mental state, and anxiety could precipitate seasickness but that experienced sailors were highly resistant (the influence of habituation) (Huppert et al. 2016, 2017). The Chinese had observed that children are particularly susceptible to motion sickness (Brandt et al. 2016). The Chinese also described different types of motion sickness, e.g., cart-sickness when traveling in carts or litter-sickness when being transported on a litter or in a sedan chair (Brandt et al. 2016).

Many Greek/Roman and Chinese sources emphasized the impact of seasickness on military actions, stressing such famous naval battles as the Battle of the

Red Cliff, which marked the end of the Han dynasty in China or – in later times – the defeat of the Spanish Armada by the English in 1588. A peculiar war-related form of motion sickness is associated with Napoleon's camel corps during the Egyptian campaign of 1798/1799, a sickness induced by riding on a camel (◘ Fig. 23.1), the "ship of the desert" (Huppert et al. 2017).

Therapeutic measures differed according to the culture (Karenberg 2009). The Western classics recommended looking at stationary contrasts on the coast, fasting or specific diets, pleasant fragrances, medicinal plants like white hellebore (containing various alkaloids but not scopolamine), or a mixture of wine and wormwood. In the East, more unusual measures were advocated, such as drinking the urine of young boys, swallowing white sand-syrup, collecting water drops from a bamboo stick, or hiding earth from the kitchen hearth under the hair (Huppert et al. 2016; Brandt et al. 2016; Huppert et al. 2017). One reason for these different therapeutic recommendations was obviously due to the different concepts of the underlying pathophysiology. The Greek view was based on the humoral theory of Empedocles and Aristotle which considered an imbalance of the four body fluids ("χολή" = yellow bile, "φλέγηα" = phlegm, "μέλαινα χολή" = black bile, "αἷμα" = blood; (Schöner 1964)) to be causative, whereas the medicine of correspondences in China attributed malfunctions to certain body substances and the life force 'Qi' (Wang 1997).

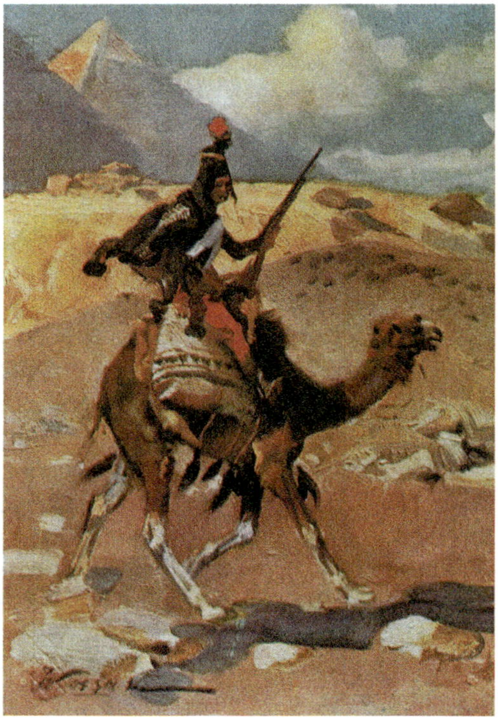

◘ **Fig. 23.1** Napoleon and the camel sickness. A soldier of Napoleon's camel (dromedary) regiment, initiated by Napoleon in 1799. Interestingly, the soldiers were considered infantry, because they dismounted to fight. Those who could not adapt to the movements of the "ship of the desert" became seasick, proving rather ineffective combatants (Un soldat du regiment dromedaries, by Wojciech Kossak, 1912; ▸ https://fr.wikipedia.org/wiki/Régiment-des-dromedares#/media/File:WKossak028.jpg)

23.5 Fear of Heights

Symptoms of fear of heights were described in ancient Roman/Greek and Chinese texts. European sources provide us with precise characterizations of the symptoms, such as worsening of eyesight and a feeling of uneasiness when walking over a bridge, the eyes being veiled with dizziness when standing on a high ladder, dizziness when gazing on high rocks, turning pale, trembling of the knees, and darkening of the eyes when looking from the heavens, or feeling dizzy when looking out high windows (Huppert et al. 2013). Chinese sources emphasize the effects of poor eyesight, confusion, and uncertainty. The Yellow Thearch observed that his fear of heights and anxiety when climbing up a watchtower were alleviated by kneeling (◘ Fig. 23.2). His observation that the severity of fear of heights depended on body position is well recognized today (Brandt et al. 1980; Bauer et al. 2012). While the Romans were aware of the triggering factor "visual height," the Chinese thought that it was the tempera-

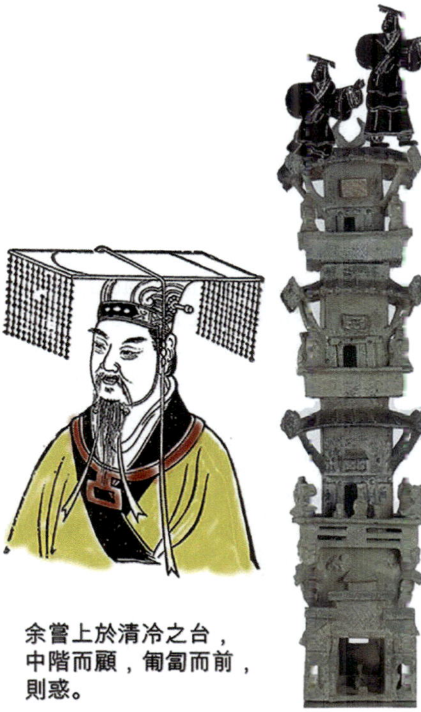

Fig. 23.2 A picture of the yellow thearch ("the yellow emperor") with a citation from the book Huangdi Neijing and a typical Chinese watchtower from the Han Dynasty, Henan Province, first to second century AD. The thearch suffered from severe symptoms of fear of heights whenever he climbed on a watchtower. He observed that he could alleviate these symptoms by kneeling down (Bauer et al 2012). This observation was later confirmed by psychophysical experiments of magnitude estimation of subjective fear of heights relative to body position (Brandt et al. 1980). Visual height intolerance is strongest during free erect stance when maintaining balance is most difficult; it becomes moderate, when the subject kneels

ture at heights which caused a "cold Qi" and was the provoking stimulus (Brandt and Huppert 2014).

23.6 Vertigo and Alcohol

Wine was an important beverage in Roman and Greek Antiquity. Mostly it was mixed with water, but mixtures with honey were also common. Thus, it is not surprising that the effects of alcohol intake were known and described in various ancient texts. In one of the first epic narrations of mankind, the *Iliad*, about 730 BC, Homer alludes to the physical effects of alcohol in the sixth book, where Hector returning home to Troy after the slaughter of battle declines his mother Hecuba's offer to bring him honey-flavored wine for reinforcement. Hector says (Homer 2018; Schadewaldt 2016):

> μή μοι οἶνον ἄειρε μελίφρονα, πότνια μῆτερ,
> μή μ' ἀπογυιώσῃς, μένεος δ' ἀλκῆς τε λάθωμαι

> Do not serve me honey-flavoured wine honourable mother.
> It lames my limbs and makes me forget courage and strength.

Juvenal describes the physical effects of rotatory alcoholic vertigo in the *Saturae* (Satires) (about 60–127 AD) (Stocker 1835; Juvenal and Persius 1918):

> *[…] quum bibitur concha, quum jam vertigine tectum ambulat et geminis exsurgit mensa lucernis.*

> […] and drinks out of perfume-bowls, while the roof spins around dizzy, the table dances, and every light is double

23.7 Allusions to Specific Vertigo Syndromes: Vestibular Migraine and Menière's Disease

In the second century AD, Aretaeus of Cappadocia describes in *De causis et signis acutorum et chronicorum morborum* a syndrome that combines hemicrania with vertigo and is associated with nystagmoid eye movements and nausea (Huppert and Brandt 2017; Hude 1958). These features resemble the symptoms of vestibular migraine, a term that was first coined only in 1999 (Dieterich and Brandt 1999). Diagnostic criteria have, in the meantime, been jointly formulated by the Committee for Classification of Vestibular Disorders of the Bárány Society and the Migraine Classification Subcommittee of the International Headache Society (HIS) (Lempert et al. 2012).

The Yellow Thearch reports in the Chinese Medical Classic *Huangdi Neijing* second century BC to the second century AD) on an episodic disorder with dizziness involving a connection between eyes and brain. The associated ringing noise in the ears strongly recalls the characteristics of a Menière's attack (Huppert and Brandt 2017). The full picture of the disease was first described and named by Prosper Menière in 1861 (Meniere 1861). He stressed the characteristic recurrent attacks of vertigo, mostly for hours, combined with unilateral hearing loss, tinnitus, and a feeling of fullness in one ear. In 2015, the diagnostic criteria for Menière's disease were reformulated by several Otolaryngological Societies, including the Committee for Classification of Vestibular Disorders of the Bárány Society (Lopez-Escamez et al. 2015).

23.8 Insights from the Eighteenth to the Twentieth Centuries on Vertigo and Motion Perception

Although the function of the vestibular organ was not yet discovered in his lifetime, Erasmus Darwin (1731–1802 AD), the grandfather of Charles Darwin, provided posterity with a rich mine of information about the emergence of dizziness syndromes and the early concepts of sensorimotor control of eye movements and multisensory actions. In his work *Zoonomia, or The Laws of Organic Life* in 1794 (Darwin 1794), he describes a plethora of physiological dizziness syndromes: those that arise when viewing moving objects, from our own motions, from riding over snow or a broad stream, dizziness when looking from a tower, when turning on one foot, walking in the dark, or resulting from the motion of a ship (seasickness). Disorders or diseases accompanied by vertigo or dizziness are also mentioned, for example, disorders resembling Mal de Debarquement syndrome, strokes of palsy with dizziness, injuries of the head, vertigo when inebriated, an upset stomach due to internal causes accompanied by vertigo, and vertiginous noises in the head (possibly Menière's disease). He also wrote about visual vertigo:

> Many people, when they arrive at 50 or 60 years of age, are affected with slight vertigo; which is generally but wrongly ascribed to indigestion, but in reality arises from a beginning defect of their sight [...] these people do not see objects so distinctly as formerly, and by exerting their eyes more than usual they perceive the apparent motions of objects, and confound them with real motions of them; and therefore cannot accurately balance themselves so as easily to preserve their perpendicularity by them.

Another example is his understanding of visual height intolerance (fear of heights):

> Anyone, who stands alone on the top of a high tower, if he has not been accustomed to balance himself by objects placed at such distances and with such inclinations, begins to stagger, and endeavours to recover himself by his muscular feelings. During this time the apparent motion of objects at a distance below him is very great and the impressions of this apparent motion continue a little time after he has experienced them; and he is persuaded to incline the contrary way to counteract their effects; and either immediately falls, or applying his hands to the building, uses his muscular feeling to preserve his perpendicular attitude, contrary to the erroneous persuasions of the eyes.

Erasmus Darwin also described rotatory vertigo due to drinking excessively alcohol:

> […] such is the vertigo of drunken people, which continues, when their eyes are closed, and themselves in a recumbent posture, as well as when they are in an erect posture, and have their eyes open.

Here Darwin observed the typical symptoms of positional alcohol nystagmus in supine position. Much later, the Nobel Prize winner Robert Bárány (1911) defined the direction-changing characteristics of positional alcohol nystagmus in humans when different head positions are assumed (nystagmus beating toward the undermost ear) (Bárány 1911). The mechanism of positional alcohol nystagmus phase I and phase II is attributed to the difference in the specific weights of endolymph and alcohol. Alcohol is lighter than endolymph, and when blood levels approach 40 mg/dl^{-1}, alcohol diffuses into the cupula, rendering it lighter than endolymph and thereby transforming the semicircular canal into gravity-sensitive receptors (Money and Myles 1974). The "morning after" drink of alcohol may re-equalize the specific gravities of alcohol and the vestibular endolymph, thus reducing the untoward symptoms (Brandt and Daroff 1980).

Although unaware of the function of vestibular semicircular canals, Wilhelm Busch (1832–1908), a German humorist, cartoonist, and poet amusingly illustrated the effects of excessive alcohol consumption: "Ein Abenteuer in der Neujahrsnacht" ("An adventure on New Year's Eve"), "Der Katzenjammer am Neujahrsmorgen" ("The hangover on New Year's Day") (Busch 1950). In the first cartoon, a rotatory vertigo is depicted with a spinning bed and room while the affected subject is lying down (Fig. 23.3). The second cartoon shows

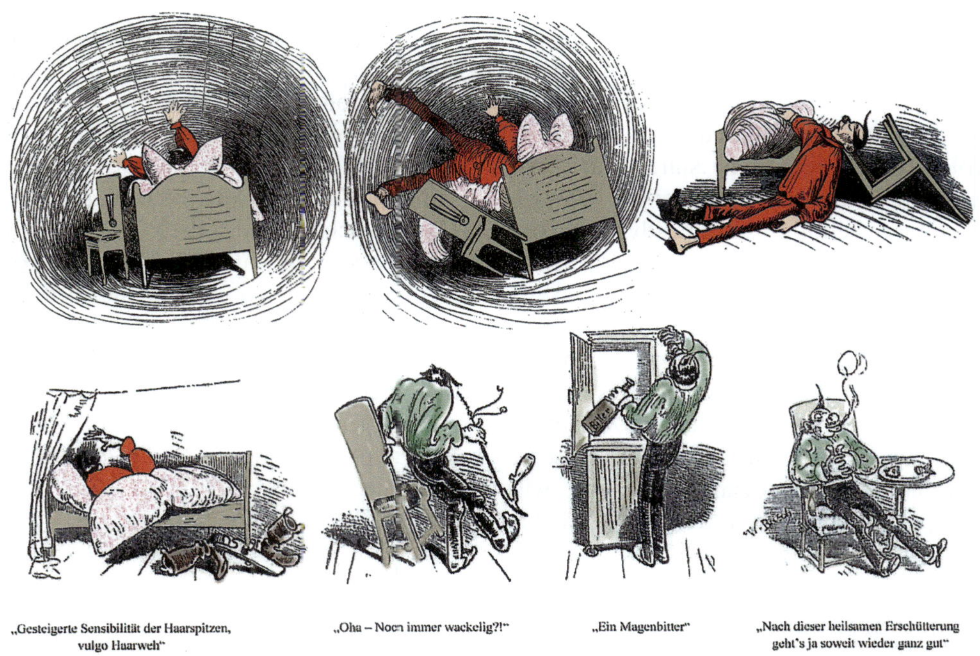

Fig. 23.3 **Upper part:** "Ein Abenteuer in der Neujahrsnacht" ("An adventure on New Year's Eve") by Wilhem Busch (Busch 1950). This funny cartoon sequence illustrates positional alcohol vertigo. **Lower part:** "Der Katzenjammer am Neujahrsmorgen" ("The hangover on New Year's Day") (Busch 1950). Wilhelm Busch illustrates vertigo and unsteadiness the morning after excessive drinking and how a "morning-after drink" has a restabilising effect

that Busch already knew about the "stabilizing morning-after drink" (■ Fig. 23.3).

Moritz Heinrich Romberg (1795–1873), an innovative German physician in Berlin, is considered to be the first clinical neurologist and the cofounder of the "German Neurological School". By publishing the first systematic textbook on neurology (Romberg 1840), his *Lehrbuch der Nervenkrankheiten des Menschen*, he revolutionized European neurology. This first textbook contains a chapter on "Vertigo, Schwindel" (Huppert and Brandt 2018). In this chapter, he delineated the symptoms, frequency, characteristics, causes, and therapeutic measures of vertigo. He emphasizes that apparent motions lead to falls and rotations, either of one's own body or of the surroundings, which cause a feeling of disturbed balance. This is often accompanied by optical or acoustical hyperesthesia (flickering before the eyes, noise in the ear – possibly allusions to vestibular migraine, and Menière's disease), double vision, painful feelings in the head, nausea and emesis, anxiety with attacks of cold sweating, trembling of the muscles, quick pulse, red or pale face, and cold feet. Moreover, he states that vertigo attacks last minutes, rarely longer. They may occur transiently or chronically. The causes are said to be a general state of weakness like convalescence, injuries and diseases of the cerebrum, especially the cerebellum and the pons, ingestion of alcohol, narcotics or nicotine, or other toxic substances like digitalis or hyoscyamus. Moreover, vertigo may occur as a prodromal state of other diseases, especially those associated with fever, when the patient assumes a certain head position over a longer time (bending down), or during unfamiliar movements such as those that occur during a sea voyage. Some of these causes can be cured, for example, vertigo induced by exhaustion or loss of body fluids (after hemorrhagias), but others like the injuries of the cerebellum cannot. His general advice is that persons suffering from vertigo and dizziness should avoid strong, sustained body rotations, heavy and warm food, baths, and lengthy sleep under a feather bed.

Although Romberg's neurological textbook provides detailed descriptions and some causes, most of the specific vertigo syndromes known nowadays are missing (Huppert and Brandt 2018). Our current knowledge of vestibular function and disorders dates back to a group of scientists who lived in the nineteenth century: among them are Jan Evangelista Purkinje, Ernst Mach, Josef Breuer, Hermann Helmholtz, and Alexander Crum-Brown. Their seminal work not only revealed the methods of sensing motion but it also laid the basis for modern vestibular and ocular motor research (Henn and Young 1975; Cohen 1984; Wade and Tatler 2005). The twentieth century witnessed another invaluable source that led to modern eye movement research. *The Moving Tablet of the Eye* (Wade and Tatler 2005) contains numerous histories of optics, ophthalmology, and eye movements. The most knowledgeable and influential contemporary physician in the study of labyrinthine malfunction was the otolaryngologist Harold Schuknecht (1917–1992). He presented controversial hypotheses and experimental evidence to explain the three most common forms of labyrinthine vertigo: benign paroxysmal positioning vertigo (first described in 1921 by Bárány), vestibular neuritis (by Ruttin in 1909), and Menière's disease (by Menière in 1861) (Brandt 1991; Schuknecht 1993; Huppert and Brandt 2018).

References

Bárány R (1911) Experimentelle Alkoholintoxikation. Monatsschr Ohrenheilkd 45:959–962

Bauer M, Huppert D, Brandt T (2012) Fear of heights in ancient China. J Neurol 259:2223–2225

Bisdorff A, von Brevern M, Lempert T, Newman-Toker DE (2009) Classification of vestibular symptoms: towards an international classification of vestibular disorders. J Vestib Res 19:1–13
Brandt T, Daroff RB (1980) The multisensory physiological and pathological vertigo syndromes. J Neurol Sci 95:3–28
Brandt T, Dieterich M (2017) The dizzy patient: don't forget disorders of the central vestibular system. Nat Rev Neurol 13:352–362
Brandt T, Huppert D (2014) Fear of heights and visual height intolerance. Curr Opin Neurol 27:111–117
Brandt T (1991) Man in motion: Historical and clinical aspects of vestibular function. A review. Brain 114:2159–2174
Brandt T, Arnold F, Bles W, Kapteyn TS (1980) The mechanism of physiological height vertigo. I. Theoretical approach and psychophysics. Acta Otolaryngol 89(5–6):513–523
Brandt T, Bauer M, Bensom J, Huppert D (2016) Motion sickness in ancient China: seasickness and cart-sickness. Neurology 87:331–335
Busch W (1950) Neues Wilhelm Busch Album. In: Klemm VH, Braunschweig VC (eds) Sammlung lustiger Bildergeschichten mit 1500 Bildern. Bertelsmann Verlag, Gütersloh
Cohen B (1984) The roots of vestibular and oculomotor research. Introduction. Hum Neurobiol 3:121
Darwin E (1794) Zoonomia, or the Laws of organic life. In: Vol 1, of Vertigo. J Johnson, London, pp 227–239
Dieterich M, Brandt T (1999) Episodic vertigo related to migraine (90 cases): vestibular migraine? J Neurol 246:883–892
Duden – Die deutsche Rechtschreibung (2017) 27th edn. Dudenverlag, Mannheim
Georges KE (2010) Ausführliches Lateinisch-Deutsches Handwörterbuch. Hahnsche Buchhandlung, Hannover, reprint
Grimm J, Grimm W (1854) Deutsches Wörterbuch. S. Hirzel Verlag, Leipzig. Neudruck und Neubearbeitung abgeschlossen 2016, S. Hirzel Verlag, Leipzig
Henn V, Young LR (1975) Ernst Mach on the vestibular organ 100 years ago. ORL J Otorhinolaryngol Relat Spec 37:138–148
Homer, Ilias 6. Gesang, 264–265. http://www.gottwein.de/Grie/hom/il106.php. Last accessed 15 Jan 2018
Hude C (ed). Areteaus (1958) Corpus Medicorum Graecorum II. Akademie-Verlag, Berlin
Huppert D, Brandt T (2017) Descriptions of vestibular migraine and Menière's disease in Greek and Chinese antiquity. Cephalalgia 37:385–390
Huppert D, Brandt T (2018) Dizziness and vertigo syndromes viewed with a historical eye. J Neurol 265(Suppl 1):127–133
Huppert D, Benson J, Krammling B, Brandt T (2013) Fear of heights in Roman antiquity and mythology. J Neurol 260:2430–2432
Huppert D, Oldelehr H, Krammling B, Benson J, Brandt T (2016) What the ancient Greeks and Romans knew (and did not know) about seasickness. Neurology 86:560–565
Huppert D, Benson J, Brandt T (2017) A historical view of motion sickness – a plague at sea and on land, also with military impact. Front Neurol 8:114
Janz RP, Stoermer F, Hiepko A (eds) (2003) Schwindelerfahrungen: Zur kulturhistorischen Diagnose eines vieldeutigen Symptoms. Editions Rodopi, Amsterdam, New York
Juvenal and Persius (1918) Satire 6. Ramsay GG (transl). Heinemann, London, Putnam's Son, New York. http://www.tertullian.org/fathers/juvenal_satires_06.htm. Last accessed 15 Jan 2018
Karenberg A (2009) Retrospective diagnosis: use and abuse in medical historiography. Prague Med Rep 110:140–145
Kluge F, Seebold E (2002) Kluge. Etymologisches Wörterbuch der deutschen Sprache, 24th edn. Walter de Gruyter, Berlin/New York
Lempert T, Olesen J, Furman J, Waterston J, Seemungal B, Carey J, Bisdorff A, Versino M, Evers S, Newman-Toker D (2012) Vestibular migraine: diagnostic criteria. J Vest Res 22: 167–172
Lopez-Escamez JA, Carey J, Chung WH, Magnusson M, Mandalà M, Newman-Toker DE, Strupp M, Suzuki M, Trabalzini F, Bisdorff A (2015) Diagnostic criteria for Menière's disease. J Vest Res 25:1–7
Menière P (1861) Mémoire sur les lesions de l'oreille interne donnant lieu à des symptômes de congestion cérébrale apoplectiforme. Gaz Méd Paris, Sér 3(16):597–601
Money KE, Myles WS (1974) Heavy water nystagmus and the effects of alcohol. Nature 247: 404–405
Romberg MH (1840) Lehrbuch der Nervenkrankheiten. Duncker, Berlin, pp 88–100
Schadewaldt W (transl.) 18th ed. (2016) Homer, Ilias. 6. Gesang, 264–265. Insel Verlag, Berlin
Schöner E (1964) Das Viererschema in der antiken Humoralpathologie. Steiner, Wiesbaden
Schuknecht H (1993) Pathology of the ear, 2nd edn. Lea and Febiger, Philadelphia

Stapleton E (2007) The dizzy clinic and the dictionary (etymology and otology). BMJ 334:361
Stevenson A (2010) The New Oxford Dictionary of English, 3rd edn. Oxford University Press, Oxford
Stocker CW (1835) The satires of Juvenal and Persius, from the texts of Ruperti and Orellius. Juvenal, Sat VI:304–305. Longman & Co, London
Wade NJ, Tatler BW (2005) The moving tablet of the eye. The origins of modern eye movement research. Oxford University Press, Oxford
Wang H (ed) (1997) Huangdi neijing yanjiu dacheng (The great compendium of the research on the Huangdi Neijing). Beijing chubanshe, Beijing

Supplementary Information

M. Strupp et al., *Vertigo and Dizziness*, https://doi.org/10.1007/978-3-030-78260-3

Index

E

F

G

H

T

U

V

W

GPSR Compliance

The European Union's (EU) General Product Safety Regulation (GPSR) is a set of rules that requires consumer products to be safe and our obligations to ensure this.

If you have any concerns about our products, you can contact us on ProductSafety@springernature.com

In case Publisher is established outside the EU, the EU authorized representative is:

Springer Nature Customer Service Center GmbH
Europaplatz 3
69115 Heidelberg, Germany

Batch number: 10621496

Printed by Printforce, the Netherlands